EMERGENCY IMAGING OF THE ACUTELY ILL OR INJURED CHILD

THIRD EDITION

EMERGENCY IMAGING OF THE ACUTELY ILL OR INJURED CHILD

THIRD EDITION

LEONARD E. SWISCHUK, M.D.

PROFESSOR OF RADIOLOGY AND PEDIATRICS
DIRECTOR, DIVISION OF PEDIATRIC RADIOLOGY
THE UNIVERSITY OF TEXAS MEDICAL BRANCH
GALVESTON, TEXAS

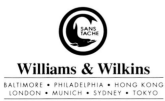

Williams & Wilkins
BALTIMORE • PHILADELPHIA • HONG KONG
LONDON • MUNICH • SYDNEY • TOKYO
A WAVERLY COMPANY

Editor: Timothy H. Grayson
Project Managers: Marjorie Kidd Keating, Kathleen Courtney Millet
Copy Editor: Carol Zimmerman
Designer: Dan Pfisterer
Illustration Planner: Ray Lowman

Accurate indications, adverse reactions, and dosage schedules for drugs are provided in this book, but it is possible that they may change. The reader is urged to review the package information data of the manufactures of the medications mentioned.

Printed in the United States of America

Chapter reprints are available from the Publisher.

Formerly titled EMERGENCY RADIOLOGY OF THE ACUTELY ILL OR INJURED CHILD

First Edition 1979
Second Edition 1986

Library of Congress Cataloging-in-Publication Data

Swischuk, Leonard E., 1937–
    Emergency imaging of the acutely ill or injured child / Leonard E. Swischuk. — 3rd ed.
        p.   cm.
    Rev. ed of: Emergency radiology of the acutely ill or injured child. 2nd ed. ©1986.
    Includes bibliographical references and index.
    ISBN 0-683-08048-2
    1. Pediatric diagnostic imaging.   2. Pediatric emergencies.
I. Swischuk, Leonard E., 1937–   Emergency radiology of the acutely ill or injured child.   II. Title.
    [DNLM: 1. Emergency Medicine.   2. Diagnostic Imaging—in infancy & childhood.   WN 240 S978e 1994]
RJ51.D5S89   1994
618.92′00754—dc20
DNLM/DLC
for Library of Congress   93-5756
                                                                       CIP

93 94 95 96 97
1 2 3 4 5 6 7 8 9 10

To Janie, my wife and very best friend

Preface to the Third Edition

As with the second edition, my aims are to retain what was useful in the previous editions, but to add newer data and to incorporate the newer imaging modalities. In this regard, many illustrations have been added or replaced. However, I have retained many illustrations of normal variations on plain films because I think these will become greater and greater problems as radiologists spend more time on the newer, more sophisticated imaging modalities. In producing this Third Edition, I am more indebted than ever to Carmen Floeck, my secretary, who played such an important part in getting the manuscript ready that it is difficult to put it in words. I would also like to thank Thelma Sanchez, her assistant, and John Ellis and Lora Hofer, our department photographers. They are true professionals and have always produced outstanding work for me.

LEONARD E. SWISCHUK, M.D.

Preface to the First Edition

I have always enjoyed the challenge of emergency medicine, for the diseases encountered are varied, and the diagnosis usually must be accomplished promptly. While many of these diagnoses can be established with the history and physical examination, in other instances they are made with the aid of roentgenograms. It is this aspect of emergency medicine to which this book is devoted, and I have attempted to present material and concepts which, over the years, have proven useful to me. In this regard, my aim was to outline general approaches to diagnostic problems, helpful rules of thumb, and specific diagnostic signs. Every so often, I felt it appropriate to delve more deeply into the pathophysiologic-roentgenographic correlations of certain diseases, but overall the main theme remained: how to approach a problem and then how to utilize the roentgenogram so as to have it yield the desired data.

The subject material in this book truly is "bread and butter" radiology, and I have tried to be as practical and clinical as possible. Most of the acute conditions commonly seen in the emergency room, outpatient clinic, or office practice have been covered, and in this regard, the main emphasis is on the evaluation of the initial films obtained. These films, of course, most often are plain films, and truly this is where the radiologist can excel. The radiologist must remain the expert on the plain film, for in spite of all of the new modalities and augmented diagnostic procedures available, the plain film remains the mainstay of the roentgenographic examination. As far as interpreting the roentgenogram, not only must one know all of the abnormal configurations encountered, but one also must be familiar with all of the normal variations which mimic pathology. In the pediatric age group, this is an especially significant problem in the skull, spine, and extremities. Because of this, I have included considerable material on normal variations causing problems, and as much as possible have placed this material next to the pathology which it mimics.

So many individuals have been of assistance to me during the time it took to write this book that it would be impossible to thank them all personally. There are many who have worked with me, many who have offered their material for inclusion, many who have offered constructive criticism and advice, and many who have offered simple encouragement. I thank all of them, and to those who allowed me to use some of their material in this book, I offer special thanks and hope that I have assigned appropriate credit in every instance. I must also thank the various residents who have passed through the Department of Radiology here in Galveston, for all of them have been most helpful in the accumulation of the material on a day-to-day basis. I hope that if they recognize a case they will take some satisfaction in seeing it being used to make a teaching point.

Two individuals, however, stand out so much that it is difficult for me to thank them enough. The first is my former secretary, Jonell Hoffman, and the second, our photographer, Milan Autengruber. Extra effort on their part became a routine daily task, and for this I am deeply indebted to both of them. I would also like to express my appreciation to Lester Murray, Mr. Autengruber's assistant; my former secretary, Cynthia Caldwell, who typed some of the early manuscript; and Donna Lofton in our Department of Medical Illustration for her assistance with the various drawings in this book. In addition, I must thank the radiology technicians who currently work for me and those who have worked for me in the past. There are too many of them to list individually, but all of them are exceptionally devoted, and needless to say, if they had not produced the roentgenograms I use, I would have nothing to illustrate with. My sincerest thanks to all of them.

I also would like to thank Dr. Robert N. Cooley, our former Chairman; and Dr. Melvyn H. Schreiber, our current Chairman, for their constant support for my various projects; and Dr. C. Keith Hayden, my very capable and helpful associate, for his daily physical and moral support. He has been of great assistance to me, and I express my sincerest appreciation to him.

Finally, I would like to express my gratitude to The Williams & Wilkins Company for their unfailing confidence and cooperation. More specifically, however, I am indebted to their astute Chief Radiology Editor, Ruby Richardson, for her perception of the tempo of medical publishing, and her overall flexibility and foresight have once again made it exceptionally easy and rewarding to compile a manuscript. She is a most dynamic and devoted individual whom I am fortunate to know and very pleased to call my friend.

LEONARD E. SWISCHUK, M.D.

Contents

CHAPTER ONE
The Chest

CHAPTER TWO
Upper Airway, Nasal Passages, Sinuses, and Mastoids

CHAPTER THREE
The Abdomen

CHAPTER FOUR
The Extremities

CHAPTER FIVE

The Head

CHAPTER SIX

The Spine and Spinal Cord

CHAPTER 1

The Chest

LOWER RESPIRATORY TRACT INFECTION (PNEUMONIA, BRONCHITIS, AND BRONCHIOLITIS)

Most childhood lower respiratory tract infections are of viral etiology (respiratory syncytial virus, parainfluenza and influenza viruses, adenovirus) and the virus-like agent, *Mycoplasma pneumoniae* (5–7). Most of these infections show distinct seasonal variation, and most usually come in epidemics (1, 7). Because of this, it is of some value to be aware of the "local virus going around the community." Knowledge of this type can aid in evaluating subsequent patients.

Bacterial lower respiratory tract infections show less seasonal variation and certainly are not prone to produce epidemics. Generally, bacterial infections result in parenchymal, alveolar pneumonias, while viral lower respiratory tract infections usually produce a bronchitis or bronchiolitis and thus remain in the interstitial space. This also is true of pertussis and *Chlamydia* infections, while *Mycoplasma* infections can behave either as viral or bacterial infections, i.e., as true alveolar consolidations or as bronchitic infections.

Bacterial infections most often are caused by the following organisms: *Streptococcus pneumoniae*, *Staphylococcus aureus*, *Haemophilus influenzae*, and hemolytic *Streptococcus*. *S. pneumoniae* (typical lobar pneumonia) infections are generally more common in older children, while *H. influenzae* infections tend to occur more commonly in infants and young children, i.e., those between the ages of 2 months and 3 years. *S. aureus* infections also are a little more common in infants and young children, but not to the same extent as *H. influenzae* infections. *M. pneumoniae* consolidative infections are more common in older children and adolescents. These age-group categorizations, of course, are merely generalizations and are not intended to be used with too much specificity or rigidity.

In addition to these features, there has been increasing attention to the problem of persistent airway hyperactivity after viral infection. This is especially prone to occur with respiratory syncytial virus-induced bronchiolitis in infants (2–4, 8, 10), but also is common with *M. pneumoniae* infections (9). Most of these studies seem to suggest that hyperactivity results from the initial infection, but there is, of course, the question of whether these individuals have hyperactive airways to begin with, and then overrespond to the infection.

Finally, it might be of some value to *review terminology used to describe pulmonary infections in children.* Certainly there is no problem with consolidation, for it infers alveolar disease. However, a problem arises when consolidation also is generically used to describe atelectasis. It is best if one can avoid this, for atelectasis is associated with marked volume loss while consolidative pneumonia is not. Consolidation produces little, if any, volume loss and infers the presence of alveolar or air space disease (Fig. 1.1A). A less common pattern of air space disease is that of patchy or fluffy alveolar infiltrates (Fig. 1.1B). Parahilar-peribronchial infiltrates (Fig. 1.1C) are synonymous with bronchitis and peribronchitis and infer that the disease process is interstitial. When peribronchial

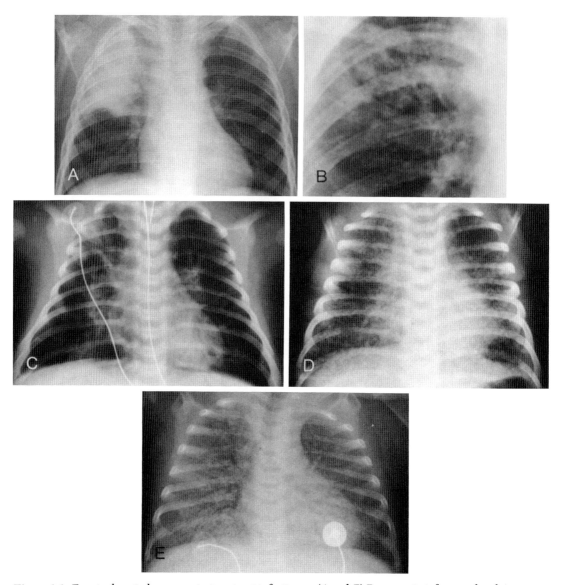

Figure 1.1. *Terminology in lower respiratory tract infections.* (**A** and **B**) Pneumonia infers an alveolar process that can manifest as lobar consolidation, patchy, fluffy infiltrates, or large nodular infiltrates. (**C**) Bronchitis-peribronchitis infers an interstitial disease process that manifests in thickening of the bronchial walls and peribronchial tissues. The resultant pattern is one of parahilar radiating infiltrates. (**D** and **E**) Pneumonitis infers an interstitial disease process that can manifest in diffuse reticulonodularity (**D**) or diffuse haziness (**E**).

inflammation becomes more pronounced and encroaches upon the adjacent alveolar parenchyma, the term ''bronchopneumonia'' could be used, but this term can be confusing, and I prefer to avoid it.

When viral infections involve the lung parenchyma beyond the immediate peribronchial space, they usually still are con-fined to the interstitium. In such cases, re-ticulonodular or diffusely hazy lungs can be seen (Fig. 1.1*D* and *E*) and the term ''pneumonitis'' rather than ''pneumonia'' is preferred. Pneumonitis, although a generic term, customarily infers an interstitial rather than an alveolar inflammatory process. ***In summary, then, consolidation*** *is equated with alveolar pneumonia, para-hilar-peribronchial infiltration with a bronchitis-peribronchitis, and reticulo-nodular or diffusely hazy infiltrates with an interstitial pneumonitis (Fig. 1.1). It is best not to use the potentially confusing term "bronchopneumonia."*

REFERENCES

1. Glezen W.B., and Denny, F.W.: Epidemiology of acute lower respiratory disease in children. N. Engl. J. Med. 288: 498–505, 1973.
2. Gurwitz, D., Mindorff, C., and Levison, H.: Increased incidence of bronchial reactivity in children with a history of bronchiolitis. J. Pediatr. 98: 551–555, 1981.
3. Horn, M.E.C., Reed, S.E., and Taylor, P.: Role of viruses and bacteria in acute wheezy bronchitis in childhood: a study of sputum. Arch. Dis. Child. 54: 587–592, 1979.
4. Kattan, M., Keens, T.G., Lapierre, J.-G., Levison, H., Bryan, A.C., and Reilly, B.J.: Pulmonary function abnormalities in symptom-free children after bronchiolitis. Pediatrics 59: 683–688, 1977.
5. Maletzky, A.J., Cooney, M.K., Luce, R., Kenny, G.E., and Grayston, J.T.: Epidemiology of viral and mycoplasmal agents associated with childhood lower respiratory illness in a civilian population. J. Pediatr. 78: 407–414, 1971.
6. McConnochie, K.M.: Bronchiolitis. Am. J. Dis. Child. 137: 11–13, 1983.
7. Mufson, M.A., Krause, H.E., Mocega, H.E., and Dawson, F.W.: Viruses, *Mycoplasma pneumoniae* and bacteria associated with lower respiratory tract disease among infants. Am. J. Epidemiol. 91: 192–202, 1970.
8. Rooney, J.C., and Williams, H.E.: Relationship between proved viral bronchiolitis and subsequent wheezing. J. Pediatr. 79: 744–747, 1971.
9. Sabato, A.P., Martin, A.J., Marmion, B.P., Kok, T.W., and Cooper D.M.: *Mycoplasma pneumoniae*: Acute illness, antibiotics, and subsequent pulmonary function. Arch. Dis. Child. 59: 1034–1037, 1984.
10. Stokes, G.M., Milner, A.D., Hodges, I.G.C., and Groggins, R.C.: Lung function abnormalities after acute bronchiolitis. J. Pediatr. 98: 871–874, 1981.

BASIC ROENTGENOGRAPHIC PATTERNS OF LOWER RESPIRATORY TRACT INFECTION

Introduction. Frequently in infants and children it is possible to differentiate viral from bacterial infection. This is possible because of the basic underlying differences in pathophysiology of the two types of infection. As noted previously, bacterial infection involves the alveoli producing a consolidating pneumonia, while viral infection involves the bronchial and peribronchial tissues resulting in a bronchitis (Fig. 1.2). *M. pneumoniae* infections can produce either form of infection (8). If no other factors were involved, differentiation between the two types of infection would be relatively simple, but unfortunately atelectasis enters the picture with viral infections. Atelectasis may be segmental or lobar and, if not handled correctly (1), can lead to erroneous roentgenographic interpretations. On the other hand, if atelectasis is handled correctly, differentiation of the two types of infection is more likely (11, 25, 26). *Therefore, it is the problem of atelectasis, and how it is managed and interpreted, that becomes the most significant factor in the analysis of chest roentgenograms in infants and children with lower respiratory tract infection.* As the child becomes older and passes into adulthood, all of this becomes less of a problem as the parahilar peribronchial pattern fails to materialize and atelectasis is far less common.

The Viral Spectrum. Any viral infection of the lower respiratory tract can produce roentgenographic patterns ranging from the infiltrate-free lungs seen with many cases of bronchiolitis, through parahilar peribronchial infiltrates with or without atelectasis, to the less commonly seen reticulonodular infiltrates, or hazy lungs (Fig. 1.3). Overall, however, the most common pattern is that of parahilar peribronchial infiltration, attesting to the fact that these infections are basically tracheobronchial. Consequently, they result in bronchitis and peribronchitis, rather than alveolar, consolidative pneumonia (2, 6, 16, 21).

Roentgenographically, so-called "parahilar peribronchial" infiltration results in

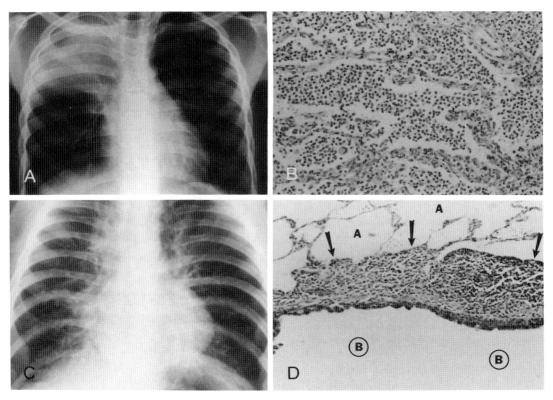

Figure 1.2. *Bacterial (alveolar) vs. viral bronchial-peribronchial (interstitial) infiltrate.* (A) Typical homogeneous bacterial consolidations in the right upper lobes. (B) Histologic material in alveolar pneumonia demonstrating the alveoli to be completely full of cells and exudate. (C) Typical viral interstitial, bronchitic-peribronchitic pattern of infiltration with streaky infiltrates radiating along the bronchovascular sheaths out toward the periphery of the lung. (D) Histologic material from a patient was viral bronchitis-peribronchitis, demonstrating that the inflammatory reaction, composed primarily of lymphocytes, lies in the immediate peribronchial area (*arrows*). The alveoli (A) are clear. Bronchus (B).

prominent and "dirty" parahilar regions (Fig. 1.4). The prominent hilar regions are due, in part, to inflammation of the bronchial walls and peribronchial tissues (2) and, in part, to associated hilar adenopathy (10). Because of the extreme variability of adenopathy, some children may present with well-circumscribed and enlarged lymph nodes, while others show no discrete adenopathy but, rather, a generalized increase in density and raggedness of the parahilar areas (Fig. 1.5). Air trapping also is a common feature of viral lower respiratory tract infections, because thickening and edema of the bronchial and peribronchial tissues predisposes the individual to more than normal narrowing of the airways during expiration. In addition, reactive bronchospasm is present and this accentuates the basic problem of air trapping. Such air trapping often is most pronounced in cases of bronchiolitis and also is a greater problem in children with asthma and infants with hyperreactive airway disease.

Clinically, infants and children with viral infections usually present with a cough, tachypnea, and a generally "miserable" picture of 2 or 3 days' duration. They look sick and feel sick. In addition, upper airway infection in the form of croup, or at least a croupy cough, nasal congestion, and coryza are common. However, most of these children do not require

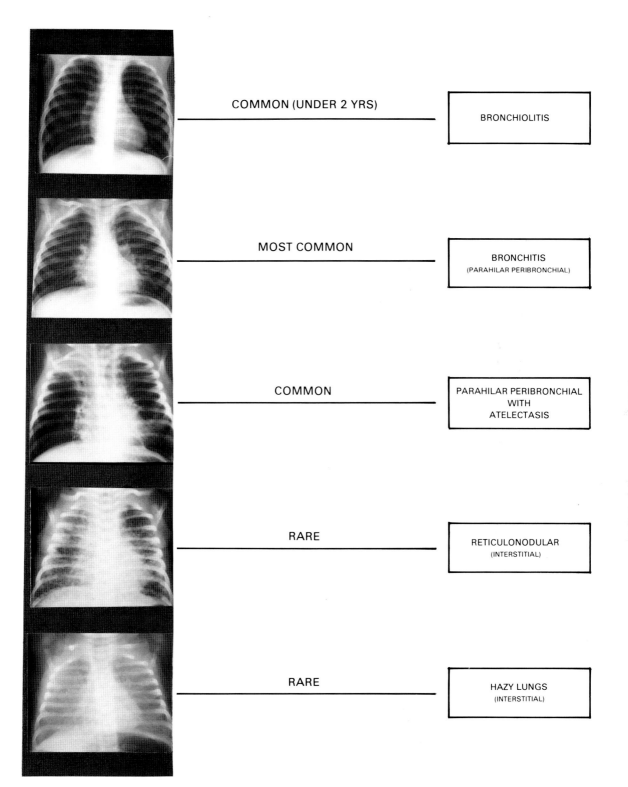

COMMON (UNDER 2 YRS) — BRONCHIOLITIS

MOST COMMON — BRONCHITIS (PARAHILAR PERIBRONCHIAL)

COMMON — PARAHILAR PERIBRONCHIAL WITH ATELECTASIS

RARE — RETICULONODULAR (INTERSTITIAL)

RARE — HAZY LUNGS (INTERSTITIAL)

Figure 1.3. *Viral lower respiratory tract infection; basic roentgenographic patterns.* Any virus can produce a number of interstitial roentgenographic patterns. The bronchitic spectrum ranges from the often infiltrate-free lungs of bronchiolitis through typical parahilar peribronchial infiltrates. Atelectasis is common and may be segmental or lobar. Less commonly diffuse reticulonodular interstitial infiltrates occur and, equally rarely, one may see diffusely hazy lungs due to interstitial parenchymal involvement. The pattern of parahilar peribronchial infiltration is the most common.

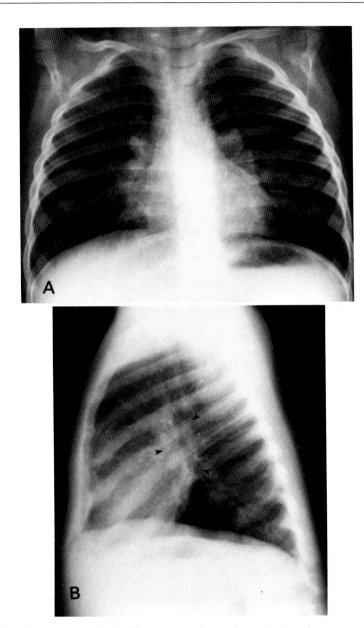

Figure 1.4. *Viral parahilar peribronchial infiltrates with adenopathy.* (*A*) Note the prominent hilar regions due in part to hilar adenopathy and in part to surrounding inflammation. The peripheral lung fields are relatively clear. (*B*) Lateral view demonstrates the characteristic increase in density and prominence of the superimposed hilar regions (*arrows*).

hospitalization, especially if they are older. Actually, what it amounts to is that they have an old-fashioned chest cold with a low-grade fever. Oral temperatures seldom exceed 102°F in these patients, although children less than 2 years of age may have higher temperatures. Even then, when corrections are made for rectal temperature readings, fevers are generally 102°F or less. On the other hand, in the early viremic stage of these infections, fevers may be higher, but chest symptoms

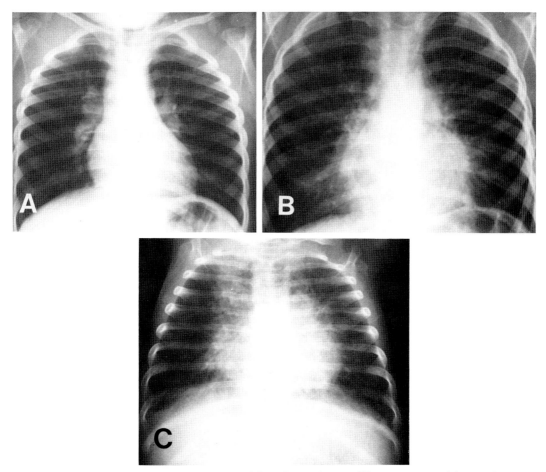

Figure 1.5. *Parahilar peribronchial infiltrates and hilar adenopathy; variable appearance.* (*A*) Note the prominent hilar regions with enlarged, readily recognizable, hilar lymph nodes. Parahilar peribronchial infiltration is minimal. (*B*) Another patient with less prominent hilar adenopathy but more extensive parahilar peribronchial infiltrates. (*C*) In this patient, note the lack of hilar adenopathy but extensive parahilar peribronchial infiltration leading to haziness of the cardiac edges or the so-called "shaggy heart" appearance.

usually are minimal or absent, and the chest x-ray is normal. Fevers also are higher in hospitalized patients (18), but this may simply be a reflection of patient selection due to severity of disease.

On auscultation, the lungs in these patients frequently are very noisy and "juicy." Although many of these noises are transmitted upper airway sounds, true rales, rhonchi, and wheezes can be heard. These sounds are variable from moment to moment, however, and generally correlate poorly with any attempts to match them, lobe for lobe, with positive roentgeno-graphic findings. The reason for this is that most of the sounds result from numerous incomplete and fleeting obstructions of the airways caused by mucous plugs and bronchospasm, while most of the densities on the chest film represent areas of atelectasis with no air flow and hence no noise.

When parenchymal involvement in viral lower respiratory tract infection occurs, usually it is widespread, and interstitial rather than alveolar. Indeed, true alveolar consolidations probably do not exist, except perhaps in very young infants and immunocompromised patients. In other patients, adenoviral infections (5, 10, 12, 13, 17) may occasionally produce consolidations, but these probably are due to a hemorrhagic bronchiolitis rather than true alveolar exudative consolidation. In most other cases, what is assumed to be a parenchymal consolidation is an area of atelectasis. The former occurs quite frequently, for atelectasis, both lobar and segmental, abounds in viral lower respiratory tract infection. Superimposed bacterial consolidations can be seen, although usually not until a week or so has passed, but true viral consolidations are rare. To be sure, I do not believe that they occur in the average, run-of-the-mill viral infection.

In terms of interstitial involvement, the most common pattern is that of streaky or reticular infiltrates, radiating outward from the hilar regions. This pattern leads to the typical "shaggy" heart, first described with pertussis infection, but actually, much more common with viral or *M. pneumoniae* infections (Fig. 1.5). With pertussis infection, the reason the "shaggy" heart is seen is that, just as with viruses, the infection is a bronchitis and not a peripheral alveolar infection. It is only later that superimposed bacterial infection may lead to consolidation.

In still other cases of viral lower respiratory tract infection, widespread reticulonodularity (Fig. 1.6) or diffuse haziness of the lungs is seen (Fig. 1.7). In some of these latter cases, the pattern of haziness involves both lungs in their entirety, while in others the findings tend to be more pronounced in the lung bases (Fig. 1.7D). The latter tends to occur with entities such as desquamative interstitial pneumonitis and other similar pneumonitides.

True alveolar infiltrates, with viral lower respiratory tract infection are uncommon, and as has been alluded to earlier, are of questionable existence in the average patient. Indeed, atelectasis is responsible for most, if not all, "apparent" consolidative infiltrates seen in children with viral lower respiratory tract infections. Roentgenographically, however, it may be difficult to always be absolutely certain that one is dealing with a viral infection only (25), for even though extensive interstitial disease always is present, the "apparent superimposed consolidation" remains difficult to evaluate.

The problem of atelectasis mimicking consolidation in viral lower respiratory tract infection is discussed in more detail at the end of this section, but for the time being, it should be realized that these patients are not as ill as the roentgenographic findings suggest. In other words, the multiple areas of segmental atelectasis do not

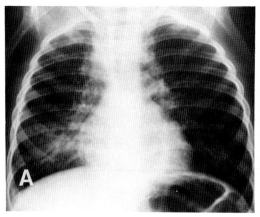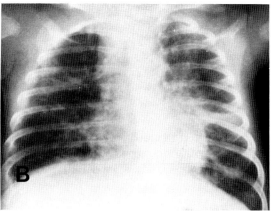

Figure 1.6. *Viral interstitial pneumonitis; reticulonodular infiltrates.* (A) Note parahilar peribronchial infiltrates with some early peripheral interstitial reticularity. (B) Another patient with more extensive reticulonodularity.

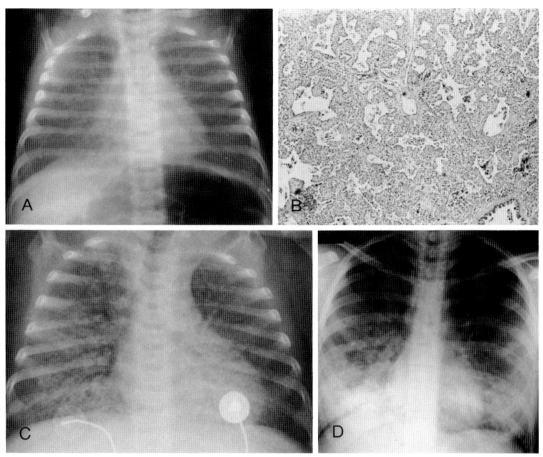

Figure 1.7. *Viral interstitial pneumonitis; hazy lungs.* (*A*) Note the diffusely hazy lungs in this infant with viral interstitial pneumonitis. The presence of air bronchograms does not necessarily infer an alveolar disease process, as demonstrated in *B*. (*B*) Histologic material from this infant demonstrates an intense interstitial infiltrate with marked thickening of the interstitium, and yet the alveoli, although severely compressed, are basically clear. Only a little cellular debris is seen here and there. (*C*) This infant with respiratory syncytial virus-induced pneumonitis also shows widespread haziness of the lungs with striking air bronchograms. (*D*) Basal distribution of hazy interstitial infiltrates in an older patient with viral pneumonitis.

render the patient toxic, and thus there often is gross discrepancy between what the roentgenograms suggest and the patient's actual clinical condition. What occurs is that the areas of atelectasis are mistakenly believed to represent pneumonic consolidations.

At the other end of the spectrum of viral lower respiratory tract infection is the young infant with bronchiolitis. Bronchiolitis is a distinct clinicoroentgenographic entity that is usually, but not exclusively, caused by respiratory syncytial virus (9,

23, 24). Its incidence peaks at around 6 months of age, but it is common in infants up to 2 years of age. As with all viral infections, parahilar peribronchial infiltrates and areas of lobar and segmental atelectasis may be seen in these infants (14, 19), but many show surprisingly clear chests (Fig. 1.8).

Pronounced overaeration as a result of air trapping always is present in bronchiolitis and, to be sure, is the hallmark of this disease. It leads to severe respiratory distress and, clinically, these infants show

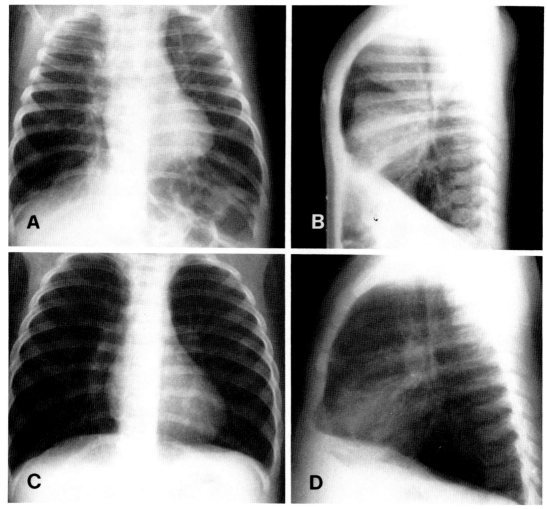

Figure 1.8. *Bronchiolitis with parahilar peribronchial infiltration.* (*A*) Note marked overaeration of both lungs and some parahilar peribronchial infiltration. (*B*) Lateral view showing marked depression and flattening of the diaphragmatic leaflets secondary to overaeration. In the upper retrosternal area, note how the marked degree of overaeration has caused the thymus gland to separate from the heart. (*C*) In this infant, note that even though there is considerable overaeration, there is minimal, if any, parahilar infiltration. (*D*) Lateral view shows marked overaeration with a characteristically bell-shaped chest and markedly depressed and flattened diaphragmatic leaflets.

marked dyspnea, tachypnea, air hunger, paroxysmal coughing, and cyanosis. Fine rales may be heard at the end of inspiration and in early expiration, and in most infants expiratory wheezes are present. However, unlike the wheezes in asthma, they do not dissipate significantly when epinephrine is administered. Bronchiolar inflammation and expiratory constriction play havoc with the already normally narrow bronchioles in these young infants, and peripheral air trapping becomes pronounced. Simply speaking, the chests in these infants are "frozen" in deep inspiration, and they do not move air.

Some infants may have multiple seasonal bouts of bronchiolitis. When this occurs, it is important to consider the possibility of underlying asthma or cystic fibrosis, for it is not unusual for infants with these diseases to first present with what appear to be repeated or especially severe and refractory bouts of bronchiolitis. Finally, it should be noted that the roentgenographic picture of severe overaeration in bronchiolitis also can be mimicked by centrally obstructing lesions such as vascular rings and mediastinal masses and cysts, and by severe dehydration and acidosis. In the latter, acidosis leads to an increase in respiratory rate and diaphragmatic excursion (to blow off excess CO_2), and the low blood volume due to the dehydration leads to a diminution in caliber of the pulmonary blood vessels and pulmonary oligemia. Together these findings result in lungs that appear overaerated and underperfused (see Fig. 1.150), a picture virtually indistinguishable from that seen with bronchiolitis when the lungs are overaerated but free of infiltrates. Clinical correlation, however, usually quickly deciphers the situation and correctly identifies the problem.

Before proceeding to a discussion of the very common problem of focal aeration disturbances associated with viral lower respiratory tract infection, it should be emphasized that the preceding categorizations of the roentgenographic patterns of viral lower respiratory tract infection are intended as anchor points only. One should not be too rigid in their application, for overlap of one pattern with another is common. In addition, all of the roentgenographic patterns discussed should be correlated with the clinical picture, for only then will they most benefit the patient and physician. If all of the clinical and laboratory parameters suggest mild disease, reassess the worrisome roentgenographic findings; do not discard them, just reassess them. In such cases what you first thought to be consolidation probably was atelecta-

sis. *One should remember that roentgenograms are for interpreting and patients are for treating. This is most important with viral infections where lobar and segmental atelectasis abound (4, 11, 19, 22, 25, 26), and tend to erroneously sway one in the direction of consolidating pneumonia.* Focal, obstructive emphysema also occurs, but not nearly as frequently as does atelectasis. However, both result from bronchial obstruction secondary to mucosal inflammation, endobronchial secretions, and mucous plugs, and the resulting roentgenographic pictures can be most misleading (Figs. 1.9 and 1.10). Areas of segmental atelectasis, in particular, have a propensity to mimic pneumonia and distract one's attention from the real problem. This can hardly be avoided, for often it is truly difficult to be sure that atelectasis only is the problem (Fig. 1.11). However, if the suspected infiltrates are streaky, linear, or wedgelike, the problem is atelectasis (Fig. 1.12). In such cases, if one still is not confident enough to withhold antibiotics, it should be realized that if they are prescribed and the infiltrates clear in just a day or two, it was not because of unusually rapid clearing of the presumed pneumonia, but rather, because of the dislodging of atelectasis-producing mucous plugs (Fig. 1.13). Once this phenomenon is appreciated, it becomes easier to understand why some children with viral lower respiratory tract infections seem to show most abnormal and disturbing roentgenographic findings in the face of surprisingly mild symptoms. The reason for this is that they do not really have pneumonia as the roentgenograms might suggest. Their basic problem still is one of bronchitis with parahilar peribronchial infiltrates; it just happens that the multiple areas of segmental atelectasis confuse the issue by mimicking alveolar consolidation. Such atelectasis is common in infants and children with viral lower respiratory tract infections, including bronchiolitis (4, 19), and occurs

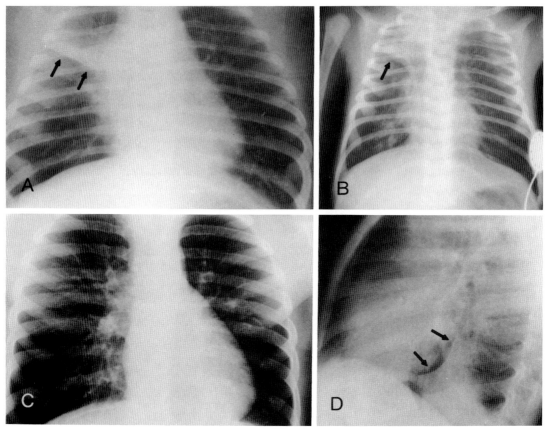

Figure 1.9. *Viral bronchitis with lobar atelectasis.*   (***A***) Note characteristic elevation of the minor fissure (*arrows*) because of partial atelectasis of the right upper lobe. Mild parahilar peribronchial infiltrates are present on both sides. (***B***) Another patient with more pronounced right upper lobe atelectasis (*arrows*). The minor fissure is elevated and there is ipsilateral shift (volume loss) of the mediastinal structures. The lungs are overaerated and extensive bilateral parahilar peribronchial infiltrates are present. (***C***) Note marked parahilar peribronchial infiltration, especially on the right. The parahilar peribronchial infiltrates are not as apparent on the left side because the left upper lobe is compensatorily overaerated (more radiolucent than the right lung) secondary to atelectasis of the left lower lobe (subtle increase in density behind the left side of the heart). The left lung is a little smaller than the right lung, suggesting overall volume loss. (***D***) Lateral view clearly demonstrates marked posterior displacement of the left major fissure (*arrows*) and elevation of the left diaphragmatic leaflet, both due to atelectasis of the left lower lobe.

Figure 1.10. *Viral bronchitis-peribronchitis with multilobar atelectasis.*   (***A***) Note bilateral parahilar peribronchial infiltrates and haziness along the right and left cardiac borders which in *B* is seen to be due to atelectasis of the right middle lobe and lingula (*arrows*). (***C***) Another patient with bilateral parahilar peribronchial infiltrates and atelectasis of the right upper and lower lobes (*arrows on the right*). In addition, note increased density behind the left side of the heart (*arrows*) due to partial atelectasis of the left lower lobe. (***D***) Lateral view demonstrates the right upper lobe atelectasis (*upper arrows*) and partial atelectasis of the left lower lobe (*arrows*). The lower thoracic vertebra are quite white because of the overlying, partially atelectatic left lung. Normally they would become blacker as one progressed downward along the thoracic spine. (***E***) Still another patient with a bizarre

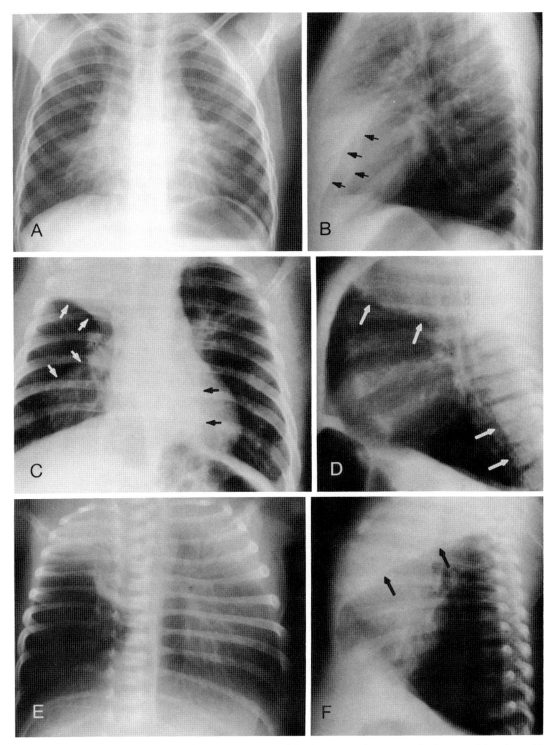

chest configuration consisting of marked overaeration of the lungs and densities in both upper lobes (*arrows*). (*F*) Lateral view demonstrates these to be due to atelectasis of the right and left upper lobes and lingula (*arrows*).

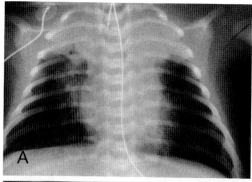

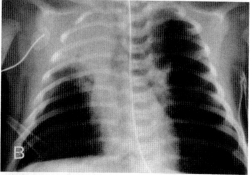

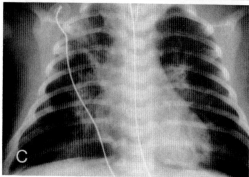

Figure 1.11. *Shifting atelectasis masquerading as lobar consolidation.* (*A*) This patient had respiratory syncytial virus infection with typical bilateral parahilar peribronchial infiltrates. The densities in both upper lobes easily could be misinterpreted for consolidating pneumonias. (*B*) On the next day, however, the left upper lobe density has disappeared. Clearly this was due to atelectasis. Now note that there is shift of the mediastinum to the right, emphasizing that the problem in the right upper lobe is one of volume loss and, hence, atelectasis. (*C*) The next day the marked degree of right upper lobe atelectasis has resolved. Only a minimal degree remains, and now typical bilateral parahilar peribronchial infiltrates consistent with a viral bronchitis-peribronchitis are seen. One must be careful not to misinterpret such lobar atelectasis, which is quite common, for areas of consolidating pneumonia.

because of inefficiency of the collateral airdrift phenomenon occurring through the ducts of Lambert and the pores of Kohn (6). In infants this mechanism is not as well developed as in adults and so areas of atelectasis tend to persist. It is important to appreciate that segmental atelectasis tends to remain somewhat central in its distribution (Fig. 1.13), a helpful finding in distinguishing these atelectatic infiltrates from the more peripheral and diffuse infiltrates seen with bacterial, alveolar infection (see Fig. 1.21).

When a major bronchus is plugged by mucus, and the entire lobe collapses, the findings often are easier to assess (Fig. 1.14). On the other hand, in some of these cases, the findings may still be puzzling, for obstructive emphysema rather than atelectasis occurs (Fig. 1.15).

Volume loss is not a prominent feature of acute consolidating pneumonia, for it is only when the pneumonia is healing and contracting (10 days or so later) that significant volume loss occurs. In the acute stages, volume loss usually is minimal (Fig. 1.16). With acute consolidating pneumonia, there is no reason for volume loss to be present, for there is no proximal airway obstruction. Consolidations begin in the periphery of a lobe and work inward. Air in the alveoli is slowly replaced by purulent exudate, the alveoli do not collapse, and volume loss is negligible. This is not so true of the right middle lobe and lingula, where volume loss may appear more pronounced (Fig. 1.16*E* and *F*). These lobes are smaller than the other lobes of the lungs and thus the minor degree of volume loss that occurs appears more pronounced than it does in the larger upper and lower lobes. Overall, however, *if volume loss is significant, atelectasis should be favored and, in addition, if multilobar involvement is present, atelectasis is more likely. To be sure, multilobar consolidation is far less common than multilobar atelectasis.* Finally, it should be noted that pleural effusions are rare with viral infections and when seen

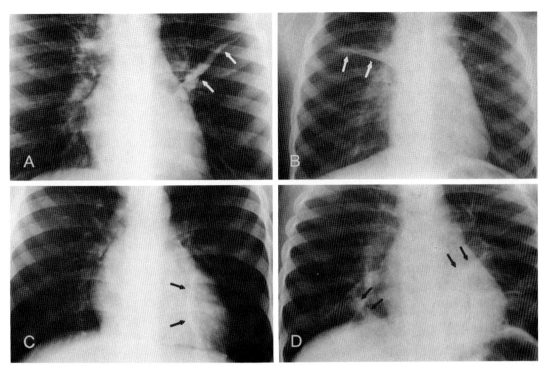

Figure 1.12. *Segmental atelectasis; varying configurations.* (*A*) Linear streak of atelectasis (*arrows*) in the left upper lobe. (*B*) Another patient with a similar streak of atelectasis in the right upper lobe (*arrows*). (*C*) Vertical (discoid) atelectasis in the left lower lobe (*arrows*). (*D*) Multiple areas of wedgelike atelectasis (*arrows*) in a patient with viral bronchitis.

usually are of very small volume. They are, of course, common with bacterial infections.

Lobar Consolidation—Bacterial Disease. Lobar consolidations most commonly are the result of *S. pneumoniae* or *H. influenzae* infections, the latter being more common in infants less than 2 to 3 years old. *M. pneumoniae* and *S. aureus* are less common causes, and consolidations secondary to *Klebsiella, Pseudomonas,* and other such infections generally are rare. *M. pneumoniae* consolidations tend to occur in older children (7). Viral consolidations, if they exist at all, are uncommon, except perhaps in the perinatal period and in immunocompromised patients. Fungal infections also can produce consolidations, with or without effusions or empyemas, and of course are more common in endemic areas.

Clinically, patients with bacterial or *M. pneumoniae* lobar consolidations present with abrupt onset of fever (usually 103°F or greater orally), lassitude, malaise, and cough. Auscultatory-roentgenographic correlation, as opposed to that with viral bronchitis, is good, and roentgenograms usually confirm the location of the clinically suspected pneumonia. Its appearance can range from a small peripheral infiltrate to a completely consolidated lobe, and its size depends on the age of the pneumonia (Fig. 1.17). The peripheral origin is important to note, for lobar atelectasis does not begin peripherally and thus it would be most unusual for it to present as a peripheral density such as is seen in Fig. 1.17A.

Multilobar consolidations, although relatively uncommon, still do occur. They can be seen in otherwise completely normal children, but also have a definite propen-

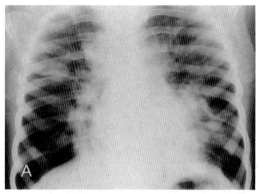

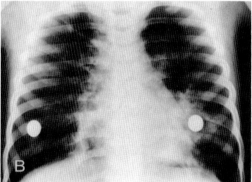

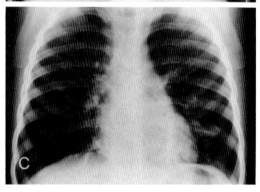

Figure 1.13. *Bronchitis with parahilar peribronchial infiltrates and patchy atelectasis.* (**A**) Note extensive bilateral parahilar peribronchial infiltrates with a predominantly central distribution. Centrally, the peribronchial inflammatory process has become a little more confluent because of peribronchial edema. Also note scattered densities in almost every lobe, due to areas of segmental atelectasis. (**B**) Eighteen hours later, after the patient was treated in a humidifying tent and antibiotics were given, considerable improvement has occurred and a more typical pattern of parahilar peribronchial infiltration is evolving. Areas of segmental atelectasis remain in both lower lobes. (**C**) Thirty-six hours after the first roentgenogram, the original changes have almost totally resolved. A residual pattern of parahilar peribronchial infiltration with

sity to occur in infants with a prior viral bronchitis and children with underlying sickle cell disease (Fig. 1.18). In the latter patients, it is not clear whether pulmonary veno-occlusive disease predisposes to the infection, but multilobar pneumonia is quite common in these patients and may, in fact, rapidly go on to involve almost all of the parenchyma of both lungs. Multilobar pneumonia, rapidly progressive, also can be seen in infants recovering from viral bronchitis, especially respiratory syncytial virus. In such cases superimposed multilobar consolidations with total opacification of both lungs are a serious complication, and frequently of precipitous onset (Fig. 1.19). Indeed, clinical deterioration accompanied by the rapid onset of a toxic, septic picture, with an increase in neutrophils and bands in the white count, occurs significantly ahead of the roentgenographic appearance of the consolidations. It is important to appreciate that the superimposed bacterial infection in these cases is a relatively late occurrence, usually becoming apparent 5 to 10 days after the initial onset of the viral infection. During this interval, fleeting areas of atelectasis are common and should not be misinterpreted as consolidations (see Fig. 1.11).

A less common pattern of alveolar consolidation is the one where the infiltrates are soft and patchy or nodular. These may be localized to one lobe or they may be diffuse (Fig. 1.20). They are also seen with fungal disease.

a few typical linear or wedgelike areas of segmental atelectasis in the lower lobes is all that remains. The original pattern of profound parahilar peribronchial infiltration with numerous superimposed areas of scattered segmental atelectasis most often is misinterpreted for widespread bacterial pneumonia. However, the central predominance, as seen in *A*, is the key to proper diagnosis. Furthermore, no bacterial infection would clear this quickly, and even though antibiotics are frequently administered in these cases, they should not be credited for the rapid clearance of what initially was misinterpreted for pneumonia.

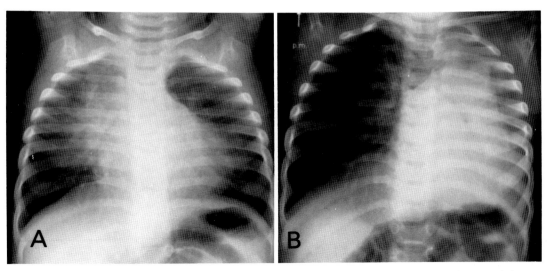

Figure 1.14. *Massive atelectasis, shifting from side to side with viral lower respiratory tract infection.* (A) Note parahilar peribronchial infiltrates and what would appear to be a large infiltrate in the right upper lobe. (B) The next day, note that the entire right lung is clear and that the apparent infiltrate in the right upper lobe has disappeared. However, the left lung has now collapsed. Such rapid clearing of the right lung is too fast for pneumonia; it represents clearing atelectasis after dislodging of a mucous plug. On this inspiratory film, the right lung also shows so-called "compensatory" overaeration; in other words, it is larger than it should be because the patient is compensating for the nonventilating left lung.

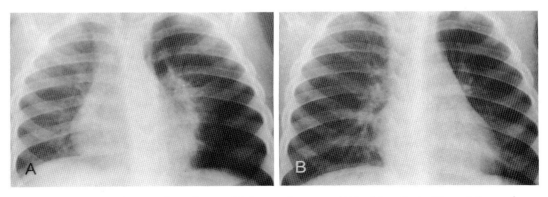

Figure 1.15. *Viral bronchitis-peribronchitis with lobar emphysema.* (A) In this patient with parahilar peribronchial infiltrates, note that the left lung is overdistended, hyperlucent, and, in fact, large. This was due to an obstructing mucous plug. (B) The next day, with the plug coughed up, only bilateral parahilar peribronchial infiltrates remain.

Finally, one or two pitfalls in the interpretation of roentgenograms in patients suspected of having consolidating pneumonia should be borne in mind. The most important of these deals with the patient who obtains the chest roentgenogram early in the course of the disease. *In such cases, because of the usual delay period of up to 12 hours from the onset of symptoms to the appearance of a roentgenographically demonstrable infiltrate, the roentgenogram can be normal.* Clinically, how-

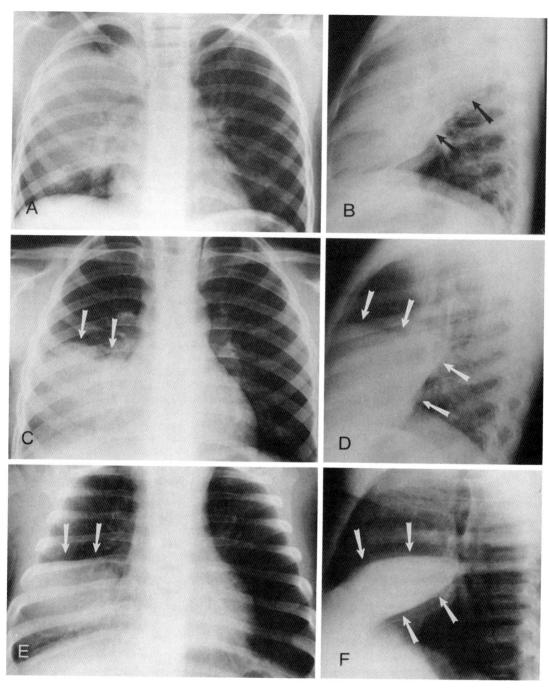

Figure 1.16. *Consolidating pneumonia (bacterial infection); various lobes.* (A) Note extensive consolidation, with clear-cut air bronchograms in the right upper and middle lobes. There is no significant volume loss and the right lung is of normal size. (B) Lateral view demonstrating the same consolidations. Again, note that there is no volume loss and that the major fissure (*arrows*) is in its normal position. (C) Classic right upper lobe consolidation in another patient. Note that there is no volume loss and that the minor fissure (*arrows*) is in its normal place. (D) Lateral view also demonstrates that the minor and major fissures (*arrows*) are in their normal place and, hence, that there is no volume loss. (E) Another patient with a right middle lobe consolidation with the minor fissure (*arrows*) in its normal place. (F) On lateral view, however, there is some volume loss of the right middle lobe (*arrows*). This occurs primarily with the right middle lobe, for the right middle lobe is smaller than the right upper and lower lobes and thus even mild degrees of volume loss tend to be exaggerated. Obviously, clinical correlation is important in these latter cases, but in all of the cases, note that even though one or two lobes are solidly consolidated, the remainder of the ipsilateral and contralateral lung remain completely clear, and that there are no parahilar peribronchial infiltrates.

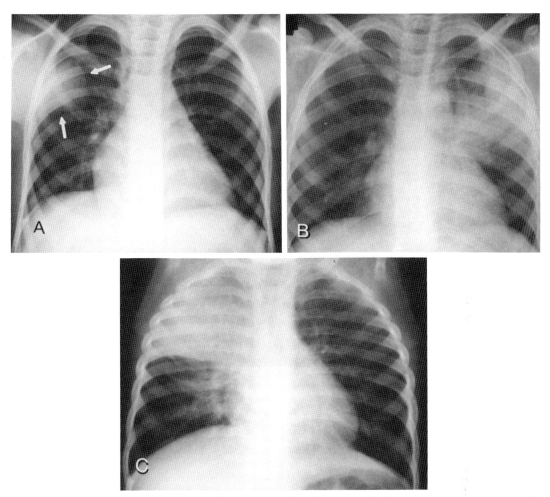

Figure 1.17. *Consolidating pneumonia: Different stages of development.*   (A) Note characteristic peripheral location of an early consolidating pneumonia in the right upper lobe (*arrows*). (B) Another patient demonstrating a more advanced consolidation in the left upper lobe. The consolidation, however, still is more dense in the periphery where it originated. (C) Well-developed consolidation of the right upper lobe demonstrates total homogeneous opacification with central air bronchograms. Note that the minor fissure is not significantly elevated. Early consolidation also is developing in the right middle lobe.

ever, fever, cough, and decreased air entry in the involved lobe are usually clearly apparent, but because the roentgenogram appears so normal one may be taken aback by the situation. At the other end of the spectrum, it is equally important to note that it is not uncommon for auscultation to fail to detect a well-developed lobar pneumonia that startlingly turns out to be present roentgenographically. These cases represent instances of advanced consolidation, and most likely breath sounds from the adjacent normal lung are so well transmitted through the consolidated lobe that they sound normal on cursory auscultation.

Mixed Viral and Bacterial Infections. With the approach just outlined and with practice, one usually can determine whether an infection is of viral or bacterial origin from the roentgenograms alone (25). Problems in interpretation usually do

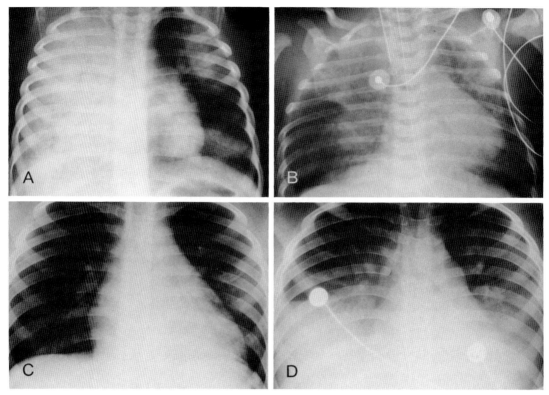

Figure 1.18. *Multilobar consolidation.* (**A**) Note the rather uncommon phenomenon of total consolidation of the right lung and early consolidations developing in the left upper and lower lobes. (**B**) Infant with extensive multilobar bacterial consolidations that developed after an initial viral infection. (**C**) Patient with sickle cell disease (note diffuse cardiomegaly) and an early consolidation on the left (*arrows*). (**D**) Less than 24 hours later, progression is rapid and extensive consolidations are present in both lower lobes. Note that, even though consolidative disease is extensive, in none of these patients is there evidence of volume loss.

not arise unless the typical parahilar peribronchial infiltrates are associated with peripheral alveolar infiltrates. The problem, then, is to decide whether these infiltrates are due to atelectasis or consolidation, and no matter how experienced one becomes, certain cases will truly remain indeterminate (25). A greater number will remain indeterminate if one deals poorly or in negative fashion with atelectasis (1) and, of course, if one deals infrequently with pediatric roentgenograms. In such cases, one must rely more on clinical correlation. This also is true when dealing with mixed infections.

In terms of such correlation, viral infections usually come to roentgenographic ex-

amination 2 or 3 days after onset of the illness, have lower presenting fevers (102°F or less orally), and usually do not produce particularly ill patients. Of course, this is a generalization and there will be those epidemics where fevers may be higher. This is especially true of young infants (18), and therefore, *degree of fever alone cannot be used to discriminate between viral and bacterial infections.* However, if white blood cell counts also are obtained, there will be a definite lymphocytosis with viral infections, while with bacterial infections there is an increase in neutrophils, a concomitant left shift, and an increase in bands. This occurs whether the bacterial infection is primary or secondarily im-

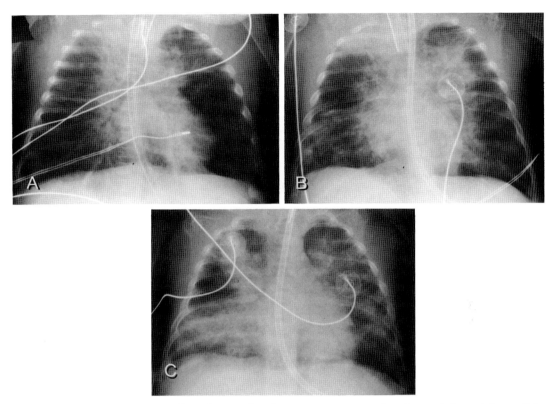

Figure 1.19. *Viral bronchitis-peribronchitis with subsequent superimposed widespread bacterial consolidation.* (*A*) Note the bilateral parahilar peribronchial infiltrates with parahilar edema and scattered segmental atelectasis in this patient with respiratory syncytial viral infection. (*B*) Five days later the basic parahilar peribronchial pattern persists. However, the patient was becoming more toxic and what was previously predominantly a lymphocytosis changed to a white blood cell count with a marked increase in segmental neutrophils and bands. (*C*) Just 18 hours later, note the development of massive bilateral consolidations involving virtually every lobe on both sides. This patient developed superimposed bacterial infection, which in these infants characteristically is precipitous.

posed on a viral problem, and thus the white blood cell count becomes an important ancillary parameter when secondary bacterial infections are suspected. Clinically, with bacterial infections there is usually abrupt onset of symptoms (in less than 24 to 36 hours) and higher fevers: 103°F or over and usually 104°–105°F orally (39°–40°C). This same abrupt onset usually also occurs in those patients who develop a bacterial infection on top of a previously existing viral infection.

When one is dealing with a viral infection and a superimposed bacterial infection, the roentgenograms may be quite confusing. One of the reasons for this is that there is a background of typical viral, parahilar, peribronchial infiltrates with areas of segmental or lobar atelectasis, and yet a consolidation also is present. In such cases, if the infiltrate in question has a smooth, homogeneous appearance rather than a streaky, linear, or wedge-like appearance, one should consider it a superimposed bacterial pneumonia (Fig. 1.21). This is especially true if the infiltrate is located far in the periphery of the lung, for it should be remembered that consolidations begin in the periphery of a lobe. Usually such superimposed consolidations involve

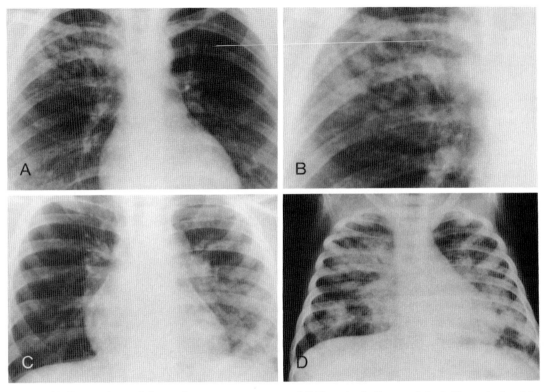

Figure 1.20. *Bacterial consolidation; less common patterns.* (**A**) Note the fluffy to nodular infiltrate in the right upper lobe. (**B**) Coned view of the right upper lobe demonstrates the soft fluffy nodules. This is relatively uncommon with bacterial infection and actually is more common with *Mycoplasma pneumoniae* infection. (**C**) Another patient with diffuse, fluffy infiltrates, short of total consolidation of the left lower lobe. (**D**) Infant with diffuse, fluffy infiltrates extending far into the periphery of both lungs. This patient had widespread staphylococcal pneumonia. Note how this pattern differs from the widespread viral pattern of radiating bronchitis-peribronchitis with scattered atelectasis seen in Figure 1.13A. There is no central predominance, with bacterial disease and the patchy infiltrates extend far into the periphery of the lung. In addition, of course, radiating parahilar peribronchial infiltrates are absent.

one lobe only, but it has been our experience that in infants, especially those with underlying respiratory syncytial virus, multilobar superimposed pneumonia is not uncommon and can develop with surprising rapidity (see Fig. 1.19).

Clinically, patients with superimposed bacterial infections usually go along for the better part of a week with signs and symptoms of a viral infection, and then rather abruptly become quite sick and toxic. This is an important clue and should signal the need for clinical reassessment and another chest roentgenogram. The reverse, that is, having a bacterial infection first and then a viral infection is not commonplace. There is good reason for this, for it has been shown that with viral infections, bronchial mucosal inflammation and edema along with increased mucus secretion and bronchospasm lead to poor tracheobronchial toilet (14). This is further aggravated by impaired ciliary cleansing action (3, 14) and overall stagnation and impaired ventilation result. Under such circumstances, chances of pathogenic bacterial growth becoming established are increased and pneumonia is more likely to develop. Such a sequence of events, in reverse, that is, viral after bacterial infection, does not occur.

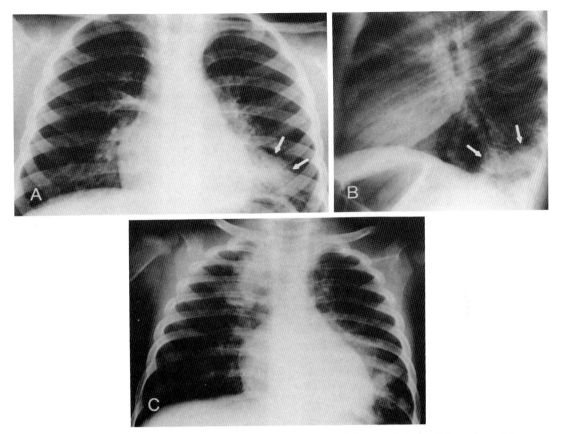

Figure 1.21. *Viral bronchitis-peribronchitis with superimposed consolidation.* (**A**) Note bilateral parahilar peribronchial infiltrates and an area of segmental atelectasis in the right upper lobe. In addition, however, note a homogeneous density, with air bronchograms just adjacent to the left cardiac border (*arrows*). (**B**) Lateral view demonstrates this latter density to be located far in the basal periphery of the lung (*arrows*). This is a superimposed consolidating pneumonia. (**C**) Another patient with parahilar peribronchial infiltrates, but with two homogeneous densities, one in the right upper lobe and one in the left lower lobe behind the heart. Neither one of these areas is associated with volume loss, and thus consolidating pneumonia should be favored.

REFERENCES

1. Bettenay, F.A.L., de Campo, J.F., and Mc-Crossin, D.B.: Differentiating bacterial from viral pneumonias in children. Pediatr. Radiol. 18: 453–454, 1988.
2. Conte, P., Heitzman, E.R., and Markarian, B.: Viral pneumonia, roentgen pathological correlations. Radiology 95: 267–272, 1970.
3. Carson, J.L., Collier, A.M., and Hu, S.S.: Acquired ciliary defects in nasal epithelium of children with acute viral upper respiratory infections. N. Engl. J. Med. 312: 463–468, 1985.
4. Eriksson, J., Nordshus, T., Carlsen, K.-H., Orstadvik, I., Westvik, J., and Eng, J.: Radiological findings in children with respiratory syncytial virus infection: Relationship to clinical and bacteriological findings. Pediatr. Radiol. 16: 120–122, 1986.
5. Gold, R., Wilt, J.C., Adhikari, P.K., and MacPherson, R.I.: Adenoviral pneumonia and its complications in infancy and childhood. J. Can. Assoc. Radiol. 20: 4, 1969.
6. Griscom, N.T., Wohl, M.E.B., and Kirkpatrick, J.A., Jr.: Lower respiratory infections: How infants differ from adults. Radiol. Clin. North Am. 16: 367–387, 1978.
7. Guckel, C., Benz-Bohm, G., and Widemann, B.: Mycoplasma pneumonias in childhood: Roentgen features, differential diagnosis, and review of literature. Pediatr. Radiol. 19: 499–503, 1989.
8. Hall, C.B., Powell, K.R., Schnabel, K.C., Gala, C.L., and Pincus, P.H.: Risk of secondary bacte-

rial infection in infants hospitalized with respiratory syncytial viral infection. Pediatrics 113:
266–271, 1988.

9. Jacobs, J.A., Peacock, Corner, B.D., Caul, E.O.,
and Clarke, S.K.R.: Respiratory syncytial and
other viruses associated with respiratory disease
in infants. Lancet 1: 871–876, 1971.

10. James, A.G., Lang, W.R., Liang, A.Y., Mackay,
R.J., Morris, M.C., Newman, J.N., Osborne,
D.R., and White, P.R.: Adenovirus type 21 bron-
chopneumonia in infants and young children. J.
Pediatr. 95: 530–533, 1979.

11. Khamapirad T. and Glezen, W.P: Clinical and radiographic assessment of acute lower respiratory
tract disease in infants and children. Semin.
Resp. Infect. 2: 130–144, 1977.

12. Kim, K.S., and Gohd, R.S.: Fatal pneumonia
caused by adenovirus type 35. Am. J. Dis. Child.
135: 473–475, 1981.

13. Lanning, P., Simila, S., and Linna, O.: Late pulmonary sequelae after Type 7 adenovirus pneumonia. Ann. Radiol. 23: 132–136, 1980.

14. Murphy, S., and Florman, A.L.: Lung defenses
against infection: A clinical correlation. Pediatrics 72: 1, 1983.

15. Odita, J.C., Nwandwo, M., and Aghahowa, J.E.:
Hilar enlargement in respiratory syncytial virus
pneumonia. Eur. J. Radiol. 9: 155–157, 1989.

16. Osborne, D.: Radiologic appearance of viral disease of the lower respiratory tract in infants and
children. A.J.R. 13: 29–33, 1978.

17. Osborne, D., and White, P.: Radiology of epidemic adenovirus 21 infection of the lower respiratory tract in infants and young children.
A.J.R. 133: 397–400, 1979.

18. Putto, A., Ruuskanen, O., and Meurman, O.:
Fever in respiratory virus infections. Am. J. Dis.
Child. 140: 1159–1163, 1986.

19. Quinn, S.F., Erickson, S., Oshman, D., and Hayden, F.: Lobar collapse with respiratory syncytial
virus pneumonitis. Pediatr. Radiol. 15: 229–
230, 1985.

20. Rice, R.P., and Loda, F.: A roentgenographic
analysis of respiratory syncytial virus pneumonia
in infants. Radiology 87: 1021–1027, 1966.

21. Scanlon, G.A., and Unger, J.D.: The radiology of
bacterial and viral pneumonias. Radiol. Clin.
North Am. 11: 317–338, 1973.

22. Shopfner, C.E.: Aeration disturbances secondary
to pulmonary infection. A.J.R. 120: 261–273,
1974.

23. Simpson, W., Hacking, P.M., Court, S.D.M., and
Gardner, P.S.: The radiological findings in respiratory syncytial virus infection in children; I.
Definitions and interobserver variation in the assessment of abnormalities on the chest x-ray. Pediatr. Radiol. 2: 97–100, 1974.

24. Simpson, W., Hacking, P.M., Court, S.D.M., and

Gardner, P.S.: The radiological findings in respiratory syncytial virus infection in children; II.
The correlation of radiological categories with
clinical and virological findings. Pediatr. Radiol.
2: 155–160, 1974.

25. Swischuk, L.E., and Hayden, C.K.: Viral vs. bacterial pulmonary infections in children (Is roentgenographic differentiation possible?). Pediatr.
Radiol. 16: 278–284, 1986.

26. Wildin, S.R., Chonmaitree, T., and Swischuk,
L.E.: Roentgenographic features of common pe-
diatric viral respiratory tract infections. Am. J.
Dis. Child. 142: 43–46, 1988.

Round Pneumonias (1–3). If you have
never seen a round pneumonia, you will
never guess what it is. Most often these so-
called round, spherical, or oval pneumonias represent pneumococcal infections in
an early consolidative phase. Some of them
appear so round that they defy distinction
from a pulmonary nodule or oval mass (Fig.
1.22). In other instances, a mediastinal
mass might be suggested (Fig. 1.23), but
the fact that one sees these pneumonias in
such a configuration is purely fortuitous. If
one could examine these patients a few
hours later, a more typical picture of consolidation would be present (Fig. 1.24).

The clue to proper diagnosis, of course,
is clinical. These children almost always
come to the attention of a physician because of abrupt onset of fever, cough, and
malaise. Usually they have a fever of between 103° and 105°F and auscultative
findings that suggest pneumonia. *Under
these circumstances, do not think of tumor
or a pulmonary nodule, think of a consolidating lobar pneumonia, usually pneumococcal in origin.*

REFERENCES

1. Greenfield, H., and Gyepes, M.T.: Oval-shaped
consolidations simulating new growth of the
lung. A.J.R. 91: 125–131, 1964.

2. Rose, R. W., and Ward, B. H.: Spherical pneumonias in children simulating pulmonary and
mediastinal masses. Radiology 106: 179–182,
1973.

3. Talner, L.B.: Pulmonary pseudotumors in childhood. A.J.R. 100: 208–213, 1967.

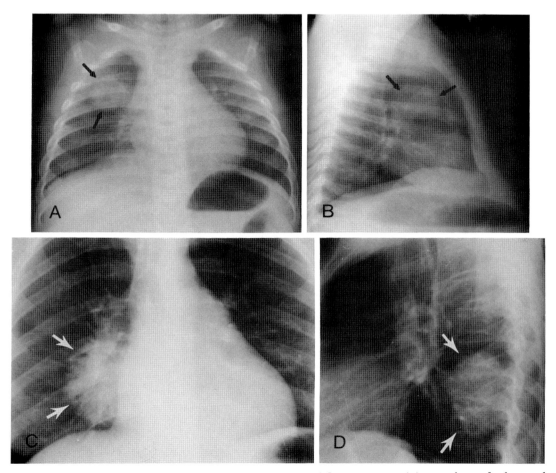

Figure 1.22. *Round or oval pneumonias; pseudopulmonary nodules or masses.* (**A**) Note the perfectly round pneumonia in the right upper lobe (*arrows*). This easily could be mistaken for a pulmonary nodule. (**B**) Lateral view demonstrates the same nodular appearance of the pneumonia (*arrows*). (**C**) Oval configuration of a lobar pneumonia in the right lower lobe (*arrows*). The configuration might suggest a mass. (**D**) Lateral view confirms the right lower lobe location of this round pneumonia (*arrows*).

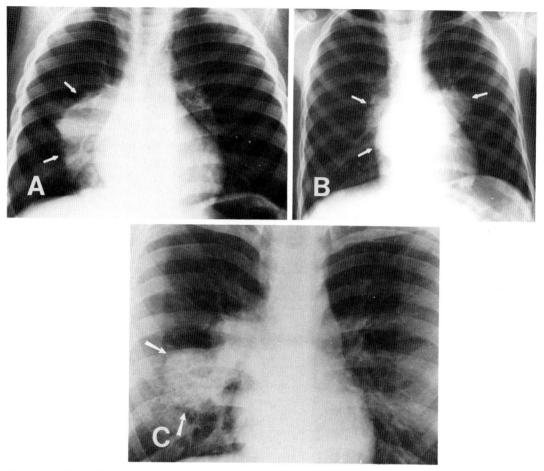

Figure 1.23. *Mass-like pneumonias.* (*A*) Note mass-like configuration of this right lower lobe pneumonia (*arrows*). (*B*) Another patient with bilateral superior segment pneumonias mimicking a paraspinal mass (*arrows*). (*C*) Round pneumonia (*arrows*) with associated adenopathy on the right.

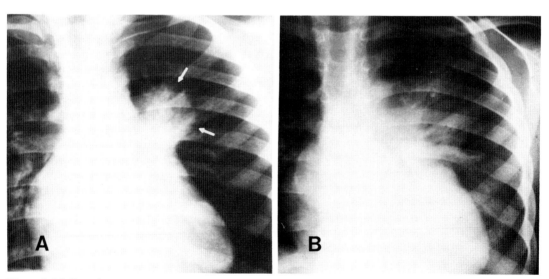

Figure 1.24. *Round pneumonia progressing to regular pneumonia.* (*A*) Note round pneumonia mimicking hilar adenopathy on the left (*arrows*). (*B*) Next day a more typical consolidation has evolved.

LOOKING FOR THE PNEUMONIA

Know Your Normal Chest First. It is most important that one be thoroughly familiar with the normal chest before one attempts to identify pneumonias, and in this regard it is a matter of studying the normal shape and densities of the various structures visualized (Fig. 1.25). For example, both hilar regions should be of relatively equal density, and the cardiac silhouette to either side of the spine should be about the same density. Indeed, analysis of the chest roentgenogram is a matter of comparing one side with the other, not only in terms of anatomic boundaries, but also in terms of comparative densities. To be sure, it is the latter comparison that often turns out to be the more useful in detecting early or hidden infiltrates.

One also should note that the margins of the heart and diaphragmatic leaflets, as they lie in juxtaposition to normally aerated lung, are crisp and distinct. This observation is useful when it comes to utilizing and understanding Felson's silhouette sign. This sign is discussed in detail in the next section, but as a preliminary consideration it should be noted that when any of the cardiac or diaphragmatic edges become hazy or fuzzy, one should suspect an adjacent abnormality such as a pulmonary infiltrate or atelectasis.

On lateral view, an important normal finding is that the space behind the heart is characteristically radiolucent (Fig. 1.25B); it represents the superimposed, normally aerated, lower lobes. Above this area, the soft tissues of the upper chest wall, axillae, and shoulder cause the lung fields to become progressively more opaque. Characteristically, then, the posterior half of the chest should become more radiolucent as one passes from top to bottom and, if it does not (i.e., the lower retrocardiac space is of equal or greater density than the superior retrocardiac space), one should suspect a pneumonia in one or other of the lower lobes (compare Fig. 1.25B with Fig.

1.32B). However in this area a pitfall to be avoided is to misinterpret normal retrocardiac lower lobe pulmonary vascular markings as being representative of an infiltrate (Fig. 1.25C). The characteristic angle and linear configuration of these pulmonary vessels are the clues to proper diagnosis. The upper retrosternal space also should be radiolucent, except in young infants, where the normal thymus gland causes the radiolucency to be replaced by radiodensity or whiteness. If this should occur in older children, look for an anterior segment, upper lobe pneumonia, or, by the same token, a superior mediastinal mass.

The right diaphragmatic leaflet normally is a little higher than the left, and because of this, it is often projected at a higher level on lateral view. Occasionally the leaflets are superimposed, but most often they appear at separate levels. The right diaphragmatic leaflet also can be identified by the fact that it usually is seen in its entirety (Fig. 1.26). In other words, it can be seen as a distinct structure right up to its insertion onto the anterior chest wall. The left leaflet, on the other hand, usually is seen only as far as the posterior cardiac wall, for at this point it blends with the cardiac silhouette (Fig.1.26). Occasionally, however, the left leaflet also can be seen in its entirety, and in such cases the usually visible gastric air bubble or inferior vena cava can be used as differentiating aids. The gastric bubble, of course, lies under the left diaphragmatic leaflet, while the inferior vena cava, being right-sided, blends with the right diaphragmatic leaflet (Fig. 1.26). All of these findings and relationships may not be present on every lateral chest film, but enough of them usually are present to enable one to determine right- or left-sidedness of a diaphragmatic leaflet, and thus, right- or left-sidedness of an adjacent lower lobe pneumonia.

Picking up Early or Minimal Infiltrates. Early infiltrates often are so subtle that they are totally overlooked or simply misinterpreted as fortuitous conglomerations

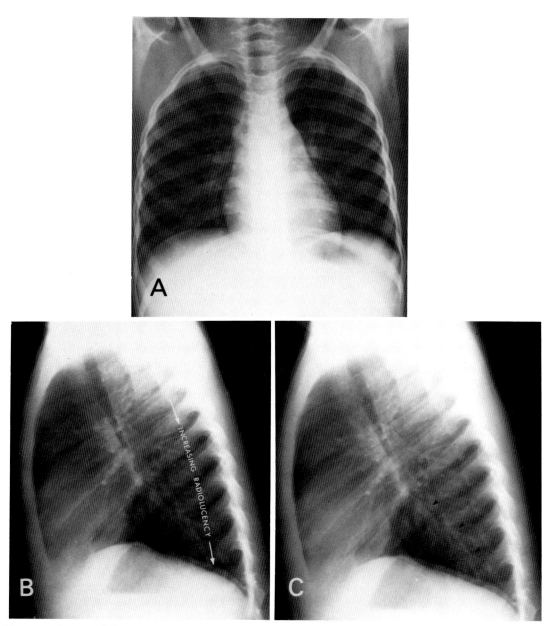

Figure 1.25. *Normal chest; pertinent roentgenographic features.* (*A*) On this frontal view, note that both lungs are of equal density and that the mediastinal, cardiac, and diaphragmatic edges are clearly demarcated. In addition, note that both sides of the heart are of equal density and that both hilar regions also appear equal in density and size. (*B*) Lateral view demonstrating increasing radiolucency from top to bottom of the retrocardiac space. Also note how sharp both diaphragmatic leaflets appear. (*C*) Same lateral view as in *B*, demonstrating normal lower lobe pulmonary vessels (*arrows*) which often are misinterpreted for pulmonary infiltrates. The characteristic sloping configuration of these vessels aids one in proper interpretation.

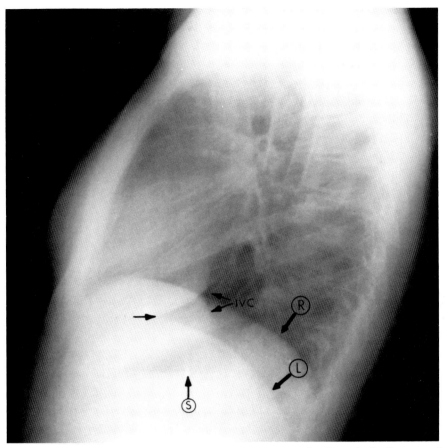

Figure 1.26. *Localizing and lateralizing the diaphragmatic leaflets.* Note that the right diaphragmatic leaflet (*R*) is higher than the left (*L*). Also note that the right diaphragmatic leaflet is seen in its entirety, while the anterior third of the left leaflet blends with the posterior aspect of the cardiac silhouette (*anteriormost arrow*). The inferior vena cava (*IVC*) blends with the right diaphragmatic leaflet, while the stomach bubble (*S*) is located immediately below the left diaphragmatic leaflet.

of rib and bronchovascular densities. The only way to diagnose such pneumonias is to be suspicious of, and then methodically substantiate, any focal area of increased density, no matter how equivocal (Fig. 1.27). If such infiltrates also happen to be adjacent to a diaphragmatic leaflet or cardiac border, the resulting positive silhouette sign (explained in detail later in this section) can aid one in their detection (Fig. 1.28).

In addition to the foregoing, one must remember to always obtain two views of the chest. One may be totally surprised as to how well a pneumonia is visible on one

view, and yet how poorly demarcated it is on the other. The reason this occurs is that while on one view the early pneumonia is seen *en face* and is "too thin" to register on the chest film, on the other view, it is visualized at 90° and now is thick enough to be seen (Fig. 1.29). Never neglect to get two views of the chest.

Using Felson's Silhouette Sign. Felson's silhouette sign (2) is a most useful sign when it comes to detecting an early or subtle infiltrate. It stems from the fact that, when two structures of equal roentgenographic density are juxtaposed, the interface between them becomes obliterated.

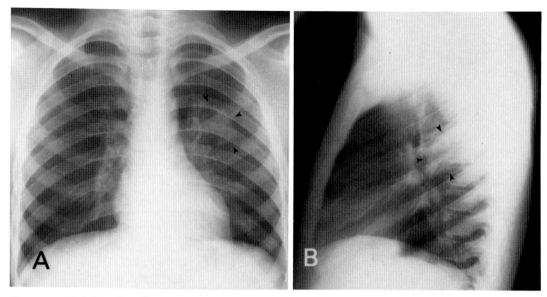

Figure 1.27. *Subtle early infiltrate.* (*A*) There is a vague area of focal infiltration in the left upper lung field, just lateral to the left hilar region (*arrows*). (*B*) Lateral view substantiates the presence of this early pneumonia, as there is a corresponding area of focally increased density in the posterior chest, superimposed over the spine (*arrows*).

In other words, if an organ such as the heart (water density) is juxtaposed against a pulmonary infiltrate (also water density), then the interface between them becomes indistinct or frankly obliterated. Normally the heart, mediastinum, and diaphragm (water density) are in juxtaposition to aerated lung (air density), and because they are of such different densities, a sharp line clearly demarcates their interfaces. However, once the density of the lung is changed from air to water (i.e., by pneumonia, hemorrhage, edema, or atelectasis), the roentgenographic interface between that portion of the lung and the adjacent mediastinum or diaphragm is obliterated and a positive silhouette sign results.

Most often the silhouette sign is applied to pneumonias in the right middle lobe and lingula. In the right middle lobe, the pneumonias that produce a silhouette sign occur in the medial segment. Those in the lateral segment are not juxtaposed to the heart, and thus do not produce a positive silhouette sign. In those cases where a medial segment pneumonia is present, the adjacent edge of the heart becomes blurred or obliterated (Fig. 1.30). When the pneumonia is in the lingula, it is the left side of the heart that becomes obliterated. Once such blurring of the cardiac silhouette is noted on frontal projection, a lateral view should be obtained for confirmation (Fig. 1.30*B*). The silhouette sign, utilized in this fashion, also is useful with pneumonias located adjacent to the superior mediastinal structures or the diaphragmatic leaflets (Fig. 1.31). In reverse, the silhouette sign also is helpful in localizing lower lobe pulmonary infiltrates. For example, if an infiltrate is present in the lower lobes, it lies behind the heart (not in juxtaposition to the lateral edge) and, consequently, the heart-lung interface is preserved (Fig. 1.32). This, then, indicates that the infiltrate is far posterior to the heart, that is, in a lower lobe.

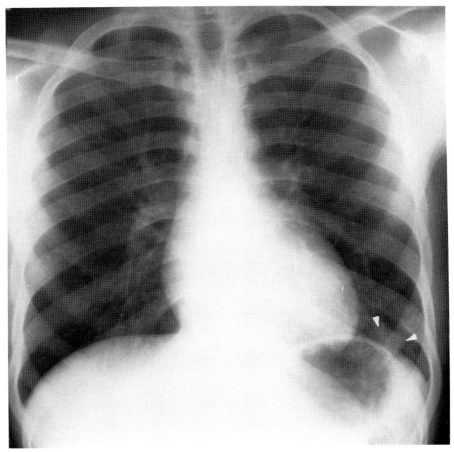

Figure 1.28. *Subtle, early infiltrate along the left diaphragmatic leaflet.* This chest could pass for normal, but on closer inspection note an early, rather subtle, infiltrate in the left lower lung field, just adjacent to the left diaphragmatic leaflet (*arrows*).

Unfortunately, the silhouette sign also occurs under some normal situations. In this regard, the most frequent site is along the right side of the heart. In many children, the bronchovascular markings adjacent to the right side of the heart are so prominent that they blend with the cardiac silhouette and result in a positive silhouette sign. *If this normal phenomenon is not appreciated, one will continually overcall right middle lobe pneumonia.* Most often this occurs when the inspiratory effort is somewhat shallow and the roentgenogram is obtained with the patient in partial lordotic position. The problem is especially prone to occur in children with parahilar peribronchial infiltrates secondary to viral lower respiratory tract infections (Fig. 1.33A) and in some cases may be due to a mild degree of atelectasis (1), not pronounced enough to be seen on lateral view. The fact that pneumonia is not present can be verified by obtaining a lateral chest roentgenogram which will show that no middle lobe infiltrate is present (Fig. 1.33B). Indeed, it would be most unusual to detect a right middle lobe, medial segment pneumonia on frontal view and not see even subtle indication of its presence on lateral view.

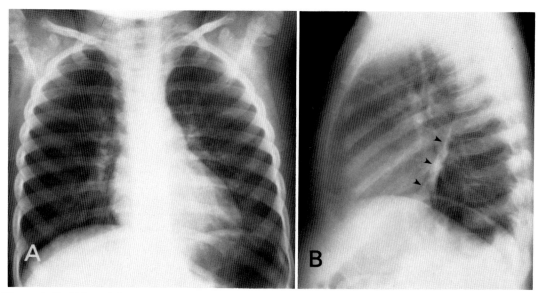

Figure 1.29. *Value of obtaining two views.* (**A**) The infiltrate is so subtle on this view that it virtually defies identification. However, on close inspection one might note that the left diaphragmatic leaflet is a little indistinct and that it is a little higher than usual (probably secondary to splinting). The left lower lobe pneumonia is seen *en face* and is too "thin" to be visible. (**B**) *Lateral view.* The pneumonia is seen at 90° to that in *A* and now is "thick" enough to register on the roentgenogram (*arrows*). In addition, note that the major fissure is in its normal position. This favors early consolidation over atelectasis, as with the latter the fissure would tend to be displaced posteriorly.

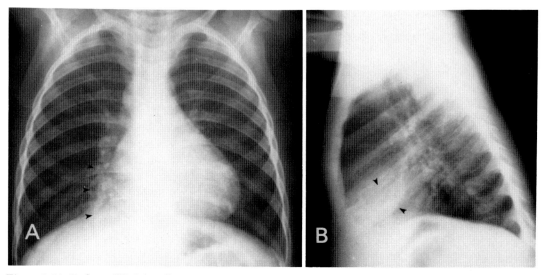

Figure 1.30. *Right middle lobe silhouette sign.* (**A**) Note that the right cardiac border is indistinct and, in fact, obliterated over its lower two-thirds by an adjacent pneumonia in the medial segment of the right middle lobe (*arrows*). The left cardiac border is sharp. (**B**) Lateral view confirms the presence of a right middle lobe pneumonia seen as an area of increased density anterioinferiorly (*arrows*).

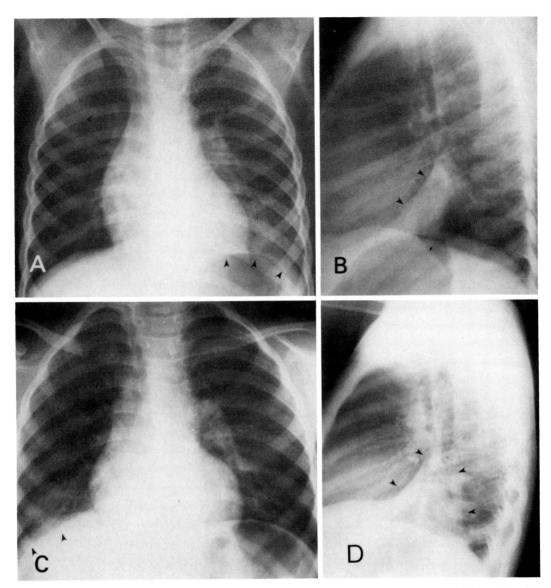

Figure 1.31. *Silhouette signs, left and right diaphragmatic leaflets.*   (*A*) The infiltrate in the left lower lung field is difficult to detect on this view, but a strong clue to its presence lies in the fact that the left diaphragmatic leaflet is indistinct (*arrows*). The gastric bubble is seen below the leaflet, but the leaflet itself is invisible (positive silhouette sign). This finding localizes the pneumonia to the left lower lobe. (*B*) Lateral view substantiates the presence of the left lower lobe pneumonia lying posterior to the major fissure (*arrows*). The portion of the diaphragmatic leaflet immediately adjacent to the pneumonia is obliterated, producing another example of a focally positive silhouette sign. (*C*) Positive silhouette sign, right diaphragm (*arrows*). A lower lobe pneumonia should be suspected. Mediastinal shift to right is due to rotation. (*D*) Lateral view confirms the right left lower lobe pneumonia (*arrows*). Note that in both cases the consolidations do not lead to any significant volume loss of the involved lobe; i.e., the major fissure in each case is in relatively normal position.

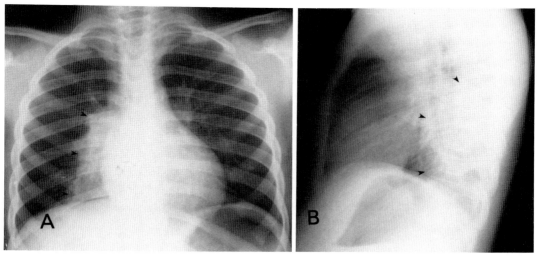

Figure 1.32. *Silhouette sign in reverse, right lower lobe localization.* (*A*) Note the rather extensive pneumonia in the right lower lobe (*arrows*). It is located behind the heart and is causing this portion of the heart to be increased in density (i.e., it is more opaque than the left side). However, because the pneumonia is behind the heart, and not in juxtaposition to its right border, the cardiac border remains distinct. If the pneumonia were in juxtaposition to the right cardiac border, that is, in the medial segment of the right middle lobe, the cardiac border would be obliterated (i.e., as in Fig. 1.30*A*). (*B*) Lateral view confirms the presence of the extensive right lower lobe pneumonia in that there is a marked increase in density of the entire posterior retrocardiac space (*arrows*). This is completely abnormal and should be compared with the normal radiolucent appearance of the lower retrocardiac space in Figure 1.25.

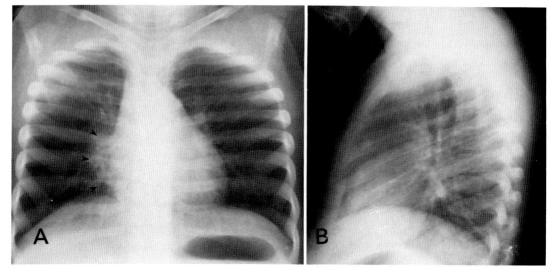

Figure 1.33. *Right middle lobe silhouette sign with parahilar peribronchial infiltrates; pseudofocal pneumonia.* (*A*) This infant has widespread parahilar peribronchial infiltrates. However, the chest film is quite lordotic (the ribs are horizontal posteriorly and slanted downward anteriorly), and this is causing the bronchovascular markings along the right cardiac silhouette to cluster even more than normal (*arrows*). Consequently, the right cardiac border is obliterated, and a right middle lobe, medial segment pneumonia is suggested. (*B*) On lateral view, however, there is no evidence of a right middle lobe infiltrate. If an infiltrate were present in the right middle lobe, it would be demonstrable on lateral view. Compare this lateral view with the lateral view in Figure 1.30, where a true right middle lobe pneumonia is present.

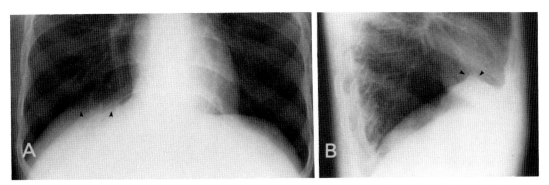

Figure 1.34. *Silhouette sign due to normal fissure insertion.* (*A*) Note focal obliteration of the right diaphragmatic leaflet (*arrows*). Is this due to an adjacent pneumonia? (*B*) Lateral view shows that the silhouette sign is produced by blending of the lower aspect of the major fissure with the right diaphragmatic leaflet (*arrows*). On frontal view, this area of blending, caught tangentially by the x-ray beam, creates a positive but normal silhouette sign. The same phenomenon can occur on the left, and also with accessory fissures.

Another instance when the silhouette sign can be seen as a normal phenomenon is when a pleural fissure blends with the upper aspect of a diaphragmatic leaflet (Fig. 1.34A). This can occur either with a major or accessory fissure, and it is only when a lateral view is obtained that this normally positive silhouette sign can be deciphered and understood (Fig.1.34B). Compare the case illustrated in Figure 1.34 with the one demonstrated in Figure 1.31D where a true right lower lobe pneumonia and a positive right diaphragmatic leaflet silhouette sign are present. *Felson's silhouette sign is an excellent sign, but one must learn to use it properly. It is always valid in principle, but at times may not be abnormal.*

REFERENCES

1. Culham, J.A.G.: The right heart border in infancy. Radiology 139: 381–384, 1981.
2. Felson, B., and Felson, H.: Localization of intrathoracic lesions by means of the posteroanterior roentgenogram: The silhouette sign. Radiology 55: 363–374, 1950.

Favorite Hiding Places of Pneumonia. There are certain areas that are notorious for hiding early pulmonary infiltrates (1). One should become familiar with all of these sites and give them a second look when inspecting the roentgenogram (Fig. 1.35). Unless one becomes thoroughly familiar with these hiding places, pulmonary infiltrates can be totally overlooked.

The first hiding place taught the radiology resident is *behind the left side of the heart* (i.e., in the left lower lobe). In most individuals the bulk of the cardiac silhouette extends to the left of the spine and thus can hide a sizable infiltrate. This is especially true if the film is too light (underpenetrated). In looking for a pneumonia in this location, one should first look for an area of focally increased density projected through the left side of the heart. A good way to check for this is to quickly compare the densities of both sides of the heart; in normal individuals they are equal, but with left lower lobe pneumonias they are not. The increase in density in cases where a pneumonia is present is due to the fact that the pneumonia is roentgenographically more dense than normal lung, and thus, when superimposed over the heart, it produces an area of increased density (Fig.1.36).

Such focal pneumonias are relatively easy to detect, but when the pneumonia is so large that it produces a generalized, rather than focal, increase in density of the entire left side of the heart, it can be missed (Fig. 1.37). In still other cases, the infiltrate may be buried deep in the phren-

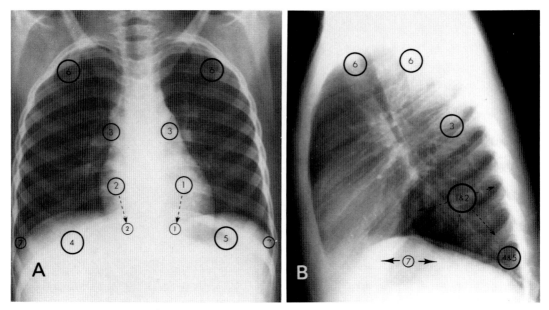

Figure 1.35. *Favorite hiding places of pneumonia.* (**A**) and (**B**) demonstrate common hiding places of pneumonia. (*1*) Behind the left side of the heart in the left lower lobe, often extending into the phrenicovertebral angle; (*2*) behind the right side of the heart in the right lower lobe, also often extending into the phrenicovertebral angle; (*3*) behind the hilar regions, in the superior segment of either lower lobe; (*4*) deep in the posterior costophrenic sulcus behind the liver; (*5*) deep in the costophrenic sulcus behind the stomach, spleen, or left lobe of the liver; (*6*) high in the upper lobes; and (*7*) deep in the lateral costophrenic sulci.

icovertebral sulci. However, when the sulci are compared one to another it becomes obvious that the abnormal one is whiter or denser than normal (Fig. 1.38). In this regard, the only pitfall to avoid is a normal increase in density in this area produced by overlapping of the cardiac silhouette and the diaphragmatic leaflet on the left (Fig. 1.38C). This usually occurs on supine films, and no such pitfall exists on the right.

So well is it ingrained in us to look behind the left side of the heart for hidden pneumonias that we forget to *look behind the right side of the heart.* Indeed, pneumonias in this area are almost always missed. The best way to recognize a pneumonia in this area again is to follow the rule that both sides of the heart should be of equal density. As on the left, right-side pneumonias may produce focal infiltrates (Fig. 1.39A) or more generalized infiltrates, resulting in a more diffuse increase

in density of all of the right side of the cardiac silhouette (Fig. 1.40A). Extension into the ipsilateral phrenicovertebral sulcus also is common (Fig. 1.40B) and should be kept in mind when perusing roentgenograms in such cases. Confirmation of all these pneumonias is once again readily accomplished with lateral chest roentgenograms (Fig. 1.39B).

Pneumonias in the superior segment of either lower lobe are notorious for hiding behind one or other of the hilar regions. In this location they cause an increase in density, and at times size, of the ipsilateral hilar region (Figs. 1.41 and 1.42). Indeed, the hilus can be so dense and prominent that lymphadenopathy is suggested (i.e., as in primary pulmonary tuberculosis). Once again, however, the lateral view clearly elucidates the problem and confirms the presence of a pneumonia in the superior segment of the involved lower lobe (Figs. 1.41 and 1.42).

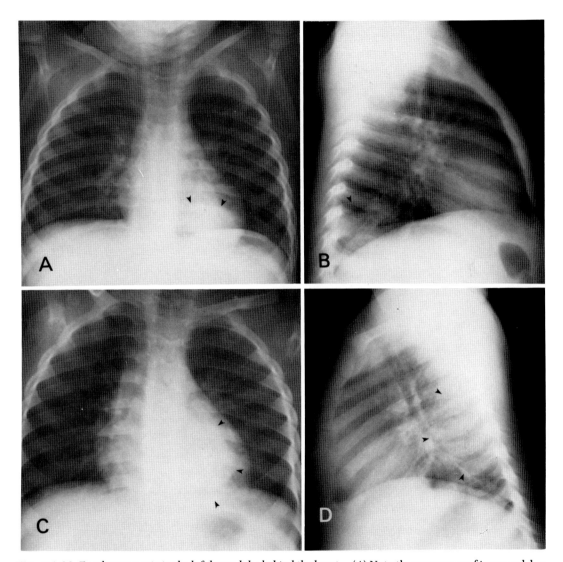

Figure 1.36. *Focal pneumonia in the left lower lobe behind the heart.* (A) Note the vague area of increased density projected through the left side of the heart (*arrows*). (B) Lateral view clearly localizes the pneumonia to the left lower lobe, deep in the costophrenic sulcus (*arrows*). Note that the adjacent part of the left diaphragmatic leaflet is obliterated, producing a positive silhouette sign. The intact leaflet visualized below this area is the right diaphragmatic leaflet. The left leaflet is higher because of splinting. (C) Note the large area of increased density behind the left side of the heart (*arrows*). (D) The lateral view demonstrates the pneumonia in the left lower lobe, but it should be noted that the finding is more subtle on this view and consists only of a diffuse increase in density of the normally radiolucent retrocardiac space (*arrows*).

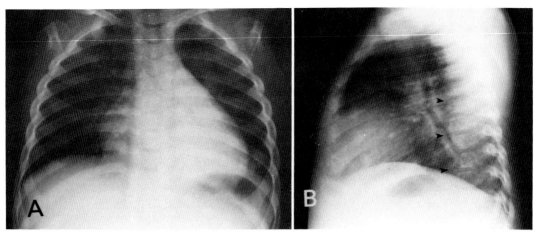

Figure 1.37. *Large left lower lobe consolidation hiding behind the heart.* (**A**) The extensive left lower lobe consolidation causes an increase in density of the entire left side of the cardiac silhouette. In spite of the size of this consolidation, it can be missed because the entire left side of the heart rather than a focal area shows increased density. A little of the consolidation projects beyond the left cardiac border, but this is a subtle finding. Of course, a lateral view should always be obtained and in *B* it clearly defines the presence of the left lower lobe consolidating pneumonia (*arrows*).

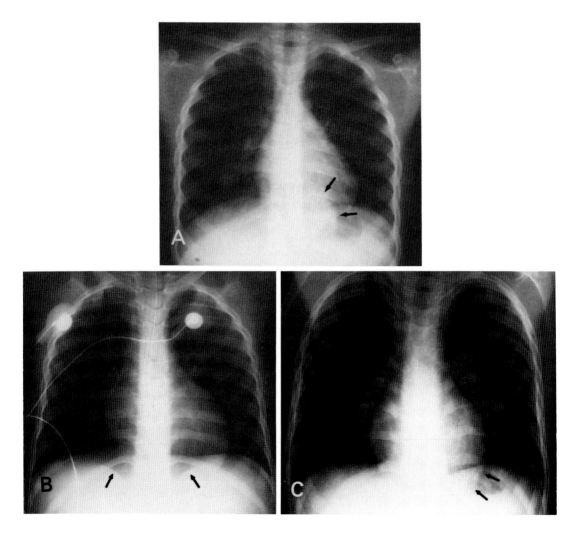

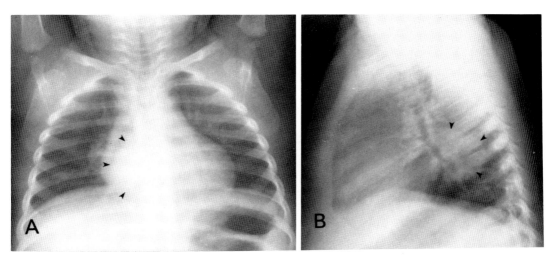

Figure 1.39. *Focal right lower lobe pneumonia behind the right side of the heart.* (*A*) Note focal area of increased density projected through the right side of the cardiac silhouette (*arrows*). (*B*) Lateral view confirms the presence of a right lower lobe pneumonia (*arrows*) located behind the heart.

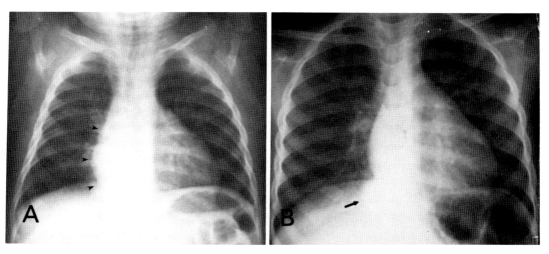

Figure 1.40. *Extensive right lower lobe pneumonia behind the right side of the heart.* (*A*) Note diffuse increase in density of that portion of the cardiac silhouette which lies to the right of the spine. This represents a pneumonia behind the right side of the heart, in the right lower lobe. (*B*) Similar finding in another patient, but in this patient there is extension of the pneumonia into the phrenicovertebral sulcus (*arrow*).

Figure 1.38. *Left lower lobe pneumonia deep in the phrenicovertebral angle.* (*A*) Note how the pneumonia in the left lower lobe extends into the phrenicovertebral angle (*arrows*). Compare this with the normal density of this angle on the other side. Also note that the diaphragmatic leaflet is obliterated in this area. (*B*) Normal chest, somewhat overaerated, showing that both phrenicovertebral angles should be of about equal radiolucency (*arrows*). (*C*) Normal pitfall wherein the left inferior cardiac border and medial left diaphragmatic leaflet overlap to produce an increase in density in the area (*arrows*).

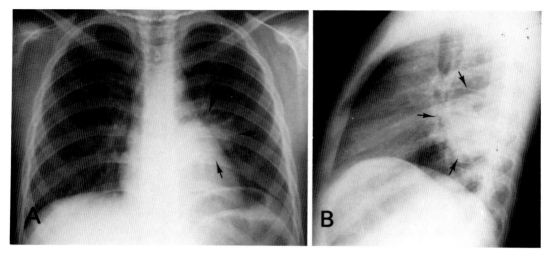

Figure 1.41. *Pneumonia behind the left hilus.* (*A*) Note that the left hilus is denser and larger than the right (*arrows*). (*B*) Lateral view shows that the pneumonia is located in the superior segment of the left lower lobe (*arrows*). If one recalls the normal position of the major fissure, it will be clearly apparent that the pneumonia must be in the superior segment of the lower lobe and not in the upper lobe.

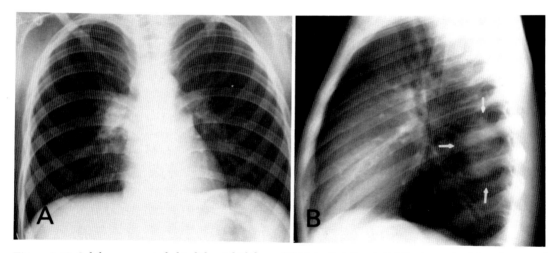

Figure 1.42. *Subtle pneumonia behind the right hilus.* (*A*) Note that the right hilus is much whiter (increased density), and slightly larger than the left hilus. At first, this might suggest unilateral hilar adenopathy. (*B*) Lateral view, however, clearly demonstrates the presence of a focal pneumonia in the superior segment of the right lower lobe (*arrows*).

Lower lobe pneumonias deep in the posterior costophrenic sulci are also frequently missed on frontal projection. On the right side these pneumonias are projected through the liver silhouette, and unless one becomes accustomed to their appearance they are most difficult to recognize (Fig. 1.43). In some cases, one may be surprised at the size of a pneumonia so hidden (Fig. 1.44). On the left side, such pneumonias can be projected through the left lobe of the liver, the stom-

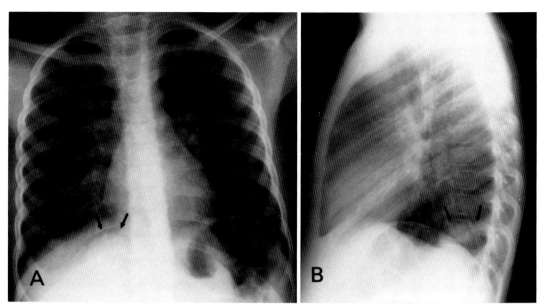

Figure 1.43. *Focal pneumonia, right lower lobe behind the liver.* (*A*) Note focal area of increased density (pneumonia) projected through the medial aspect of the liver silhouette (*arrows*). (*B*) Lateral view showing how deep this pneumonia lies in the posterior costophrenic sulcus (*arrows*). The right diaphragmatic leaflet (*lower leaflet*) is partially obliterated by the adjacent infiltrate (*arrows*), while the left diaphragmatic leaflet is clearly visualized through the infiltrate.

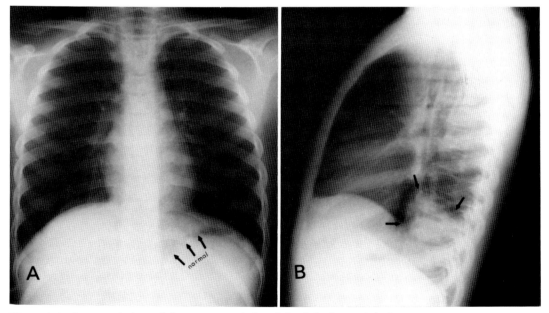

Figure 1.44. *Large right lower lobe pneumonia hiding behind the liver.* (*A*) This pneumonia is so large that it could be missed for that reason. However, note that there is a general increase in density of the entire area below the right diaphragmatic leaflet, but, more importantly, that there is increased density of the phrenicovertebral sulcus. It should be radiolucent, just like the normal one on the left (*arrow*). (*B*) Lateral view shows that this increase in density is due to a large consolidating right lower lobe pneumonia (*arrows*). The portion of the right diaphragmatic leaflet just below and adjacent to the infiltrate is completely obliterated (positive silhouette sign).

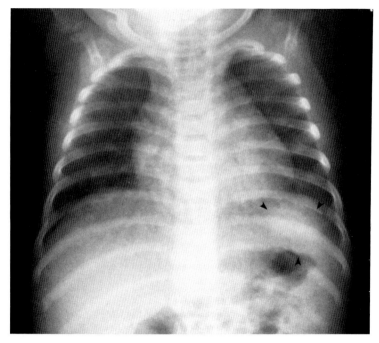

Figure 1.45. *Subtle focal pneumonia behind left diaphragmatic leaflet.* Note vague area of increased density projected through the left diaphragmatic leaflet (*arrows*). This was an early consolidating pneumonia of the left lower lobe, deep in the posterior costophrenic sulcus.

ach bubble, or the spleen (Fig. 1.45). On lateral view, these pneumonias usually lie deep in the posterior costophrenic sulcus and frequently obliterate the adjacent portion of the diaphragmatic leaflet (i.e., positive silhouette sign).

Two other places where pneumonias can hide are high in the upper lobe and deep in the lateral costophrenic sulcus. In the former instance, the pneumonia is often confused with normal overlying soft tissues (Fig. 1.46). In such cases, one should compare the densities of both apices (actually one should do this for all areas of the chest) and check the lateral view for confirmation. In checking the apices for subtle infiltrates, it is worthwhile to "black-out" the remainder of the chest with an opaque piece of cardboard. When this maneuver is performed, comparison of the apices is easier, and subtle infiltrates stand out with more clarity. Pneumonias deep in the lateral costophrenic sulci are usually missed because one simply does not look in this re-

gion. These pneumonias are truly subtle and are usually seen on frontal projection only (Fig. 1.47).

REFERENCE

1. Burko, H.: Considerations in the roentgen diagnosis of pneumonia in children. A.J.R. 88: 555–565, 1962.

Other Pulmonary Infections. The preceding sections dealt mainly with the usual bacterial and viral infections presenting in the acute care setting, but a few points regarding other pulmonary infections that can be encountered are in order. First, one might consider *pertussis infection*, which is still relatively common. For the most part, patients with pertussis present with viral-like parahilar peribronchial infiltrates (Fig. 1.48A) (5, 9). This should not be a surprise as pertussis infection is a bronchitis and peribronchitis, which, in the past, led to the so-called "shaggy heart" appearance (1). Interestingly enough, however, although parahilar peri-

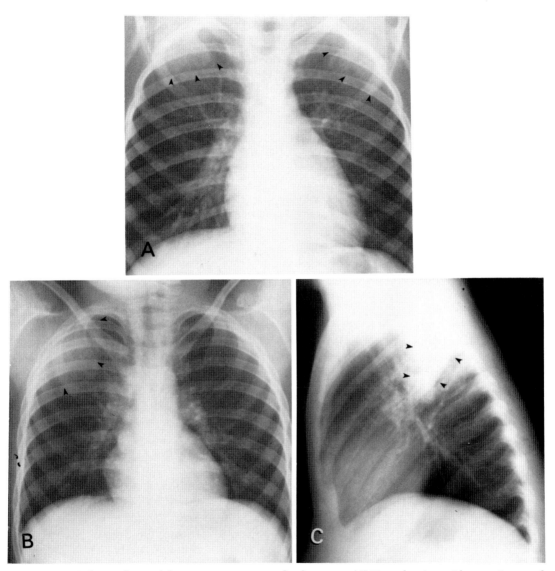

Figure 1.46. *High apical upper lobe pneumonia vs. normal soft tissues.* (*A*) Normal patient with vague increased density high in the apices due to normal overlying soft tissues (*arrows*). (*B*) Patient with unilateral increase in density in the same area (*arrows*) representing a pneumonia. This pneumonia could easily be overlooked or mistaken for normal soft tissue density. (*C*) On lateral view, however, the pneumonia is clearly visualized in the posterior segment of the right upper lobe (*arrows*).

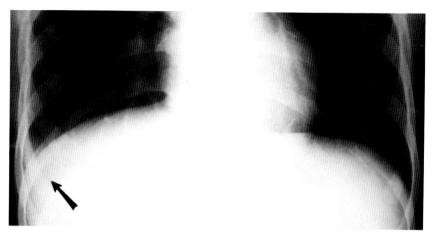

Figure 1.47. *Costophrenic sulcus pneumonia.* Note the early infiltrate deep in the right costophrenic sulcus (*arrow*) of this patient who had chest pain over the right lower chest, laterally. These pneumonias are commonly overlooked and are not usually seen on lateral view. Consequently, they must be picked up on the frontal projection.

bronchial infiltrates are common, it is also common to see completely clear, but over-aerated, lungs (2). Indeed, over the years we have found this pattern to be more common, an important point to appreciate. The shaggy heart appearance results from parahilar peribronchial infiltratives blurring the usually sharp cardiac and mediastinal edges. Currently, of course, the shaggy heart most commonly is seen with viral or *Mycoplasma* infections, but it also is seen with pertussis and *Chlamydia* infections.

With pertussis, it should be remembered that since the basic problem is a bronchitis-peribronchitis, consolidations occur only in those few cases where superimposed bacterial infection is seen. Therefore, in the usual case of pertussis, the lungs are overaerated and either completely clear or demonstrative of parahilar peribronchial infiltrates. Segmental and lobar atelectasis also are common and, interestingly enough, a similar appearance usually is seen with *Chlamydia* infections (Fig. 1.48B). This infection also is a bronchial-peribronchial infection, and in the past was referred to as "pertussoid" pneumonia.

Mycoplasma pneumoniae infections are extremely variable in their clinical and roentgenographic presentation (3, 4, 6, 7, 12, 13, 16), but still the most common presentation is that of a widespread viral-like bronchitis-peribronchitis with or without associated segmental or lobar atelectasis (14) (see Fig. 1.51A). On the other hand, *M. pneumoniae* infections also can present with consolidations (6, 7), and, as has been noted earlier in this chapter, the clinical picture then is not unlike that seen with pneumococcal pneumonia. However, when diffuse parahilar peribronchial infiltrates are seen, the clinical picture more closely resembles that of a viral infection. Another interesting pattern of infiltration in patients with *M. pneumoniae* infection, especially in older children or adolescents, is that of unilobar, or basically unilobar, distribution of reticulonodular or reticular infiltrates (Figs. 1.49 and 1.50). Associated atelectasis is common in these patients (Fig. 1.49) and in the purest sense they represent patients with so-called "walking pneumonia." They usually have symptoms for 1 to 2 weeks before they finally come to the physician's attention. Occasionally one is fortunate enough to witness a transition of the infection from this basically interstitial phase to one more alveolar (Fig. 1.51).

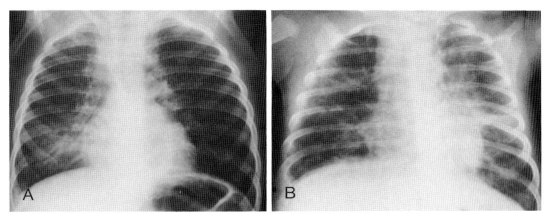

Figure 1.48. *Pertussis infection.* (**A**) Note typical parahilar peribronchial infiltrates similar to those seen with viral disease. The lungs are overaerated. (**B**) *Chlamydia infection.* The findings are very similar to those seen with pertussis and viral infection. Note an area of segmental atelectasis in the left mid lung field. *Mycoplasma* infections also commonly present with this type of infiltrative pattern.

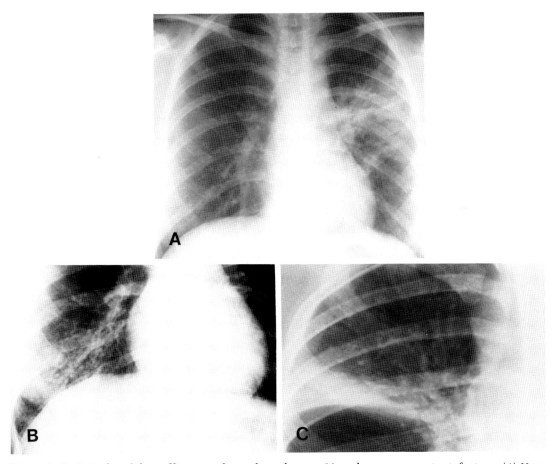

Figure 1.49. *Reticulonodular infiltrates with streaky atelectasis: Mycoplasma pneumoniae infection.* (**A**) Note streaky, reticular infiltrate in the left upper lobe. (**B**) Reticulonodular infiltrate in the right upper lobe. (**C**) Reticulonodular infiltrate in the right upper lobe, associated with early atelectasis. All of these patients had *Mycoplasma pneumoniae* infection.

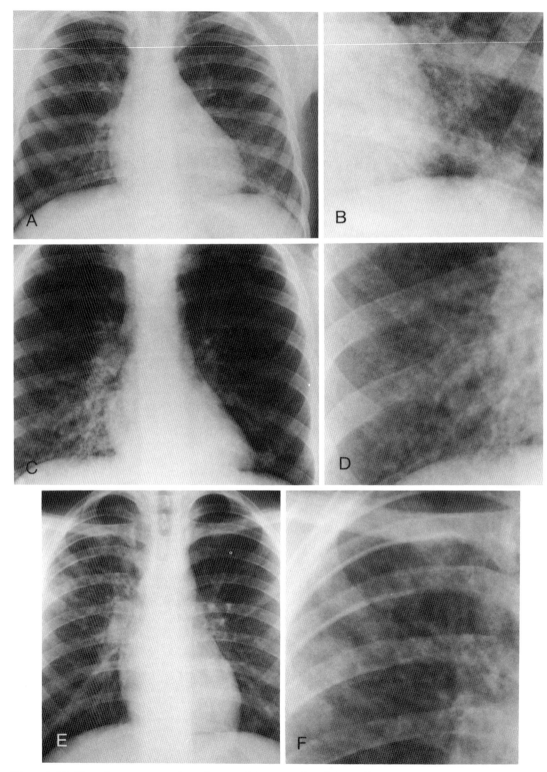

Figure 1.50. *Mycoplasma pneumoniae infections; lobar reticulonodular infiltrates.* (*A*) Note the subtle, hazy infiltrate in the left lower lobe. (*B*) Coned view demonstrates its delicately reticular interstitial pattern. (*C*) Another patient with a more coarse appearing reticular infiltrate in the right lower lobe. Note associated right hilar adenopathy. (*D*) Coned view of the infiltrate. (*E*) A third patient with a more nodular infiltrate in the right upper lobe. (*F*) Coned view demonstrates the relatively large nodules, suggesting that the disease process now may have extended in the adjacent alveoli.

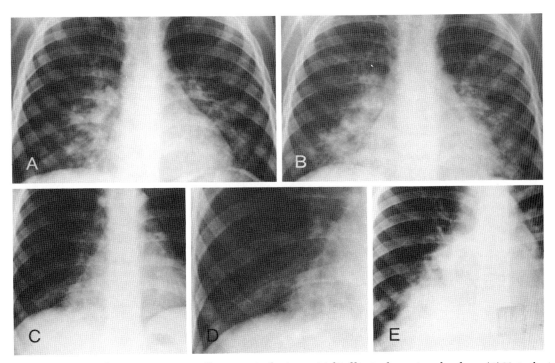

Figure 1.51. *Mycoplasma pneumoniae infection; reticular interstitial infiltrates becoming alveolar.* (*A*) Note the bilateral reticulonodular, but basically reticular, infiltrates with a typical central predominance. (*B*) By the next day, the infiltrates, especially on the right, have become more confluent and involve the adjacent parenchyma. (*C*) Another patient with a reticular infiltrate in the right middle lobe, obliterating the right cardiac border. (*D*) Coned view demonstrates the reticular nature of the infiltrate. (*E*) Next day, note how the infiltrate, now in the right middle and lower lobes, has become consolidated. There is no volume loss and therefore atelectasis is not the problem.

However most patients retain their original interstitial pattern of reticulonodular infiltration.

Primary pulmonary tuberculosis also still is common and can present with a wide variety of roentgenographic findings (10, 18). However, most often one will be confronted with unilateral hilar or paratracheal adenopathy and some other finding in the lung (Fig. 1.52), the most common of which is lobar or segmental atelectasis (10, 11, 18–20) (Fig. 1.52). Occasionally, a consolidation is encountered (Fig. 1.52D) and, rarely, a focal, nodular, fluffy parenchymal infiltrate may be seen. Cavitation is not a common problem in primary pulmonary tuberculosis (16) and, when seen, probably is more a problem of pneumatocele formation (11) than actual ab-

scess formation. Obstructive emphysema of a lobe also occasionally can be seen with tuberculosis (Fig. 1.52C), but unilateral hilar or paratracheal adenopathy and associated ipsilateral atelectasis remain the hallmarks of this infection (Fig. 1.52A and see Figs. 1.80 and 1.81). Bilateral hilar adenopathy is relatively uncommon (see Fig. 1.78B).

Both atelectasis and emphysema usually are due to endobronchial granuloma formation rather than external bronchial compression by enlarged nodes, no matter how prominent the nodes appear. Indeed, atelectasis can be seen with little in the way of adenopathy (Fig.1.52B). Pleural effusions are not as common as in adults but still at times can be massive. In summary, then, a good rule of thumb for suspecting

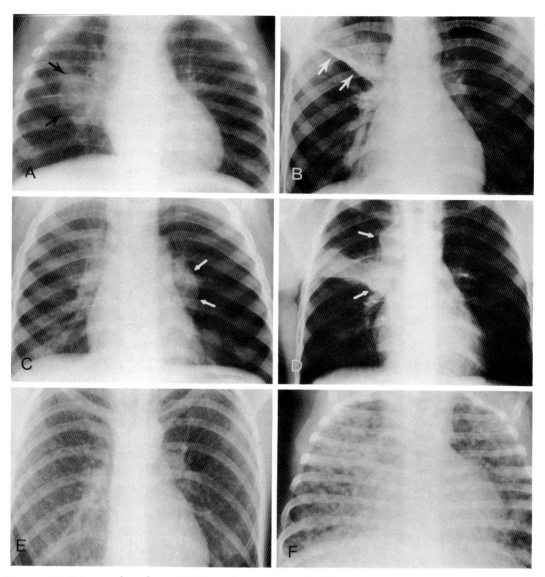

Figure 1.52. *Primary tuberculosis.* (**A**) Note characteristic right hilar and paratracheal adenopathy (*arrows*). (**B**) Another patient with atelectasis of the right upper lobe (*arrows*) and little in the way of hilar or paratracheal adenopathy. (**C**) Left hilar adenopathy (*arrows*) with obstructive emphysema of the left lung. A minimal reticular infiltrate is present throughout the right lung and hilar adenopathy also is present on the right. (**D**) Right hilar and paratracheal adenopathy (*arrows*) with early consolidation of the right upper lobe. (**E**) Diffuse miliary infiltrates throughout both lungs. There is no hilar adenopathy. (**F**) Infant with more coarse-appearing reticulonodular infiltrates.

primary pulmonary tuberculosis in infancy and childhood is: *unilateral hilar or paratracheal adenopathy, with or without parenchymal change (almost any type), should be presumed tuberculous in origin until proven otherwise.* Even though these findings can be mimicked by atypical tuberculous, fungal, and some cases of *M.*

pneumoniae infection, tuberculosis will most often be the cause and should be the primary diagnosis until proven otherwise.

Miliary tuberculosis occasionally also can be seen, and while in older children the infiltrates are truly miliary (Fig. 1.52E), in infants the individual nodules are larger and not as miliary. They appear

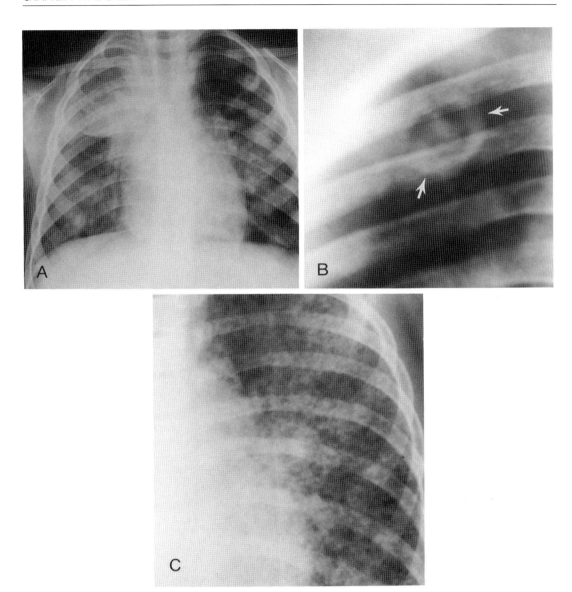

Figure 1.53. *Fungal disease.* (*A*) Actinomycosis presenting with consolidation of the right upper lobe and nodules scattered throughout both lungs. (*B*) Aspergillosis with characteristic fungal ball (*arrows*). Note the nidus in the center. (*C*) Acute disseminated histoplasmosis presenting a diffused reticulonodular pattern. (From S.D. John and L.E. Swischuk: Fungus infections of the chest in infants and children. J. Thorac. Imaging 7: 91–98, 1992).

more reticulonodular (Fig. 1.52*F*). In many of these latter cases, it is difficult to detect underlying adenopathy or any other pulmonary change, while in others one may see associated adenopathy, atelectasis, and even the peripheral Ghon lesion.

Fungal infections are not particularly common in childhood, except in the so-

called "fungus belts." If one resides in such an area, it soon becomes apparent that the roentgenographic findings are very variable (8), ranging from acute disseminated reticulonodular or fluffy infiltrates through lobar consolidations (Fig. 1.53). In still other cases, findings not unlike those seen with primary pulmonary tu-

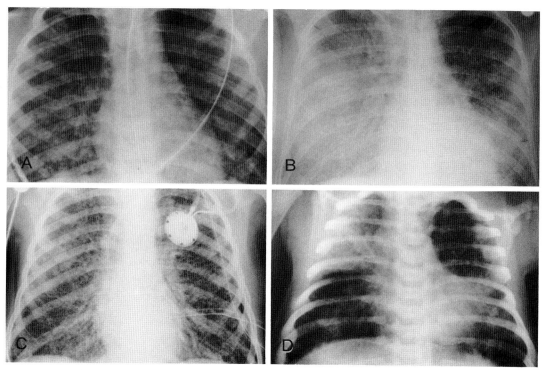

Figure 1.54. *Infection in immunocompromised patients.* (*A*) Typical reticulonodular infiltrate throughout both lungs. This can be seen with viral infections, *Pneumocystis carinii* infections, tuberculosis, and with nonspecific, reactive lymphoid tissue proliferation. (*B*) Diffuse, interstitial haziness of both lungs, most characteristic of *P. carinii* infection, but also seen with viral infection. (*C*) Diffuse, reticular interstitial infiltrates due to *Herpes pneumonitis.* (*D*) Another patient, a very young infant with *H. pneumonitis* showing alveolar involvement with consolidation of the right upper lobe and early consolidation of the lingula. Underlying, note the basic pattern of interstitial infiltration.

berculosis are encountered. This being the case, one soon will elevate fungal infections from the bottom of the list of diagnostic possibilities to a higher, more realistic, position. So-called "fungus balls" (Fig. 1.53*B*) are most often seen with aspergillosis.

Immunocompromised patients respond differently to infections and human immunodeficiency virus (HIV)-infected patients are in this category. Basically, however, these patients are chronically ill and tend to have chronic, smoldering infections. For the most part, they do not present with "clean" consolidations or typical parahilar-peribronchial infiltrates. Most often they present with chronic, reticulonodular interstitial infiltrates or patchy alveolar infiltrates (Fig. 1.54), which usually are due to infection by an opportunistic organism such as cytomegalic inclusion virus (CMV) or *Pneumocystis carinii*. However, infections due to almost any virus, fungus, tuberculosis, atypical tuberculosis, or other indolent infectious agent can be seen. In advanced cases, extensive consolidations, pleural effusions, and empyemas occur. Finally, it might be noted that patients with sickle cell disease are especially prone to develop pneumococcal and *M. pneumoniae* infections (13, 14), and in many cases these can be rather profound and rampant infections (Fig. 1.18*C* and *D*). There is, of course, always the added problem of veno-occlusive disease due to sludging in these patients, and this may prove to be important in these patients (i.e., infarction may precede infection).

REFERENCES

1. Barnhard, H.J., and Kniker, W.T.: Roentgenologic findings in pertussis with particular emphasis on the "shaggy heart" sign. A.J.R. 84: 445–450, 1960.
2. Bellamy, E.A., Johnston, I.D.A., and Wilson, A.G.: The chest radiograph in whooping cough. Clin. Radiol. 38: 39–43, 1987.
3. Clyde, W.A., Jr., and Denny, M. W.: *Mycoplasma* infections in childhood. Pediatrics 40: 669–684, 1967.
4. Cordero, L., Cuadrado, R., Hall, C.B., and Horstmann, D.M.: Primary atypical pneumonia: An epidemic caused by *Mycoplasma pneumoniae.* J. Pediatr. 71: 1–12, 1967.
5. Fawcitt, J., and Parry, H.E.: Lung changes in pertussis and measles in childhood: A review of 1894 cases with a followup study of the pulmonary complications. Br. J. Radiol. 30: 76–82, 1957.
6. Fernald, G.W., Collier, A.M., and Clyde, W.A., Jr.: Respiratory infections due to *Mycoplasma pneumoniae* in infants and children. Pediatrics 55: 327–335, 1975.
7. Herbert, D.H.: The roentgen features of Eaton agent pneumonia. A.J.R. 98: 300–304, 1966.
8. John, S.D., and Swischuk, L.E.: Fungus infections of the chest in infants and children. J. Thorac. Imaging 7: 91–98, 1992.
9. Kohn, J.L., Schwartz, I., Greenbaum, J., and Daly, M.M.I.: Roentgenograms of the chest taken during pertussis. Am. J. Dis. Child. 67: 463, 1944.
10. Leung, A.N., Müller, N.L., Pineda, P.R., and FitzGerald, J.M.: Primary tuberculosis in childhood: Radiographic manifestations. Radiology 152: 87–91, 1992.
11. Matsaniotis, N., et al.: Bullous emphysema in childhood tuberculosis. J. Pediatr. 71:703, 1967.
12. Putman, C.E., Curtis, A. McB., Simeone, J.F., and Jensen, P.: *Mycoplasma* pneumonia: Clinical and roentgenographic patterns. A.J.R. 124: 417–422, 1975.
13. Sabato, A.R., Martin, A.J., Marmion, B.P., Kok, T.W., and Cooper, D.M.: *Mycoplasma pneumoniae:* Acute illness, antibiotics, and subsequent pulmonary function. Arch. Dis. Child. 59: 1034–1037, 1984.
14. Seeler, R.A., Metzger, W., and Mufson, M.A.: *Diplococcus pneumoniae* infections in children with sickle cell anemia. Am. J. Dis. Child. 123: 8–10, 1972.
15. Shulman, S.T., et al.: The unusual severity of mycoplasma pneumonia in children with sickle cell disease. N. Engl. J. Med. 287: 164–167, 1972.
16. Solomon, A., and Rabinowitz, L.: Primary cavitating tuberculosis in childhood. Clin. Radiol. 23: 483–485, 1972.
17. Stallings, M.W., and Archer, S.B.: Atypical mycoplasma pneumonia. Am. J. Dis. Child. 126: 837–838, 1973.
18. Stansberry, S.D.: Tuberculosis in infants and children. J. Thorac. Imaging 5: 17–27, 1990.
19. Veneeklas, G. M. H.: Cause and sequelae of iatropulmonary shadows in primary tuberculosis. Am. J. Dis Child. 83: 271–273, 1952.
20. Weber, A.L., Bird, K.T., and Janover, H.L.: Primary tuberculosis in childhood with particular emphasis on changes affecting the tracheobronchial tree. A.J.R. 103: 123–132, 1968.

PLEURAL FLUID COLLECTIONS AND EMPYEMA

The types of fluid which can collect in the pleural space include: (a) pus (empyema, pyothorax), (b) serous fluid (hydrothorax), (c) blood (hemothorax), and (d) chyle (chylothorax). *Empyema* is usually a complication of an underlying pneumonia and in this regard in the past was seen most commonly with *S. aureus* infections (7, 10, 12, 13, 25), but this infection is not as common now (27). Currently, under the age of 3 years, *H. influenzae* most often is the causative organism (11, 22, 31), and in the older child, *S. pneumoniae* (pneumococcus) is more common. Empyema also can be seen with hemolytic streptococcal pulmonary infections (14) and secondary to osteomyelitis of the spine or subdiaphragmatic infections such as hepatic or subphrenic abscess. However, most occur secondary to pneumonias caused by *S. aureus*, *S. pneumoniae*, and *H. influenzae*.

Empyemas can develop rapidly and progression from a subtle collection of fluid to a full-blown empyema in less than 24 hours is not uncommon. Most of these patients, of course, are quite ill, but it is surprising how relatively asymptomatic some of them appear. The roentgenographic changes depend on the size of the pyogenic fluid collection and may range from complete opacification of a hemithorax with massive mediastinal shift (Fig. 1.55A) to less strik-

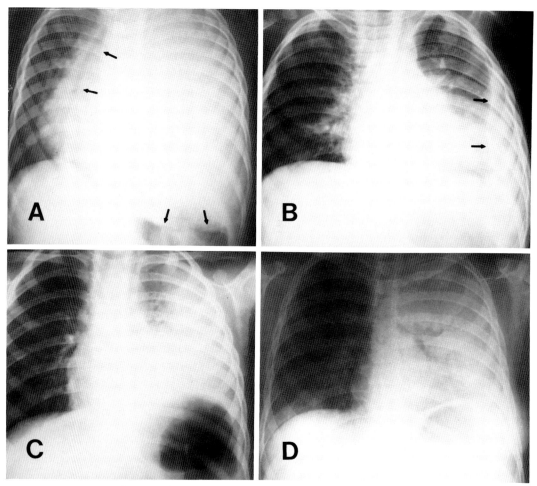

Figure 1.55. *Empyema; classic configuration and atypical patterns.* (*A*) Classic massive empyema with contralateral mediastinal displacement and ipsilateral diaphragmatic leaflet depression (*arrows*). (*B*) Another typical case, but with a smaller empyema (*arrows*). (*C*) *Empyema with no shift.* The developing empyema is not large enough to produce mediastinal shift. (*D*) *Pneumonia or empyema?* The air bronchogram would at first suggest consolidating pneumonia. However, one should ask the question, "How many times have I seen a consolidating pneumonia involving the entire lung?" This would be unusual and furthermore, the air bronchogram does not extend to the periphery. The problem here is a developing empyema, partially compressing the ipsilateral lung.

ing and perhaps more puzzling changes. In this regard, it should be remembered that the empyema must first compress the lung and then shift the mediastinum. Consequently, at certain stages of the development of an empyema, shift may be minimal or absent and the incompletely compressed lung can be identified by its air bronchogram (Fig. 1.55C and D). However, the air bronchogram does not extend far into the periphery, for the peripheral

portion of the lung is compressed and surrounded by exudate. Currently, ultrasound is very useful in delineating the fluid in such cases. Indeed, ultrasound is most useful in detecting empyemas in general, whether the fluid collection is free flowing or loculated. When loculated, the fluid collections may be unilocular, or multilocular with many septae (Figs. 1.56 and 1.57). The latter collections, of course, are difficult to drain. Pulmonary infiltrates are

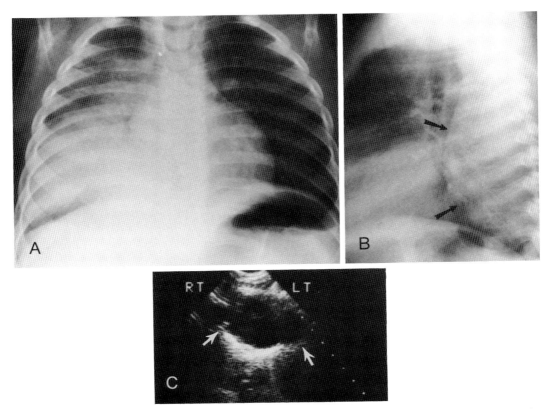

Figure 1.56. *Empyema; ultrasonographic detection.* (*A*) Patient with a consolidation of the right middle lobe and a density projected over the lower portion of the upper lobe. (*B*) Lateral view demonstrating increased density in the region of the right middle lobe but a mass located posteriorly (*arrows*). The upper portion of this mass is causing the area of increased density in the lower portion of the right upper lobe on the frontal view. (*C*) Sonogram demonstrates the density to be a hypoechoic, loculated empyema (*arrows*).

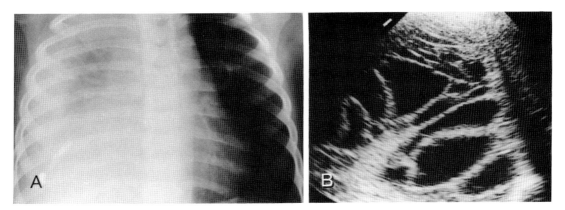

Figure 1.57. *Empyema; ultrasonographic confirmation.* (*A*) Note the totally opacified hemithorax and a little aeration of the right upper lung. There is contralateral mediastinal shift, and a space-occupying problem is present on the right. Pleural fluid or a frank empyema compressing the lungs circumferentially should be suspected. (*B*) Ultrasonogram demonstrates the presence of a multiloculated empyema.

variable, and in many cases once the purulent fluid is removed, the lungs turn out to be surprisingly clear. This is a common paradox and difficult to explain. One would presume that a consolidating pneumonia would be seen in all these cases. However, it may be that the peripheral pneumonia in such cases, rather than extending into the adjacent lung as usual, causes more inflammation of the pleural space and an empyema develops. This, however, is only conjecture.

If *empyema is accompanied by pneumothorax* so that pyopneumothorax results, one can be almost completely certain that *S. aureus* is the offending organism. The thick, tenacious secretions characteristic of this infection lead to air trapping secondary to endobronchial obstruction, and as a result complicating pneumothorax is common. In many cases, the free air is loculated into numerous compartments, and a multitude of air-fluid levels are seen on the upright film (Fig. 1.58). However, whether this occurs or not, the presence of free air and fluid in the pleural space, in the absence of trauma, should suggest *S. aureus* infection with pyopneumothorax. Every so often, some other organism will produce the same picture, but in the long run it will be *S. aureus*.

Simple pleural effusions, of course, can be seen with pneumonias produced by the same organisms producing empyemas (Fig. 1.59), including *M. pneumoniae* infections (5). Pleural effusions also can be seen with primary tuberculous and fungal infections, but are rare with viral infections (1, 5). Simple pleural effusions also are commonly seen with kidney disease such as the nephrotic syndrome and acute glomerulonephritis, chest and abdominal tumors such as neuroblastoma and lymphosarcoma, subphrenic or hepatic inflammatory processes, chest wall or spine lesions, pancreatitis, congestive heart failure, and the collagen vascular diseases. All pleural effusions are readily demonstrable with CT and ultrasound, but the latter is more expedient (15, 16) (Fig. 1.60).

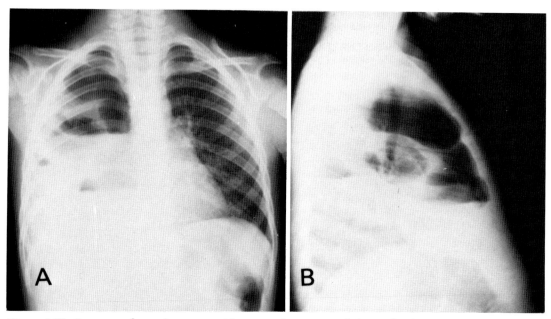

Figure 1.58. *Pyopneumothorax (empyema with pneumothorax in staphylococcal infection).* (**A**) Note the numerous air-fluid levels on the right. This finding is characteristic of staphylococcal infections. Some of the air collections also could be pneumatoceles. (**B**) Lateral view showing similar findings.

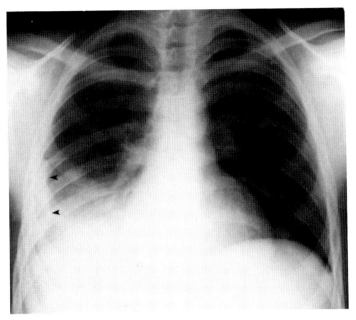

Figure 1.59. *Pneumonia with pleural effusion.* This patient has a right lower lobe consolidating pneumococcal pneumonia, but in addition there is a pleural effusion on the right (*arrows*).

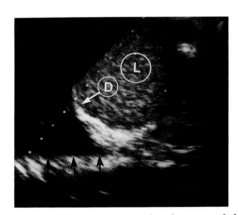

Figure 1.60. *Value of ultrasound in detection of pleural fluid.* Note typical sonolucent fluid in the posterior sulcus (*arrows*). Diaphragm (*D*), liver (*L*).

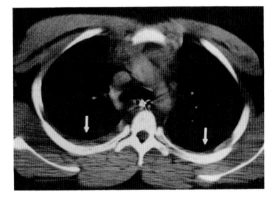

Figure 1.61. *Pleural fluid; CT demonstration.* Note bilateral small posterior pleural effusions (*arrows*).

With CT on axial views, pleural fluid is best seen along the posterior and lateral walls of the chest (Fig. 1.61). When such fluid is deep in the costophrenic sulcus, it may be difficult to differentiate it from abdominal fluid. It is here that ultrasound is most useful, as it clearly identifies the diaphragm (15) (Fig. 1.60).

Most often the first roentgenographic sign of a pleural effusion consists of blunting of the costophrenic angles so as to produce wedgelike menisci which extend upward along the lateral chest wall (Fig.1.62A). Similar collections with characteristically curved or sloping menisci are seen in the posterior costophrenic angles on lateral view (Fig. 1.62B), while larger volumes of pleural fluid can be seen to extend up the entire lateral chest wall and

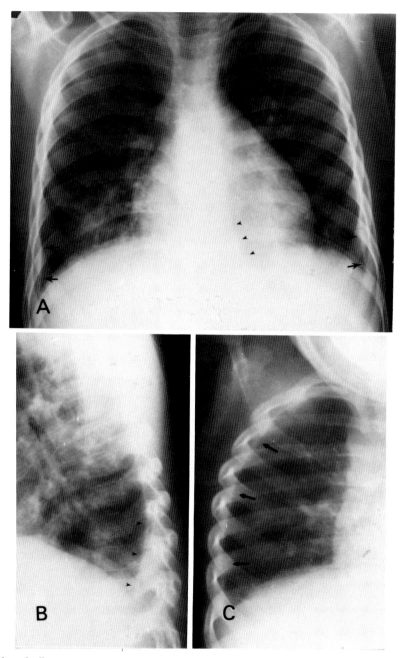

Figure 1.62. *Pleural effusions; common presenting configurations.* (**A**) Note characteristic early accumulations of pleural fluid in both costophrenic angles (*large arrows*). In addition, there is accumulation of fluid in the left paraspinal gutter, just barely visible through the cardiac silhouette (*small arrows*). (**B**) Lateral view demonstrating characteristic sloping or curving configuration of fluid in the posterior costophrenic angles (*arrows*). (**C**) Larger volume pleural effusion layered along the entire right lateral chest wall and extending over the apex (*arrows*).

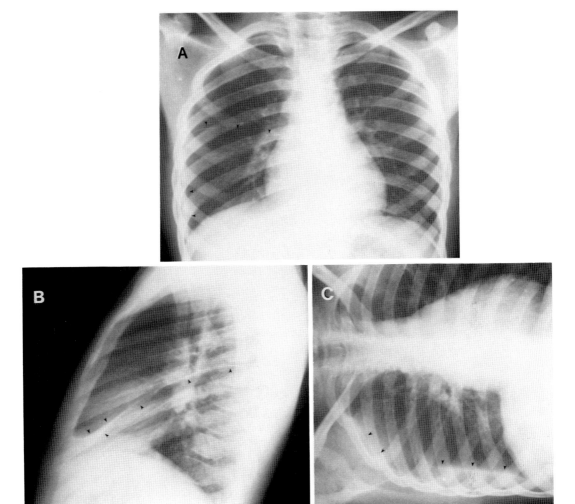

Figure 1.63. *Early, subtle pleural effusions.* (A) The pleural effusion on the right might be overlooked in this child who eventually was determined to have a collagen vascular disease. However, note that there is fluid along the right lateral chest wall (*lateral arrows.*) and some fluid in the right minor fissure (*upper arrows*). (B) Lateral view showing thin layers of fluid in all the interlobar fissures, but note specifically the typical tapering wedgelike configuration of fluid in the anteriormost portion of the right major fissure (*arrows*). A layer of fluid is also present retrosternally. (C) Decubitus film with the right side down demonstrates how much fluid actually is present on the right (*arrows*). Decubitus views are invaluable in demonstrating actual volumes of known pleural effusions and confirming the presence of subtle ones.

eventually over the apex of the lung (Fig. 1.62C). A similar layering phenomenon can occur retrosternally (Fig. 1.63B). In other instances, early pleural effusions may present with what at first appears to be unusual prominence or thickening of the interlobar fissures or with wedgelike tapering accumulations of the fluid at either end of these fissures (Fig. 1.63). Fluid accumulations in the right or left major fissures characteristically appear as a thick, sloping line (Fig. 1.64), the so-called vertical fissure (3, 29).

Pleural effusions in the supine position frequently are overlooked. Most often, one encounters such effusions in a critically ill or severely injured child where a supine, instead of an upright, chest film is ob-

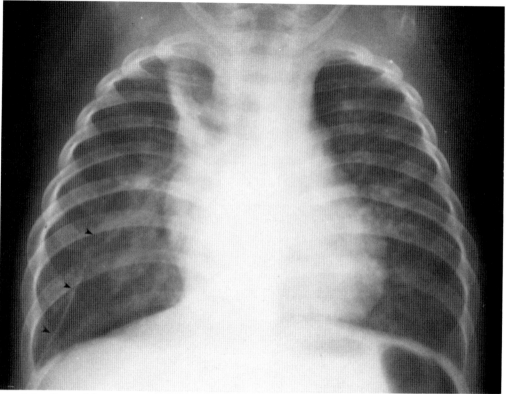

Figure 1.64. *Vertical fissure.*   When fluid accumulates in the major fissure, its lowermost portion can be seen as a sloping, but basically vertical, line on frontal view (*arrows*). In this case, it is on the right but it can also be seen on the left. This patient has congestive heart failure, secondary to congenital heart disease (endocardial cushion defect with left to right shunt). Atelectasis of the right upper lobe also is present.

tained. In such cases, fluid layers beneath the lung (6), and rather than conforming to one of its more typical configurations, it simply produces a generalized increase in density of the involved hemithorax (Fig. 1.65). If this is the only sign present, one can see why the pleural effusion can be missed. If, on the other hand, other more classic signs of pleural effusion are present, the diagnosis is easier to establish.

Subpulmonic pleural effusions also are often difficult to detect and, in fact, may completely elude the unwary observer. These effusions are free flowing (6, 18, 20, 24) and in the upright position collect between the lung and the diaphragmatic leaflet. In some cases, the fluid so conforms to the normal curvature of the diaphragm

that one is led to believe that the diaphragmatic leaflet is elevated (Fig. 1.66). However, if *telltale subtle signs are sought for*, these effusions can be detected with greater certainty. Specifically, *these signs consist of:* (a) unusual flatness of the apparently high diaphragmatic leaflet, (b) a sharp drop-off of the diaphragmatic leaflet laterally, (c) obliteration of the adjacent portion of the cardiac silhouette, (d) increased density of the posterior phrenicovertebral sulcus, (e) paraspinal collections of fluid, especially on the left (26), (f) peculiar bumps and humps of the apparently high diaphragmatic leaflet, (g) an increase in the space between the top of the apparently elevated diaphragmatic leaflet and stomach bubble, (h) loss of visualization of

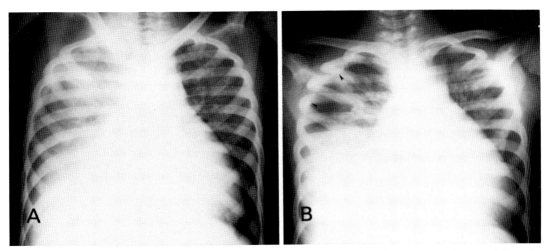

Figure 1.65. *Pleural effusion; supine film findings.* (**A**) Note the generalized increase in density of the right hemithorax. Cardiomegaly and pulmonary edema also are present in this patient who suffered a severe fluid overload. The fact that a large volume of fluid is layered behind the right lung might be overlooked if this were the only film obtained. (**B**) An upright view, however, shows clearing of the right upper lung field secondary to the fluid shifting downward. It now totally opacifies the lower lung field and mimics a consolidation. Some fluid remains in the apex (*arrows*).

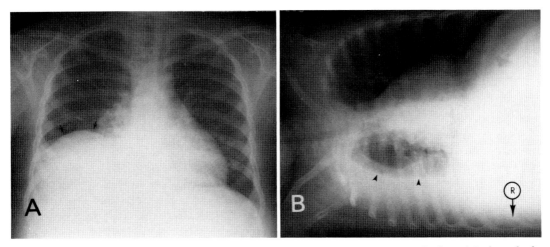

Figure 1.66. *Subpulmonic effusion presenting as an apparently elevated diaphragmatic leaflet.* (**A**) The right diaphragmatic leaflet appears elevated (*arrows*). However, the finding actually represents a subpulmonic effusion. (**B**) Decubitus view with right side down confirms the presence of the large pleural effusion. This patient had nephrotic syndrome.

the normal blood vessels of the lung through the uppermost part of the apparent diaphragmatic leaflet (24), and (i) evidence of pleural fluid collecting in more familiar sites with more familiar configu-

rations. All of these aspects of subpulmonic effusions are illustrated in Figure 1.67.

In terms of apparent elevation of the diaphragmatic leaflet with subpulmonic effusions and the sharp drop-off laterally, an

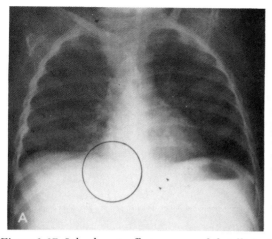 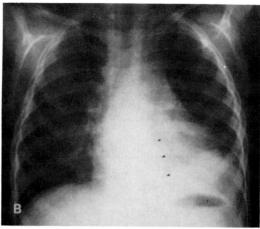

Figure 1.67. *Subpulmonic effusion; some subtle telltale signs.* (*A*) There is a subpulmonic effusion on the right. Telltale signs include: (a) slight elevation and flattening of the right diaphragmatic leaflet; (b) a sharp drop-off of the lateral aspect of the diaphragmatic leaflet; (c) minimal fluid along the lateral chest wall extending into the minor fissure (*arrows on the right*); (d) obliteration of the right cardiac border (positive silhouette sign); and (e) opacification of the right phrenicovertebral angle (*circle*). The normal, radiolucent left phrenicovertebral angle is defined by the arrows just to the left of the lower thoracic spine. (*B*) Subpulmonic effusion on the left causes apparent elevation of the diaphragmatic leaflet. However, note the increased distance between the top of the apparent diaphragmatic leaflet and the stomach bubble and the triangular collection of fluid in the paraspinal gutter (*arrows*). Both of these findings should alert one to the presence of a subpulmonic effusion, but in addition it should be noted that while the pulmonary vascular markings can be seen through the top of the right diaphragmatic leaflet, they are not as easily visible through the top of the apparently high left diaphragmatic leaflet. Such obliteration of the vascular markings by the presence of subpulmonic fluid is another subtle telltale finding of such effusions. In other cases, peculiar bumps along the diaphragmatic leaflets serve to alert one to the presence of a subpulmonic effusion (i.e., Fig. 1.68).

explanation involving the pulmonary ligament has been offered (23). Evidently the pulmonary ligament more or less tethers the lung medially and does not allow it to be elevated to the same degree as its lateral counterpart. Consequently, when fluid collects between the lung and the diaphragm, the lateral portion of the lung is elevated to a greater degree, and the step-off occurs.

In addition to the foregoing considerations regarding subpulmonic effusions, it should be remembered that right-sided subpulmonic effusions can depress the liver downwardly so as to render it palpable clinically, while those on the left can depress the diaphragm and gastric bubble to such an extent that a masslike configuration results (Fig. 1.68). Indeed, one may be surprised at how much fluid can accumulate in the subpulmonic space.

On lateral view, subpulmonic effusions often are easier to detect, for they fill the posterior costophrenic sulcus in the characteristic meniscoid or sloping fashion of any pleural effusion (Fig. 1.69), but of course if one still is uncertain, a decubitus view almost always clarifies the situation (Fig. 1.69). Indeed, with the decubitus view and with the patient in the Trendelenburg position, effusions as small as 5 to 25 ml can be demonstrated (2, 17, 21).

Mediastinal and paraspinal gutter effusions also often elude detection. Posteriorly, in the paraspinal gutter, these effusions usually assume a variably long, tapering, triangular or wedgelike paraspinal configuration (see Figs. 1.62A and 1.67B), while anteriorly or in the middle mediastinum, these effusions may appear masslike (19) or triangular (Fig. 1.70). Large pleural effusions occasionally can

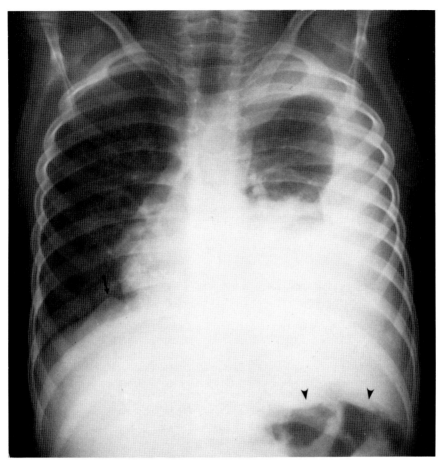

Figure 1.68. *Massive pleural effusion with large subpulmonic component.*   Note the large effusion on the left. It virtually encircles the aerated lung. However, there also is a large subpulmonic component that depresses the stomach and splenic flexure to such a degree that a mass might be suggested (*arrows on left*). The *arrow on the right* points to the telltale bump of a subpulmonic effusion, simultaneously present on the right.

mimic a lobar consolidation (Fig. 1.71), and, unquestionably, decubitus views are the answer here. In still other cases, pleural effusions, or empyemas, may become loculated in the various interlobar fissures (Fig. 1.72). Characteristically, these accumulations are round, oval, or spindle-shaped, but some may appear as large pulmonary masses (Fig. 1.73) and others as irregular infiltrates (Fig. 1.74). However, many are more typical and show characteristically tapering ends as they lie along the axis of the involved fissure (Fig. 1.75). In this regard, it might also be noted that while on one projection these effusions

may appear characteristic, on the other they usually appear atypical. Pleural effusions or empyemas that loculate laterally or posteriorly are less of a problem (Fig. 1.76). Those effusions or empyemas, which loculate along the lung base and thus become difficult to differentiate from a subphrenic abscess, can be identified with confidence using ultrasonography.

Finally, before leaving the discussion of pleural effusions, it should be noted that many normal children have minimal collections of pleural fluid in their costophrenic angles (4). This is entirely normal and common (Fig. 1.77), and the findings

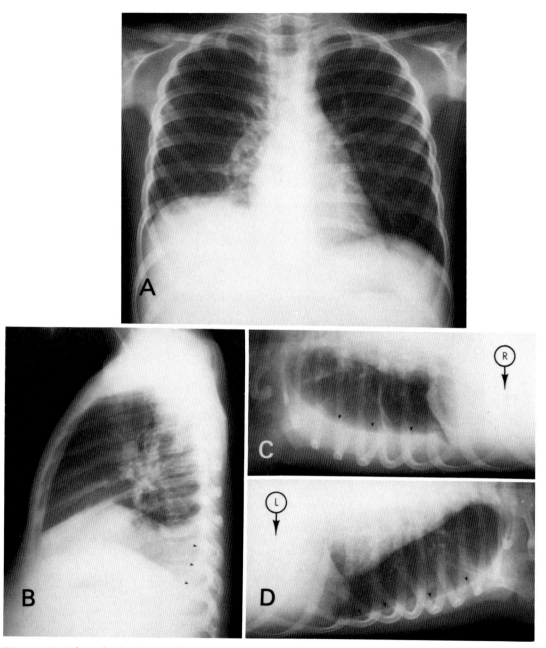

Figure 1.69. *Bilateral subpulmonic effusions; value of lateral and decubitus films.* (**A**) Both diaphragmatic leaf-lets appear elevated in this patient with nephrotic syndrome. Bilateral subpulmonic pleural effusions are present. (**B**) Lateral view demonstrates characteristic blunting and obliteration of both posterior costophrenic angles, and a typical sloping edge of one of the posterior collections of pleural fluid (*arrows*). (**C**) Right lateral decubitus film shows how the fluid layers along the right lateral wall. (**D**) Left lateral decubitus view shows similar findings on the left (*arrows*).

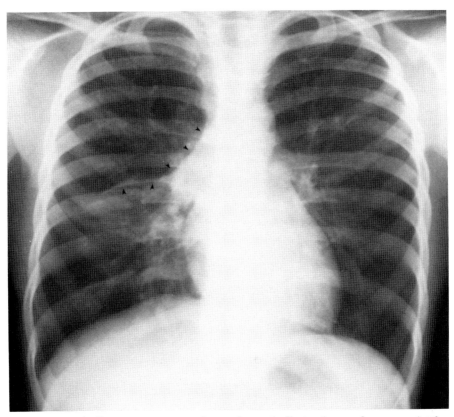

Figure 1.70. *Mediastinal effusion.* Note triangular mediastinal effusion (*upper three arrows*). The triangular configuration could be confused with the sail sign of the normal thymus gland in a younger infant, or an area of segmental atelectasis. However, if it is noted that fluid also extends into the minor fissure (*lower two arrows*), an effusion should be favored.

should not be misinterpreted as a pathologic pleural effusion.

Chylothorax is not a common problem in childhood, but occasionally can be seen with rupture of the thoracic duct secondary to blunt chest trauma. It also has been described in the battered child syndrome (8). Otherwise, chylothorax is a problem of newborn and young infants (28, 30), and of the post-thoracotomy patient. Occasionally, the thoracic duct can be obstructed by a hidden mediastinal tumor or cyst and chylothorax can be the presenting problem, but this is a rare situation.

Other pleural fluid collections can be seen with spontaneous or traumatic esophageal rupture (9), bronchial tears following blunt chest trauma, and with bleeding secondary to rib fractures or post-traumatic great vessel rupture. With esophageal perforations and bronchial tears, both air and fluid are seen in the pleural space (i.e., hemopneumothorax or hydropneumothorax). With esophageal perforations, these changes usually occur on the left side in older children and adults, but on the right in neonates (9). These perforations are believed to result from an acute increase in intraesophageal pressure secondary to traumatic compression of the abdomen and lower chest, or in some cases from profound vomiting.

Finally, it should be noted that a picture suggesting a large pleural effusion can re-

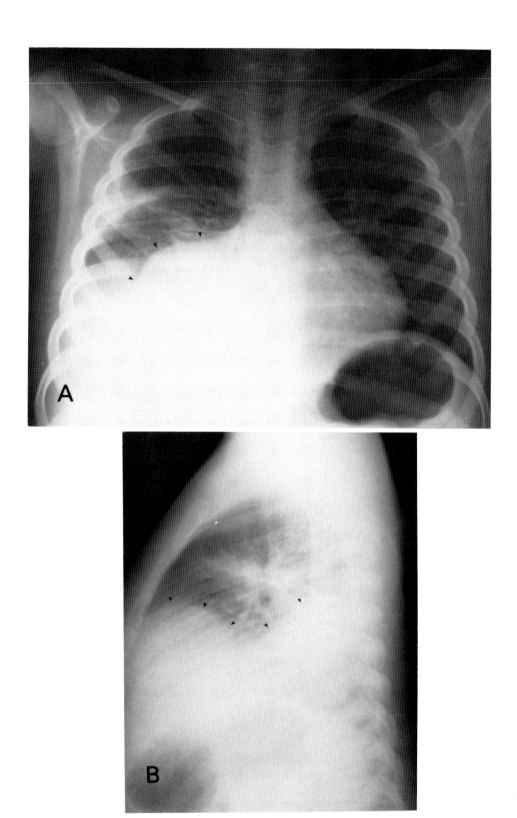

Figure 1.71. *Pleural effusion mimicking lobar pneumonia.* (*A*) The pleural effusion on the right could be misinterpreted for a consolidating pneumonia (*arrows*). Note fluid along the right lateral chest wall and some fluid extending into the minor fissure. (*B*) On lateral view, subpulmonic fluid collections are outlined *by the arrows.* Either one of these configurations could be misinterpreted as a consolidating lobar pneumonia.

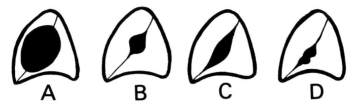

Figure 1.72. *Loculated interlobar fissure effusions; diagrammatic representations.* (*A*) Large loculated effusion. The characteristic tapering, spindled ends often are not present with effusions this large. (*B*) Classic appearance of loculated interlobar effusion presenting as a rounded or oval mass with characteristic tapering, spindle-shaped ends trailing into the fissure. (*C*) Similar configuration but with a longer, more oval effusion. (*D*) Less characteristic, irregular collection of loculated pleural fluid.

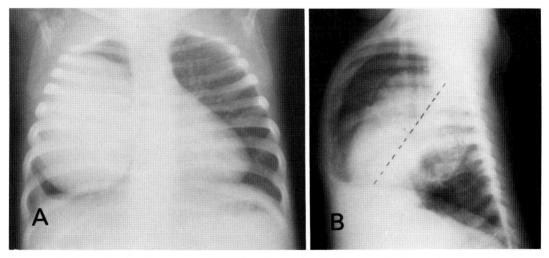

Figure 1.73. *Large loculated empyema.* (*A*) This patient originally had a staphylococcal pneumonia with empyema. This roentgenogram was obtained 3 weeks after treatment and shows how the empyema has loculated into a large, perfectly oval, mass-like lesion. The findings defy distinction from a cyst or tumor. (*B*) Lateral view shows the location of the apparent mass. Although the characteristic tapering ends of a loculated pleural effusion are not present, the main axis of the lesion still conforms to the axis of the greater fissure (*dotted line*), and is the clue to correct diagnosis.

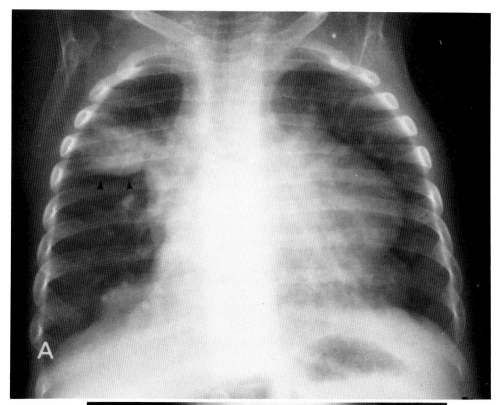

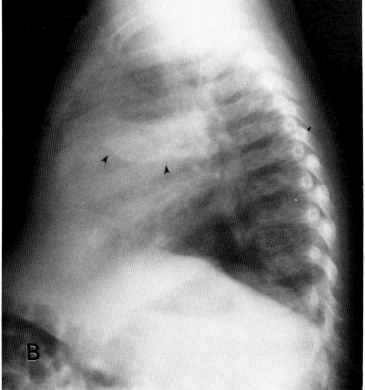

Figure 1.74. *Loculated pleural effusion; irregular configuration.* (**A**) On frontal view, this loculated effusion could be misinterpreted for an early consolidating pneumonia (*arrows*). This patient also has an underlying left to right shunt, some congestion, and bilateral eventrations. (**B**) Lateral view delineates the somewhat irregular appearing loculated pleural effusion in the right minor fissure (*arrows*).

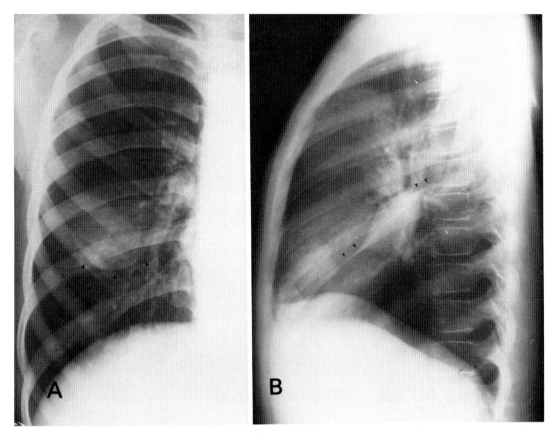

Figure 1.75. *Classic loculated pleural effusion.* (A) Note the area of increased density in the right mid lung field and especially note the sharp rounded lower edge (*arrows*). (B) Lateral view clearly establishes that a loculated effusion is present in the right major fissure. Notice the characteristic tapering, spindle-shaped ends of this pseudomass (*arrows*). It lies along the fissure and its tapering ends trail into the fissure. Because these effusions tend to disappear rapidly and unexpectedly, they have been termed vanishing tumors.

sult in those cases where there is massive unilateral atelectasis and pronounced contralateral compensatory emphysema (see Fig. 1.87*B*). It is most important that this pitfall be appreciated so as to avoid needless thoracentesis. The same precaution should be observed in those cases of atypical upper lobe atelectasis mimicking apical pleural effusions (see Fig. 1.91).

REFERENCES

1. Cho, C.T., Hiatt, W.O., and Behbehani, A.M.: Pneumonia and massive pleural effusion associated with adenovirus type 7. Am. J. Dis. Child. 126: 92–94, 1973.
2. Collins, J.D., Burwell, D., Furmanski, S., Lorber, P., and Steckel, R.J.: Minimal detectable pleural effusions. A roentgenpathology model. Radiology 105: 51–53, 1972.
3. Davis, L.A.: Vertical fissure line. A.J.R. 84: 451–453, 1960.
4. Ecklof, O., and Torngren, A.: Pleural fluid in healthy children. Acta Radiol. 11: 346–349, 1971.
5. Fine, N.L., Smith, L.R., and Sheedy, P.F.: Frequency of pleural effusions in mycoplasma and viral pneumonias. N. Engl. J. Med. 283: 790–793, 1970.
6. Fleischner, F.G.: Atypical arrangement of free pleural effusion. Radiol. Clin. North Am. 1: 347–361, 1963.
7. Forbes, G.B., and Emerson, G.L.: Staphylococcal pneumonia and empyema. Pediatr. Clin. North Am. 4: 215–229, 1957.

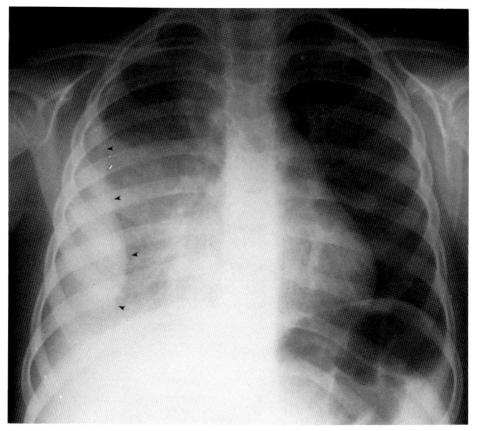

Figure 1.76. *Loculated fluid (empyema); lateral chest wall.* This patient had a pneumococcal pneumonia and eventually developed an empyema which then finally loculated laterally (*arrows*). Such loculations are common in the resolving stage of any type of empyema.

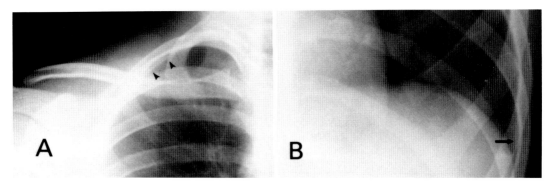

Figure 1.77. *Normal pleural reflections mimicking pleural effusions.* (**A**) Apparent fluid over the apex of the right lung (*arrows*). This finding is commonly seen in children and is due to normal soft tissues between the lung and ribs. (**B**) Pleural reflection in the left costophrenic angle of a normal child (*arrows*). There is some debate as to whether this finding represents the pleural reflection alone, or a minimal amount of normal pleural fluid. Whichever explanation is correct, the finding is normal, but probably it reflects the presence of a small amount of normal fluid (4).

8. Green, H.G.: Child abuse presenting as chylothorax. Pediatrics 66: 620–621, 1980.

9. Harell, G.S., Friedland, G.W., Daily, W.J., and Cohn, R.B.: Neonatal Boerhaave's syndrome. Radiology 95: 665–668, 1970.

10. Highman, J.H.: Staphylococcal pneumonia and empyema in childhood. A.J.R. 106: 103–108, 1969.

11. Honig, P.J., Pasquariello, P.S., Jr., and Stool, S.E.: H Influenzae pneumonia in infants and children. J. Pediatr. 83: 215–219, 1973.

12. Huxtable, K.A., Tucker, A.S., and Wedgewood, R.J.: Staphylococcic pneumonia in childhood: Longterm follow-up. Am. J. Dis. Child. 108: 262–269, 1964.

13. Kanof, A., Epstein, B., Kramer, B., and Mauss, I.: Staphylococcal pneumonia and empyema in childhood. N. Engl. J. Med. 264: 738–743, 1961.

14. Kevy, S.V., and Lowe, B.A.: Streptococcal pneumonia and empyema in childhood. N. Engl. J. Med. 264: 738–743, 1961.

15. Landay, M., and Harless, W.: Ultrasonic differentiation of right pleural effusion from subphrenic fluid on longitudinal scans of the right upper quadrant: Importance of recognizing the diaphragm. Radiology 123: 155–158, 1977.

16. Martinez, O.C., Serrano, B.V., and Romero, R.R.: Real-time ultrasound evaluation of tuberculous pleural effusions. J. Clin. Ultrasound 17: 407–410, 1989.

17. Moskowitz, H., Platt, R.T., Schachar, R., and Mellins, H.: Roentgen visualization of minute pleural effusion: Experimental study to determine the minimal amount of pleural fluid visible on a radiograph. Radiology 109: 33–35, 1973.

18. Peterson, J.A.: Recognition of infrapulmonary pleural effusion. Radiology 74: 34–41, 1960.

19. Pines, A., Kaplinsky, N., Rubinstein, Z., Bregman, J., Meytes, D., and Frankl, O.: Massive loculated pleural effusion simulating mediastinal masses. Br. J. Radiol. 55: 240–242, 1982.

20. Rigler, L.G.: Roentgen diagnosis of small pleural effusions: A new roentgenographic position. J.A.M.A. 96: 104–108, 1931.

21. Rigler, L.G.: Roentgenologic observations of the movement of pleural effusions. A.J.R. 25: 220–230, 1931.

22. Riley, H.D., and Bracken, E.C.: Empyema due to Haemophilus influenzae in infants and children. Am. J. Dis. Child. 110: 24–28, 1965.

23. Rudikoff, J.C.: The pulmonary ligament and subpulmonic effusion. Chest 80: 505–507, 1981.

24. Schwartz, M., and Marmorstein, B.: New radiologic sign of subpulmonic effusion. Chest 67: 176–178, 1975.

25. Smith, P.L., and Gerald, B.: Empyema in childhood followed roentgenographically: Decorti-

cation seldom needed. A.J.R. 106: 114–117, 1969.

26. Trackler, R.T., and Brinker, R.A.: Widening of the left paravertebral pleural line on supine chest roentgenograms in free pleural effusions. A.J.R. 96: 1027–1034, 1966.

27. Turner, J.A.P.: Staphylococcal pneumonia, a contemporary rarity. Clin. Pediatr. 11: 69–71, 1972.

28. Watson, E.G., and Foster, L.F.: Spontaneous chylothorax in infancy: Prognosis and management. Am. J. Dis. Child. 72: 89–94, 1946.

29. Webber, M.M., and O'Loughlin, B.J.: Variations of pleural vertical fissure line. Radiology 82: 461–462, 1964.

30. Wessel, M.A.: Chylothorax in two-week-old infant with spontaneous recovery. J. Pediatr. 25: 201–210, 1944.

31. Vinik, M., Altman, D.H., and Parks, R.E.: Experience with Haemophilus influenzae pneumoniae. Radiology 86: 701–706, 1966.

HILAR AND PARATRACHEAL ADENOPATHY

Enlarged lymph nodes in the hilar or paratracheal regions are most often inflammatory in nature, and, in this regard, bilateral hilar adenopathy most often is seen with viral lower respiratory tract infections (see Fig. 1.4). Of course, bilateral hilar and paratracheal adenopathy also can be seen with conditions such as sarcoidosis (Fig. 1.78A), histoplasmosis, and other fungal disease, histiocytosis X, sinus histiocytosis (1), and even on occasion with tuberculosis (Fig. 1.78B). Discrete hilar adenopathy secondary to lymphoma or leukemia is not as common a presenting feature in children as is coalescent mediastinal adenopathy.

Unilateral hilar or paratracheal adenopathy occasionally occurs with bacterial and *Mycoplasma* infections (Fig. 1.79), but more often such adenopathy is the hallmark of primary pulmonary tuberculosis in childhood. There is good reason for this to occur, for if one considers the basic pathology in tuberculosis, one will recall that adenopathy is secondary to the peripheral Ghon lesion, and that this lesion usually is

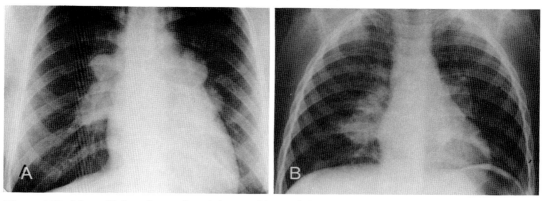

Figure 1.78. *Bilateral hilar adenopathy.* (*A*) Typical lumpy bilateral hilar adenopathy in patient with sarcoid. (*B*) Tuberculosis with bilateral hilar adenopathy. Most often in tuberculosis, hilar adenopathy is unilateral.

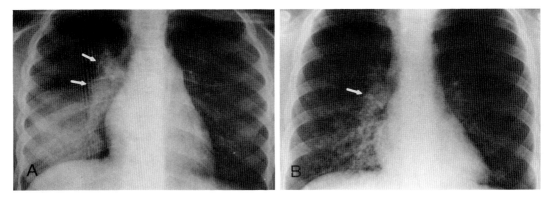

Figure 1.79. *Unilateral adenopathy with pulmonary infection.* (*A*) Note the classic consolidation with no significant volume loss in the right lower lobe. There is ipsilateral hilar adenopathy (*arrows*). (*B*) Reticulonodular pattern characteristic of *Mycoplasma pneumoniae* infection in the right lower lobe and associated ipsilateral hilar adenopathy (*arrow*).

single. Because of this, hilar or paratracheal lymph node involvement usually is unilateral. Indeed, *a good rule to follow is that unilateral hilar or paratracheal adenopathy, with or without associated change in the lungs, should be considered tuberculous in origin until proven otherwise.* Occasionally, *M. pneumoniae* infections can produce similar findings, but primary pulmonary tuberculosis should be the first consideration in any patient presenting with such a picture. Adenopathy in these cases may be discrete and smooth-edged or fuzzy because of associated, adjacent edema (Fig. 1.80).

Atelectasis is a common associated finding in tuberculosis and usually is secondary to endobronchial disease, and not the adenopathy (see p. 47). However, the associated atelectosis may obscure the fact that hilar adenopathy is present (Fig. 1.81*A* and *B*). This is less of a problem when obstructive emphysema is present (Fig. 1.81*C*), but emphysema is far, far less common than atelectasis.

Before leaving the subject of hilar ade-

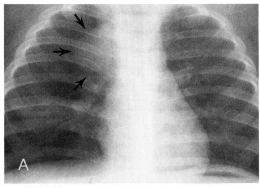

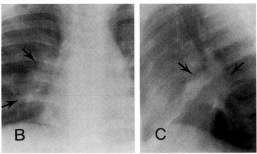

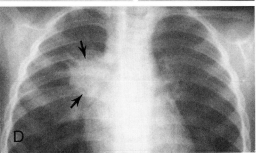

Figure 1.80. *Hilar and paratracheal adenopathy.* (*A*) Note smooth-edged right paratreacheal adenopathy (*arrows*) in patient with tuberculosis. (*B* Less distinct but nonetheless clearly evident and prominent right hilar adenopathy (*arrows*) in a patient with tuberculosis. (*C*) Note the paracarinal location on lateral view. (*D*) Another patient with right hilar adenopathy but with fuzzy edges (*arrows*) due to adjacent inflammatory edema. Also note an early consolidation developing in the right middle lobe.

nopathy, one should recall that its presence can be mimicked, on frontal view, by superior segment lower lobe pneumonias. However, no such problem should last for long, for on lateral view it will be clearly seen that hilar adenopathy is central (par-acarinal) while superior segment lower lobe pneumonias lie posterior to the carina (Fig. 1.82). Large pulmonary arteries, such as might be seen with pulmonary hypertension mimicking hilar adenopathy, are not as great a problem in childhood as in the adult.

REFERENCE

1. Siegel, M.J., Shackelford, G.D., and McAlister, W.H.: Sinus histiocytosis: Some radiologic observations. A.J.R. 132: 783–785, 1979.

ATELECTASIS AND EMPHYSEMA

Which Side Is Abnormal? Among the most troublesome problems with unilateral, total lung, atelectasis or emphysema is trying to decide which side of the chest is abnormal. In this regard, there is no question that an inspiratory-expiratory sequence of chest roentgenograms is the ultimate answer, but there are *certain rules that can be utilized in determining which side is abnormal* before these are obtained. More specifically, these include: (a) in obstructive emphysema, the large, hyperlucent lung usually shows diminished pulmonary vascularity; (b) in compensatory emphysema, the large emphysematous, radiolucent (nonobstructed) lung usually shows normal or engorged pulmonary vascularity; and (c) an obstructed, emphysematous lung, no matter how large, cannot compress the other lung to the point of total atelectasis or opacity (Fig. 1.83).

Of course, not every initial film reveals the foregoing findings with clarity, and thus an inspiratory-expiratory film sequence should be obtained. The most important point to note on this study is that usually *the abnormal lung, no matter what its appearance, does not significantly change its size from inspiration to expiration.* In other words, the lung that changes size most is the normal lung (Fig. 1.83C and *D*). For the most part, these rules suf-

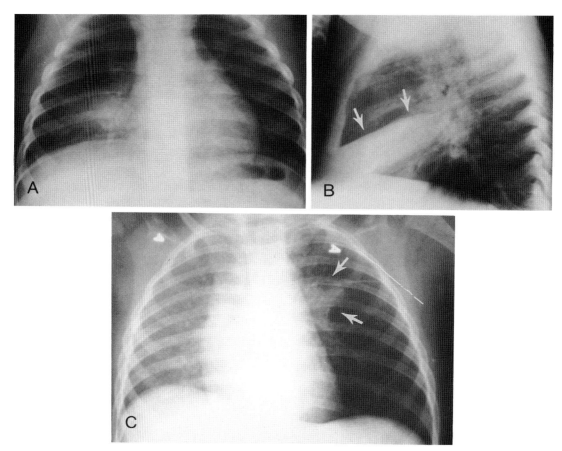

Figure 1.81. *Tuberculous adenopathy with associated aeration abnormalities.* (*A*) Note the density in the region of the right middle lobe. Hilar adenopathy is not easy to detect. (*B*) Lateral view demonstrates that the density is due to classic right middle lobe atelectasis (*arrows*). Note the prominent hilar region attesting to the presence of hilar adenopathy. (*C*) Another patient with left hilar adenopathy (*arrows*) associated with obstructive emphysema of the left lung. Both of these patients had primary pulmonary tuberculosis.

fice for almost any aeration disturbance encountered except, perhaps, that with a congenitally hypoplastic lung. A hypoplastic lung is small and hyperlucent (decreased vascularity), but shows significant change in volume on inspiratory-expiratory film studies.

Atelectasis is a common roentgenographic finding and can involve an entire lung, lobe, or just a portion of a lung. Indeed, sublobar or segmental atelectasis is quite common in children and, for the most part, occurs with viral lower respiratory tract infections and asthma. To be sure, these areas of atelectasis often are con-

fused with true pulmonary infiltrates (Fig. 1.84). The reason for such atelectasis being common in children is that the collateral air drift phenomenon, through the pores of Kohn and ducts of Lambert, is not as efficient in children as in adults (7). Consequently, whereas in the adult atelectasis, especially segmental, does not last very long, it does tend to linger in children. If such atelectasis is widespread and patchy, it is indeed difficult to differentiate from pulmonary infiltration (Fig. 1.84C). On the other hand, when such atelectasis produces vertical, horizontal, or oblique streaks or wedges, it is easier to appreciate

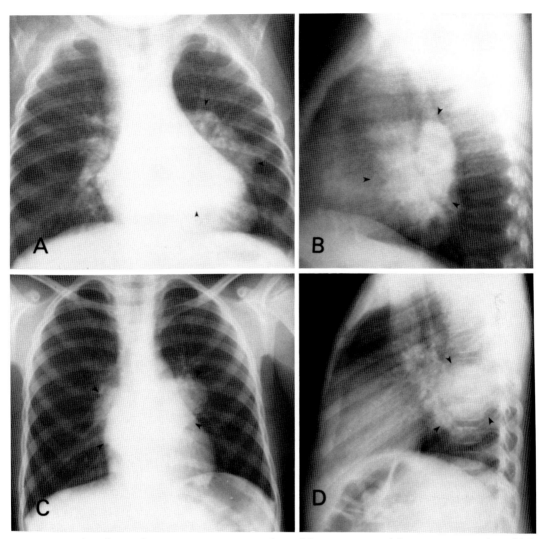

Figure 1.82. *Hilar adenopathy versus superior segment lower lobe pneumonia.* (**A**) Note massive unilateral left hilar adenopathy in this patient with primary pulmonary tuberculosis (*arrows*). (**B**) Lateral view shows typical central, paracarinal location of hilar adenopathy (*arrows*). (**C**) Patient in whom findings might at first suggest bilateral hilar adenopathy or a posterior mediastinal mass (*arrows*). (**D**) Lateral view shows that the findings represent bilateral superior segment lower lobe pneumonias (*arrows*). Characteristically, these pneumonias lie high in the lower lobes, behind the major fissure, and, unlike enlarged hilar lymph nodes, behind the carina. In most cases, they overlie the spine. This patient had pneumococcal "double" pneumonia with consolidations in the superior segment of both lower lobes.

these densities for what they are (Fig. 1.85). Such atelectasis often is referred to as discoid, plate-like, or vertical atelectasis.

Atelectasis also can produce a confusing picture when a lobe is just beginning to collapse. The problem arises when the lobe collapses against a major fissure (Fig. 1.86). In such cases, the outer edge of the slightly elevated or inwardly displaced fissure remains sharp, while the inner edge is somewhat indistinct. Indistinctness results from the fact that aeration of the lung still occurs, perhaps through the collateral air

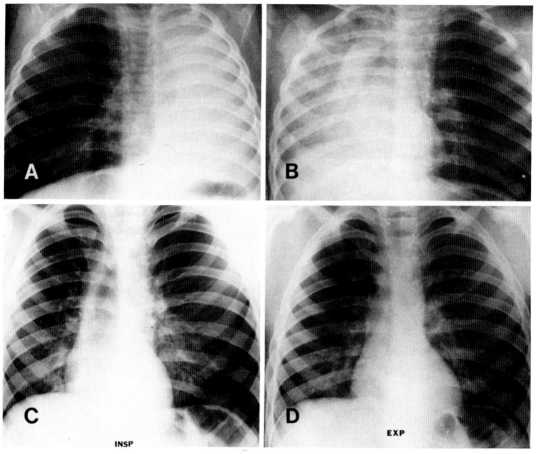

Figure 1.83. *Atelectasis and emphysema; which side is abnormal?* (*A*) Note complete opacification of the left lung. The right lung shows compensatory emphysema and relatively normal vascularity. The fact that the left lung is totally opacified suggests that the problem is atelectasis on the left. An enlarged lung, due to obstructed emphysema, no matter how large it gets, seldom, if ever, totally compresses the other lung. (*B*) The right lung is small in this case, but not totally opacified and airless. The problem here is obstructive emphysema on the left. The vascularity may be slightly decreased, but an expiratory view would be necessary for final diagnosis. (*C*) Large left lung. Note that vascularity is normal or even slightly engorged in the left lung, suggesting compensatory emphysema. (*D*) Expiratory film shows the left lung to empty well, but the right lung to change little in size. It is the right lung that is abnormal and, indeed, was obstructed by an endobronchial mucous plug in an asthmatic.

drift, which even though less efficient in children, still occurs. Overall, then, aeration of the collapsing lobe still is present, and thus while the outer edge of the lung abutting the fissure is sharp, the inner aspect is indistinct.

Atelectasis of an entire lung, or a lobe thereof, is most often seen with asthma, viral lower respiratory tract infection, primary tuberculosis, and foreign bodies. In the classic case of total lung atelectasis, the findings are clearly apparent, for the entire hemithorax becomes opacified, the mediastinum shifts to the ipsilateral side, and the heart virtually disappears into the atelectatic lung (Fig. 1.87A). However, because the other lung becomes overaerated (compensatory emphysema), one very often misinterprets the findings as being abnormal on the wrong side (i.e., obstruc-

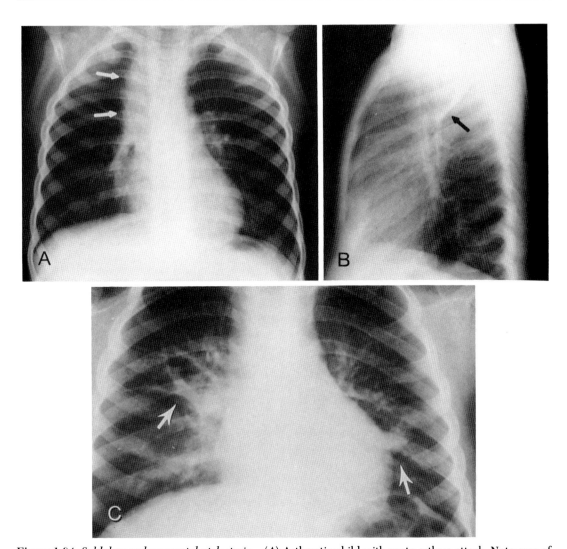

Figure 1.84. *Sublobar and segmental atelectasis.* (*A*) Asthmatic child with acute asthma attack. Note area of apparent consolidation in the right paratracheal region (*arrows*). This represents collapse of a portion of the right upper lobe. A more subtle finding, assisting in one's interpretation, is the fact that there slight right mediastinal shift. (*B*) Lateral view demonstrates early atelectasis (*arrows*). With such minimal degrees of atelectasis, the fissures may not be markedly displaced and differentiation from pneumonia more difficult. (*C*) Widespread parahilar peribronchial infiltrates due to viral bronchitis with scattered linear, wedgelike and patchy areas of segmental atelectasis (*arrows*).

tive emphysema with mediastinal shift). Expiratory films are the answer here, but before they are obtained one should also evaluate the pulmonary vascularity. In compensatory emphysema, the vascularity in the overaerated lung usually is normal or accentuated, while in obstructive em-

physema usually it is decreased. Furthermore, it should be noted that in total lung atelectasis the collapsed lung is totally opaque, even down into the costophrenic angle. This can happen only with atelectasis or agenesis, for an overaerated lung alone, no matter how large, cannot com-

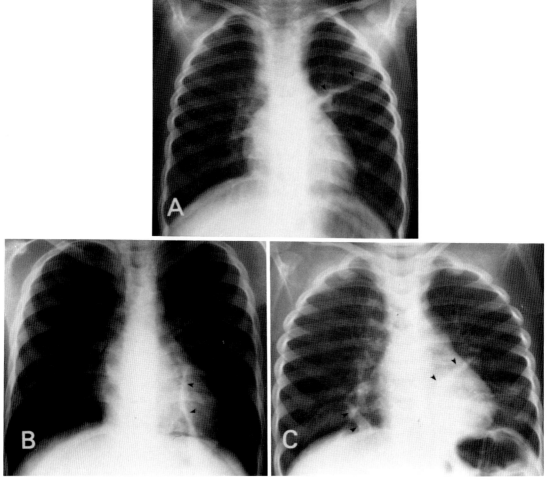

Figure 1.85. *Discoid, "plate-like" or vertical atelectasis.* (**A**) Segmental discoid atelectasis in the left upper lobe (*arrows*). (**B**) Another patient demonstrating so-called vertical discoid atelectasis (*arrows*). (**C**) Multiple oblique densities are seen throughout both lung fields, representing multiple areas of segmental, wedgelike atelectasis (*arrows*).

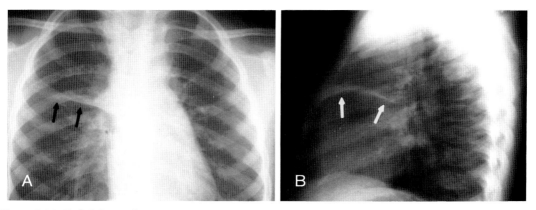

Figure 1.86. *Early lobar atelectasis.* (**A**) Note slight elevation of the minor fissure (*arrows*) and that its inferior edge is sharp, while its superior edge is fuzzy. (**B**) Lateral view showing similar findings (*arrows*). Without close inspection, these findings often are misinterpreted for small interlobar effusions, but pleural effusions demonstrate sharp edges on both sides.

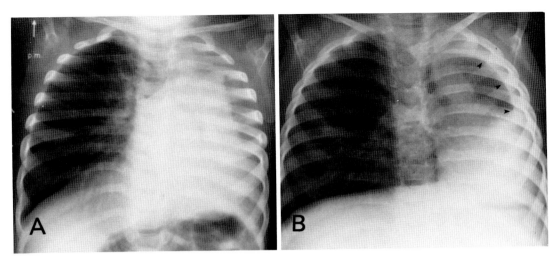

Figure 1.87. *Total atelectasis of a lung.* (**A**) In this infant atelectasis was due to an obstructing mucous plug. Note the marked loss of volume on the left, pronounced shift of the mediastinum to the left, and overexpansion of the right lung. However, the pulmonary vascularity in the right lung is normal or, in fact, a little increased. This rules against obstructive emphysema of the right lung. With obstructive emphysema the vascularity is diminished. (**B**) Another patient with complete atelectasis of the left lung and pronounced compensatory emphysema of the right lung. Indeed, the right lung has herniated across the mediastinum to produce a configuration erroneously suggesting a left pleural effusion (*arrows*). This is not pleural fluid; it merely represents the interface between the overaerated, herniated right lung as it is superimposed on the collapsed left lung. The pulmonary vascularity in the right lung is not markedly diminished, and this identifies the problem as one of compensatory, rather than obstructive emphysema. In other words, blood from the atelectatic left lung is shunted to the right lung. If the right lung were distended because of obstructive emphysema, the vascularity would be diminished.

press the other lung to the point of complete opacity. Some aeration will remain, and will be most evident in the costophrenic angle.

Classic atelectatic patterns (4, 8, 9) for collapse of the various lobes are demonstrated in Figure 1.88, but from the onset it should be stressed that while on one view the atelectatic lobe may be clearly visualized, on the other it may be difficult to perceive. This occurs because on one view the lobe is seen on edge (easier to see), while on the other, it is seen *en face* (more difficult to see). Indeed, atelectatic lobes visualized *en face* often are so ill-defined that they are misinterpreted as pulmonary infiltrates. It is only when one notes that there is associated volume loss and, on the other view, a typical lobar collapse pattern that one comes to the conclusion that atelectasis only is present.

The pattern of collapse of the upper lobes is different from side to side. This is explained by the fact that on the right the minor fissure separates the right and middle lobes, while on the left the lingula functions as part of the left upper lobe. On the right, on frontal projection, the elevated minor fissure is characteristic (Fig. 1.89A). On lateral view, the minor and major fissures often outline the collapsed right upper lobe as a "V" (Fig. 1.89B), but it is not always easy to see the "V" in its entirety. On the left side, since no minor fissure is present, one sees only a vague area of increased density over the left upper and mid lung fields (Fig. 1.89C). On lateral view, the left upper lobe and lingula collapse anteriorly and are demarcated posteriorly by the forwardly displaced major fissure (Fig. 1.89D). In most of these cases, the displaced major fissure tends to parallel the anterior chest wall. On the right, a similar configuration results only when the

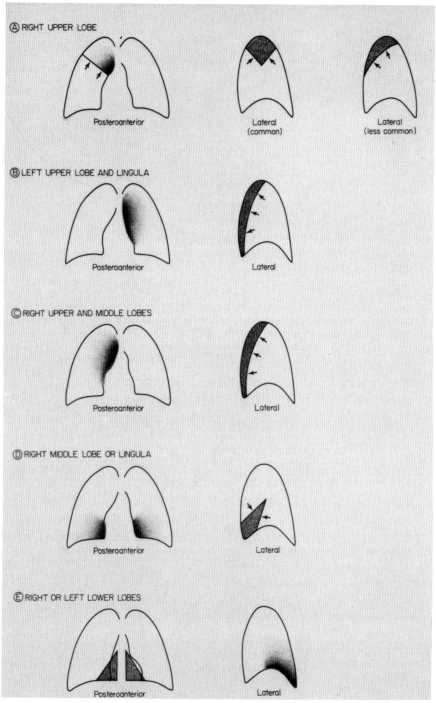

Figure 1.88. *Lobar atelectasis; diagrammatic representation of classic patterns.* (*A*) Right upper lobe atelectasis. (*B*) Left upper lobe and lingular atelectasis. (*C*) Right upper and right middle lobe atelectasis. (*D*) Right middle lobe or lingular atelectasis. (*E*) Right lower lobe or left lower lobe atelectasis. *Arrows* indicate direction of collapse and displacement of the involved major fissures. Roentgenographic examples of the above patterns are presented in Figures 1.89–1.95.

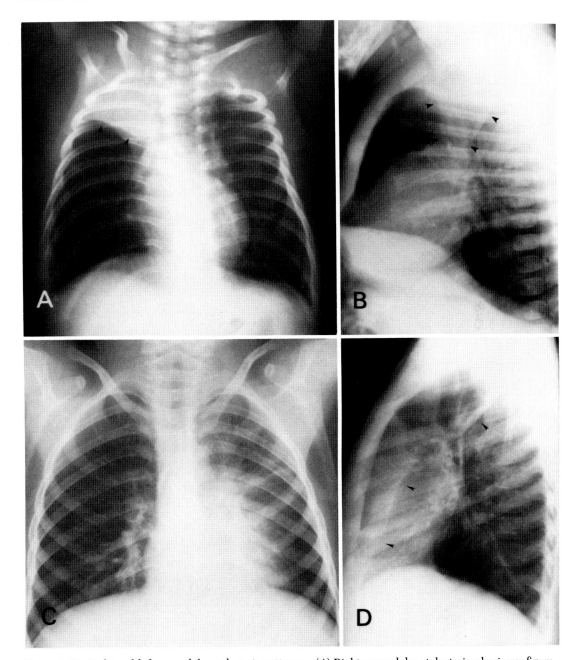

Figure 1.89. *Right and left upper lobe atelectatic patterns.* (*A*) Right upper lobe atelectasis, classic configuration. The minor fissure (*arrows*) is elevated, and the collapsed upper lobe is dense and triangular. In addition, there is some mediastinal shift to the right. This patient had bronchiolitis with a complicating mucous plug in the right upper lobe. (*B*) Lateral view of right upper lobe atelectasis demonstrating a characteristic V-shaped configuration (*arrows*). The minor fissure delineates the collapsed lobe anteriorly, and the major fissure delineates it posteriorly. (*C*) Left upper lobe and lingular atelectasis. First note that there is mediastinal shift to the left, and then that the entire left cardiac border is obliterated (positive silhouette sign). In addition, note diffuse central haziness in the left lung field. (*D*) Lateral view shows characteristic configuration of the collapsed left upper lobe and lingula. The major fissure is displaced anteriorly and more or less parallels the anterior chest wall (*arrows*).

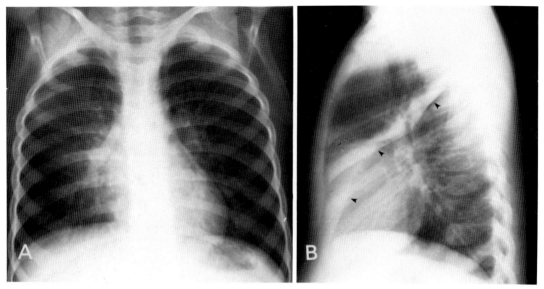

Figure 1.90. *Right upper and middle lobe atelectasis.* (***A***) Note diffuse haziness over the medial portion of the right lung field. An adjacent positive silhouette sign obliterates the entire right mediastinal edge, and the right hemithorax is slightly smaller than the left. There is some ipsilateral mediastinal shift and slight elevation of the right diaphragmatic leaflet (secondary signs of collapse). (***B***) Lateral view showing characteristic forward displacement of the major fissure as it outlines the collapsed upper and middle lobes (*arrows*).

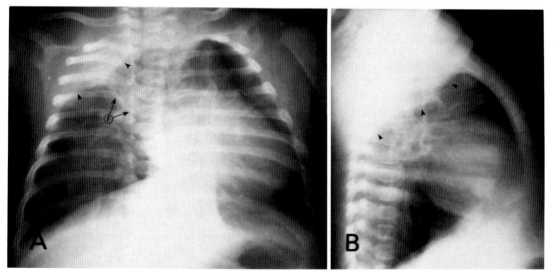

Figure 1.91. *Atypical right upper lobe atelectasis.* (***A***) Note the atelectatic right upper lobe compressed toward the apex of the right hemithorax (*arrows*). The minor fissure (*F*) is barely visible but elevated. Since the right upper lobe has collapsed, the right middle lobe has become overaerated and has herniated across the anterior mediastinum to the left side. This patient also has left lower lobe atelectasis as demonstrated by the dense area behind the left side of the heart. (***B***) Lateral view demonstrating the atypically collapsed right upper lobe in the apex of the thorax (*arrows*).

middle and upper lobes are collapsed together (Fig. 1.90).

Finally, it should be noted that either
the right or left upper lobe can collapse in
atypical fashion (5) and in so doing produce a pleural effusion-like picture (Fig.
1.91). To the unwary, the findings will
strongly suggest a pleural effusion, and an

unwarranted thoracentesis may even be
performed. This can be avoided, however,
by becoming familiar with this type of
upper lobe collapse.

Right middle lobe and lingular collapse
produce focal areas of increased density
along the lower right or left cardiac borders (Fig. 1.92). In many cases, these find-

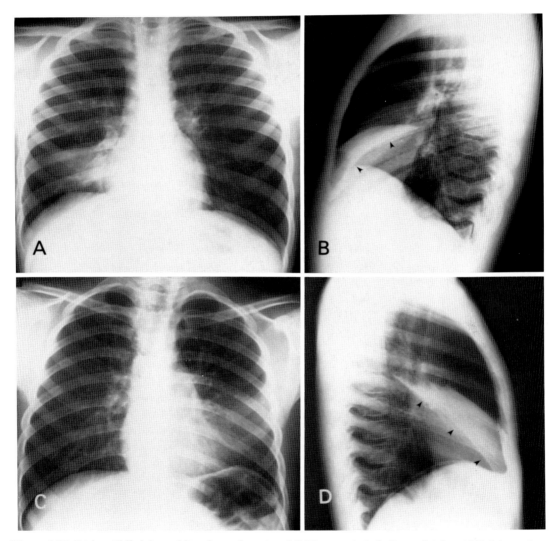

Figure 1.92. *Right middle lobe and lingular atelectasis.* (**A**) Characteristic findings of right middle lobe atelectasis consisting of an area of increased density just to the right of the lower cardiac border, obliteration of the
adjacent portion of the cardiac border (positive silhouette sign), elevation of the diaphragmatic leaflet, and depression of the right hilum. The latter two findings, plus the slight mediastinal shift to the right, are secondary
signs which indicate that a volume loss problem is present. (**B**) Lateral view shows the typical V-shaped configuration of the collapsed right middle lobe (*arrows*). (**C**) Lingular atelectasis producing findings similar to those
of right middle lobe atelectasis but on the left side. (**D**) *Arrows* delineate the characteristically triangular collapsed lingula.

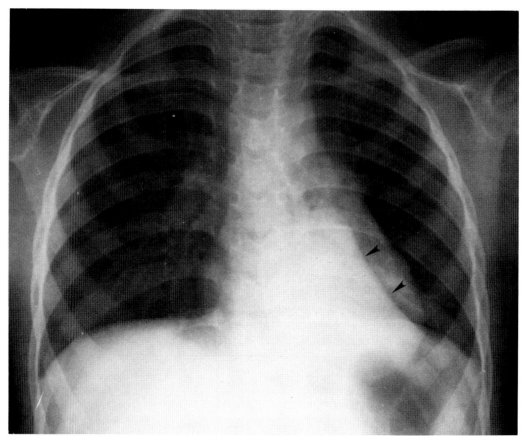

Figure 1.93. *Left lower lobe atelectasis.*   Note the characteristic triangular area of increased density behind the left side of the heart adjacent to the spine (*arrows*). In less pronounced cases, the triangular configuration is not as distinct and a vague area of increased density only is seen.

ings may at first suggest pneumonia, but the characteristic V-shaped configuration on lateral view should enable one to make the proper diagnosis. However, it should be mentioned that some variation in the discretness and density of the V-shaped collapse pattern should be expected, for it is entirely dependent on the degree of atelectasis present.

Lower lobe collapse is best appreciated on frontal view (Figs. 1.93 and 1.94), for on lateral view it may be totally invisible. At most, the lateral view may reveal a diffuse increase in density over the lower posterior half of the chest, and in some cases, loss of visualization of the adjacent diaphragmatic leaflet (i.e., positive silhouette

sign; see Fig. 1.94*B*). Only rarely will the edge of the major fissure be seen demarcating the lower lobe anteriorly.

On frontal view, differentiation of lower lobe collapse from right middle lobe or lingular collapse is accomplished by noting the presence or absence of an adjacent positive silhouette sign. With right middle lobe or lingular atelectasis, the ipsilateral cardiac border is obliterated, while with lower lobe atelectasis it is not (compare Fig. 1.92 with Fig. 1.93). Classically, left lower lobe collapse produces a triangular area of increased density confined, more or less, to the area behind the left side of the heart (Fig. 1.93). On the right, because there is less cardiac mass, the triangular

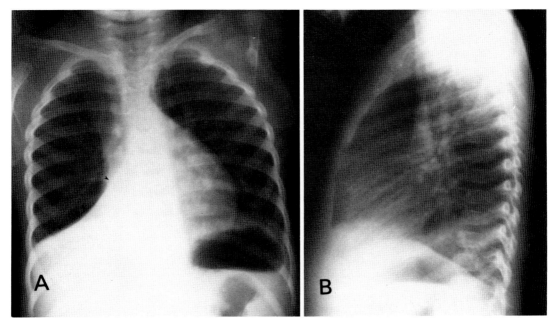

Figure 1.94. *Right lower lobe atelectasis.* (*A*) Note the dense triangular configuration of the collapsed right lower lobe (*arrows*) extending beyond the right cardiac border. In addition, the right cardiac leaflet is obliterated and elevated and there is slight mediastinal shift to the right. (*B*) Lateral view shows only a vague area of increased density over the spine. The left diaphragmatic leaflet is clearly visualized (note the stomach bubble beneath it), but the right is obliterated because of a positive silhouette sign.

density of the collapsed right lower lobe often extends beyond the right cardiac border (Fig. 1.94). On the left, if the lower portion of the inferior pulmonary ligament is congenitally defective, anchoring of the left lower lobe is less than normal, and the lobe collapses against the spine in a rounded fashion (6). A paraspinal mass is then suggested, for the characteristic triangular shape of left lower lobe collapse is absent.

When more than one lobe is collapsed in a patient and the lobes are adjacent, problems in interpretation can arise. Peculiar patterns result and usually reflect a combination of the findings seen when each of the lobes collapses separately (Figs. 1.89C and D and 1.95).

All of the foregoing patterns of lobar atelectasis are understandably somewhat variable from patient to patient, for they depend to a large extent on the degree of atelectasis present. Because of this, it is of

value to be familiar with certain accessory signs that become useful in subtle cases. For example, elevation or depression of a hilus from its usual location (remember that the left hilus is normally a little higher than the right) suggests that there is atelectasis of the upper (elevated hilus) or lower (depressed hilus) lobe. By the same token, elevation of the ipsilateral diaphragmatic leaflet usually is present with lower lobe atelectasis and with all types of lobar collapse there is the inevitable ipsilateral shift of the mediastinum. This latter finding, however, may not always be striking and often becomes more convincing with inspiratory-expiratory film sequences. So-called "round atelectasis" in adults (2, 11) is not commonly seen in children. Atelectasis may appear so round in these patients that a pulmonary nodule or mass is erroneously suggested.

Before leaving the subject of atelectasis, a comment regarding the so-called *right*

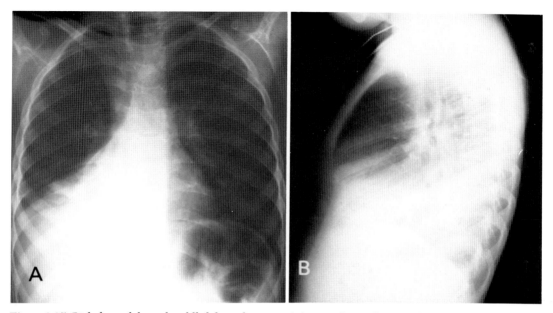

Figure 1.95. *Right lower lobe and middle lobe atelectasis.* (**A**) Frontal view showing characteristic configuration of the collapsed right lower and middle lobes. The triangular configuration suggests lower lobe collapse and the fact that the cardiac border is obliterated indicates that, in addition, the right middle lobe is collapsed. (**B**) Lateral view showing a large area of increased density behind and over the heart due to the atelectatic right lower and middle lobes.

middle lobe syndrome (1, 3) is worthwhile. This is a poorly defined "syndrome" which simply reflects that the right middle lobe is chronically or recurrently atelectatic. Because this phenomenon occurs more commonly in the right middle lobe, the term "right middle lobe syndrome" has been coined.

There is no specificity with regard to etiology of the right middle lobe syndrome. It can be seen as the aftermath of viral or tuberculous infections and in some cases be a feature of asthma. The presence of the right middle lobe syndrome suggests a chronic aeration disturbance and, eventually, further investigation is required. Most often, this consists of bronchoscopy whereupon proximal, inflammatory narrowing of the right middle lobe bronchus may be delineated. If repeated pulmonary infections are a problem, the right middle lobe may well require surgical removal. However, in most cases only expectant treatment is necessary.

Emphysema can be generalized or lobar. Generalized emphysema is seen with central obstructing lesions such as foreign bodies in the trachea, multiple peripheral foreign bodies, paratracheal masses, vascular rings, diffuse peripheral small airway disease with air trapping (i.e., viral or thermal injury-induced bronchitis or bronchiolitis), and with bronchospasm secondary to asthma and cystic fibrosis (Fig. 1.96). A similar problem has been noted in some children with $\alpha 1$-antitrypsin deficiency (12).

Emphysema due to tracheal obstruction is often accompanied by expiratory wheezing and stridor. The roentgenographic findings may not be striking, for the only feature may be what would initially be considered an apparently "overexuberant" normal inspiration. However, when it is remembered that it is difficult to obtain a film in deep inspiration in young infants, this finding alone should alert one to the fact that generalized air trapping is present.

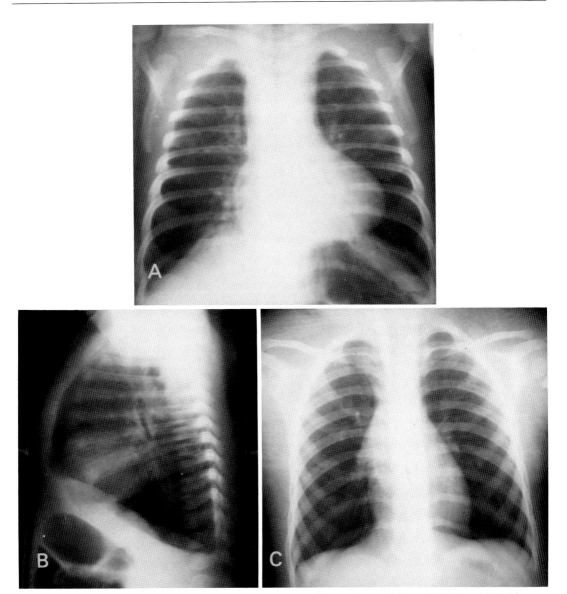

Figure 1.96. *Obstructive emphysema; generalized.* (*A*) Note the overdistended lungs in this patient with a vascular ring producing expiratory air trapping. (*B*) Lateral view showing marked overdistension of the chest with a typical bell-shaped configuration and flat diaphragmatic leaflets. (*C*) Marked overaeration secondary to thermal injury induced bronchiolitis. This patient suffered from smoke inhalation and expired shortly thereafter. Note how depressed the diaphragmatic leaflets are. The soft tissues of the chest wall show extensive edema secondary to widespread skin burns.

Thereafter, one should look for more specific findings such as: (a) abnormal tracheal deviation, (b) a right-side aortic arch (indicating a vascular ring problem), (c) a mediastinal mass, or (d) opaque airway foreign bodies.

Lobar emphysema is best known in its congenital form and, in this regard, most often involves the left upper lobe (Fig. 1.97A). The right upper lobe and right middle lobe (Fig. 1.97B) also are frequently involved, but lower lobe involve-

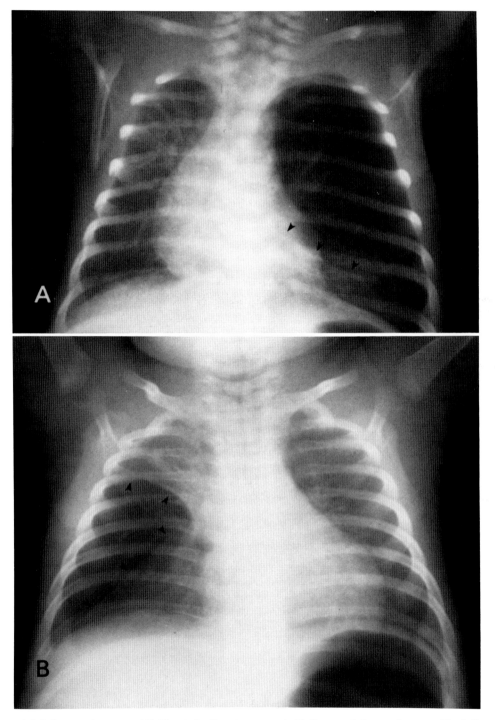

Figure 1.97. *Lobar emphysema.* (A) Classic findings in congenital left upper lobe emphysema. The left upper lobe is hyperlucent, the left lower lobe collapsed in a small triangle (*lower arrows*), and the mediastinum shifted to the right. (B) Right middle lobe emphysema producing an overaerated right middle lobe defined by the upwardly displaced minor fissure (*upper arrows*), and the downwardly and medially displaced major fissure (*lower arrows*). The right upper and lower lobes show slight increase in density because they are partially compressed.

ment is rare. Many of these patients present in the newborn period, while others are asymptomatic into adulthood. Still others can come to the attention of the physician when a superimposed lower respiratory tract infection aggravates the air-trapping problem and renders the patient symptomatic. The whole problem can wax and wane (10) and frequently is dependent on whether or not an associated viral bronchitis is present. Transient lobar emphysema secondary to endobronchial mucus plugging as seen in asthma and viral lower respiratory tract infections also is frequently encountered, and surely is a common problem with obstructing endobronchial foreign bodies. In addition, lobar emphysema can be seen with other obstructing lesions such as the pulmonary sling (aberrant left pulmonary artery) syndrome, mediastinal masses or cysts, and in infants with bronchopulmonary dysplasia.

Most instances of well-developed lobar emphysema pose no real problem as far as roentgenographic interpretation is concerned, but a modification might be made in those cases where the right middle lobe alone is involved. In such cases, the unwary observer may be fooled and pick the right middle lobe as being normal (but compensatorily overinflated) and the right upper and right lower lobes as showing primary collapse. In these cases, it is only when one realizes that the combination of right upper lobe and lower lobe atelectasis is rather uncommon, that one begins to focus attention on the right middle lobe as the one abnormally overaerated (Fig. 1.97*B*). Of course, if still in doubt and as part of a general policy of confirming a suspected abnormality of aeration, inspiratory-expiratory film sequences should be obtained.

In the odd case, congenital lobar emphysema will be mimicked by cystic disease of the lung (i.e., congenital adenomatoid malformation). In these cases, air trapping in the multiple cysts becomes so profound that the septa between the cysts

are almost obliterated and a picture of lobar emphysema or even pneumothorax is suggested.

Before leaving the topic of emphysema, a note might be made regarding those times when bilateral obstructive emphysema is mimicked by overaeration of the lungs due to some other nonpulmonary problem. In this regard, the most common situation is that of overaeration of the lungs secondary to dehydration and acidosis as seen with viral gastroenteritis (see Fig. 1.150). The clinical picture in these infants, of course, usually quickly clarifies the situation. The other time when lungs appear overdistended and suggest obstructive emphysema is when a child takes an overexuberant inspiration for the roentgenographic examination. All that is required here is that one be aware of this pitfall and remember not to interpret the roentgenograms in the absence of clinical history.

REFERENCES

1. Billig, D.M., and Darling, D.B.: Middle lobe atelectasis in children. Clinical and bronchographic criteria in the selection of patients for surgery. Am. J. Dis. Child. 123: 96–98, 1972.
2. Cho, S.R., Henry, D.A., Beachley, M.C., and Brooks, J.W.: Round (helical) atelectasis. Br. J. Radiol. 54: 643–650, 1981.
3. Dees, S.C., and Spock, A.: Right middle lobe syndrome in children. J.A.M.A. 197: 8–14, 1966.
4. Felson, B.: *Chest Roentgenology*, pp. 92–142. W.B. Saunders, Philadelphia, 1973.
5. Franken, E.A., Jr., and Klatte, B.C.: Atypical (peripheral) upper lobe collapse. Ann. Radiol. 20: 87–93, 1977.
6. Glay, J., and Palayew, M.J.: Unusual pattern of left lower lobe atelectasis. Radiology 141: 331–333, 1981.
7. Griscom, N.T., Wohl, M.E.B., and Kirkpatrick, J.A., Jr.: Lower respiratory infections: How infants differ from adults. Radiol. Clin. North Am. 16: 367–387, 1978.
8. Krause, G.R., and Lupert, M.: Gross anatomico-spatial changes occurring in lobar collapse: A demonstration by means of three-dimensional plastic models. A.J.R. 79: 258–268, 1958.
9. Lubert, M., and Krause, G.R.: Patterns of lobar collapse as observed radiographically. Radiology 56: 165–182, 1951.
10. Morgan, W.J., Lemen, R.J., and Rojas, R.: Acute

worsening of congenital lobar emphysema with subsequent spontaneous improvement. Pediatrics 71: 844–848, 1983.

11. Schneider, H.J., Felson, B., and Gonzalez, L.L.: Rounded atelectasis. A.J.R. 134: 225–232, 1980.

12. Talamo, R.C., Levison, H., Lynch, M.J., Hercz, A., Hyslop, N.E., Jr., and Bain, H.W.: Symptomatic pulmonary emphysema in childhood associated with hereditary α1-antitrypsin and an elastase inhibitor deficiency. J. Pediatr. 79: 20–26, 1971.

PNEUMATOCELES AND PULMONARY ABSCESS

A *pneumatocele* is an air-filled cyst, variable in size, usually thin-walled, fluid-free, and most frequently seen as a complication of a staphylococcal pulmonary infection. Pneumatoceles may be single or multiple, but most often rather than being the presenting feature of the pulmonary infection they tend to develop during the course of the disease. Some pneumatoceles are subject to rapid changes in size (Fig. 1.98), and may rupture to produce complicating pneumothoraces, but most remain relatively static for extended periods of time.

Eventually, they disappear (3), and overall the vast majority are asymptomatic.

In addition to being seen with *S. aureus* infection, pneumatoceles can be seen with other bacterial pneumonias (1, 6) and occasionally with tuberculosis. They also have been documented with hydrocarbon pneumonia (9), hyperimmunoglobulinemia E syndrome (5, 8), and are a common feature of closed, or blunt chest trauma. For the most part, little needs to be done about a pneumatocele, for regardless of the cause, it is only when complications such as pneumothorax or infection arise that definitive therapy is required.

Various etiologies have been considered in the development of pneumatoceles and, in this regard, it has been suggested that pneumatoceles represent subpleural blebs, rather than intraparenchymal blebs (2). This seems a reasonable explanation but probably does not account for all pneumatoceles, and some most likely are truly intraparenchymal. However, whatever the precise location or terminology, most agree that pneumatoceles result from alveolar or bronchiolar rupture secondary to

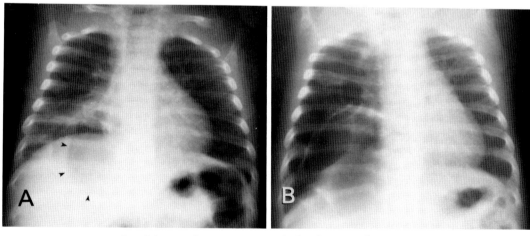

Figure 1.98. *Pneumatocele.* (A) Note a large pneumatocele developing in the right lower lung of an infant with staphylococcal pneumonia (*arrows*). A smaller pneumatocele is seen just lateral to the large one. (B) Seven days later, note how large the pneumatoceles have become. Indeed, there is a tension phenomenon present with the mediastinum being shifted to the left. Eventually, some 30 days later, the chest film in this infant was completely normal.

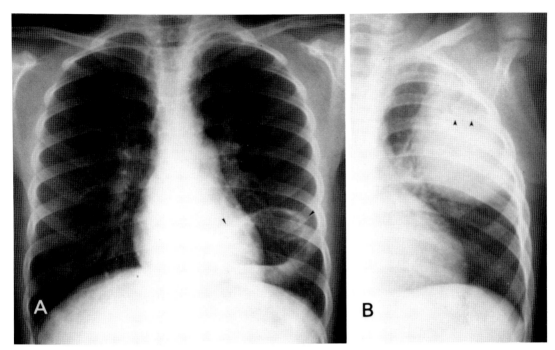

Figure 1.99. *Pulmonary abscess.*   (*A*) Note the rather thick-walled, irregular-appearing abscess cavity in the left lower lobe (*arrows*). There is an air-fluid level at the bottom of the abscess. (*B*) Another patient with an abscess in the left upper lung. Its hazy margin reflects adjacent inflammatory change. The abscess is nearly full of fluid with only a small air-fluid level noted at the top (*arrows*).

air trapping distal to areas of small airway obstruction (4).

Pulmonary abscesses are a complication of lobar pneumonia or chronic bronchial obstructions (7). They are easily recognized by their round or oval configuration, air-fluid levels, and relatively thick walls (Fig. 1.99). Overall, most pulmonary abscesses tend to appear different from pneumatoceles, primarily in that they contain fluid and that their walls are thicker and more irregular. Of course, if infection supervenes in a pneumatocele, differentiation may be more difficult, but this is not a particularly common occurrence.

Acute cavitating pneumonias usually are bacterial in origin, but also have been reported with *M. pneumoniae* infections (6). In any of these cases, it is not always possible to determine whether one is dealing with an infected pneumatocele or ab-

scess. CT is excellent in providing final anatomic data in all of these lesions (9), but is no better than the chest film in differentiating one from another (Fig. 1.100).

REFERENCES

1. Asmar, B.I., Thirumoorthi, M.C., and Dajani, A.S.: Pneumococcal pneumonia with pneumatocele formation. Am. J. Dis. Child. 132: 1091–1093, 1978.
2. Boissett, G.F.: Subpleural emphysema complicating staphylococcal and other pneumonias. J. Pediatr. 8: 259–266, 1972.
3. Caffey, J.: On the natural regression of pulmonary cysts during early infancy. Pediatrics 11: 48, 1953.
4. Conway, D.J.: The origin of lung cysts in childhood. Arch. Dis. Child. 26: 504, 1951.
5. Hill, H.R.: The syndrome of hyperimmunoglobulinemia E and recurrent infections. Am. J. Dis. Child. 136: 767–771, 1982.
6. Johnson, F.: Cavitating lesions in a cold agglutinin positive pneumonia. Pediatr. Radiol. 6: 181–182, 1977.

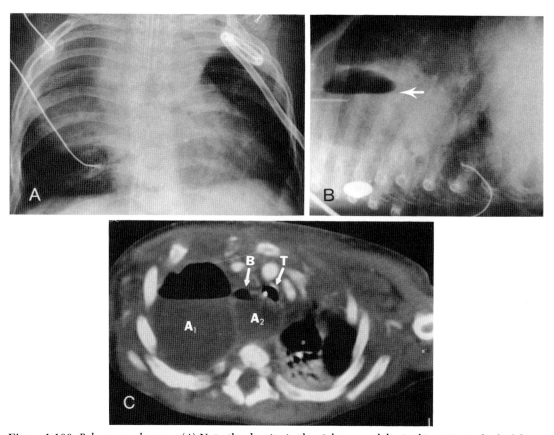

Figure 1.100. *Pulmonary abscess.* (*A*) Note the density in the right upper lobe in this patient who had fever after tracheoesophageal fistula repair. (*B*) Cross-table lateral view demonstrates an air-fluid level (*arrow*) within the abscess. (*C*) CT study demonstrates a multicompartmentalized (A1, A2) pulmonary abscess that has displaced the right mainstem bronchus (*B*) and trachea (*T*) forward.

7. Marks, P.H., and Turner, J.A.P.: Lung abscesses in childhood. Thorax 23: 216, 1968.
8. Merten, D.F., Buckley, R.H., Pratt, P.C., Eff-mann, E.L., and Grossman, H.: Hyperimmuno-globulinemia E syndrome: Radiographic observations. Radiology 132: 71–78, 1979.
9. Stones, D.K., van Niekerk, C.H., and Cilliers, C.: Computerized tomography in pneumatoceles after paraffin ingestion. Pediatr. Radiol. 17: 443–446, 1987.
10. Warner, J.O., and Gordon, I.: Pneumatoceles following haemophilus pneumonia. Clin. Radiol. 32: 99–105, 1981.

PNEUMOMEDIASTINUM, PNEUMOTHORAX, AND PNEUMOPERICARDIUM

Pneumomediastinum and pneumothorax in childhood can be seen with closed or penetrating chest or neck trauma (3), asthma, pulmonary infections with air trapping (10), airway foreign bodies (2), and occasionally with other obstructing lesions of the airway. Spontaneous pneumothorax and pneumomediastinum are not as common in children as in adults (5, 12, 19). A rather rare cause of pneumothorax or pneumomediastinum is diabetic ketoacidosis (22, 24). In these cases it is the "overbreathing" associated with acidosis that leads to airway rupture. Finally, pneumomediastinal air can be seen after abruptly increased intrathoracic pressures, as can occur with violent coughing episodes and after retching with vomiting (15) (Fig. 1.101).

Pneumomediastinal air collections are central in location (4) and of an endless as-

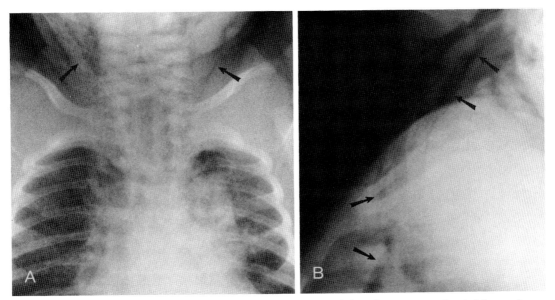

Figure 1.101. *Mediastinal emphysema due to spasmodic coughing.* (*A*) In this patient with parahilar peribronchial infiltrates and a viral bronchitis, note considerable free air in the soft tissues of the neck (*arrows*). This was induced by spasmodic coughing. (*B*) Lateral view demonstrates free air in the mediastinum anterior to the trachea (*lower arrows*) and in the retropharyngeal space (*upper arrows*).

sortment of shapes and sizes. They tend to outline, and surround, the various mediastinal structures such as the thymus, the aorta, and the pulmonary artery. In some cases, the free air extends upward to outline the great vessels and soft tissues of the superior mediastinum and neck, and in other cases the air may outline the heart (Fig. 1.102). In the latter case, the findings should not be confused with a medial pneumothorax (see Fig. 1.104), or pneumopericardium (see Fig. 1.108). In addition, one should be aware of the fact that pneumomediastinal air can collect subpleurally along the diaphragm (9, 14), and may even extend across the mediastinum to result in the "continuous diaphragm sign" of Levin (8). In these latter cases, the heart virtually is lifted off the diaphragm so that the diaphragm is seen in its entirety (Fig. 1.102*B*). So gross is the finding that it may be missed for this reason alone. In those cases where air collects subpleurally, that is, beneath the visceral pleura of the diaphragm, a variably thick strip of air is seen along the diaphragmatic leaflet. Clinically, mediastinal air often produces so-called crunching or crackling noises. Seldom is simple pneumomediastinum a cause for alarm, for even extensive air collections are relatively, if not entirely, asymptomatic. Only occasionally will one encounter such severe pneumomediastinum that surgical intervention might be required (17).

Pneumothorax, on the other hand, usually is accompanied by pain on inspiration and, if large enough and under tension, by respiratory distress. Auscultatory findings include decreased air entry or muffled breath sounds on the involved side, contralateral shift of the cardiac apical impulse, and in some cases of left-side pneumothorax, a "click" that might be confused with the crunch of a pneumomediastinum (23).

The job of the radiologist, in cases of pneumothorax, is not so much to detect the large one, for this is relatively easy, but rather to detect the one under tension or the one so subtle that it would otherwise be missed. In this regard, in the patient in

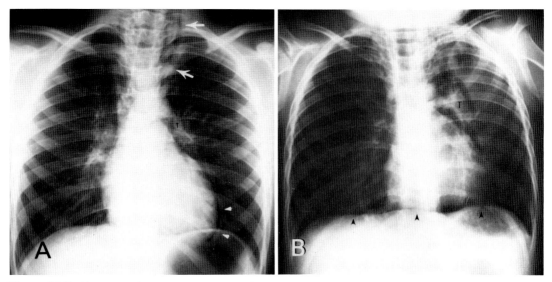

Figure 1.102. *Pneumomediastinum; varying configurations.* (*A*) Asthmatic child with pneumomediastinum showing air: (a) surrounding the small triangular thymus gland (*T*); (b) extending as linear sheaths into the neck and superior mediastinum (*upper arrows*); and (c) extending along the lower left cardiac edge (*lower arrows*). (*B*) Another asthmatic child with pneumomediastinal air outlining the thymic gland on the left (*T*) and producing the continuous diaphragm sign (*arrows*). The diaphragm is seen in its entirety from side to side, including that portion just beneath the cardiac silhouette. A similar configuration can be seen on lateral view. Smallness of the left hemithorax and increased density over the left upper lobe are due to partial atelectasis of the left upper lobe and lingula.

the supine position, since air collects anterior to the lung, a free lung edge may not be visualized. However, certain telltale signs are usually present (18, 21) and should be sought for. They include: (a) increased lucency, and often, size of the involved hemithorax (air under tension over the anterior surface of the lung); (b) contralateral shift of the mediastinum (tension phenomenon); and (c) increased sharpness or crispness of the ipsilateral mediastinal edge (Fig. 1.103). The latter finding results from the fact that free air rather than aerated lung abuts the heart, *and because of this the edge of the heart and other mediastinal structures become more clearly demarcated; i.e., they appear "sharper" or "crisper."* The same phenomenon occurs over the diaphragmatic leaflets if air happens to accumulate solely along the bottom of the lung. In addition, the diaphrag-

matic leaflet may be depressed or show a double contour (16, 25). In still other cases, air may accumulate deep in the costophrenic or paravertebral sulci (7) and produce increased radiolucency in this area (Fig. 1.103D).

For the most part, the foregoing findings are quite dependable in allowing one to detect an anterior pneumothorax on supine films. *However, it should be remembered that increased "sharpness" or "crispness" of the mediastinal edge or diaphragmatic leaflet also can be seen when a lung becomes overdistended, either because of obstruction or because of compensatory emphysema.* Consequently, if one suspects an anterior or basal pneumothorax on a supine film, some other film should be obtained for confirmation. For the most part this can be a cross-table lateral (11), regular lateral, decubitus, or expiratory

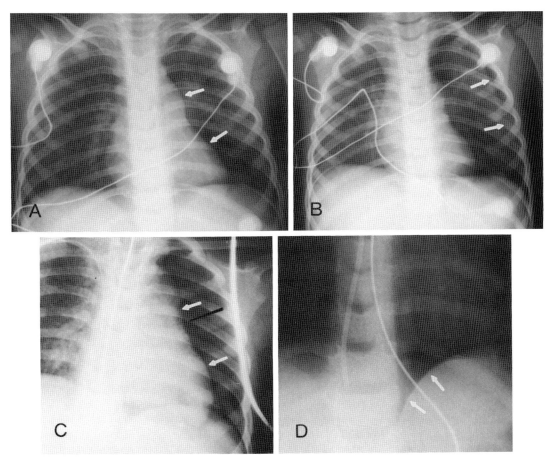

Figure 1.103. *Pneumothorax; supine film findings.* (***A***) The fact that a pneumothorax is present on the left might be missed. However, note that the left mediastinal edge is "sharper" or "crisper" than on the right (*arrows*). This sign indicates that free air is present, lying anterior to the lung and against the heart. (***B***) Moments later, an expiratory film more clearly demonstrates the pneumothorax. The free lung edge on the left is now clearly visualized (*arrows*) and the compressed left lung, virtually bathed in an envelope of free air, is easy to detect. Note that the trapped air on the left causes the left hemithorax to remain large and hyperlucent, and that the left cardiomediastinal edge is still sharper than its mate on the right. (***C***) Another patient with similar findings due to an anterior pneumothorax on the left (*arrows*). (***D***) Deep sulcus sign (7) in the same patient consisting of increased radiolucency of the left paravertebral sulcus (*arrows*).

phase roentgenogram. During expiration, the lungs empty and become smaller but the free air of the pneumothorax does not. One can use any or all of these views as an aid in detecting a subtle pneumothorax, and actually one should not limit oneself to a single additional view. Another misleading configuration of pneumothorax occurs when air collects along the medial aspect of the lung so as to mimic a pneumomediastinum or pneumopericardium (Fig. 1.104). In such cases, an expiratory, regular or cross-table lateral, or decubitus view once again becomes useful for differentiation (13, 18).

On upright view, large pneumothoraces are not difficult to detect; the free lung edge is usually readily discernable, and the

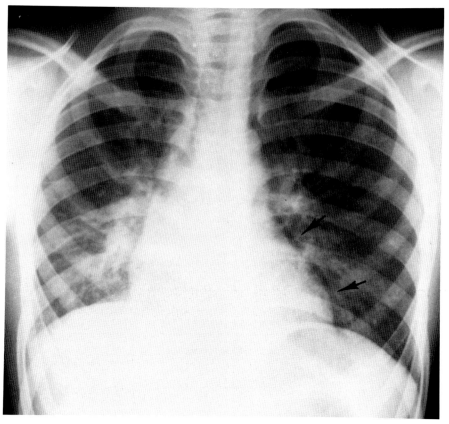

Figure 1.104. *Medial pneumothorax.*   Note the thin strip of free air along the left cardiac border (*arrows*). The finding represents a medial pneumothorax and should not be confused with pneumomediastinum or pneumo-pericardium.

area lateral to it appears blacker than usual and free of vascular markings (Fig. 1.105). However, smaller pneumothoraces require astute inspection and careful scrutiny of the lung over its apex and in the costophrenic angle. In the costophrenic angle, one should look for the typical, laterally pointing, V-shaped air fluid level. If you see this finding, look harder for a pneumothorax for it will be there (Fig. 1.106). The V-shaped configuration results from the fact that fluid lies both in the anterior and posterior pleural space, and as the x-ray beam travels through the chest, these two fluid levels are traversed at two different angles and appear as the two

limbs of the "V." Over the apex of the lung, free air is seen as a slender, radiolucent apical cap, and finally when a localized pneumothorax is seen next to a collapsed lobe (1), bronchial obstruction should be considered (Fig. 1.107). Ordinarily, pneumothorax does not compress a single lobe.

Pneumopericardium usually is traumatic in origin and not particularly difficult to recognize. It can be seen with penetrating chest trauma or blunt chest trauma. The latter, of course, is less common. In addition, it has been noted with airway foreign bodies (20), and it has been suggested that air enters the pericardium through

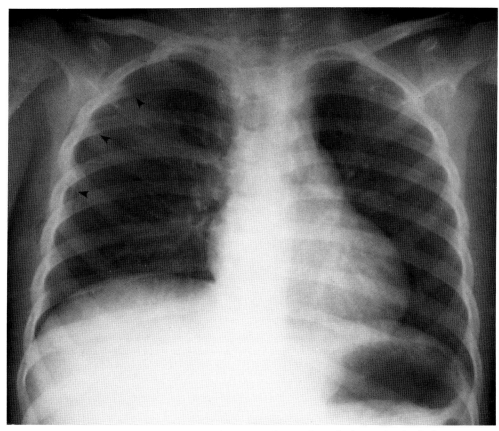

Figure 1.105. *Typical pneumothorax.* Note the free lung edge on the right (*arrows*). The findings are typical of pneumothorax in that there are no vascular markings beyond the free lung edge.

tears between it and the adjacent connective tissue attachments to the pleura.

Pneumopericardium is identified by noting free air around the heart (Fig. 1.108). However, more often than not it is some other roentgenographic finding that usually is misinterpreted as being representative of pneumopericardium; i.e., medial pneumothorax, pneumomediastinum, and the artifactual Mach effect (6, 18) enhancement of a normal pericardial radiolucency occurring between the cardiac edge and the adjacent lower lobe pulmonary artery branches (Fig. 1.109B).

In terms of pneumopericardium, the key to distinguishing it from these other entities is to actually note the fine white

line of the pericardium as it is separated from the heart by air (Fig. 1.108). Unfortunately, this configuration also can be seen with pneumomediastinum. However, pneumomediastinal air usually outlines one side of the heart only (Fig. 1.109A), while with pneumopericardium, air usually outlines the entire heart (Fig. 1.108). Nonetheless, in cases where air collections are minimal, if no other signs of pneumomediastinum are present, it may be difficult to make the distinction.

Finally, a note regarding air in the inferior pulmonary ligament is in order. Most often seen with blunt chest trauma (see Fig. 1.138), it also can occur with mediastinal air from other causes. Its character-

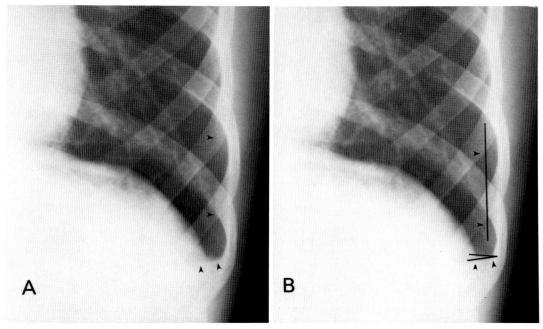

Figure 1.106. *Horizontal V sign in pneumothorax.* (A) At first the V-shaped collection of fluid in the left costophrenic angle might be overlooked (*lower two arrows*). The free lung edge is barely discernable (*upper two arrows*). (B) Diagrammatic representation of the horizontal V-sign and the free lung edge.

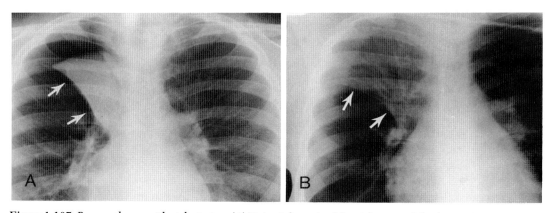

Figure 1.107. *Pneumothorax with atelectasis.* (A) Note atelectasis of the right upper lobe (*arrows*) and increased lucency in the area. This is due to an associated pneumothorax. (B) After the pneumothorax clears, residual atelectasis of the right upper lobe (*arrows*) is seen.

Figure 1.108. *Pneumopericardium.* (A) Traumatic pneumopericardium. Note the halo of free air around the heart and the clearly visualized pericardial sac (*large arrows*). Air also extends along the aorta (*small arrows*). (B) Note air in the pericardial sac posteriorly (*arrows*), but also note that air clearly outlines both the pulmonary artery (*PA*) and aorta. The pericardium attaches onto the base of the great vessels, and with larger volume pericardial air collections, the aorta and pulmonary artery are outlined by the air.

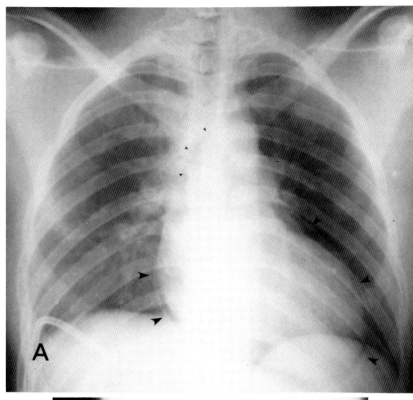

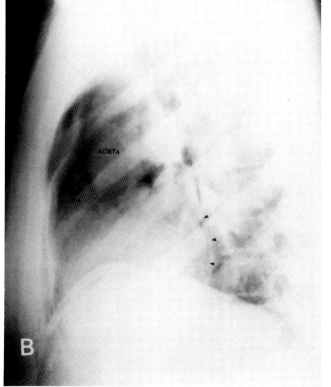

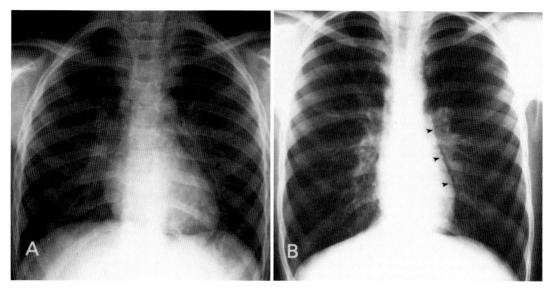

Figure 1.109. *Pseudopneumopericardium.* (*A*) Pneumomediastinum mimicking pneumopericardium. Note what appears to be the pericardial sac on the left (*arrows*). However, if this truly were the pericardial sac, enough air is present so that it should surround the entire cardiac silhouette. Furthermore, the thymus gland (*T*) usually would not be elevated and visualized as a separate structure with pneumopericardium. (*B*) *Mach effect.* Note what would appear to be free air along the left cardiac border (*arrows*). The artifact is produced by a thin strip of normally aerated lung being projected between the cardiac border and the descending left lower lobe pulmonary artery. In such cases, radiolucency of the apparent stripe of pneumopericardial air is enhanced by the Mach effect.

istic location and usually somewhat oval configuration just along the spine on frontal view are the keys to proper diagnosis.

REFERENCES

1. Berdon, W.E., Dee, G.J., Abramson, S.J., Altman, R.P., and Wung, J.-T.: Localized pneumothorax adjacent to a collapsed lobe: A sign of bronchial obstruction. Radiology 150: 691–694, 1984.
2. Burton, E.M., Riggs, W., Jr., Kaufman, R.A., and Houston, C.S.: Pneumomediastinum caused by foreign body aspiration in children. Pediatr. Radiol. 20: 45–47, 1989.
3. Eklof, O., and Thomasson, B.: Subcutaneous emphysema, pneumomediastinum and pneumothorax secondary to blunt injury to the throat. Ann. Radiol. 23: 169–173, 1980.
4. Evans, J., and Smalldon, T.: Mediastinal emphysema. A.J.R. 64: 375–389, 1950.
5. Feldman, R.W., Oram-Smith, J.C., Manning, L.G., and Buckley, C.J.: Spontaneous mediastinal emphysema. J. Pediatr. Surg. 15: 648–650, 1980.
6. Friedman, A.C., Lautin, E.M., and Rothenberg, L.: Mach bands and pneumomediastinum. J. Can. Assoc. Radiol. 32: 232–235, 1981.
7. Gordon, R.: The deep sulcus sign of pneumothorax. Radiology 136: 25–27, 1980.
8. Levin, B.: Continuous diaphragm sign: Newly recognized sign of pneumomediastinum. Clin. Radiol. 24: 337–338, 1973.
9. Lillard, R.L., and Allen, R.P.: The extrapleural air sign in pneumomediastinum. Radiology 85: 1093–1098, 1965.
10. Lipinski, J.K., and Goodman A.: Pneumothorax complicating bronchiolitis in an infant. Pediatr. Radiol. 9: 244–246, 1980.
11. MacEwan, D.W., Dunbar, J.S., Smith, R.D., and St. Brown, B.: Pneumothorax in young infants: Recognition and evaluation. J. Can. Assoc. Radiol. 22: 264–269, 1971.
12. McSweeney, W.J., and Stempel, D.A.: Non-iatrogenic pneumomediastinum in infancy and childhood. Pediatr. Radiol. 1: 139–144, 1973.
13. Moskowitz, P.S., and Griscom, N.T.: The medial pneumothorax. Radiology 120: 143–147, 1976.
14. O'Gorman, L.D., Cottingham, R.A., Sargeant, E.N., and O'Laughlin, B.J.: Mediastinal emphysema in the newborn: Review and description of the new extrapleural gas sign. Dis. Chest 53: 301–308, 1968.

15. Overby, K.J., and Litt, I.F.: Mediastinal emphysema in an adolescent with anorexia nervosa and self-induced emesis. Pediatrics 81: 134–136, 1988.
16. Rhea, J.T., van Sonnenberg E., and McLoud, T.C.: Basilar pneumothorax in the supine adult. Radiology 133: 593–595, 1979.
17. Stiegmann, G.V., Brantigan, C.O., and Hopeman, A.R.: Tension pneumomediastinum. Arch. Surg. 112: 1212–1215, 1977.
18. Swischuk, L.E.: Two lesser known but useful signs of neonatal pneumothorax. A.J.R. 127: 623–627, 1976.
19. Sturtz, G.S.: Spontaneous mediastinal emphysema. Pediatrics 74: 431–432, 1984.
20. Tjen, K.Y., Schmaltz, A.A., Ibrahim, A., and Nolte, K.: Pneumopericardium as a complication of foreign body aspiration. Pediatr. Radiol. 7: 121–123, 1978.
21. Tocino, I.M., Miller, M.H., and Fairfax, W.F.: Distribution of pneumothorax in the supine and semi-recumbent critically ill adult. A.J.R. 144: 901–905, 1985.
22. Toomey, F.B., and Churnock, R.F.: Subcutaneous mediastinum and pneumothorax in diabetic ketoacidosis. Radiology 116: 543, 1975.
23. Wright, J.T.: The radiological sign of "clicking" pneumothorax. Clin. Radiol. 16: 292–294, 1965.
24. Zahller, M.C., Skoglund, R.R., and Larson, J.M.: Pneumomediastinum associated with diabetic ketoacidosis. J. Pediatr. 93: 529–530, 1978.
25. Ziter, F.M.H., Jr., and Westcott, J.L.: Supine subpulmonary pneumothorax. A.J.R. 137: 699–701, 1981.

PULMONARY CONGESTION AND EDEMA

Pulmonary congestion, and eventually frank pulmonary edema, can arise from a number of cardiac and extracardiac causes. However, before discussing the roentgenographic features of pulmonary congestion and edema, it would be wise to first address the problem of *"pneumonia" versus congestion.* Indeed, I suspect that this is the most frequently asked question by the clinician of the roentgenologist. Unfortunately, there is no simple answer to the problem, for the solution comes only through experience, but there are one or two points that might be utilized to differentiate the two problems.

First, one should be aware that problems arising in the differentiation of pulmonary congestion from "pneumonia" are most frequently encountered in young infants. Almost always the problem is one of differentiating the findings of a viral lower respiratory tract infection with a parahilar-peribronchial, pattern of infiltration from true congestion (25). Indeed, in some of these cases the roentgenographic patterns virtually defy distinction from one another, and if one were to limit the examination to the lung fields alone, it certainly would be nearly impossible to differentiate the two. However, one should look at the heart too, for if cardiomegaly is present, cardiac disease is most likely, and if it is not, viral pulmonary infection should be one's choice (Fig. 1.110). In this regard, it might be remembered that these patients have a viral bronchitis, and not a true pneumonia, and that their disease process is in the interstitial compartment, just as is early pulmonary edema.

Pulmonary vascular congestion can be divided into two broad groups, active and passive (Fig. 1.111). Active congestion is most often seen with underlying left to right shunts and admixture lesions, and thus, its presence virtually assures that a congenital heart lesion is present. In such cases, more blood flows through the lungs than normal, and because of this, the pulmonary vessels enlarge, become more tortuous, and, as opposed to normal vessels, are visualized far into the periphery (outer third) of the lung (Fig. 1.111A). Once this pattern of pulmonary congestion is appreciated, one can go on to differentiate one lesion from another, but a discussion of this finding is beyond the scope of this book.

Passive congestion, on a purely cardiac basis, infers the presence of an obstructing lesion on the left, and/or a failing left heart. This can occur with obstructing lesions such as aortic stenosis and coarctation of the aorta, but more often it occurs with myocardial dysfunction such as is present with left-side overload heart lesions, acute myocarditis, or some form of cardiomyopathy. The roentgenographic pattern of pas-

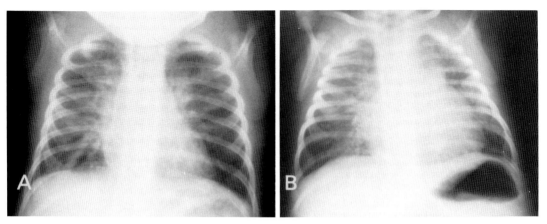

Figure 1.110. *Pneumonitis vs. congestion.* (*A*) The parahilar distribution of infiltrates in this infant with a viral lower respiratory tract infection might be mistaken for pulmonary congestion. However, the heart is not enlarged. (*B*) Contrarily, the parahilar pattern of pulmonary congestion secondary to heart disease in this patient might be misinterpreted for parahilar-peribronchial infiltration except that the heart is enlarged.

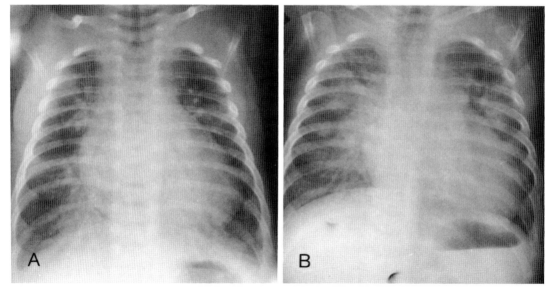

Figure 1.111. *Active vs. passive congestion.* (*A*) In this patient with a large ventricular septal defect, note cardiomegaly and prominent pulmonary vessels bilaterally. Although the vessels are a little indistinct, they still are identifiable as individual structures. (*B*) Same patient now with myocardial decompensation and passive congestion. Note that the parahilar regions are prominent and hazy because of pulmonary edema. The individual vessels, as identified in *A*, are no longer discretely visible.

sive congestion differs completely from that of active congestion, for in the former, the volume of blood flowing through the lungs is not increased. Rather, since pulmonary venous pressures are elevated, blood flow through the lungs is impeded, the pulmonary veins distend, fluid oozes out into the perivascular interstitium (transudate), and an overall fuzzy appearance of the vessels results (Fig. 1.111*B*). Actually, what one is witnessing is the development of interstitial pulmonary edema.

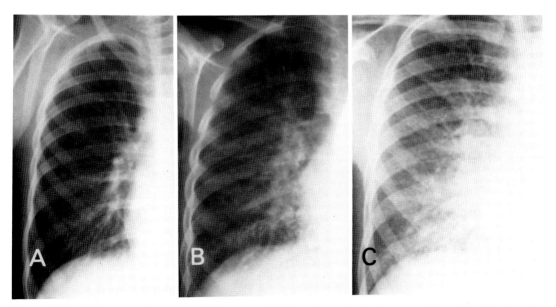

Figure 1.112. *Pulmonary edema; interstitial stage.*   (*A*) Note the early development of streaky white lines (interstitial septal edema) radiating from the hilar region. In this case, the lines primarily are Kerley "A" lines. This patient had acute glomerulonephritis. (*B*) More extensive reticular pattern of pulmonary interstitial edema in a patient with cardiac failure secondary to aortic stenosis. (*C*) Very extensive interstitial edema producing pronounced reticulation throughout the lung and some underlying parenchymal haziness. Kerley A and B lines are present. This patient had acute glomerulonephritis.

Pulmonary edema results from increased permeability of the pulmonary capillaries, either due to increased pulmonary venous pressures secondary to a failing left heart or to direct damage to the capillaries. In the latter case, pulmonary vascular pressures usually are normal, but in either instance, when fluid first seeps out of the vessels, it accumulates in the pulmonary interstitium. This being the case, one first will note the development of stringy or reticular white lines in the chest and then increasing opacity or haziness of the lungs (Fig. 1.112 and 1.113). The white lines represent fluid in the interstitial septa of the lungs and commonly are referred to as Kerley "A" and "B" lines (10). The B lines are the small, transverse lines usually best seen in the costophrenic sulci, while the A lines are the longer lines, generally running outward from the hilar regions (Figs. 1.112 and 1.113). The hazy appearance that eventually develops may at first suggest alveolar fluid accumulation,

but actually, it still probably represents fluid in the interstitial space (Fig. 1.113C). Alveolar fluid is much more dense and usually is patchy, fluffy, or totally confluent (Fig. 1.113D).

Once fluid saturates the interstitium, alveolar pulmonary edema begins to develop. In other words, fluid then oozes out into the alveolar space and it is at this point that the various alveolar patterns mentioned develop. In a few instances, edema fluid collects more centrally in the parahilar regions, leaving the periphery of the lungs relatively clear and producing the typical "butterfly" configuration (Fig. 1.113D). In many of these cases, the patchy and asymmetric nature of the infiltrate makes it most difficult to differentiate from widespread pneumonia, but the basically central predominance favors edema.

One of the most common causes of pulmonary edema in childhood is *acute glomerulonephritis* (9, 16, 19, 33). These pa-

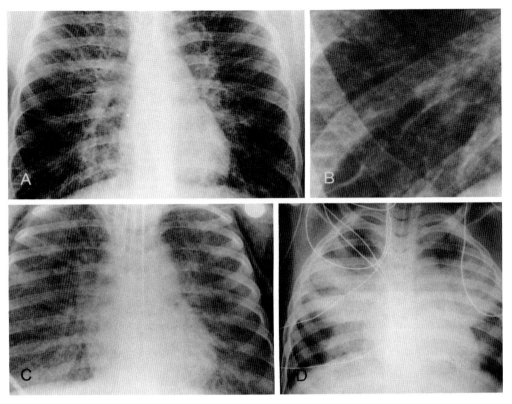

Figure 1.113. *Pulmonary edema: various interstitial through fluffy alveolar configurations.* (**A**) Widespread interstitial pulmonary edema leading to a streaky parahilar pattern with Kerley A and B lines in a patient suspected of inhaling a noxious substance. (**B**) Coned view of the right base demonstrates the Kerley A and B lines characteristic of an interstitial disease process. (**C**) Another patient with extensive pulmonary edema, primarily interstitial, leading to hazy lungs. Patient with adult respiratory distress syndrome. (**D**) Alveolar pulmonary edema in a typical butterfly configuration. Note that the densities due to the edema now are very confluent and very opaque. Edema in this case was due to fluid overload.

tients often demonstrate a combination of interstitial and alveolar edema and, overall, the findings frequently first suggest myocarditis with cardiac failure. Indeed, the pattern of congestion, including the presence of Kerley's B lines and pleural effusions, is virtually indistinguishable from that seen with acute myocarditis (Fig. 1.112C). At first, this roentgenographic picture may seem strange for the disease, but it is more common than generally believed and actually quite typical. The most likely cause for pulmonary congestion and cardiomegaly in these patients is circulatory overload (hypervolemia) secondary to sodium and fluid retention (19). No cardiac disease has been demonstrated in these patients, and, indeed, once the fluid overload

is corrected, the chest findings return to normal. Some of these patients may demonstrate a little cardiomegaly, but normal heart size is more often the rule.

It is most important to appreciate this roentgenographic manifestation of glomerulonephritis, for not only will it be seen in clinically apparent cases, but it may be the first clue to the diagnosis in clinically atypical patients. I have seen children with little, if any, facial puffiness and peripheral edema, who visit the emergency room for a cough and shortness of breath and whose roentgenograms demonstrate findings typical of glomerulonephritis.

Other causes of pulmonary edema include iatrogenic fluid overload, smoke or hot air inhalation (5, 13, 21, 30, 36), noxious fume inhalation, near-drowning (12, 29, 32, 40), neurogenic pulmonary edema secondary to increased intracranial pressure (4, 7, 11, 22), rheumatic pneumonia (33), collagen vascular disease, massive aspiration (17), fat embolism (2, 6, 8, 20), allergic pneumonitis (39), and the shocked lung syndrome (1, 9, 18, 24–27). In addition, pulmonary edema has been demonstrated with poisoning by the following chemicals or drugs: cocaine, heroin (15), methadone (38), salicylates (37), Librium (31), carbon monoxide (34), and insecticides (3, 14). In many of these conditions, cardiomegaly is minimal or absent, and this finding serves to alert one to the extracardiac origin of the pulmonary edema in these cases. Edema, in such cases, often results from the damaging of capillaries, with resultant increased permeability and the extravasation of fluid into the interstitial and alveolar spaces. In other instances, cardiac failure occurs, but often the underlying mechanisms are more complicated or incompletely understood.

Neurogenic pulmonary edema occurs as the aftermath of an acute rise in intracranial pressure, but its precise etiology is incompletely understood. Generally, however, it has been noted that these patients demonstrate bradycardia, peripheral vasoconstriction, lowered cardiac output, and elevated pulmonary venous pressures (7, 22). Because of this, hydrostatic pressure across the pulmonary capillaries becomes excessive and fluid extravasates into the surrounding lung tissue. Hyperactivity of the vagus nerve has been incriminated as leading to bradycardia and lowered cardiac output in these patients, but, overall, the precise etiology is unclear.

Near-drowning is not so much a matter of pulmonary edema as one of aspirating water into the lungs. As far as the roentgenographic findings are concerned, it makes little difference as to whether one aspirates salt or fresh water (29). Only the volume is important, for the more water aspirated, the more striking the roentgenographic findings. The chest film in these patients usually shows patchy alveolar infiltrates and serves as a baseline study (see Fig. 1.146B). It must be stressed, however, that clinical assessment, with serial blood gas determinations, is more important than judging the patient's condition from the roentgenograms. Fluid aspirated into the lung usually clears quickly, but if asphyxia also occurs, neurogenic pulmonary edema and even shock lung can develop. In these cases, the patchy pattern of alveolar fluid often gives way to one of diffuse interstitial edema.

Pulmonary edema secondary to smoke inhalation or noxious fume inhalation is self-explanatory. However, it should be noted that if smoke or hot air inhalation has caused bronchiolar damage, the chest film may show pronounced air trapping rather than pulmonary edema. These changes may clear after 1 or 2 days and later be replaced by nonspecific infiltrates caused by edema and microatelectasis secondary to pulmonary microemboli (13, 35). In severe cases, a necrotizing bronchiolitis with widespread patchy atelectasis and hemorrhage can develop. Very often these latter patients go on to rapid demise.

Fat embolism with subsequent pulmonary congestion results from the trapping of fat droplets in the pulmonary circulation after they have been dispersed into the bloodstream by the fracturing of a long bone such as the femur. However, it is not a common complication in childhood, and, overall, while many patients with fractures have evidence of fat droplets in the bloodstream, only a few develop pulmonary complications.

Shock lung or adult respiratory distress syndrome (9, 18, 26) occurs after profound hypoxia and hypotension, and the latter is seen with any number of conditions leading to these complications: i.e., trauma, severe burns, blood loss, septic shock, neurogenic shock, etc. (18). The roentgenographic findings (Fig. 1.113B) develop after the shock state has resolved. The etiology of shock lung is unknown, but a central neurologic origin has been suggested (23, 24). In this regard, it has been suggested that cerebral hypoxia leads to reactive arterial spasm in the lungs and, hence, hypoxia of the lungs. The net result is a loss of surfactant, increased cell wall permeability, and small vessel thrombosis (28). Roentgenographically, this results in interstitial and then alveolar pulmonary edema and scattered areas of segmental atelectasis and hemorrhage. The problem, in reality, is similar to that seen in newborns with hyaline membrane disease or the respiratory distress syndrome, and hence the term "adult respiratory distress syndrome."

REFERENCES

1. Adrens, J.F.: Shock lung. South. Med. J. 65: 206–208, 1972.
2. Berrigan, T.J., Carsky, E.W., and Heitzman, E.R.: Fat embolism. Roentgenographic-pathologic correlation in 3 cases. A.J.R. 96: 967–971, 1966.
3. Bledsoe, F.H., and Seymour, E.Q.: Acute pulmonary edema associated with parathion poisoning. Radiology 103: 53–56, 1972.
4. Chang, C.H., and Smith, C.A.: Postictal pulmonary edema. Radiology 89: 1087–1089, 1967.
5. Cudmorer, R.E., and Virom, E.: Inhalation injury to respiratory tract of children. Prog. Pediatr. Surg. 14: 173, 1981.
6. Feldman, F., Ellis, K., and Green, W.: Fat embolism syndrome. Radiology 114: 535–542, 1975.
7. Felman, A.H.: Neurogenic pulmonary edema: Observations in 6 patients. A.J.R. 112: 393–396, 1971.
8. Goodwin, N.M.: Fat embolus—the post-traumatic syndrome. S. Afr. Med. J. 48: 998–1000, 1976.
9. Greene, R: Adult respiratory distress syndrome: Acute alveolar damage. Radiology 163: 57–66, 1987.
10. Heitzman, E.R., Ziter, F.M., Markarian, B., McClennan, B.L., and Sherry, H.S.: Kerley's interlobar septal lines: Roentgen pathologic correlation. A.J.R. 100: 578–582, 1967.
11. Huff, R.W., and Fred, H.L.: Postictal pulmonary edema. Arch. Intern. Med. 117: 824–825, 1966.
12. Hunter, T.B., and Whitehouse, W.M.: Freshwater near drowning: radiological aspects. Radiology 112: 51–56, 1974.
13. Kangarloo, H., Beachley, M.C., and Ghahremani, G.G.: The radiographic spectrum of pulmonary complications in burn victims. A.J.R. 128: 441–445, 1977.
14. Kass, J.B., Khamapirad T., and Wagner, M.L.: Pulmonary edema following skin absorption of organo-phosphate insecticide, Pediatr. Radiology 7: 113–114, 1978.
15. Katz, S., Aberman, A., Frand, U.I., Stein, I.M., and Funlop, M.: Heroin pulmonary edema, evidence for increased pulmonary capillary permeability. Am. Rev. Respir. Dis. 106: 472–474, 1972.
16. Kirkpatrick, J.A., and Fleisher, D.S.: Roentgen appearance of chest in acute glomerulonephritis in children. J. Pediatr. 64: 492–498, 1964.
17. Landay, M.J., Christensen, E.E., and Bynum, L.J.: Pulmonary manifestations of acute aspiration of gastric contents. A.J.R. 131: 587–592, 1978.
18. Lyrene, R.K., and Truog, W.E.: Adult respiratory distress syndrome in a pediatric intensive care unit: Predisposing conditions, clinical course, and outcome. Pediatrics 67: 790–795, 1981.
19. Macpherson, R.I., and Banerjee, A.J.: Acute glomerulonephritis: A chest film diagnosis? J. Can. Assoc. Radiol. 25: 58–64, 1974.
20. Marayama, Y., and Little, J.B.: Roentgen manifestations of traumatic pulmonary fat embolism. A.J.R. 79: 945–952, 1962.
21. Mellins, R.B., and Park, S.: Respiratory complications of smoke inhalation in victims of fire. J. Pediatr. 87: 1–7, 1975.
22. Milley, J.R., Nugent, S.K., and Rogers, M.C.: Neurogenic pulmonary edema in childhood. J. Pediatr. 94: 706–709, 1979.
23. Moss, G.: The role of the central nervous system in shock: The centroneurogenic etiology of the respiratory distress syndrome. Crit. Care Med. 4: 181–185, 1974.
24. Moss, G., Staunton, C., and Stein, A.A.: Cerebral etiology of the "shock lung syndrome." J. Trauma 12: 885–890, 1972.
25. Munk, J.: The radiological differentiation between acute diffuse interstitial pneumonia and pulmonary interstitial edema in infancy and early childhood. Br. J. Radiol. 47: 752–757, 1974.
26. Ostendorf, P., Birzle, H., Vogel, W., and Mittermayer, C.: Pulmonary radiographic abnormalities in shock: Roentgen-clinical-pathological correlation. Radiology 115: 257–263, 1975.
27. Pfenninger, J., Gerber, A., Tshappeler, H., and Zimmerman, A.: Adult respiratory distress syndrome in children. J. Pediatr. 101: 352–357, 1982.
28. Pinet, F., Tabib, A., Clermont, A., Loire, R., Motin, J., and Artru, F.: Post-traumatic-shock lung: Post-morten microangiographic and pathologic correlation. A.J.R. 139: 449–454, 1982.
29. Putman, C.E., Tummillo, A.M., Myerson, D.A., and Myerson, P.J.: Drowning: Another plunge. A.J.R. 125: 543–548, 1975.

30. Putman, C.E., Loke, J., Matthay, R.A., and Ravin, C.E.: Radiographic manifestations of acute smoke inhalation. A.J.R. 129: 865–870, 1977.

31. Richman, S., and Harris, R.D.: Acute pulmonary edema associated with librium abuse, a case report. Radiology 103: 57–58, 1972.

32. Rosenbaum, H.T., Thompson, W.L., and Fuller, R.H.: Radiographic pulmonary changes in near-drowning. Radiology 83: 306–312, 1964.

33. Serlin, S.P., Rimza, M.E., and Gay, J.H.: Rheumatic pneumonia: The need for a new approach. Pediatrics 56: 1075–1077, 1975.

34. Sone, S., Higashihara, T., Kotake, T., Morimoti, S., Miura, T., Ogawa, M., and Sugimoto, T.: Pulmonary manifestations in acute carbon monoxide poisoning. A.J.R. 120: 865–871, 1974.

35. Stone, H.H.: Pulmonary burns in children. J. Pediatr. Surg. 14: 48–52, 1979.

36. Teixidor, H.S., Rubin, E., Novick, G.S., and Alonso, D.R.: Smoke inhalation: Radiologic manifestations. Radiology 149:383–387, 1983.

37. Walters, J.S., Woodring, J.H., Stelling, C.B., and Rosenbaum, H.D.: Salicylate-induced pulmonary edema. Radiology 146: 289–293, 1983.

38. Wilen, S.B., Ulreich, S., and Rabinowitz, J.G.: Roentgenographic manifestations of methadone-induced pulmonary edema. Radiology 114: 51–55, 1975.

39. Wolf, S.J., Stillerman, A., Weinberger, M., and Smith, W.: Chronic interstitial pneumonitis in a 3-year-old child with hypersensitivity to dove antigens. Pediatrics 79: 1027–1029, 1987.

40. Wunderlich, P., Ruprecht, E., Treffz, F., Thomsen, H., and Burhardt, J: Chest radiographs of near-drowned children. Pediatr. Radiol. 15: 297–299, 1985.

PERICARDIAL FLUID AND MYOCARDITIS

Myocarditis and pericardial effusions can occur together, and differentiation of the two may be difficult. However, in their pure forms the major difference between them is that with myocarditis passive vascular congestion is present, while with pericardial effusion it is not (Fig. 1.114). Of course, if both are present the findings may well overlap. Pericardial fluid accumulations can occur with rheumatic, viral,

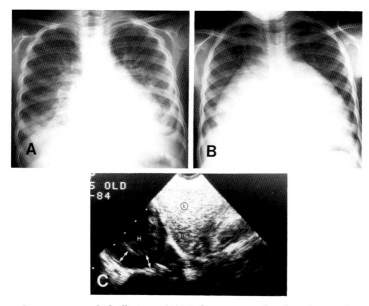

Figure 1.114. *Myocarditis vs. pericardial effusion.* (**A**) Moderate generalized cardiomegaly and marked passive congestion of the pulmonary vasculature in this patient with myocarditis. However, the superior mediastinum, in the region of the aorta and pulmonary artery, is not widened. Bilateral pleural effusions also are present. (**B**) Pericardial effusion producing diffuse globular enlargement of the cardiac silhouette. Note that the superior mediastinum is widened and that the aorta and pulmonary artery are completely obscured. The pulmonary vasculature, however, is not congested. (**C**) Ultrasound study demonstrating pericardial effusion (*arrows*). Heart (*H*), diaphragm (*D*), liver (*L*).

bacterial, or tuberculous pericarditis, kidney disease (glomerulonephritis and the nephrotic syndrome), collagen vascular diseases, and as hemopericardium with chest trauma (9, 11). Chylopericardium is very rare.

The roentgenographic identification of pericardial effusions of enough volume to cause cardiac enlargement entails study of the superior mediastinum. When such effusions are present, the great vessel silhouettes (aorta and pulmonary artery) become obliterated, for fluid accumulates in that portion of the pericardial sac which extends over their bases (7). This is, perhaps, the most important roentgenographic finding to detect, for enlargement of the cardiac silhouette is relatively nonspecific. Displacement of the epicardial fat pad has also been described with pericardial effusion (6, 10), but in my experience this finding is difficult to utilize in most cases. Actually, *when one suspects a pericardial effusion one should turn to ultrasonography for diagnosis* (1–5, 8) (Fig. 1.114C). Myocarditis most often is of viral origin, but bacterial and even tuberculous infection also can lead to myocardial inflammation. In the past, rheumatic myocarditis was the most common form of carditis in childhood. The roentgenographic features of myocarditis, with passive pulmonary vascular congestion and interstitial pulmonary edema are seen in Figure 1.114A.

REFERENCES

1. Abbasi, A.S., Ellis, N., and Flynn, J.J.: Echocardiographic M-scan technique in diagnosis of pericardial effusion. J. Clin. Ultrasound 1: 300–305, 1973.
2. Ellis, K., and King, D.L.: Pericarditis and pericardial effusion: Radiologic and echocardiographic diagnosis. Radiol. Clin. North Am. 11: 393–413, 1973.
3. Feigenbaum, H.: Echocardiographic diagnosis of pericardial effusion. Am. J. Cardiol. 26: 475–479, 1970.
4. Feigenbaum, H., Waldhausen, J.A., and Hyde, L.P.: The ultrasound diagnosis of pericardial effusion. J.A.M.A. 191: 711–714, 1965.
5. Goldberg, B.B., Ostrum, B.J., and Isard, H.J.: Ul-
trasonic determination of pericardial effusion. J.A.M.A. 202: 927–930, 1967.
6. Lane, E.J., Jr., and Carsky, E.W.: Epicardial fat: Lateral plain film analysis in normals and in pericardial effusion. Radiology 91: 1–5, 1968.
7. Soulen, R.L., Lapayowker, M.S., and Cortex, F.M.: Distribution of pericardial fluid: Dynamic and static influences. A.J.R. 103: 583–588, 1968.
8. Soulen, R.L., Lapayowker, M.S., and Gimenez, J.L.: Echocardiography in the diagnosis of pericardial effusion. Radiology 86: 1047–1051, 1966.
9. Stolz, J.L., Borns, P., and Schwade, J.: The pediatric pericardium. Radiology 112: 159–165, 1974.
10. Torrance, D.J.: Demonstration of subepicardial fat as an aid in diagnosis of pericardial effusion or thickening. A.J.R. 74: 850–855, 1955.
11. Van Reken, D., Strauss, A., Hernandez, A., and Feigin, R.D.: Infectious pericarditis in children. J. Pediatr. 85: 165–169, 1974.

ASTHMATIC CHILD

The child with asthma comes to the emergency room, not so much for the diagnosis of asthma, but for the diagnosis or exclusion of one of its complications. On a practical basis, the problem often boils down to the following: (a) Is infection present and, if so, what kind? (b) Are there any focal aeration disturbances (i.e., atelectasis or obstructive emphysema)? (c) Is there evidence of pneumomediastinum or pneumothorax? In this regard, the value of chest roentgenograms for patients with their first attack of asthma has been questioned (7), but on a practical basis it is difficult to deny a chest roentgenogram for these patients.

In answer to the question of whether infection is present in a patient with asthma, one should note that, although asthmatic children are more susceptible to lower respiratory tract infections, these more often are viral than bacterial (15, 18–20). This is especially true if increased wheezing accompanies the infections (20), for bacterial infections usually do not cause increased wheezing in asthmatic children (15). There is good reason for this to be so, for bacterial infections usually are parenchymal (alveolar) infections with little in the way of associated bronchitis. Viral infections, on the other hand, manifest as a widespread bronchitis-peribronchitis, and it is this aspect of these infections that predisposes to bronchospasm, mucous plug formation, and aggravation of the basic pathophysiology of asthma. This, of course, is not to say that bacterial infections with parenchymal consolidations do not occur in asthmatic children, for indeed they do, but only to emphasize that such infections are much less common than generally believed. Bacterial infections generally do not aggravate asthmatic symptoms, for they do not have a significant bronchitic component. For the most part, they present just as they do in nonasthmatics.

In asthmatics, therefore, most of the time what is at first suspected to be a parenchymal infiltrate turns out to be an area of segmental atelectasis (Fig. 1.115). The problem here is much the same as in those patients with viral bronchitis and areas of atelectasis. Segmental and lobar atelectasis are extremely common in asthma, and, once this is appreciated, one will come to the realization that the single most common cause of pulmonary density on the chest films of asthmatic children is transient atelectasis secondary to endobronchial mucous plugging and not pneumonia (6). Furthermore, such changes are much more common in children than in adults (28).

In many asthmatic children, a characteristic baseline roentgenogram is seen (6, 8).

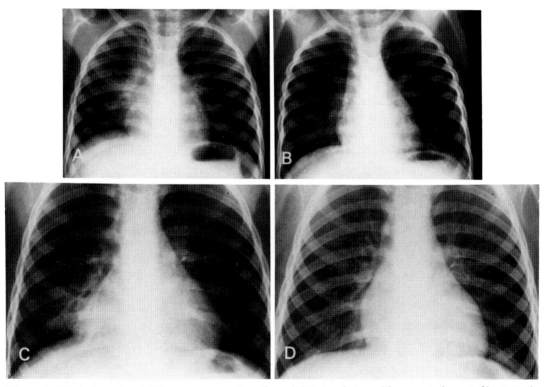

Figure 1.115. *Atelectasis mimicking pneumonia in asthma.* (A) Note what would appear to be an infiltrate in the right upper lobe (*arrows*). (B) Less than 24 hours later the infiltrate has disappeared. It was due to partial atelectasis of the right upper and middle lobes. Such areas of atelectasis are common in asthma and are frequently misinterpreted for patchy pneumonia. (C) Another patient with an apparent right middle lobe infiltrate (*arrows*) that suggests a pneumonia. Also note generalized overaeration. (D) Twenty-four hours later, the chest film is normal. No pneumonia would clear this rapidly. The findings were due to transient middle lobe atelectasis.

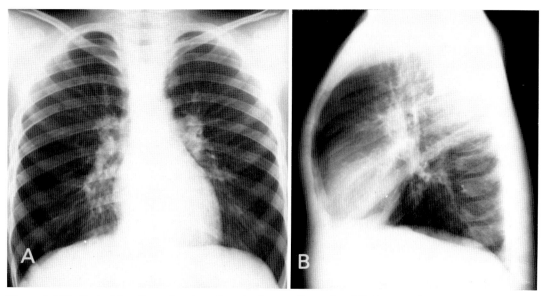

Figure 1.116. *Typical baseline, chronic asthmatic chest radiograph.* (*A*) Note moderate overaeration, pronounced parahilar peribronchial infiltration, some bronchial cuffing, and hilar adenopathy. (*B*) Lateral view showing overdistended chest. Note how the heart is pushed away from the sternum.

It consists of widespread overaeration, parahilar peribronchial infiltration with bronchial cuffing, and an overall picture very similar to that seen with viral lower respiratory tract infections (Fig. 1.116). To be sure, so similar are the findings that it is often difficult to determine whether or not an asthmatic child has a superimposed viral lower respiratory tract infection. All of these findings may at first appear relatively nonspecific, but familiarity with them soon leads to a typical template for the so-called "asthmatic chest" in childhood. Histologically, in these children there is thickening of the bronchi and peribronchial tissues (9, 10), and, bronchographically, the following changes have been demonstrated: (a) spasm of the bronchi at their bifurcations, (b) increased secretions, (c) increased bronchial dilatation, (d) mucosal irregularities and dilated mucous glands, and (e) mucous plugs (24).

It must be noted, however, that not all asthmatic patients have this typical baseline chest appearance. Indeed, there are those who merely show overaeration and never really develop a pattern of chronic, parahilar peribronchial infiltration. It is not completely understood why this should occur, but it does, and in addition to these considerations there is the problem of hyperactive airway disease (5, 25). This latter condition is somewhat nebulous and often, in the long run, it is difficult to completely separate the two conditions. However, patients with asthma are severely afflicted and require more treatment and hospital visits.

The generalized air trapping commonly seen in asthmatics is, of course, secondary to bronchospasm. During acute attacks such air trapping may be profound, and it is at these times that there is a greater tendency for complications such as pneumomediastinum and pneumothorax to occur (2, 11, 12, 14, 16, 17, 21, 22). Pneumomediastinum, however, is by far the more common of the two (Fig. 1.117*A* and *B*), and in some of these cases the mediastinal air can leak into the interstitial tissues of the neck and chest wall (Fig. 1.117*C* and *D*). Most often, pneumomediastinum is

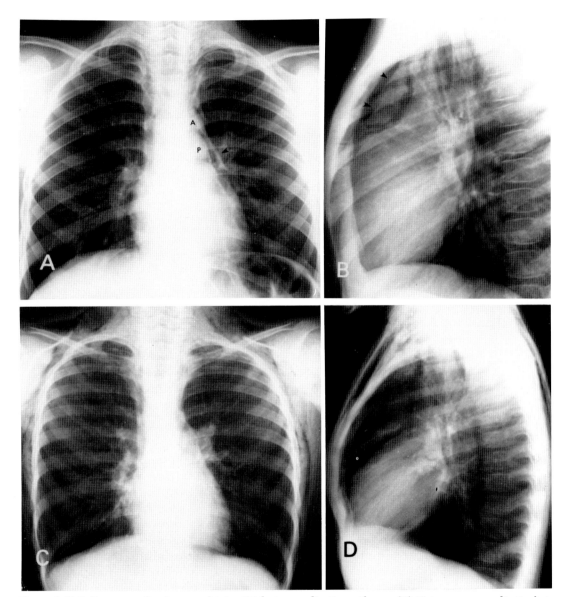

Figure 1.117. *Pneumomediastinum and interstitial air complicating asthma.* (*A*) Note pneumomediastinal air outlining the aorta (*A*), pulmonary artery (*P*), and a slender left thymic lobe (*arrow*). (*B*) Lateral view in another patient demonstrating a small thymus gland (*arrows*) surrounded by pneumomediastinal air. (*C*) Note the typically overdistended chest with chronic parahilar peribronchial infiltrates in this child with an acute asthmatic attack. A little air is present in the superior mediastinum, but most has escaped into the soft tissues of the neck and chest wall. (*D*) Lateral view. Note interstitial air in the soft tissues of the chest wall, both anteriorly and posteriorly. Some air is seen in the mediastinum.

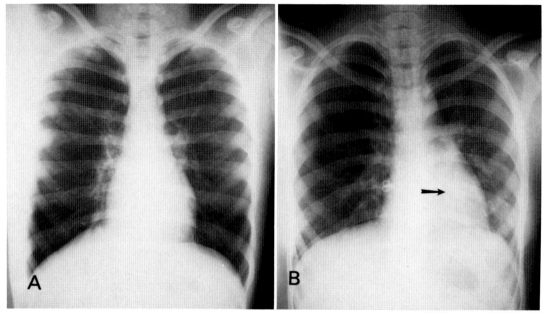

Figure 1.118. *Mucous plug causing unsuspected obstructive emphysema.* (**A**) On this inspiratory chest film, the lungs are markedly overdistended, but apart from this, the roentgenogram would most likely be interpreted as normal. One would not suspect that any focal aeration disturbance was present, and yet, as is seen in **B**, an obstructing mucous plug is present on the right. (**B**) On expiration, note that the mediastinum has shifted to the left (*arrow*), and that while the left lung has emptied partially, the right lung remains large and radiolucent, attesting to the fact that obstructive emphysema is present. In such cases, obstruction is of such a degree that enough air escapes during expiration to keep the obstructed lung from getting overly large.

treated conservatively, but occasionally surgical decompression has been required (16).

Endobronchial mucous plugs, as has been noted earlier, are common in asthmatic children and may lead either to atelectasis or obstructive emphysema (7), but atelectasis is much more common. The presence of these plugs may not be appreciated until expiratory films are obtained (Figs. 1.118 and 1.119).

Other findings seen in acute asthma include prominence of the pulmonary artery and elongation of the entire cardiac silhouette (Fig. 1.120). The latter finding is explained by the fact that the diaphragm is depressed downward, and the heart is elongated and squeezed by the overdistended lungs. Prominence of the pulmonary artery usually is explained on the basis of transient pulmonary hypertension

secondary to increased pulmonary vascular resistance produced by the profound degree of emphysema and sludging of the blood in the pulmonary arteries.

In other cases of asthma, when the antibody-antigen reaction occurs on the tracheobronchial mucosal surfaces, there is a release of the so-called primary mediators which act on the lung to produce (a) bronchospasm, (b) increased sludging of the blood, and (c) breakdown of the cellular membranes with the exudation of fluid into the interstitium to produce pulmonary edema, even to the point of producing Kerley's B lines (23). However, this pattern is rare and usually not seen until initial bronchospasm has been broken, and thus is usually not a presenting picture of the disease.

Chronic mucous plugging with superimposed aspergillosis infection (3, 13, 26) is not particularly common in childhood

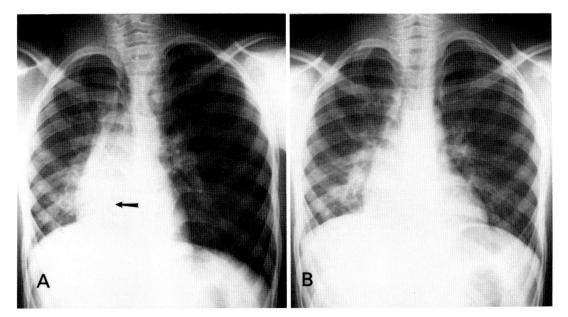

Figure 1.119. *Mucous plug with distracting contralateral compensatory emphysema.* (A) On this inspiratory view, there is marked mediastinal shift to the right (*arrow*), and the left lung might be suspected of being abnormal. However, as is shown in *B*, it is normal and on this view merely shows compensatory overaeration on inspiration. (B) *Expiratory films showing that the problem lies on the right.* Note that the left lung has emptied but that the right lung has not changed in size. A little mediastinal shift to the right persists, attesting to the fact that the problem is one of an obstructing mucous plug on the right. The thin radiolucent band outlining the left pericardial border represents a small medial pneumothorax.

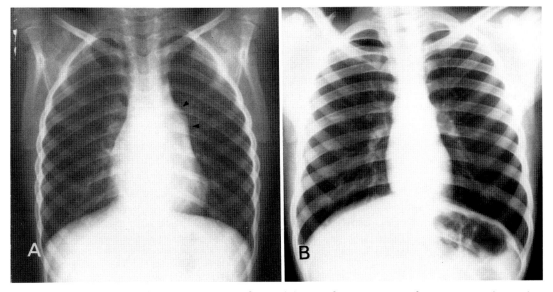

Figure 1.120. *Prominent pulmonary artery in asthma.* (A) Note the prominent pulmonary artery (*arrows*) in this patient with an acute asthmatic attack. This is a common finding in asthmatic children and is a reflection of acute pulmonary hypertension. (B) *Elongated small heart in asthma.* Note the long thin cardiac silhouette in this asthmatic child suffering from status asthmaticus. Such stretching of the heart with resultant smallness of the cardiac silhouette (microcardia) is not uncommon in asthma. If dehydration is present in these patients, it further accentuates the findings of microcardia. Note that in this patient perihilar peribronchial infiltrates are virtually absent, which demonstrates that not all asthmatic children show the degree of perihilar peribronchial infiltration seen in Figure 1.116.

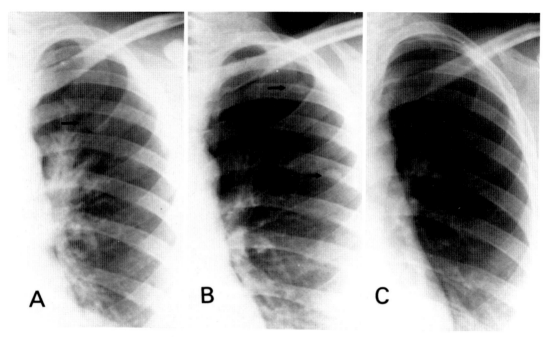

Figure 1.121. *Transient peripheral mucous plugs.* (*A*) Adolescent asthmatic with round nodule in left upper lobe (*arrow*). (*B*) During another admission the previous nodule disappeared but two new ones appeared (*arrows*). (*C*) At a later date, no nodules are present. These nodules represent transient peripheral mucous plugs, probably with focal, subsegmental atelectasis.

asthma, but it can occur. In these cases, the mucous plugs can be seen as oval or elongated, sometimes Y-shaped densities in the lung field. Distal to these areas, one usually sees focal air trapping and increased lucency of the involved lobe. Transient mucous plugs without superimposed aspergillosis infection also occur and probably are more common than generally realized (Fig. 1.121).

Before leaving the topic of asthma, a note might be in order regarding chronic gastroesophageal reflux and asthma (1, 4, 27). Although much publicized in recent years, and probably responsible for a few cases of asthma, the problem probably arises much less frequently than was first believed. In addition, these patients usually are not so much emergency problems as chronic pulmonary problems. On an emergency basis, one is much more likely to see an asthmatic in trouble because of contact with some antigen or contracting a

viral lower respiratory tract infection. Finally, there also is the question of hyperactive baroreceptors in the lungs of these patients. Although poorly understood, hyperactive baroreceptors could explain why many asthmatics seem to have difficulty when barometric pressure is changing rapidly (i.e., a moving weather front) and no other triggering factors are apparent.

REFERENCES

1. Berquist, W.E., Rachelefsky, G.S., Kadden, M., Siegel, S.C., Katz, R.M., Fonkalsrud, E.W., and Ament, M.E.: Gastroesophageal reflux—associated recurrent pneumonia and chronic asthma in children. Pediatrics 68: 29–35, 1981.
2. Bierman, C.W.: Pneumomediastinum and pneumothorax complicating asthma in children. Am. J. Dis. Child. 114: 42–50, 1967.
3. Carlson, V., Martin, J., Keegan, J., and Dailey, J.: Roentgenographic features of mucoid impaction of the bronchi. A.J.R. 96: 947–952, 1966.
4. Christie, D.L., O'Grady, L.R., and Mack, D.V.: Incompetent lower esophageal sphincter and gastroesophageal reflux in recurrent acute pul-

monary disease of infancy and childhood. J. Pediatr. 93: 23–27, 1978.

5. Cloutier, M.M., and Loughlin, G.M.: Chronic cough in children: A manifestation of airway hyperreactivity. Pediatrics 67: 6–12, 1981.

6. Eggleston, P.A., Ward, B.H., Pierson, W.E., and Bierman, C.W.: Radiographic abnormalities in acute asthma in children. Pediatrics 54: 442–449, 1974.

7. Gershel, J.C., Goldman, H.S., Stein, R.E.K., Shelov, S.P., and Ziprokowski, M.: The usefulness of chest radiographs in first asthma attacks. New Engl. J. Med. 336–340, 1983.

8. Gillies, J.D., Reed, M.H., and Simons, F.E.R.: Radiologic assessment of severity of acute asthma in children. J. Can. Assoc. Radiol. 31: 45–47, 1980.

9. Hodson, C.J., and Trickey, S.E.: Bronchial wall thickening in asthma. Clin. Radiol. 11: 183, 1960.

10. Hungerford, G.D., Williams, H.B.L., and Gandevia, B.: Bronchial walls in radiologic diagnosis of asthma. Br. J. Radiol. 50: 783–787, 1977.

11. Jorgensen, J., Falliers, C., and Bukantz, S.: Pneumothorax and mediastinal and subcutaneous emphysema in children with bronchial asthma. Pediatrics 31: 824–832, 1963.

12. Kirsh, M., and Orvald, T.: Mediastinal and subcutaneous emphysema complicating acute bronchial asthma. Chest 57: 580–581, 1970.

13. McCarthy, D., Simon, G., and Hargreave, F.: The radiological appearances in allergic bronchopulmonary aspergillosis. Clin. Radiol. 21: 366–375, 1970.

14. McGovern, J.P., Ozkaragoz, K., Roett, K., Haywood, T.J., and Hensel, A.E., Jr.: Mediastinal and subcutaneous emphysema complicating atopic asthma in infants and children. Pediatrics 27: 951–960, 1961.

15. McIntosh, K., Ellis, E.F., Hoffman, L.S., Lybass, T.G., Eller, J.J., and Fulginiti, V.A.: The association of viral and bacterial respiratory infections with exacerbations of wheezing in young asthmatic children. J. Pediatr. 82: 578–590, 1973.

16. McNicholl, B.: Pneumomediastinum and subcutaneous emphysema in status asthmaticus, requiring surgical decompression. Arch. Dis. Child. 35: 389–392, 1960.

17. McSweeney, W.J., and Stempel, D.A.: Non-iatrogenic pneumomediastinum in infancy and childhood. Pediatr. Radiol. 1: 139–144, 1973.

18. Minor, T.E., Baker, J.W., Dick, E.C., DeMeo, A.N., Ouellette, J.J., Cohen, M., and Reed, C.E.: Greater frequency of viral respiratory infections in asthmatic children as compared with their non-asthmatic siblings. J. Pediatr. 85: 472–477, 1974.

19. Minor, T.E., Dick, E.C., DeMeo, A.N., Ouellette, J.J., Cohen, M., and Reed, C.E.: Viruses as precipitants of asthmatic attacks in children. J.A.M.A. 227: 292–298, 1974.

20. Mitchell, I., Inglis, H., and Simpson, H.: Viral infection in wheezy bronchitis and asthma in children. Arch. Dis. Child. 51: 707–711, 1976.

21. Ozonoff, M.: Pneumomediastinum associated with asthma and pneumonia in children. A.J.R. 95: 112–117, 1965.

22. Payne, T., and Geppert, L.: Mediastinal and subcutaneous emphysema complicating bronchial asthma in a nine-year-old male. J. Allergy 32: 135–138, 1961.

23. Prossor, I.M., and Thurley, P.: Case report, septal lines in a case of asthma with eosinophilia. Br. J. Radiol. 49: 176, 1976.

24. Robinson, A.E., and Campbell, J.B.: Bronchography in childhood asthma. A.J.R. 116: 559–566, 1972.

25. Sibbald, B., Horn, M.E.C., and Gregg, I.: A family study of genetic basis of asthma and wheezy bronchitis. Arch. Dis. Child. 55: 354–357, 1980.

26. Wang, J.L.F., Patterson, R., Mintzer, R., Roberts, M., and Rosenberg, M.: Allergic bronchopulmonary aspergillosis in pediatric practice. J. Pediatr. 94: 376–381, 1979.

27. Winterleitner, H., Eipl, M., Jarisch, R., et al.: Bronchial asthma and gastroesophageal reflux in childhood. Z. Kinderchir. 27: 216–226, 1979.

28. Zieverink, S.E., Harper, A.P., Holden, R.W., Klatte, E.C., and Brittain, H.: Emergency room radiography of asthma: An efficacy study. Radiology 145: 27–29, 1982.

FOREIGN BODIES IN THE LOWER AIRWAY

Small infants are virtual vacuum cleaners, for anything they see goes into their mouths and foreign body aspirations into the airway are as common as ever. Clinically, the problem often is clearly apparent, for the aspiration, followed by coughing, gagging, vomiting, varying degrees of respiratory distress, and even cyanosis all are clearly documented. *Interestingly enough, however, these symptoms often subside quickly, and the patient may appear surprisingly well and even asymptomatic (7) shortly after the acute problem.* The reason for this is that the endobronchial receptors responsible for producing the initial symptoms soon lose their sensitivity and react less to the foreign body (1). However, do not be fooled by this lull in the clinical picture, for the foreign body is still present and, if not detected, may lead to the development of recurrent pneumonias or wheezing suggestive of asthma. *Indeed, wheezing in the absence of known pulmonary disease such as asthma, especially if it is unilateral, should be considered due to a foreign body until proven otherwise.*

Once foreign body aspiration is suspected, the roentgenographic workup should be thorough and undertaken immediately. The patterns of aeration disturbance are varied; many are subtle and many are missed. Indeed, even the experienced observer cannot let his guard down when a foreign body problem is being investigated; every possible clue should be sought. Of course, if the foreign body is opaque (i.e., teeth, pebbles, metal tacks, etc.), the problem is lessened (8), but most foreign bodies are nonopaque and thus one must rely on an evaluation of disturbances of aeration. Unfortunately, these may not always be apparent, and in one series, 31% of patients studied had normal initial chest x-rays (7).

Before embarking on a discussion of the aeration disturbances, a few general considerations might be in order. First, it should be noted that there is a difference between tracheal (central) and bronchial (peripheral) foreign bodies. The latter, of course, are much more common (1, 9), and there is a slight preponderance of right bronchial foreign bodies (1, 9). At first, one might expect that the overwhelming majority of aspirated foreign bodies would settle in the right bronchus, but it has been shown that in infants and young children the right and left bronchial angles are rather symmetric, and it is only in the older child and adult that the right bronchus offers a more direct route for aspirated foreign bodies (5).

Central foreign bodies located in the trachea, but below the larynx, can be difficult to diagnose and *plain films can be deceptively normal* (Fig. 1.122). The reason for this is that the aeration disturbance is

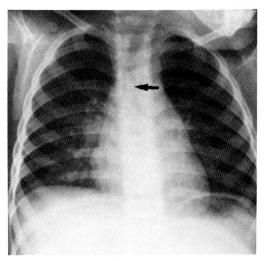

Figure 1.122. *Tracheal foreign body.* This is an inspiratory film and easily could be passed for normal. One might note that the lungs are not as large as one would expect for a full inspiration, but almost always the film would be read as normal. However, a peanut (*arrow*), just barely visible, was present in the trachea. The trachea is well distended, confirming that the film is an inspiratory film and not an expiratory film. The trachea normally narrows on expiration.

generalized and not lateralized to one or other of the lungs. Furthermore, the problem more often is one of inspiratory underaeration rather than overaeration. In other words, restricted air entry more than air exit and obstructive emphysema is the pathophysiologic malady. At the same time there may be paradoxical enlargement of the cardiac and mediastinal silhouettes (4, 6). Ordinarily, with inspiration, as the lungs enlarge and diaphragmatic leaflets become depressed, heart size diminishes. However, with central obstruction, be it in the trachea or the larynx, intrathoracic pressures become more negative during inspiration and the heart and mediastinum enlarge. This certainly is a useful sign, but not one easy to detect.

As far as endobronchial foreign bodies are concerned, the plain chest film frequently demonstrates the unilateral aeration abnormality, but if it does not the mandatorily obtained expiratory chest film will do so. If this fails, fluoroscopy can be performed, but usually is not necessary.

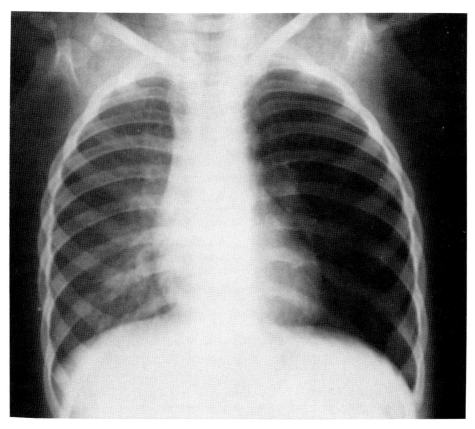

Figure 1.123. *Foreign body in the left main stem bronchus with obstructive emphysema.* Note the large hyperlucent, underperfused (oligemic) left lung. Such underperfusion is characteristic obstructive emphysema and is not seen with compensatory emphysema. The mediastinum is shifted to the right, and the left diaphragmatic leaflet is displaced downward. The findings are classic for a check valve foreign body producing obstructive emphysema on the left.

Indeed, plain films are quite accurate (11), and, in terms of abnormalities encountered, the most common is obstructive emphysema. In advanced cases, obstructive emphysema is not difficult to identify (Fig. 1.123). Obstructive emphysema develops because, during inspiration, there is enough physiologic dilatation of the bronchus to allow some air to get around the foreign body and enter the lung. On expiration, however, physiologic narrowing of the bronchus occurs, and in the presence of an occluding foreign body a check-valve phenomenon develops and air is trapped in the lung. Ensuing mucosal edema aggravates the problem, and these events, cycled over and over, eventually lead to progressive air trapping and overdistension of the involved lung or lobe. In these children, such a lobe or lung appears larger and more radiolucent than the other lung (Fig. 1.123). Largeness is explained on the basis of chronic air trapping, while hyperlucency occurs because more air than normal is present in the lung, and because pulmonary blood flow is diminished. Indeed, this latter finding is the hallmark of obstructive, emphysematous overdistension of a lung, and as such can be used to differentiate obstructive emphysema from compensatory emphysema. With compensatory emphysema, although the lung may appear large during inspiration, pulmonary blood flow is not compromised. Decreased blood flow in an obstructed lung is due in part to compression of the vessels, and in part to hypoxia- induced vasospasm.

In other cases of obstructive emphysema, the findings may not be so obvious. In these cases, entry and exit of air is abnormal but neither predominates to the point where frank obstructive emphysema or total atelectasis results. Consequently, the lung may be of normal or nearly normal size, and it is only during expiration that one notes that the involved lung does not deflate and is pathologically obstructed. In many of these cases, a clue to the fact that some degree of obstructive emphysema exists is that the pulmonary vascularity in the involved lung or lobe is somewhat diminished (Fig. 1.124). Indeed, *a good rule*

to follow is that the lung with diminished blood flow is the abnormal lung whether it is large and hyperlucent or small and hyperlucent. In this regard, *another good rule to follow is that the lung that changes shape least or not at all between inspiration and expiration is the abnormal lung.*

Clearly, inspiratory-expiratory film sequences are the key to identifying obstructed lungs. However, in some cases one may resort to decubitus films (3), for with lateral decubitus positioning, a normal lung, if it is the dependent lung, empties and becomes smaller (i.e., it is compressed). With an obstructed lung, however, the trapped air prevents it from collapsing and becoming smaller in the dependent, decubitus position (Fig. 1.125).

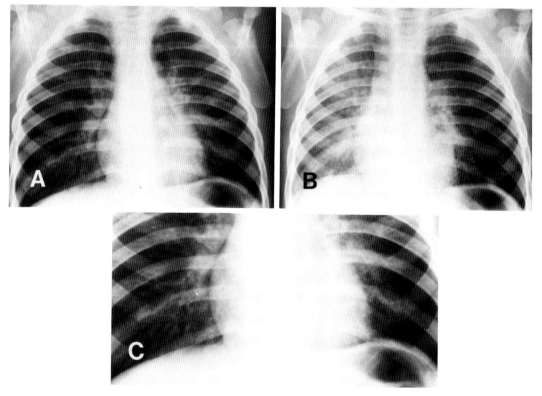

Figure 1.124. *Obstructed lung, subtle findings.* (*A*) On this inspiratory film, note that, even though the right lung is a little larger than the left, it is the left lung that shows decreased vascularity. (*B*) Subsequent expiratory film shows that the right lung empties normally (i.e., changes size dramatically), while the left lung retains its original size and does not empty. A foreign body was present in the left main bronchus. (*C*) Coned view of the lungs as shown in *A* demonstrates the decrease in vascularity in the left base to better advantage.

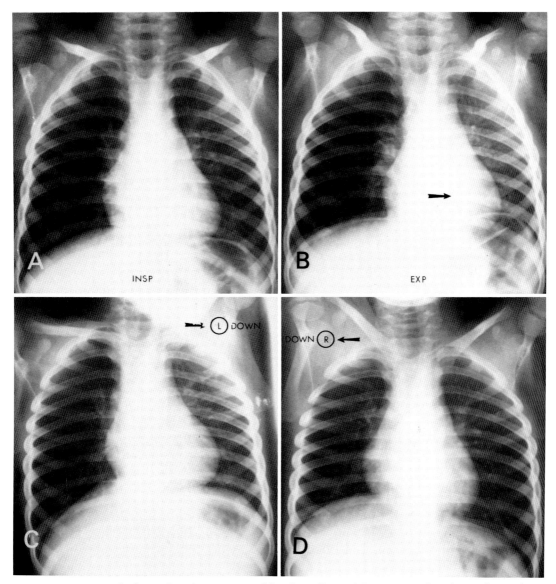

Figure 1.125. *Foreign body—value of expiratory and decubitus films.* (*A*) Inspiratory (*INSP*) view shows a large, hyperlucent right lung. An obstructing foreign body in the right main bronchus should be suspected. (*B*) Expiratory film (*EXP*) accentuates the hyperlucent large right lung. Note how air has emptied from the normal left lung and that the mediastinum is now clearly shifted to the left (*arrow*). (*C*) Left lateral decubitus film. The left side is down, and the left lung is partially deflated (compressed). This is normal in the left side down decubitus position. The right lung is relatively overinflated. (*D*) Right lateral decubitus. This time the right side is down and the right lung should have deflated. However, because it is obstructed it remains radiolucent and large (i.e., the presence of obstructive emphysema does not allow it to deflate). The decubitus films in *C* and *D* are illustrated in the upright position for ease of comparison.

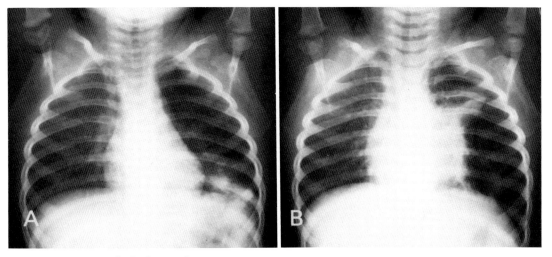

Figure 1.126. *Foreign body disguised as pneumonia.* (**A**) Note the infiltrate in the left lower lung field. Clinically, pneumonia was suspected. The overaerated left upper lobe was believed to represent compensatory emphysema. (**B**) However, on the next day, note how obstructive emphysema has developed in the left lower lobe. There was an underlying foreign body (peanut fragments) in the left lower lobe.

Simply speaking, the obstructed lung acts as an air cushion or inflated balloon and will not deflate on compression. These points notwithstanding, however, almost always with regular inspiratory-expiratory films, one can identify the abnormal lung, and while fluoroscopic examination of the chest may more vividly demonstrate findings such as contralateral mediastinal shift and fixation of the involved diaphragmatic leaflet, seldom is it necessary.

When patchy atelectasis or pneumonic infiltrates are associated with obstructing foreign bodies, they may distract one away from the actual problem (10). Indeed, it is not unusual for such children to be treated for a presumed pneumonia for a number of days or even weeks and yet in the final analysis to be determined to have an obstructing foreign body (Fig. 1.126). In other instances, if the foreign body is not recognized, emphysema eventually is replaced by atelectasis. This is especially likely to occur with a foreign body of low irritation such as a piece of plastic, metal, or bone. Peanuts and popcorn, on the other hand, because of their fat content, produce a more pronounced and rapidly

ensuing local inflammatory reaction. Because of this, the obstructive problem is accelerated and the patient comes to the attention of the physician sooner. Unrecognized foreign bodies also eventually may present as chronic infections, including pulmonary abscess and bronchiectasis. However, after emphysema, atelectasis is the most common manifestation of a bronchial foreign body (Fig. 1.127).

Foreign bodies that totally occlude a bronchus can produce lobar or total lung atelectasis (Fig. 1.128). In some of these cases, occlusion of the bronchus may occur so rapidly that cyanosis and syncope are surprisingly rapid in onset. In these cases, the abrupt mediastinal shift leads to syncope by producing acute kinking and obstruction of the inferior and superior vena cavae, and also by rendering one lung abruptly functionless. Some foreign bodies produce such gross aeration disturbances that complicating pneumomediastinum (2) and pneumothorax can result. In such cases, the roentgenographic findings may be very puzzling, for the presence of the mediastinal air often distracts one's attention from the basic underlying problem

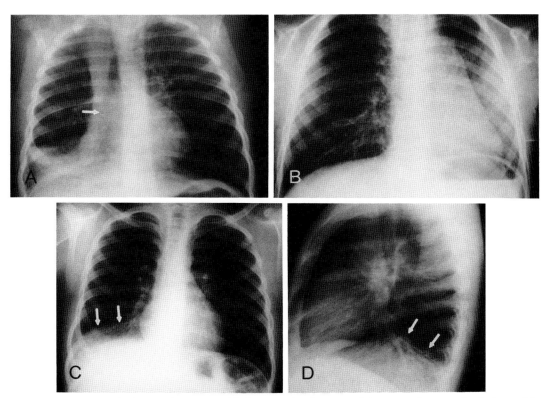

Figure 1.127. *Foreign bodies producing variable degrees of atelectasis.* (*A*) Note atelectasis of right lower lobe and compensatory emphysema of the right upper lobe and entire left lung. Also, note tack (*arrow*) in the right main bronchus. If this tack were not seen, a foreign body might not be suspected. (*B*) Another patient with partial collapse of the left lung due to carrot particles in the left bronchus for 3 days. There is marked shift of the mediastinum to the left, and the right lung is overdistended. However, since the blood vessels still are prominent, one should consider overdistension of the right lung to be due to compensatory, and not obstructive, emphysema. If the problem was one of obstructive emphysema of the right lung, the vessels would be less prominent and, indeed, attenuated. (*C*) Chronic foreign body in the right lower lobe producing basilar atelectasis (*arrows*). (*D*) Lateral view demonstrating the atelectasis (*arrows*) to better advantage.

(Fig. 1.129). These complications usually result from rupture of the lung that is obstructed, but occasionally from overdistension and rupture of the compensatorily overdistended normal lung.

Finally, it should be noted that not all foreign bodies need remain lodged in any one position for the entire time they are in the tracheobronchial tree. Indeed, some foreign bodies tend to move back and forth, and in this regard may even move from one bronchus to another. If this is the case, they will produce confusing clinical and roentgenographic findings. By the

same token, one should not be surprised to encounter a patient who, on his own, coughs up the foreign body and becomes symptom-free, while awaiting initial or further diagnostic studies (Fig. 1.130). Still another peculiarity of endobronchial foreign bodies is that dealing with multiple foreign bodies. Very often the aspirated material has been chewed or partially chewed and numerous fragments are aspirated. Many times, such fragments are small and cause little in the way of additional difficulty, but if the fragments are incompletely chewed and rather large, dif-

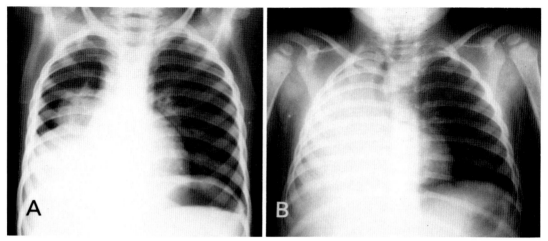

Figure 1.128. *Foreign body causing total massive atelectasis.* (*A*) Note right lower lobe and right middle lobe atelectasis resulting from a long-standing foreign body of low irritation (plastic bottle cap). The findings, except that there is marked volume loss, could be misinterpreted for a simple pneumonia. (*B*) Massive, total atelectasis of the right lung. This infant inhaled a pinto bean in the right main bronchus. In less than 60 minutes, total atelectasis of the right lung occurred with pronounced respiratory distress, cyanosis, and syncope.

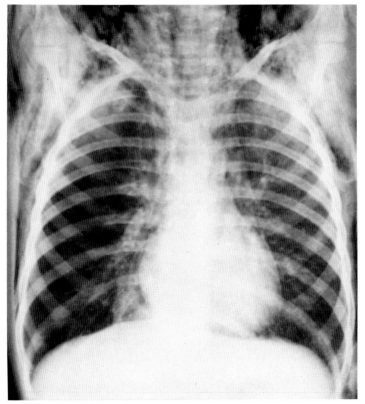

Figure 1.129. *Foreign body with mediastinal and interstitial air.* Note extensive free air in the mediastinum and soft tissues of the neck and chest. So striking are the findings that one might miss the fact that the right lung is a little more radiolucent than the left. The reason for this discrepancy in radiolucency is that a foreign body was present in the right bronchus and the right lung was trapping air. (Courtesy of Webster Riggs, M.D.)

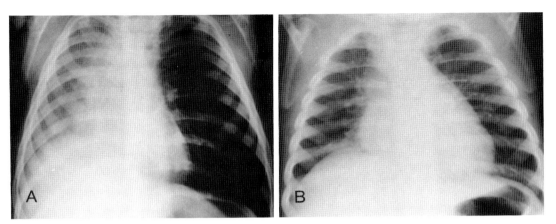

Figure 1.130. *Foreign body; coughed up.* (**A**) Note classic obstructive emphysema of the left lung. (**B**) This patient had a coughing spell and coughed up the foreign body; the left lung now is nearly normal. However, a little emphysema remains, probably secondary to some residual mucosal edema. This is not an uncommon finding just after foreign bodies are dislodged or removed.

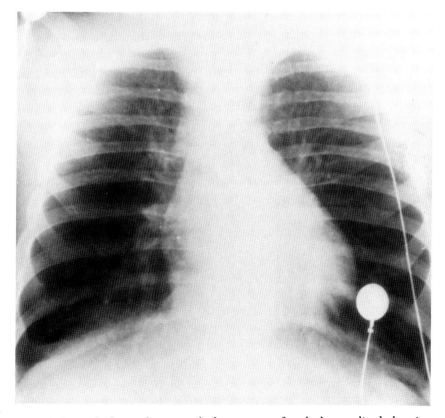

Figure 1.131. *Multiple foreign bodies.* This patient had acute onset of marked generalized wheezing and severe respiratory compromise. History of foreign body aspiration was vague, but the patient's condition deteriorated rapidly and bronchoscopy was performed. Numerous peanut fragments were found scattered throughout the bronchi of both lungs.

fuse, and catastrophic, air trapping with numerous peripheral obstructions can be seen (Fig. 1.131).

REFERENCES

1. Blazer, S., Naveh, Y., and Friedman, A.: Foreign body in the airway: Review of 200 cases. Am. J. Dis. Child. 134: 68–71, 1980.
2. Burton E.M., Riggs, W., Jr., Kaufman, R.A., and Houston, C.S.: Pneumomediastinum caused by foreign body aspiration in children. Pediatr. Radiol. 20: 45–47, 1989.
3. Capitanio, M.A., and Kirkpatrick, J.A.: The lateral decubitus film, and aid in determining air-trapping in children. Radiology 103: 460–462, 1972.
4. Capitanio, M.A., and Kirkpatrick, J.A.: Obstructions of the upper airway in children as reflected on the chest radiograph. Radiology 107: 159–161, 1973.
5. Cleveland, R.H.: Symmetry of bronchial angles in children. Radiology 133: 89–93, 1979.
6. Grunebaum, M., Adler, S., and Varsano, I.: The paradoxical movement of the mediastinum: A diagnostic sign of foreign body aspiration during childhood. Pediatr. Radiol. 8: 213–218, 1979.
7. Laks Y., and Barzilay, Z.: Foreign body aspiration in childhood. Pediatr. Emerg. Care 4: 102–106, 1988.
8. Pochaczevsky, R., Leonidas, J.C., Feldman, F.,

Naysan, P., and Ratner, H.: Aspirated and ingested teeth in children. Clin. Radiol. 24: 349–353, 1973.
9. Reed, M.H.: Radiology of airway foreign bodies in children. J. Can. Assoc. Radiol. 28: 111–118, 1977.
10. Seibert, R.W., Seibert, J.J., and Williamson, S.L.: The opaque chest: When to suspect a bronchial foreign body. Pediatr. Radiol. 16: 193–196, 1986.
11. Svedstrom, E., Puhakka, H., and Kero, P.: How accurate is chest radiography in the diagnosis of tracheobronchial foreign bodies in children? Pediatr. Radiol. 19: 520–522, 1989.

PENETRATING AND NONPENETRATING (BLUNT) CHEST TRAUMA

Blunt chest trauma is more common than penetrating trauma, but assessing either is not an easy task. There are many subtle findings to look for, and the thoracic cage, cardiovascular structures, pleural space, and pulmonary parenchyma must be examined quickly and carefully. Plain films suffice in many cases but CT is required in more severe or puzzling cases (33). In terms of the thoracic cage, although rib

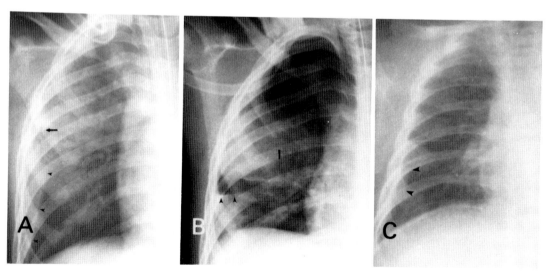

Figure 1.132. Rib fractures. (**A**) Rib fracture with pneumohemothorax. Note the rib fracture involving the fifth rib on the right (*upper large arrow*). Diffuse haziness of the right lung is due to blood in the pleural space (*lower small arrows*), and an associated pulmonary contusion. (**B**) Upright view showing an air fluid level (*arrows*) substantiating the presence of a pneumohemothorax. The pulmonary contusion is more clearly visualized on this view, and, in addition, fractures of the posterior third, fourth, and fifth ribs now are visible. (**C**) Rib fracture with subpleural hematoma. There is a small subpleural hematoma (*arrows*) in this patient who was sat upon by his older sibling. He had chest pain and point tenderness over the area. Although a rib fracture is not visualized, it should be suspected when a subpleural hematoma is identified.

fractures are common, unless they are grossly displaced or multiple, they are not particularly easy to detect on initial films. However, this is not such a great drawback, for it is much more important to determine whether complications such as pneumothorax or hemothorax are present (Fig. 1.132A and B). In other cases, a rib fracture may be detected by the presence of a local subpleural hematoma (Fig. 1.132C), but most often rib fractures are more easily detected later, when they are healing.

Rib fractures also aid in directing one's attention to more serious intrathoracic or abdominal injuries. For example, anterior or lateral rib fractures over the lower thoracic area should cause one to look more earnestly for evidence of splenic or liver trauma. Low posterior rib fractures should alert one to the possibility of underlying renal trauma, and fractures of the first three ribs should obligate one to rule out great vessel injury (11, 25, 41). However, by no means does fracturing of these ribs mean that vascular injury is inevitable. Indeed, most often it is not present (44). Nonetheless, the possibility must be kept in mind, and when searching for rib fractures in this area, one should look for collections of fluid (blood) over the apex of the lung (Fig. 1.133).

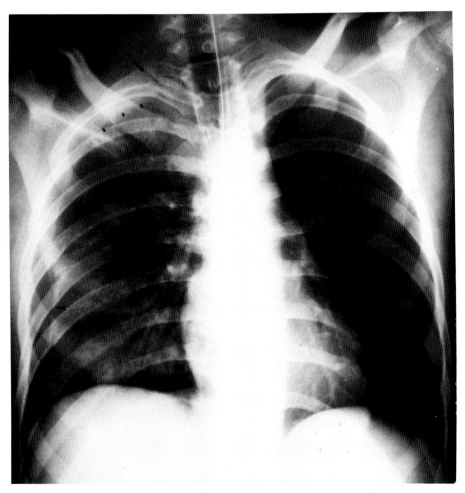

Figure 1.133. *Fracture of the first rib with apical blood.* Note the fracture of the first rib on the right (*upper large arrow*). Just beneath it note blood over the apex of the right lung (*upper three small arrows*). A pneumothorax also is delineated (*lower arrows*).

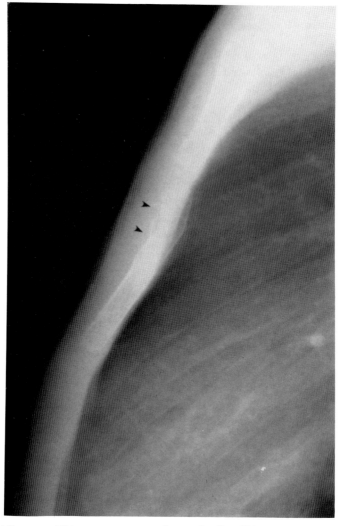

Figure 1.134. *Sternal fracture.*   This patient was wrestling and suffered blunt chest trauma. The sternum is fractured (*arrows*), and there is a little pre- and retrosternal soft tissue swelling.

Fractures of the sternum are best visualized on the lateral view and, of course, on CT scans. They usually result from blunt trauma to the chest such as occurs with steering wheel injuries or other direct, severe, blows to the chest (Fig. 1.134). Retro- and presternal soft tissue swelling from associated edema and bleeding are commonly noted, but the most important aspect of sternal fractures is that they frequently are associated with underlying cardiac injury. Consequently, if the injury

is severe, the cardiac silhouette should be inspected closely, but even more importantly, an ECG should be obtained.

Pulmonary parenchymal manifestations of blunt trauma are numerous and include pulmonary contusion (38, 39, 43), pulmonary hematoma (23, 36, 42), and traumatic pneumatoceles (1, 4–7, 24, 26, 34). Pulmonary contusions produce pneumonia-like areas of homogeneous or nodular consolidation (Fig. 1.135), which usually become larger and denser during the first

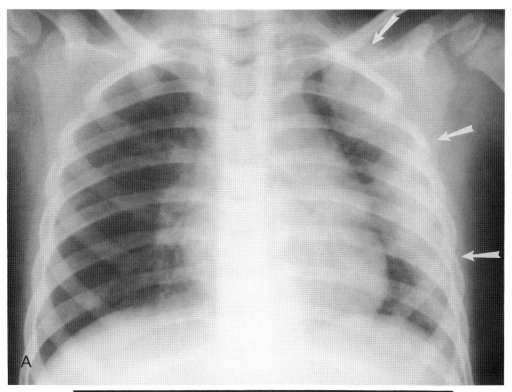

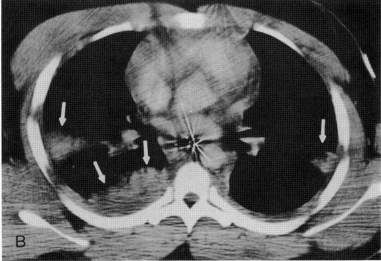

Figure 1.135. *Pulmonary contusion.* (**A**) Young patient with an extensive contusion in the left lung (*arrows*). (**B**) CT study in another patient demonstrating multiple contusions (*arrows*) and bilateral pleural effusions.

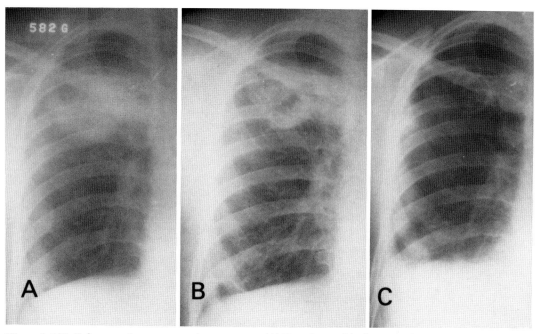

Figure 1.136. *Pulmonary hematoma with cavitation.* (*A*) Note a mass-like lesion in the right upper lobe. (*B*) A few days later, note that a cavity is developing in this hematoma. (*C*) More than a month later, a thin-walled cavity remains. (Reprinted with permission from C.J. Fagan and L.E. Swischuk: Traumatic lung and paramediastinal pneumatoceles. Radiology 120: 11–18, 1976.)

24–48 hours after injury. Pulmonary contusions clear slowly and eventually may contract to the point of suggesting a pulmonary mass. Densities that appear round or oval from the onset probably represent pulmonary hematomas. Usually they are slow to resolve and may cavitate during the course of their resolution (Fig. 1.136).

Traumatic pneumatoceles or air cysts frequently occur with blunt chest trauma and may be seen either in the pulmonary parenchyma or in the mediastinum (5, 6, 7, 16, 26). They usually are seen with other manifestations of pulmonary injury and develop within minutes or hours of the injury. These air cysts or pneumatoceles may be round or oval, single or multiple, and some may contain blood (Fig. 1.137). Generally, they are thin-walled and may increase in size rather rapidly after they first appear. Similar air collections in the mediastinum tend to be more elongated and

paraspinal in position (Fig. 1.138). These air collections are believed to lie in the inferior pulmonary ligament (6, 7, 26), although similar collections can occur in the retroesophageal ligament. Overall, traumatic pneumatoceles are relatively innocuous, for seldom do they rupture or become infected. For the most part, they slowly become smaller and disappear over a 2- to 3-week period. To the uninitiated, however, they frequently constitute a problem of distraction from other potentially more serious problems that might also be present.

More catastrophic injuries to the respiratory system include bronchial and tracheal fracture or tear (2, 3, 14, 15, 19, 27) and torsion of the lung (8, 22). Torsion of the lung, with subsequent infarction, is often difficult to diagnose roentgenographically, but it has been pointed out that since such a lung makes a 180° turn

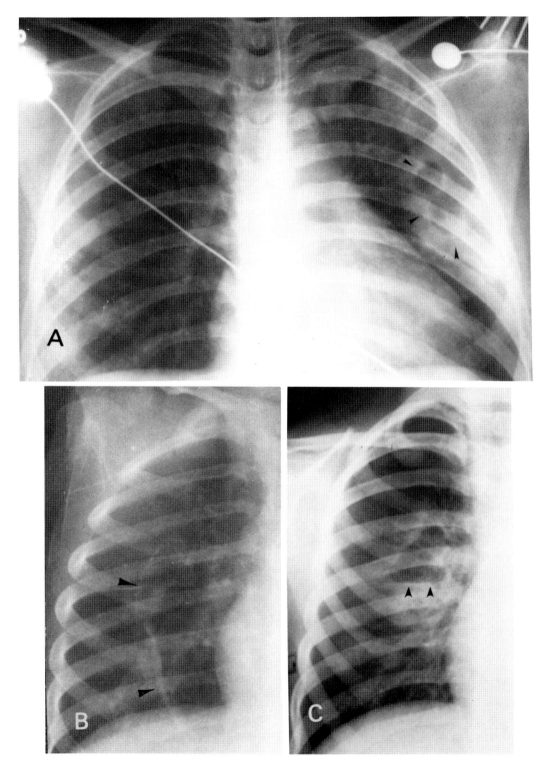

Figure 1.137. *Traumatic pneumatoceles.* (*A*) Note the two spherical, thin-walled pneumatoceles (*arrows*) in the contused left lung of this child run over by a truck. (*B*) Large post-traumatic pneumatocele on the right side (*arrows*). (*C*) Another patient with a traumatic pneumatocele demonstrating an air-fluid level (*arrows*) on upright view. The air-fluid level represents air and blood in the pneumatocele. (Reprinted with permission from C.J. Fagan and L.E. Swischuk: Traumatic lung and paramediastinal pneumatoceles. Radiology 120: 11–18, 1976.)

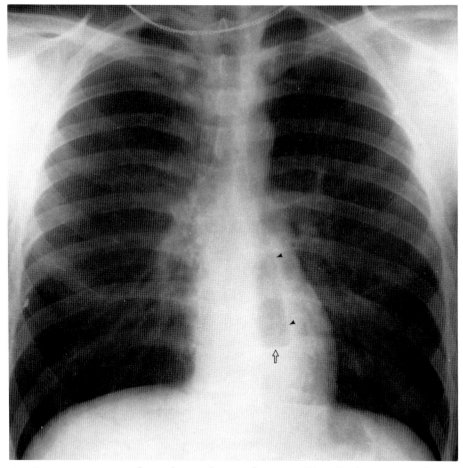

Figure 1.138. *Traumatic pneumatocele in inferior pulmonary ligament.*   Note the characteristic elongated, paraspinal air collection (*small arrows*) characteristic of a pneumatocele in the inferior pulmonary ligament. The *lower arrow* points to an air-fluid (blood) level. (Reprinted with permission from C.J. Fagan and L.E. Swischuk: Traumatic lung and paramediastinal pneumatoceles. Radiology 120: 11–18, 1976.)

around its hilus, the vascular pattern of the upper and lower lobes is inverted (8, 22). This finding, however, first requires awareness of its existence and then close scrutiny of the roentgenogram for its presence.

With *bronchial fracture* one may see massive pneumothorax and/or massive atelectasis (Fig. 1.139A), and, indeed, with blunt chest trauma, *massive atelectasis should be presumed secondary to bronchial fracture until proven otherwise.* With tracheal lacerations, pneumomediastinum

is more common than pneumothorax, and if bleeding occurs into the mediastinum, it will appear widened. When a pneumothorax results from a bronchial tear, it usually is massive, and when the lung is completely detached from its bronchus, upright views will show it to fall to the bottom of the hemithorax (14) (Fig. 1.139B). In other cases of bronchial fracture, the air column in the proximal portion of the fractured bronchus appears tapered or beveled, and, in still other instances, air may be seen tracking along the bronchial or tra-

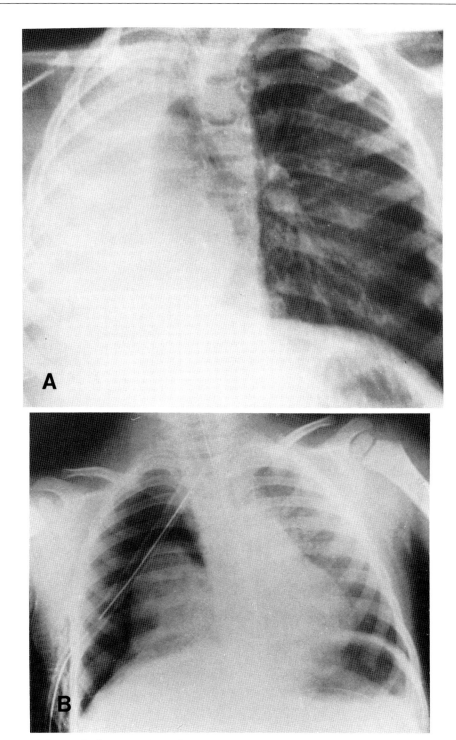

Figure 1.139. *(A) Bronchial rupture of right lung manifesting as total atelectasis of the right lung.* Rib fractures are present on the other side. (Reprinted with permission from S. Mahboubi, and A.E. O'Hara: Bronchial rupture in children following blunt chest trauma. Pediatr. Radiol. 10: 133–138, 1981.) *(B) Avulsion of the bronchus.* Note the massive pneumothorax and collapsed, dropped right lung. (Reprinted with permission from F.L. Grover, et al.: Diagnosis and management of major tracheobronchial injuries. Ann. Thorac. Surg. 28: 385–391, 1979.)

cheal wall itself (15, 27). If bleeding also occurs, fluid will be seen in the ipsilateral hemithorax. With tracheal tears, the endotracheal tube may lie outside the trachea, and the balloon, because it is not contained by the ruptured trachea, may be overdistended (27). Unfortunately, however, many cases of fractured bronchi are cases of incomplete fracture, and neither atelectasis nor pneumothorax is present at the onset. It is only later when a frank tear occurs that these complications develop.

Cardiovascular manifestations of blunt chest trauma also are varied and include bloody or serious pericardial effusions, myocardial contusions (13, 17, 35), and traumatic aneurysms of the heart or aorta. Of course, in the more severe cases, frank tears or ruptures of these latter structures can occur (9, 21, 32, 35, 37). In addition, aortic insufficiency associated with traumatic aneurysms of the ascending aorta can be encountered (28). Minimal myocardial injuries are best detected with electrocardiograms or with myocardial scintograms

(13), or perhaps **MRI**. Such myocardial injuries are not detectable roentgenographically, but with more extensive contusions nonspecific cardiomegaly will be seen. Pericardial effusions, if large enough, produce enlargement of the cardiac silhouette, but with smaller effusions, ultrasonography is the diagnostic procedure of choice.

Injury to the aorta and great vessels is most important to detect, but unfortunately the roentgenographic findings often tend to elude one's initial observation. Because of this, one must constantly be on guard for signs of superior mediastinal widening (21, 30, 31, 37) or the collecting of blood over the apex of the left lung (Fig. 1.140A). This latter finding has been termed the left apical extrapleural cap sign (32), and results from leaking of blood from a ruptured aortic arch into the pleural space over the left lung. There is a normal defect in the pleural covering over the aorta in this area (transverse arch), and mediastinal blood can track directly into the

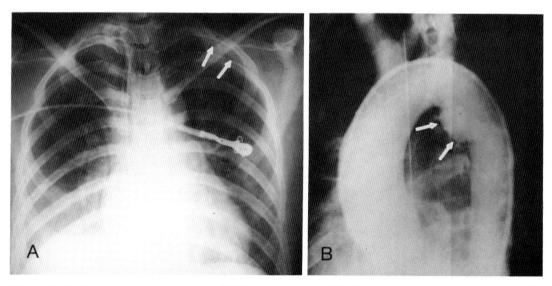

Figure 1.140. *Traumatic aortic aneurysm.* (*A*) Note a collection of fluid over the left lung apex (*arrows*). This constitutes the apical cap sign. There is a posterior fracture of the right third rib. The superior mediastinum is slightly widened, but more importantly, the endotracheal and esophageal tubes are shifted to the right. These findings substantiate the fact that a mediastinal hematoma is present. (*B*) Subsequent aortogram demonstrates a traumatic aortic aneurysm (*arrows*).

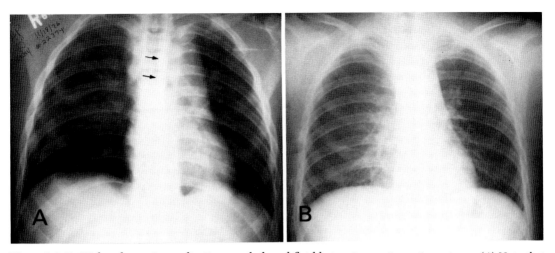

Figure 1.141. *Widened superior mediastinum and pleural fluid but no traumatic aortic rupture.* (A) Note that there is a pneumothorax on the right and that there is blood layered over the apex of the left lung. The superior mediastinum is widened, but note that the tube in the esophagus is in a normal location(*arrows*). It is not shifted to the right. (B) Repeat film the next day with the patient in an upright position shows persistence of the right pneumothorax but a normal appearing superior mediastinum. Some fluid is still present on the left. The findings in A were due to supine positioning, and not a periaortic hematoma due to aortic rupture.

left apical pleural space. The finding is subtle but important and should be sought for with diligence. Unfortunately, however, it is not always present, and also can be seen with nonaortic trauma. For this reason, it is not specific, but in combination with other signs of aortic rupture, especially mediastinal widening (30, 31), should be treated with considerable suspicion. Thereafter, if aortic or great vessel injury is suspected, immediate CT, or preferably aortography (37), is required (Fig. 1.140).

Mediastinal widening as it is seen with aortic rupture must be differentiated from widening secondary to the presence of normal thymus and supine positioning. Most injured patients are examined in the supine position and the superior mediastinum may appear wide. In this regard, it has been noted that with widening due to aortic rupture the trachea and esophagus are displaced to the right (12, 21, 37, 40) (Fig. 1.140). If widening is due to thymus gland and supine positioning, these structures are not displaced to the right (Fig. 1.141). This is an important observation to make,

and frequently it is facilitated by the fact that these patients have indwelling tubes in either the trachea or esophagus, or in both of these structures. Recently, it has been noted that if these midline structures are not displaced, one can confidently exclude aortic injury (20, 37). This is important in confusing cases (Fig. 1.142), where a simple mediastinal hematoma may mimic aortic rupture (10).

Pneumopericardium is not particularly common with blunt chest trauma, but does occur. It is, of course, more common with penetrating wounds to the chest, and roentgenographically, it is identified by air surrounding the cardiac silhouette. In these cases, the pericardium itself is usually visible, and it is most important than a pneumopericardium not be confused with a medial pneumothorax or pneumomediastinum (see Figs. 1.102 and 1.104). An uncommon injury is rupture of the pericardium. In such cases, the heart is displaced or dislocated to the left (18), and because of this the findings resemble those seen with unilateral congenital absence of the

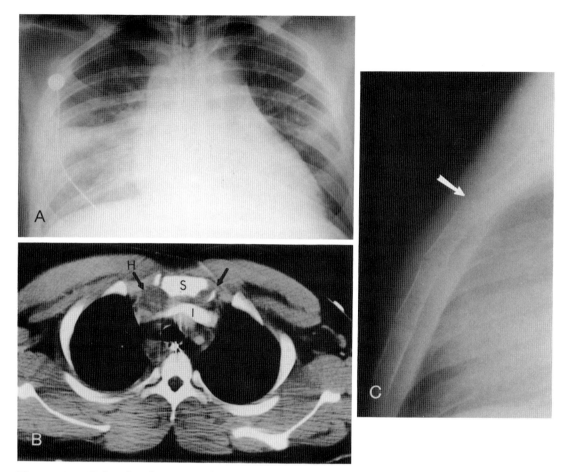

Figure 1.142. *Widened mediastinum without traumatic aortic aneurysm.* (*A*) Note the wide mediastinum in this patient. However, the esophageal tube and trachea are not displaced to the right. There is a contusion on the right. (*B*) CT scan with contrast identifies the innominate vein (*I*) and sternum (*S*), and in between these two structures, a hematoma (*H*). Mediastinal widening was due to this hematoma. Note the displaced sternal fracture fragment (*arrow*). (*C*) Lateral view of the sternum demonstrates the fracture through the sternomanubrial junction (*arrow*).

left pericardium, or shifting of the heart to the left by a pronounced pectus excavatum deformity of the chest.

Penetrating injuries to the chest, heart, and great vessels can produce all of the findings seen with closed (blunt) chest trauma, but, in addition, one can see air in the heart and great vessels (Fig. 1.143). Delayed complications such as cardiac or great vessel tears with hemopericardium also can be encountered, and with metallic foreign bodies such as bullets one may see the bullet in one of the chambers of the heart or great vessels. In other instances, the bullet may be lodged in the mediastinum, lung, or spine (Fig. 1.143).

REFERENCES

1. Blane, C.E., White, S.J., Wesley, J.R., et al.: Immediate traumatic pulmonary pseudocyst formation in children. Surgery 90: 872–875, 1981.
2. Burke, J.F.: Early diagnosis of traumatic rupture of the bronchus. J.A.M.A. 181: 682–686, 1962.
3. Chesterman, J.T., and Satsangi, P.N.: Rupture of the trachea and bronchi by closed chest injury. Thorax 21: 21–27, 1966.
4. Cochlin, D.L., and Shaw, M.R.P.: Traumatic lung

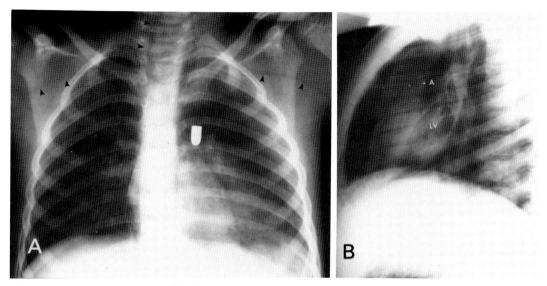

Figure 1.143. *Penetrating injury of the heart with free air.* (*A*) Note the bullet lodged in the back of this patient. Also note: (a) contusion of the left lung; (b) air in the heart; (c) air in the pericardium (best seen on the right); and (d) air in the subclavian and carotid arteries (*upper arrows*). (*B*) Lateral view demonstrates air in the left ventricle (*LV*) and aorta (*A*). The patient soon died. The bullet is not seen on this view but was lodged in the soft tissues of the back. (Courtesy of Virgil B. Graves, M.D.).

cysts following minor blunt chest trauma. Clin. Radiol. 29: 151–154, 1978.

5. Elyaderani, M.K., and Gabriele, O.F.: Traumatic paramediastinal air cysts. Br. J. Radiol. 52: 458–460, 1979.

6. Fagan, C.J., and Swischuk, L.E.: Traumatic lung and paramediastinal pneumatoceles. Radiology 120: 11–18, 1976.

7. Felman, A.H., Rogers, B.M., and Talbert, J.L.: Traumatic mediastinal air cyst: A case report. Pediatr. Radiol. 4: 120–121, 1976.

8. Felson, B.: Lung torsion: Radiographic findings in nine cases. Radiology 162: 631–638, 1987.

9. Fishbone, G., Robbins, D.I., and Osborn, D.J.,: Trauma to the thoracic aorta and great vessels. Radiol. Clin. North Am. 11: 543–554, 1973.

10. Fleisher, A.G., David, I., Hilfer, C., Mekhjian, H.A., and Stanley-Brown, E.G.: Mediastinal hematoma mimicking aortic rupture. J. Pediatr. Surg. 21: 445–446, 1986.

11. Galbraith, N.F., Urschel, H.C., Jr., Wood, R.E., et al.: Fracture of the first rib associated with laceration of the subclavian artery. J. Thorac. Cardiovasc. Surg. 65: 649–652, 1973.

12. Gerlock, A.J., Jr., Muhletaler, C.A., Coulam, C.M., and Hayes, P.T.: Traumatic aortic aneurysm: Validity of esophageal tube displacement sign. A.J.R. 135: 713–718, 1980.

13. Go, R.T., Doty, D.B., Chiu, C.L., and Christie, J.H.: A new method of diagnosing myocardial

contusion in man by radionuclide imaging. Radiology 116: 107–110, 1975.

14. Grover, F.L., Ellestad, C., Arom, K.V., Root, H.D., Cruz, A.B., and Trinkle, J.K.: Diagnosis and management of major tracheobronchial injuries. Ann. Thorac. Surg. 28: 385–391, 1979.

15. Harvey-Smith W., Bush, W., and Northrop, C.: Traumatic bronchial rupture. A.J.R. 134: 1189–1193, 1980.

16. Hyde, I.: Traumatic paramediastinal air cysts. Br. J. Radiol. 44: 380–383, 1971.

17. Ildstad, S.T., Tollerud, D.J., Weiss, R.G., Cox, J.A., and Martin, L.W.: Cardiac contusion in pediatric patients with blunt thoracic trauma. J. Pediatr. Surg. 25: 287–289, 1990.

18. Kermond, A.J.: The dislocated heart: An unusual complication of major chest injury. Radiology 119: 59–60, 1976.

19. Lynn, R.B., and Iyengar, K.: Traumatic rupture of the bronchus. Chest 61: 81–83, 1972.

20. Mahboubi, S., and O'Hara, A.E.: Bronchial rupture in children following blunt chest trauma. Pediatr. Radiol. 10: 133–138, 1981.

21. Marnocha, K.E., and Maglinte, D.D.T.: Plain-film criteria for excluding aortic rupture in blunt chest trauma. A.J.R. 144: 19–22, 1985.

22. Moser, E.S., Jr., and Proto, A.V.: Lung torsion: Case report and literature review. Radiology 162: 639–643, 1987.

23. Parsai, D., Nussle, D., and Cuendet, A.: Presen-

tation of two cases of pulmonary hematoma in child after closed chest trauma, and review of literature. Ann. Radiol. 17: 831–836, 1974.

24. Pearl, M., Milstein, M., and Rook, G.D.: Pseudocyst of the lung due to traumatic nonpenetrating lung injury. J. Pediatr. Surg. 8: 967–968, 1973.

25. Pierce, G., Maxwell, J., and Boggan, M.: Special hazards of 1st rib fractures. J. Trauma 15: 264–267, 1975.

26. Ravin, C., Smith, G.W., Lester, P.D., McLoud, T.C., and Putman, C.E.: Post-traumatic pneumatocele in the inferior pulmonary ligament. Radiology 121: 39–41, 1976.

27. Rollins, R.J., and Tocino, I.: Early radiographic signs of tracheal rupture. A.J.R. 148: 695–698, 1987.

28. Rowland, T.W.: Traumatic aortic insufficiency in children: Case report and reviews of the literature. Pediatrics 60: 893–895, 1977.

29. Savastano, S., Feltrin, G.P., Miotto, D., and Chiesura-Corona, M.: Value of plain chest film predicting traumatic aortic rupture. Ann. Radiol. 32: 196–200, 1989.

30. Sefczek, D.M., Sefczek, R.J., and Deeb, Z.L.: Radiographic signs of acute traumatic rupture of the thoracic aorta. A.J.R. 141: 1259–1262, 1983.

31. Seltzer, S.E., Orsi, C.D., Kirshner, R., and DeWeese, J.A.: Traumatic aortic rupture: Plain radiographic findings. A.J.R. 137: 1011–1014, 1981.

32. Simeone, J.F., Minagi, H., and Putman, C.E.: Traumatic disruption of the thoracic aorta: Significance of the left apical extrapleural cap. Radiology 117: 265–268, 1975.

33. Sivit, C.J., Taylor, G.A., and Eichelberger, M.R.: Chest injury in children with blunt abdominal trauma: Evaluation with CT. Radiology 171: 815–818, 1989.

34. Sorsdahl, O.A., and Powell, J.W.: Cavitary pulmonary lesions following non-penetrating chest trauma in children. A.J.R. 95: 118–124, 1965.

35. Soulen, R.L., and Freeman, E.: Radiologic evaluation of traumatic heart disease. Radiol. Clin. North Am. 19: 285–297, 1971.

36. Specht, D.E.: Pulmonary hematoma. Am. J. Dis. Child. 111: 559–563, 1966.

37. Spouge, A.R., Burrows, P.E., Armstrong, D., and Daneman, A.: Traumatic aortic rupture in the pediatric population: Role of plain film, CT and angiography in the diagnosis. Pediatr. Radiol. 324–328, 1991.

38. Stephens, E., and Templeton, A.W.: Traumatic nonpenetrating lung contusion. Radiology 85: 247–252, 1965.

39. Ting, Y.M.: Pulmonary parenchymal findings in blunt trauma to the chest. A.J.R. 98: 343–349, 1966.

40. Tisnado, J., Tsai, F.Y., Als, A., and Roach, J.F.: A new radiographic sign of acute traumatic rupture of the thoracic aorta: Displacement of the nasogastric tube to the right. Radiology 125: 603–608, 1977.

41. Weiner, D.S., and O'Dell, H.W.: Fractures of the first rib associated with injuries to the clavicle. J. Trauma 9: 412–422, 1969.

42. Williams, J.R., and Bonte, F.J.: Pulmonary hematoma secondary to non-penetrating injury. South. Med. J. 55: 622–625, 1962.

43. Williams, J.R., and Stembridge, V.A.: Pulmonary contusion secondary to non-penetrating chest trauma. A.J.R. 91: 284–290, 1964.

44. Woodring, J.H., Fried, A.M., Hatfield, D.R., Stevens, R.K., and Todd, E.P.: Fractures of first and second ribs: Predictive value for arterial and bronchial injury. A.J.R. 138: 211–215, 1982.

MISCELLANEOUS CHEST PROBLEMS

Hydrocarbon Pneumonitis. The most commonly ingested hydrocarbons include furniture polish, gasoline, kerosene, and charcoal lighter fluid, and the most important aspect of these hydrocarbons is that the lower their viscosity and surface tension, the greater is the likelihood that they will be diffusely aspirated into the tracheobronchial tree. In this regard, it is mineral seal oil in certain furniture polishes (i.e., red furniture polish) that causes most of the difficulty, for it is one of the lightest of hydrocarbon distillates (13, 14). Consequently, an infant does not have to aspirate a large volume of a hydrocarbon-containing mineral seal oil to be in serious difficulty.

There often still is some controversy as to whether the pneumonitis resulting from ingestion of hydrocarbons occurs because of aspiration or because of absorption of the hydrocarbon from the stomach, but most authorities now favor aspiration as the major mechanism (6, 12, 14, 16). Although a small amount of the hydrocarbon probably is absorbed from the gastrointestinal tract and expelled through the lungs, it is not enough to explain the pulmonary changes. It may explain the cerebral depression that some of these children demonstrate after such ingestion, but unless the ingestion is massive, damage to the lungs from hydrocarbons circulating in the bloodstream is negligible.

Characteristically, with hydrocarbon ingestion and inhalation, roentgenographic pulmonary changes are absent for the first 6–12 hours, that is, unless massive aspiration occurs. Consequently, a normal chest film during this lag period can be misleading, and, indeed, it is much more important to evaluate the patient clinically and to obtain blood gas values early. Often the values will be abnormal, for the local effects of lipid dissolution, (i.e., surfactant destruction and the development of microatelectasis) lead to serious gas exchange

problems (6, 7). In addition, cell membrane destruction occurs, and all of this, along with small vessel thrombosis, soon leads to bronchiolar necrosis and a necrotizing bronchopneumonia (6).

After the usual clear lung period, infiltrates quickly develop in the lung bases (Fig. 1.144). This characteristic location in itself supports aspiration as the cause of hydrocarbon pneumonitis, and the changes can range from minimal fluffy infiltrates to dense, confluent infiltrates involving a good portion of the lungs bilaterally. In the latter cases, focal emphysema and pneumatocele formation (Fig. 1.145) are not

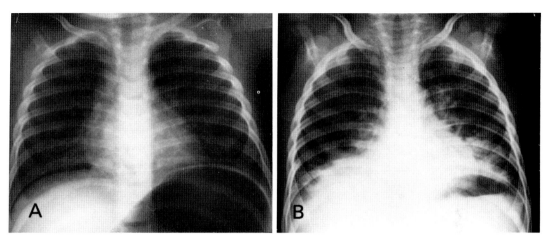

Figure 1.144. *Hydrocarbon pneumonitis.* (*A*) This patient aspirated red furniture polish, but 2 hours after ingestion, the lungs are clear. (*B*) By 12 hours, however, note extensive infiltrates in the lung bases.

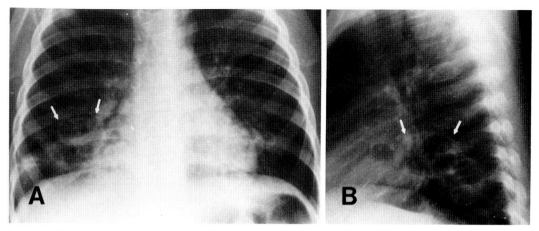

Figure 1.145. *Pneumatoceles with hydrocarbon aspiration.* (*A*) Frontal view demonstrating bilateral, basal, medial infiltrates and pneumatoceles in the right lower lobe (*arrows*). (*B*) Lateral view demonstrates these pneumatoceles (*arrows*) to better advantage.

uncommon and most likely result from air trapping from the damaged small bronchi and bronchioles (1–3, 10, 11). All of these changes are slow to clear, often taking up to 2–3 weeks to completely disappear (4, 6, 8, 14). Indeed, long-term pulmonary function abnormalities have been noted in some patients (9). Currently, in addition to regular therapy in these patients, extracorporeal membranous oxygenation (ECMO) has been advocated in severe cases (15).

One other roentgenographic finding has been described in the early stages of hydrocarbon ingestion, and that is the double gastric fluid level. This sign was described with kerosene ingestion (5) and results from the fact that hydrocarbons float on top of the gastric secretions and appear as a more radiolucent fluid layer. Consequently, the presence of both liquids can be seen, but I have not been able to personally witness this finding, and I believe it to be rare.

REFERENCES

1. Baghassarian, O.M., and Weiner, S.: Pneumatocele formation complicating hydrocarbon pneumonitis. A.J.R. 95: 104–111, 1965.
2. Bergeson, P.S., Hales, S.W., Lustgarten, M.D., and Lipow, H.W.: Pneumatoceles following hydrocarbon ingestion. Am. J. Dis. Child. 129: 49–54, 1975.
3. Campbell, J.B.: Pneumatocele formation following hydrocarbon ingestion. Am. Rev. Respir. Dis. 101: 414–418, 1970.
4. Daeschner, C.W., Jr., Blattner, R.J., and Collins, V.P.: Hydrocarbon pneumonitis. Pediatr. Clin. North Am. 4: 243–253, 1957.
5. Daffner, R.H., and Jiminez, J.P.: The double gastric fluid level in kerosene poisoning. Radiology 106: 383–384, 1973.
6. Eade, N.R., Taussig, L.M., and Marks, M.I.: Hydrocarbon pneumonitis. Pediatrics 54: 351–357, 1974.
7. Giamonna, S.T.: Effects of furniture polish on pulmonary surfactant. Am. J. Dis. Child. 113: 658–663, 1967.
8. Griffin, J.W., Daeschner, C.W., Collins, V.P., and Eaton, W.L.: Hydrocarbon pneumonitis following furniture polish ingestion: Report of fifteen cases. J. Pediatr. 45: 13–26, 1954.
9. Gurwitz, D., Kattan, M., Levison, H., and Culham, J.A.G.: Pulmonary function abnormalities in asymptomatic children after hydrocarbon pneumonitis. Pediatrics 62: 789–794, 1978.
10. Gwinn, J.L., Lee, F.A., Weinberg, H.D., and Beam, C.W.: Radiological case of the month (pneumatocele formation following hydrocarbon pneumonitis). Am. J. Dis. Child. 127: 875–876, 1974.
11. Harris, V.J., and Brown, R.: Pneumatoceles as a complication of chemical pneumonia after hydrocarbon ingestion. A.J.R. 125: 531–537, 1975.
12. Heinisch, H.M., and Levejohann, R.: The pathogenesis of radiological changes in the lungs after ingestion of petroleum distillates: An experimental study in rabbits and extrapolation of the results in children. Ann. Radiol. 16: 263–266, 1973.
13. Huxtable, K.A., Bolande, R.P., and Klaus, M.: Experimental furniture polish pneumonia in rats. Pediatrics 34: 228–235, 1964.
14. Jimenez, J.B., and Lester, R.G.: Pulmonary complications following furniture polish ingestion: A report of 21 cases. A.J.R. 98: 323–333, 1966.
15. Scalzo, A.J., Weber, T.R., Jager, R.W., Connors, R.H., and Thompson, M.W.: Extracorporeal membrane oxygenation for hydrocarbon aspiration. Am. J. Dis. Child. 144: 867–871, 1990.
16. Wolfe, B.M., Brodeur, A.E., and Shields, J.B.: The role of gastrointestinal absorption of kerosene in producing pneumonitis in dogs. J. Pediatr. 76: 867–873, 1970.

Other Pulmonary Aspiration Problems. Aspiration of gastric contents into the tracheobronchial tree with resultant pneumonia can be focal or widespread (5), and the findings depend on the volume of fluid aspirated and the patient's position during the aspiration episode. In small infants, aspiration often occurs into the right upper lobe and results in right upper lobe atelectasis. Presumably, aspiration occurs into the right upper lobe of these infants because they are fed in the recumbent position on their right side. Aspiration in the upright position leads to medial, lower lobe infiltrates, and the roentgenographic findings are not unlike those seen with hydrocarbon pneumonitis. With massive aspiration, the findings may mimic those of pulmonary edema or widespread bacterial pneumonia. Severe cases are referred to as Mendelson's syndrome (5, 7–9). In these cases, a severe chemical pneumonitis sec-

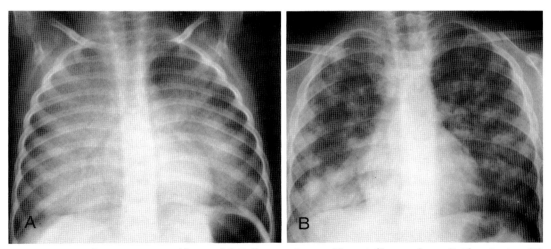

Figure 1.146. *Other aspiration problems.* (A) Diffuse, widespread hazy infiltrates due to lipid aspiration. (B) Diffuse fluffy nodular infiltrates due to aspiration of water in near- drowning.

ondary to the aspiration of acid gastric contents occurs, and the roentgenographic findings reflect extensive pulmonary edema. Chronic aspiration problems lead to pulmonary fibrosis, bronchitis, and even bronchiectasis. Infiltrates secondary to significant aspirations usually take weeks, or even months, to completely clear. This is especially true of lipid aspiration, which often leads to very dense, hazy lungs (Fig. 1.146A). Aspiration of detergents also can lead to serious damage to the lungs (3).

Causes of aspiration are numerous (2) and include swallowing mechanism defects, tracheoesophageal fistulae, aspiration during episodes of seizure activity or unconsciousness, drowning, and, as mentioned earlier, incidental aspiration during normal feeding of young infants. In addition, aspiration can occur secondary to gastroesophageal reflux. Occasionally, such reflux has been incriminated in the sudden infant death syndrome (3, 4). Massive aspiration of particulate matter such as dirt and sand (1, 2) also usually leads to sudden death. If the foreign material contains calcium carbonate (2), it can be seen as opaque material filling the bronchi on chest films.

Near-drowning presents another com-

mon aspiration problem. In this regard, it makes no difference whether salt or fresh water is aspirated (6), for it is the volume of water that makes the difference. Usually the aspirated water clears quickly, although if a patient aspirates a great deal of associated debris, problems may be more prolonged and certainly infection then becomes a common complication. The findings in near-drowning are usually nonspecific and consist of a variable degree of patchy, fluffy alveolar pulmonary infiltration (Fig. 1.146B). With near-drowning, it should be noted that many of these patients also are asphyxiated. As a result, they develop brain edema and in some cases neurogenic pulmonary edema. In addition, they may develop, as they recover from the initial aspiration, superimposed adult respiratory distress syndrome.

REFERENCES

1. Bergeson, P.S., Hinchcliffe, W.A., Crawford, R.F., Sorenson, M.J., and Trump, D.S.: Asphyxia secondary to massive dirt aspiration. J. Pediatr. 92: 506–507, 1978.
2. Bonilla-Santiago J., and Fill, W.L.: Sand aspiration in drowning and near drowning. Radiology 128: 301–302, 1978.
3. Einhorn, A., Horton, L., Altieri, M., Ochsenschlager, D., and Klein, B.: Serious respiratory

consequences of detergent ingestions in children. Pediatrics 84: 472–474, 1989.

4. Herbst, J.J., Book, L.S., and Bray, P.F.: Gastroesophageal reflux in the "near miss" sudden infant death syndrome. J. Pediatr. 92: 73–75, 1978.

5. Mendelson, C.L.: The aspiration of stomach contents into the lungs during obstetric anaesthesia. Am. J. Obstet. Gynecol. 52: 191–204, 1946.

6. Putman, C.E., Tummillo, A.M., Myerson, D.A., and Myerson, P.J.: Drowning: Another plunge. A.J.R. 125: 543–548, 1975.

7. Richman, H., and Abramson, S.F.: Mendelson's syndrome. Am. J. Surg. 120: 531–536, 1970.

8. Teabeaut, J.R., II: Aspiration of gastric contents: An experimental study. Am. J. Pathol. 28: 51–63, 1952.

9. Wilkins, R.A., Lacey, G.J., Flor, R., and Taylor, S.: Radiology in Mendelson's syndrome. Clin. Radiol. 27: 81–85, 1976.

Delayed Diaphragmatic Hernia. Occasionally, an older child can present with acute respiratory distress secondary to herniation of the abdominal viscera into the thoracic cavity. Indeed, such occurrences in older children are being documented more often (1–3, 5–16). These patients frequently present with acute respiratory distress, which may or may not be preceded by vomiting. The resulting roentgenographic findings may be startling and puzzling, and unless the possibility of delayed diaphragmatic hernia is kept in mind, the proper diagnosis may elude the initial observer. Indeed, misinterpretation for a large pneumothorax or pulmonary cyst is usual (Fig. 1.147). In those cases where the stomach contains fluid, the findings may be misinterpreted as an intrathoracic mass. Rarely, gastric rupture or small bowel necrosis can occur (4, 17).

An upper gastrointestinal (GI) series may be needed for verification that the stomach or other portion of the GI tract is in the chest, but, if gastric volvulus also is present, barium may not pass from the esophagus to the stomach. If volvulus is not present, barium will be seen to pass from

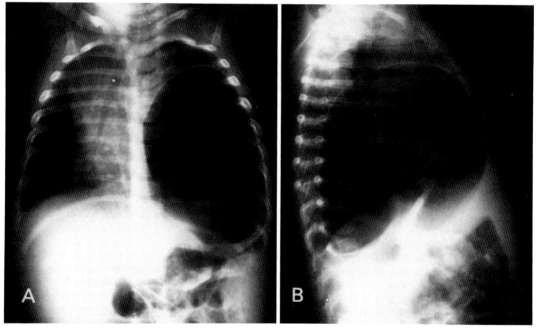

Figure 1.147. *Diaphragmatic hernia, delayed presentation in older child.* (**A**) Note a large cyst-like lesion in the left hemithorax. It displaces the heart and mediastinum to the right. The findings might be misinterpreted as a large lung cyst or pneumothorax. However, note that there is no gastric bubble visualized in the abdomen. (**B**) Lateral view shows the incarcerated, dilated stomach herniated into the chest of this young child who presented with an acute vomiting episode followed by severe respiratory distress. (Courtesy of Virgil B. Graves, M.D.).

the esophagus upward into the stomach which, of course, is in the chest cavity. Most of these cases are presumed to be instances of delayed herniation through a congenital diaphragmatic defect, but it also should be noted that such hernias can occur after blunt abdominal trauma either on an acute or delayed basis. In addition, rupture of the diaphragm has been documented in association with coughing in pertussis (6).

REFERENCES

1. Berman, L., Stringer, D., Ein, S.H., and Shandling, B.: The late presenting pediatric Bochdalek hernia: A 20-year review. J. Pediatr. Surg. 23: 735–739, 1988.
2. Booker, P.D., Meerstadt, P.W.D., and Bush, G.H.: Congenital diaphragmatic hernia in the older child. Arch. Dis. Child. 56: 253–257, 1981.
3. Brill, P.W., Gershwind, M.E., and Krasna, I.H.: Massive gastric enlargement with delayed presentation of congenital diaphragmatic hernia: Report of three cases and review of the literature. J. Pediatr. Surg. 12: 667–674, 1977.
4. Byard, R.W., Bourne, A.J., and Cockington, R.A.: Fatal gastric perforation in a 4-year-old child with a late presenting congenital diaphragmatic hernia. Pediatr. Surg. Int. 6: 44–46, 1991.
5. Day, B.: Late appearance of Bochdalek hernia. Br. Med. J. 1: 786, 1976.
6. Dutta, T.: Spontaneous rupture of diaphragm due to pertussis. J. Pediatr. Surg. 10: 147–148, 1975.
7. Faure, C., Sauvegrain, J., and Bomsel, F.: Right-sided congenital diaphragmatic hernia with delayed radiologic manifestations. Ann. Radiol. 14: 305–313, 1971.
8. Gaisie, G., Young, L.W., and Oh, K.S.: Late onset Bochdalek's hernia with obstruction: Radiographic spectrum of presentation. Clin. Radiol. 34: 267–270, 1983.
9. Glasson, M.J., Barter, W., Cohen, D.H., and Bowdler, J.D.: Congenital left posterolateral diaphragmatic hernia with previously normal chest x-ray. Pediatr. Radiol. 3: 201–205, 1975.
10. Golladay, E.S., Katz, J.R., Katz, H., and Haller, J.A., Jr.: Delayed presentation of congenital posterolateral diaphragmatic hernia: A dramatic cause of failure to thrive. J. Pediatr. Surg. 16: 503–505, 1981.
11. Hurdiss, L.W., Taybi, H., and Johnson, L.M.: Delayed appearance of left-sided diaphragmatic hernia with infancy. J. Pediatr. 88: 990–992, 1976.
12. Kenny, J.D., Wagner, M.L., Harberg, F.J., Corbet, A.J., and Rudolph, A.J.: Right-sided diaphragmatic hernia of delayed onset in the newborn infant. South. Med. J. 70: 373–374, 1977.
13. Kirchner, S.G., Burko, H., O'Neill, J.A., and Stahlman, M.: Delayed radiographic presentation of congenital right diaphragmatic hernia. Radiology 115: 155–156, 1975.
14. MacPherson, R.I.: "Acquired" congenital diaphragmatic hernia. J. Pediatr. Surg. 12: 657–666, 1977.
15. Malone, P.S., Brain, A.J., Kiely, E.M., et al.: Congenital diaphragmatic defects that present late. Arch. Dis. Child. 64: 1542–1544, 1989.
16. McCue J., Ball, A., Brereton, R.J., Wright, V.M., and Shaw, D.: Congenital diaphragmatic hernia in older children. J.R. Coll. Surg. Edinb. 30: 305–310, 1985.
17. Woolley, M.M.: Delayed appearance of a left posterolateral diaphragmatic hernia resulting in significant small bowel necrosis. J. Pediatr. Surg. 12: 673–674, 1977.

Delayed Congenital Lobar Emphysema. Congenital lobar emphysema is usually considered a neonatal problem, but this condition occasionally can present at a later point in childhood (1). Indeed, a superimposed viral infection can convert or aggravate a relatively asymptomatic case into one with full-blown symptoms (Fig. 1.148). The problem most often in-

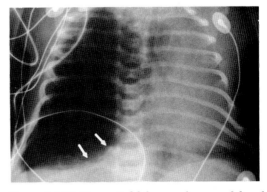

Figure 1.148. *Congenital lobar emphysema; delayed presentation.* In this patient with a superimposed respiratory syncytial viral infection, emphysema in the right upper lobe is very profound. Note the collapsed right lower lobe (*arrows*). The right lung is so overdistended that it is herniating to the left across the upper mediastinum. There is contralateral shift of the heart to the left. Note that there are virtually no lung markings in the emphysematous right upper lobe.

volves the upper lobes, with the left being involved more than the right. The next most common lobe to be involved is the right middle lobe, and in some series right middle lobe involvement is a little more common than right upper lobe involvement. Lower lobe involvement is virtually unheard of. With upper lobe emphysema, the key to proper diagnosis is visualization of the compressed, triangular appearing lower lobe deep in the costovertebral angle (Fig. 1.148). In many of these cases, the lung is so overdistended that parenchymal markings, for the most part, are invisible, and the findings are misinterpreted

for massive tension pneumothorax. With middle lobe involvement, the upper and lower lobes become atelectatic, and usually the atelectatic lobes are erroneously believed to be primarily atelectatic rather than compressed by the overdistended middle lobe.

REFERENCE

1. Taber, P., Benveniste, H., and Gans, S.L.: Delayed infantile lobar emphysema. J. Pediatr. Surg. 9: 245–246, 1974.

Allergic Pneumonitis. Allergic manifestations in a lung can occur with toxic

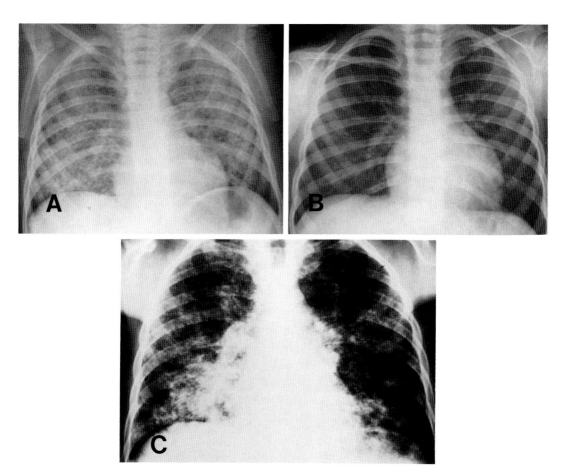

Figure 1.149. *Allergic lung.* (A) Note extensive infiltrates scattered throughout both lungs of this child with an allergic manifestation due to cytotoxic drug administration for treatment of leukemia. (B) Twenty-four hours later, after steroid administration, the lungs are clear. (C) Patchy infiltrates in another patient with an "allergic lung" secondary to inhaled fungal antigens. Farmer's lung is the term often applied to these cases. (Courtesy of A. Selke, M.D.)

substances that are either inhaled or ingested (2, 6–9). The resultant infiltrates may be widespread (Fig. 1.149) or focal. When such infiltrates come and go rapidly in different areas of the lung, the terms Löffler's pneumonia or pulmonary infiltrates with eosinophilia (PIE) often are applied (2, 7). A detailed discussion of all of the causes of allergic pneumonitis is beyond the scope of this book, *but it should be stressed that proper questioning of the patient regarding the intake of any medication or drugs is mandatory when unexplained infiltrates are seen on chest roentgenograms.* Nonspecific pulmonary infiltrates also are seen in the milk allergy or Heiner's syndrome (1, 3–5). In most instances, the findings are nonspecific.

REFERENCES

1. Chang, C.H., and Wittig, H.J.: Heiner's syndrome. Radiology 92: 507–508, 1969.
2. Citro, L.A., Gordon, M.E., and Miller, W.T.: Eosinophilic lung disease (or how to slice P.I.E.). A.J.R. 117: 787–797, 1973.
3. Diner, W.C., Knicker, W.T., and Heiner, D.C.: Roentgenologic manifestations in the lungs in milk allergy. Radiology 77: 564–572, 1961.
4. Heiner, D.C., and Sears, J.W.: Chronic respiratory disease associated with multiple circulating precipitins to cow's milk. Am. J. Dis. Child. 100: 500–502, 1960.
5. Heiner, D.C., Sears, J.W., and Knicker, W.T.: Multiple precipitins to cow's milk in chronic respiratory disease: A syndrome involving poor growth, gastrointestinal symptoms, evidence of allergy, iron deficiency anemia, and pulmonary hemosiderosis. Am. J. Dis. Child. 103: 634–654, 1962.
6. Katz, R.M., and Kniker, W.T.: Infantile hypersensitivity pneumonitis as a reaction to organic antigens. N. Engl. J. Med. 288: 233–237, 1973.
7. Levin, D.C.: The P.I.E. syndrome—pulmonary infiltrates with eosinophilia: A report of 3 cases with lung biopsy. Radiology 89: 461–465, 1967.
8. Singleton, E.B., and Wagner, M.L.: *Radiologic Atlas of Pulmonary Abnormalities in Children,* pp. 130–131, W.B. Saunders, Philadelphia, 1971.
9. Unger, G.F., Scanlon, G.T., Fink, J.N., and Unger, J.D.: A radiologic approach to hypersensitivity pneumonias. Radiol. Clin. North Am. 11: 339–356, 1973.

Dehydration, Acidosis, Overaeration, and Microcardia. Dehydration with acidosis commonly reflects itself on the chest roentgenograms of young infants (3). In such cases, the findings result from dehydration secondary to vomiting and/or diarrhea, and the patient's lungs appear overaerated and undervascularized (Fig. 1.150). In addition, the cardiac silhouette often is small, and the findings frequently are confused with those of bronchiolitis. Decreased vascularity and smallness of the cardiac silhouette (microcardia) result from hypovolemia, while overaeration results from the metabolic acidosis present. These infants attempt to blow off carbon dioxide, and in so doing, overaerate. Microcardia, with overdistended lungs, also can be seen with acute, large-volume blood loss, and with more severe asthmatic attacks. In the latter instance, the overdistended lungs depress the diaphragmatic leaflets downward, and this causes the heart to be stretched. In addition, the heart is compressed by the emphysematous lungs.

Other causes of microcardia include Addison's disease, anorexia nervosa, and, of course, a normal long thin heart in an asthenic individual (usually a young female patient). Microcardia secondary to cardiac atrophy, with actual loss of muscle bulk (protein), as a result of long-standing debilitating disease (malignancy, malnutrition, severe burns, chronic infection, etc.) is a less common cause of a small cardiac silhouette (1, 2, 4).

REFERENCES

1. Altemus, L.R.: Malnutrition with microcardia. A.J.R. 99: 674–680, 1967.
2. Hellerstein, H.J., and Santiago-Stevenson, D.: Atrophy of heart: Correlative study of eighty-five proved cases. Circulation 1: 93–126, 1950.
3. Nathan, M.H.: Diagnosis of dehydration, acidosis, and gastroenteritis in infants from chest radiograph. Radiology 83: 297–305, 1964.
4. Swischuk, L.E.: Microcardia: An uncommon diagnostic problem. J. Radiol. 103: 115–118, 1968.

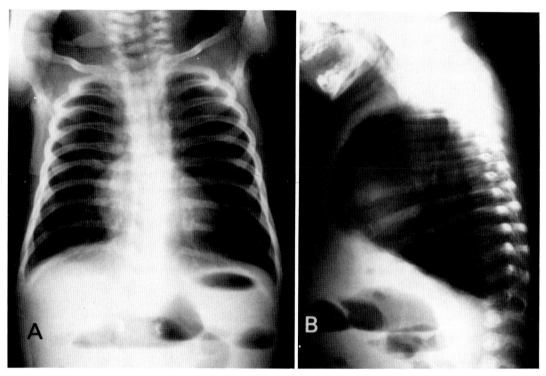

Figure 1.150. *Dehydration and overaeration.* (*A*) Note the overdistended hyperlucent appearance of the lungs in this infant with severe gastroenteritis, diarrhea, and dehydration. The vascularity is diminished and the heart somewhat small in size. Air-fluid levels scattered throughout the abdomen indicate the presence of gastroenteritis. In other cases, the cardiac silhouette is even smaller than in this infant. (*B*) Lateral view showing emphysematous appearance of the lungs, not unlike that seen with bronchiolitis.

Hypoplastic-Agenetic Lung. Lung hypoplasia or agenesis of a lung generally are asymptomatic problems (1, 2), except when they declare themselves in the neonatal period. Hypoplasia of the lung results in a small, hyperlucent lung with diminished pulmonary blood flow, for the pulmonary artery also is hypoplastic (Fig. 1.151). The small, hyperlucent lung ventilates normally, that is, there is normal decrease in size with expiration and therefore such lungs are not predisposed to infection. Pulmonary angiography, pulmonary perfusion and ventilation scintigraphy studies, and even CT scans have been utilized in the evaluation of these patients, but all of these studies are superfluous as they lend nothing more to the information obtained from the plain films. Simply speaking, these patients have a small lung that has decreased pulmonary blood flow, and thus the lung appears small and hyperlucent. Ventilatory excursion is relatively normal, but because of the decreased pulmonary blood flow the lung is basically less efficient in terms of gas exchange. Only severe cases require workup.

With lung agenesis, if the entire lung is agenetic, the problem usually declares itself in the neonatal period. In such cases, the involved hemithorax is small and completely opaque, and there is marked shift of the mediastinum to the ipsilateral side. Concomitantly, there is overdistension (compensatory emphysema) of the other lung, and because the agenetic lung cannot

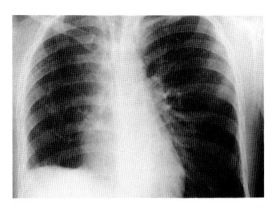

Figure 1.151. *Hypoplastic lung.* Note that the right lung is smaller than the left. In addition, note that vascularity is diminished on the right and a little increased on the left.

receive blood from the right ventricle, all of the blood is diverted to the normal lung and vascularity in the normal lung appears increased. A more difficult problem arises when only one or two lobes are agenetic. Most often, this occurs on the right and has been termed the "hypogenetic right lung syndrome" (3). The lobes involved usually are the upper and middle lobes, and when involved, they lead to decreased volume of the hemithorax. At the same time, there is increased density of the involved hemithorax and a very confusing picture results, which often is misinterpreted as pneumonia (Fig. 1.152). The key deterrent to this misinterpretation should be the fact that these patients demonstrate significant volume loss, and as has been reiterated many times, consolidating pneumonias generally are not associated with any significant volume loss.

Hemoptysis in Childhood. Hemoptysis in childhood is not as common as in the adult but it can occur with hemangiomas in the hypopharynx or upper airway, bacterial pneumonias, other acute and chronic pulmonary infections (5), cystic fibrosis (5), bronchial adenomas (6), and intrathoracic gastroenteric cysts (1, 2). Pulmonary infections and foreign bodies, however, have been shown to account for approximately half of the cases (5).

With gastroenteric cysts, pulmonary changes may range from discrete cystic masses to nonspecific, consolidative-like lesions. If ulceration of the cysts leads to perforation, blood and free air also will be seen in the thoracic cavity (2). With bronchial adenoma, the findings vary from a solitary pulmonary nodule to focal atelectasis or emphysema caused by airway obstruction by the nodule. In children, however, bronchial adenomas are rare.

Pulmonary hemosiderosis also is a cause of hemoptysis in childhood (3, 4), and then the condition is associated with iron deficiency anemia, variable respiratory distress, oxygen diffusion difficulties, and a wide variety of roentgenographic findings. In acute cases, parenchymal bleeding leads to fluffy, bilateral parenchymal infiltrates (Fig. 1.153A), but with repeated bleeding, chronic fibrosis ensues and pulmonary changes may consist of hazy lungs to lungs with miliary-like reticulonodularity (Fig. 1.153B). In any given patient the findings may be different from time to time but chronic, progressive fibrosis eventually ensues (3, 4).

REFERENCES

1. Currarino, G., and Williams, B.: Causes of congenital unilateral pulmonary hypoplasia: A study of 33 cases. Pediatr. Radiol. 15: 15–24, 1985.
2. Cremin, B.J., and Bass, E.M.: Retrosternal density; a sign of pulmonary hypoplasia. Pediatr. Radiol. 3: 145–147, 1975.
3. Felson, B.: Pulmonary agenesis and related anomalies. Semin. Roentgenol. 7: 17–30, 1972.

REFERENCES

1. Chang, S.H., Morrison, L., Shaffner, L., and Crowe, J.E.: Intrathoracic gastrogenic cysts and hemoptysis. J. Pediatr. 88: 594–596, 1976.
2. Macpherson, R.I., Reed, M.H., and Ferguson, C.C.: Intrathoracic gastrogenic cysts: Cause of lethal pulmonary hemorrhage in infants. J. Can. Assoc. Radiol. 24: 362–369, 1973.
3. Matsaniotis. N., Karpouzas, J., Apostolopoulou, E., and Messaritakis, J.: Idiopathic pulmonary

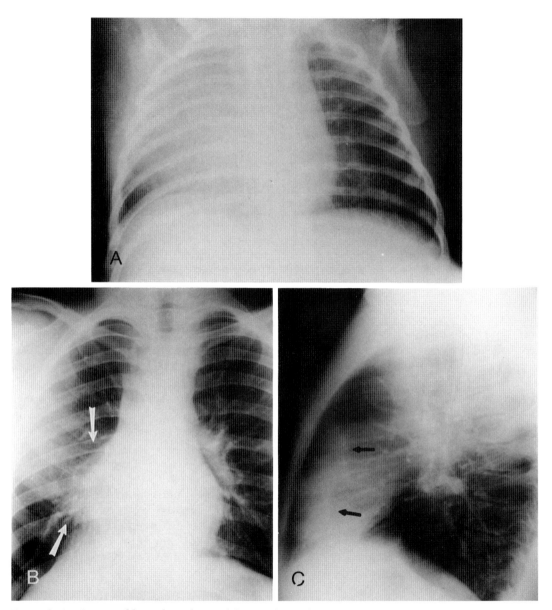

Figure 1.152. *Congenital hypoplastic lung.* (*A*) Note the small, semiopaque right hemithorax with ipsilateral mediastinal shift. The density of the right lung often is misinterpreted as pneumonia. However, volume loss should steer one away from this diagnosis. (*B*) Another patient with agenesis of the right middle lobe producing increased density (*arrows*) along the right cardiac border. One might interpret the findings as a right middle lobe pneumonia. However, note that overall there is volume loss on the right. (*C*) Lateral view demonstrates a vague, lower retrosternal density (*arrows*), but no evidence of a right middle lobe consolidation.

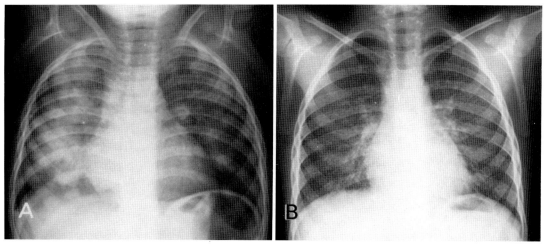

Figure 1.153. *Pulmonary hemosiderosis; varying configurations.* (*A*) Fluffy, asymmetric infiltrates, resembling widespread pneumonia or even pulmonary edema. (*B*) Another child showing diffuse miliary infiltrates not unlike those seen with miliary tuberculosis.

hemosiderosis in children. Arch. Dis. Child. 43: 307–309, 1968.

4. Repetto, G., Lisboa, C.M., Emparanza, E., Ferretti, R., Neira, N., Etchart, M., and Maneghello, J.: Idiopathic pulmonary hemosiderosis. Pediatrics 40: 24–32, 1967.

5. Tom, L.W.C., Weisman, R.A., and Handler, S.D.: Hemoptysis in children. Ann. Otol. Rhinol. Laryngol. 89: 419–424, 1980.

6. Wellons, H.A., Eggleston, P., Golden, G.T., and Allen, M.: Bronchial adenoma in childhood. Am. J. Dis. Child. 130: 301–304, 1976.

Anterior Chest Pain. Anterior chest pain is a common complaint of children, but most often it is musculoskeletal and frequently secondary to overexercising or viral infections. In this regard, it can result from Tietze's syndrome, a costochondritis of the upper costochondral junctions of presumed viral origin. In other cases, it may be pleuritic, but anterior chest pain in children seldom is due to heart disease (1).

REFERENCE

1. Driscoll, D.J., Glicklich, L.B., and Galen, W.J.: Chest pain in children: A prospective study. Pediatrics 57: 648–651, 1976.

Rapidly Expanding Chest Masses and Cysts. A complete discussion of pulmonary and mediastinal masses is beyond the scope of this book and not particularly relevant to its theme of emergency medicine. Only one or two points need be made regarding a child who might present with a chest mass in the emergency room. Such children can present with chest pain, respiratory distress, wheezing, or asthma-like symptoms (1). One of the more common masses is a mediastinal lymphoma or a thymus gland infiltrated with leukemic cells. Both have a similar appearance, and the roentgenographic findings are quite characteristic (Fig. 1.154*A*). Other tumors also can be encountered and pulmonary cysts that become infected also can compress the airway and cause respiratory distress (Fig. 1.154*B* and *C*). Tumors can expand rapidly because of rampant malignant growth or hemorrhage, while pulmonary cysts usually become larger because of supervening infection, or occasionally, hemorrhage.

REFERENCE

1. Swischuk, L.E.: Acute respiratory distress in the infant. Radiol. Clin. North Am. 16: 77–90, 1977.

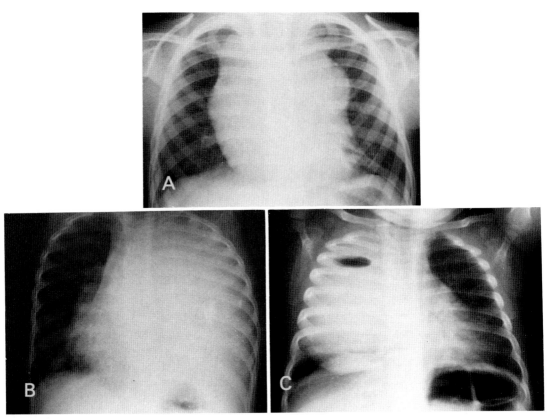

Figure 1.154. *Rapidly expanding masses and cysts.*   (**A**) Note the large mediastinal mass in this child presenting with a 4-day history of wheezing and respiratory distress, suggesting a pulmonary infection. Biopsy-proven lymphoma. (**B**) This child presented with asthma-like symptoms. Note the large mass with calcification in the left chest. It was a teratoma. (**C**) Infant presenting with respiratory distress. Note the large infected bronchogenic cyst in the right chest. It is compressing the trachea and right bronchus.

NORMAL FINDINGS CAUSING PROBLEMS

Technically Poor Examination. The fallacy of assessing a chest roentgenogram obtained during expiration is well known, and cannot be overstressed. On the expiratory film, the normal lungs and heart may erroneously appear totally abnormal (Fig. 155A), and it is only after proper inspiration is accomplished that this is appreciated. Rotation of the chest to one side or another causes obvious problems, and lordotic position can throw the heart and pulmonary vessel into such projection that abnormality is suggested. In this regard, lordotic positioning tends to accentuate the hilar regions and upper lobe vascularity, and cause the heart to assume a right ventricular hypertrophy configuration.

Normal Thymus Gland. The normal thymus gland is notorious for mimicking pathology. Detailed dissertations on the thymus gland are available elsewhere (1–3), and only a few puzzling configurations are illustrated here. The normal thymus gland usually covers the superior aspect of the heart like an umbrella and blends imperceptibly with the cardiac silhouette (Fig. 1.156A). Subtle notches may delineate its inferiormost extent, and on lateral view it will occupy the anterior, superior mediastinal compartment, and be delin-

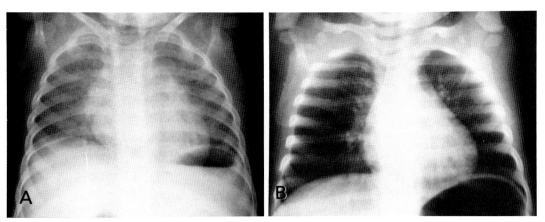

Figure 1.155. *Technically poor films.* (*A*) Expiratory view causes the lungs to appear infiltrated and the heart enlarged. The thymus gland drapes the superior cardiac silhouette, and on the right might suggest hilar adenopathy or a mediastinal mass. (*B*) Same infant with deeper inspiration but lordotic positioning. Lordotic positioning is manifested by horizontal positioning of the posterior ribs, downward pointing anterior ribs, and accentuation of the vascular markings in the upper lobes. This infant was normal.

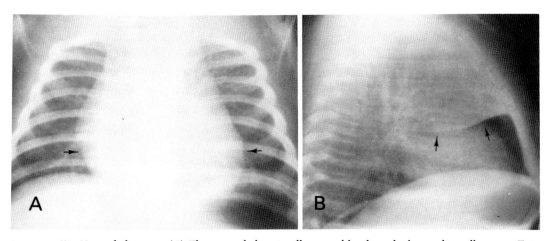

Figure 1.156. *Normal thymus.* (*A*) The normal thymic silhouette blends with the cardiac silhouette. Faint notches are seen at the junction of the thymic lobes and heart (*arrows*). The great vessels are difficult to find. (*B*) Lateral view showing the normal position of the thymus gland, and its undulating lower edge (*arrows*). (From L.E. Swischuk: *Radiology of the Newborn and Young Infant,* Williams & Wilkins, Baltimore, 1973.)

eated by a straight or undulating line along its inferior border (Fig. 1.156*B*). In other cases, the thymus (right lobe especially) may be very large and erroneously suggest a mediastinal or cardiac mass (see Fig. 1.159*B*). An important feature of the normal thymus gland is that no matter how large it is, it does not displace the trachea.

The normal thymus gland now also is readily imaged with ultrasound, CT, or magnetic resonance imaging (MRI) (Fig. 1.157).

In some cases, the thymus gland is triangular in shape, producing the so-called sail sign (Fig. 1.158*A*). If rotation is present in these patients, the sail-like lobe of

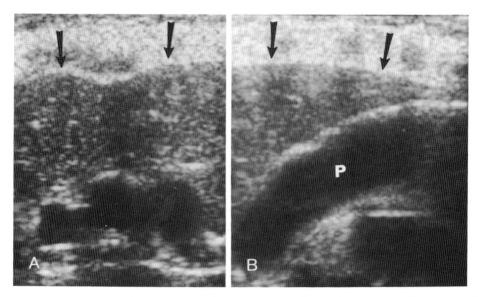

Figure 1.157. *Normal thymus; ultrasonographic findings.* (*A*) Axial view demonstrates characteristic thymic texture of this large but normal thymus gland (*arrows*) in an infant with a cardiac murmur. Note the great vessels behind the thymus. (*B*) Midsagittal view demonstrates the characteristic sail-like configuration of the normal thymic gland (*arrows*). It lies just over the pulmonary artery (*P*).

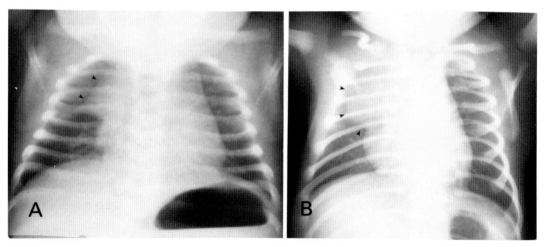

Figure 1.158. *Thymus "sail" sign and pseudopneumonia.* (*A*) Typical sail sign of normal thymus (arrows). (*B*) Rotation to the right in this infant causes the normal thymus to appear as though it were a consolidating pneumonia of the right upper lobe (*arrows*).

the thymus may be thrown into such projection that a consolidating upper lobe pneumonia is suggested (Fig. 1.158*B*). In older children, residual normal thymus also may erroneously suggest a mediastinal mass (Fig. 1.160). *In such cases one should*

remain practical and calm, and one should ask oneself the question, "Why was this child examined?" If the answer is because of possible pneumonia, chest cold, routine chest, preoperative chest, etc., then one should ask oneself the next question,

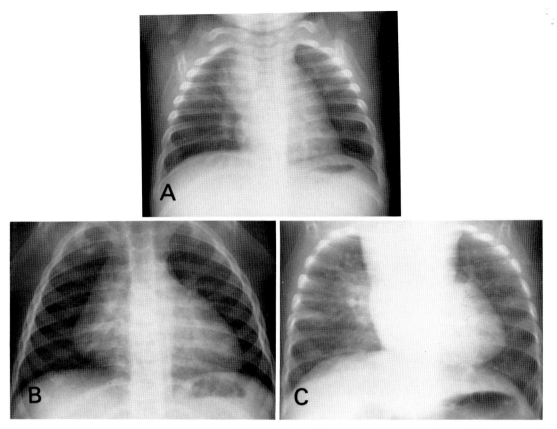

Figure 1.159. *Mass-like configuration of normal thymus gland.* (*A*) Bilateral superior mediastinal fullness caused by normal thymus gland. (*B*) Large right thymic lobe suggesting a mass. (*C*) Peculiar superior medial widening, secondary to incomplete descent of normal thymus gland and lordotic positioning.

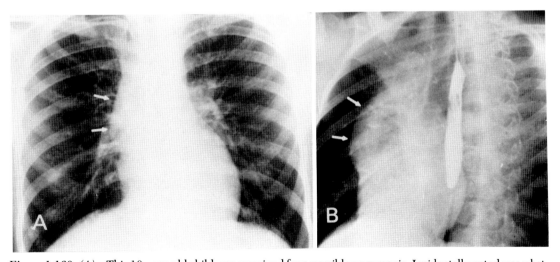

Figure 1.160. (*A*)   This 10-year-old child was examined for a possible pneumonia. Incidentally noted was what at first was interpreted to be a superior mediastinal mass (*arrows*). (*B*) Oblique view with barium demonstrates the same mass (*arrows*). It was normal thymus gland.

"Could I be dealing with normal thymus?" Certainly a normal thymus would be the most likely possibility, and thereafter a repeat chest film in 30 days would be in order. A mass such as one due to a lymphoma would not remain the same size, while normal thymus would almost invariably remain the same in size and configuration. Taking a little time to assess the findings may be more productive than going on to CT or MRI examination. The reason for this is that very often even on these studies the thymic gland has a peculiar configuration and the problem is not solved.

Normal thymus is most commonly seen in patients under the age of 2 years, but it can be seen in older children. Indeed, one can see normal thymus in children even up to the age of 10–14 years, not routinely, but not so uncommonly that the possibility should be discounted completely.

REFERENCES

1. Caffey, J.: *Pediatric X-Ray Diagnosis*, ed. 6, p. 443. Year Book, Chicago, 1972.
2. Swischuk, L.E.: *Radiology of the Newborn and Young Infant*, p. 9. Williams & Wilkins, Baltimore, 1973.
3. Tausend, M.E., and Stern, W.Z.: Thymic patterns in the newborn. A.J.R. 95: 125–130, 1965.

CHAPTER 2

Upper Airway, Nasal Passages, Sinuses, and Mastoids

NORMAL ANATOMY OF UPPER AIRWAY

One must be thoroughly familiar with the normal anatomy of the upper airway before attempting to identify pathology. Fortunately, this is not too difficult a task, for air in the airway provides one with an ideal contrast agent. However, unless a proper roentgenogram is obtained one will be seriously compromised. The upper airway roentgenogram must be obtained during inspiration, with the patient in true lateral position, and, preferably, with the neck extended (Fig. 2.1). This, of course, requires some degree of technical expertise, but if the study is obtained during expiration, or with forward flexion of the neck, an endless number of peculiar, misleading, or virtually noninterpretable configurations of the buckled upper airway result (Fig. 2.2). This also results in problems with the retropharyngeal soft tissues, where they may erroneously appear pathologically thickened. Frontal views of the upper airway also are helpful, but they do not provide as much information as do lateral views.

In terms of normal retropharyngeal soft tissues, there is a normal increase in thickness at the level of the larynx, producing a step-off of the posterior wall of the airway. In other words, the fully distended hypopharynx extends further posteriorly than does the subglottic trachea (Fig. 2.2B and D). With true retropharyngeal soft tissue thickening this step-off usually is obliterated and the airway is displaced anteriorly in a smoothly curving fashion (see Fig. 2.20). This usually does not occur with normal buckling, for even though gross distortions occur (Fig. 2.2A), the step-off, on full inspiration, is preserved (Fig. 2.2B). In these cases, part of the problem is that normal lymphoid tissue may extend into the retropharynx and cause the normal soft tissues to appear disturbingly thick and lumpy (see Fig. 2.21).

Normal adenoidal and tonsillar tissue can pose another problem in evaluation of the upper airway, for in some children the adenoids and tonsils are large (Fig. 2.3). However, the question is whether they present a clinical problem. Indeed, in some older children, normal adenoidal tissue can be very abundant. Under 3 months of age, however, adenoidal tissue is normally quite sparse (1).

REFERENCE

1. Capitanio, M.A., and Kirkpatrick, J.A.: Nasopharyngeal lymphoid tissue. Roentgen observations in 257 children two years of age or less. Radiology 96: 389–391, 1970.

UPPER AIRWAY OBSTRUCTION AND ACUTE STRIDOR

Stridor is descriptive of noisy breathing and usually infers the presence of a lesion in the upper airway. However, *before one embarks on an imaging workup of patients with stridor, the clinical features should be reviewed to determine whether the stridor is:* (a) inspiratory or expiratory, (b) associated with wheezing, (c) associated with voice alterations, or (d) associated with dysphagia (Fig. 2.4). If it is inspiratory, or both inspiratory and expiratory, chances

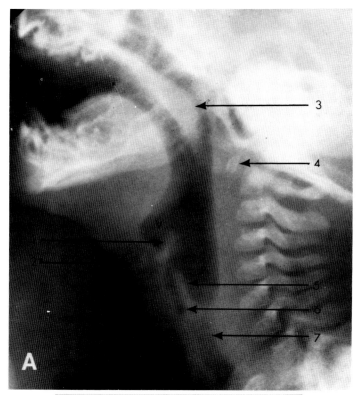

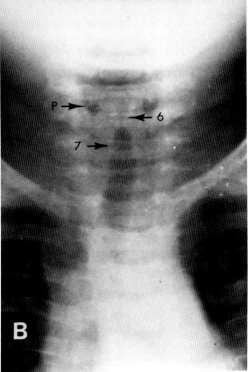

Figure 2.1. (*A and B*) *Normal upper airway.* Note the following structures: (*1*) epiglottis, (*2*) body of the hyoid bone, (*3*) uvula, (*4*) anterior arch of C_1, (*5*) aryepiglottic folds, (*6*) ventricle of glottis, (*7*) subglottic portion of trachea, (*V*) vallecula, and (*P*) piriform fossa.

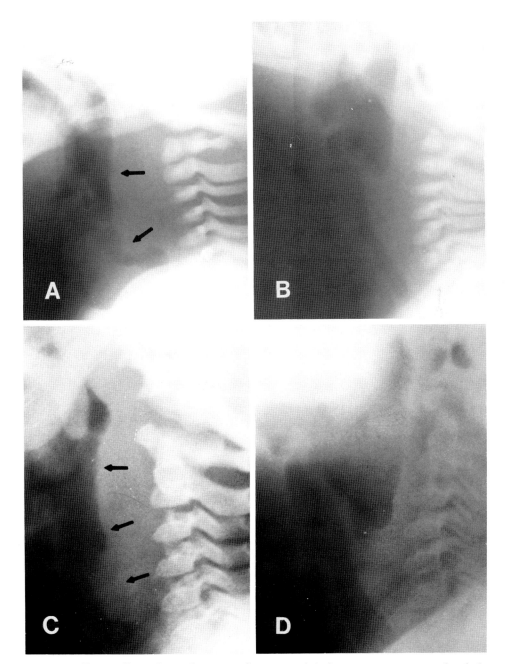

Figure 2.2. *Technically poor film with pseudomass configuration.* (*A*) This patient was examined with the neck flexed forward and the airway incompletely distended. A retropharyngeal mass (*arrows*) is suggested. (*B*) With proper positioning, however, note that no mass is present and the step-off between the hypopharynx and subglottic trachea is preserved. (*C*) Another patient showing what would appear to be a lumpy retropharyngeal mass (*arrows*). Lumpiness favors adenoidal tissue. (*D*) Properly obtained film with full distension of the airway shows no mass.

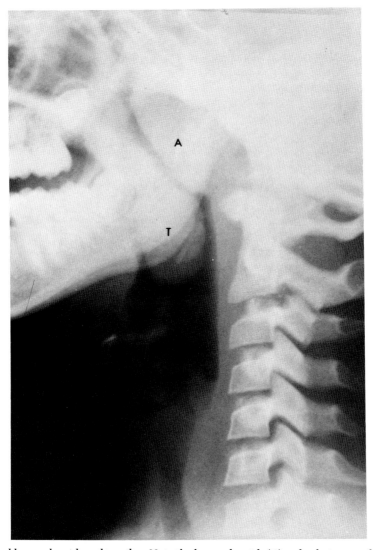

Figure 2.3. *Normal large adenoids and tonsils.* Note the large adenoids (*A*) and palatine tonsils (*T*) in this child.

are that the lesion is in the glottic or paraglottic region, but if it is purely expiratory, the lesion probably exists below the glottis, often in the chest. In these latter cases, expiratory wheezing also is present and may predominate. Voice or cry alterations associated with stridor almost always place the lesion in the glottis, while dysphagia with stridor usually is seen with lesions in the hypopharynx (i.e., epiglottitis, retropharyngeal abscess, hypopharyngeal tumors or cysts). Dysphagia also can

be seen with problems in the chest (i.e., vascular rings or mediastinal masses or cysts).

After one's clinical assessment of the patient with stridor, the next investigative procedure should be a lateral roentgenogram of the upper airway, and not endoscopy. With a proper lateral neck roentgenogram, there hardly is a lesion that will go undetected, and when a chest film and an occasional barium swallow also are obtained, virtually nothing should escape de-

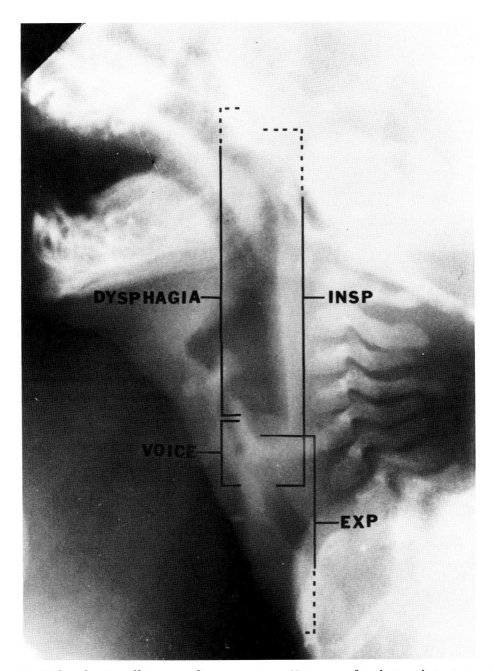

Figure 2.4. *Stridor—location of lesion according to symptoms.*   Note zones of predominantly inspiratory or expiratory stridor and the area of overlap. Also note the area for dysphagia and voice problems.

tection (2, 8, 19, 42). In this regard, improved visualization of the airway, both on frontal and lateral views, can be accomplished by combining increased filtration of the x-ray beam, a higher kilovoltage technique, and magnification (22). However, I have not personally found these measures necessary.

Epiglottitis.   Epiglottitis usually affects older children, with the peak incidence occurring between 3 and 6 years. More recently, however, its more common occurrence in younger children has been documented (2, 10, 11). Epiglottitis usually presents abruptly with variable inspiratory stridor and dysphagia and is caused by *Haemophilus influenzae* infection (8, 20, 21, 30, 36), but viral epiglottitis also can occur (12). Other causes of epiglottitis include thermal injury due to ingestion of hot fluids (26), angioneurotic edema (15), and chronic *Monilia* infection (1, 18).

Dysphagia in epiglottitis is secondary to the marked degree of supraglottic inflammation and edema present and, clinically, the cherry red epiglottis is classic. However, most physicians still are cautious regarding examination of the oropharynx in these patients because of the possibility of inducing glottic spasm. For this reason, the roentgenogram has become a more popular method of diagnosing epiglottitis, and, indeed, this relatively innocuous study can clearly demonstrate its presence (3, 8, 9,

14, 31, 36, 37, 41, 43). However, it should be stressed that *these patients should not be sent to the x-ray examination room unattended,* for the possibility of acute airway obstruction is always present and can be precipitated by neck extension necessary for the radiographic study.

In the classic case of epiglottitis, on lateral view, the roentgenographic findings of epiglottitis are typical, and consist of thickening and edema of the aryepiglottic folds and epiglottis (Fig. 2.5A). In advanced cases, the swollen epiglottis appears as an upward-pointing thumb and, hence, reference is made to the "thumb" sign. With more extensive disease, a supraglottic mass may be suggested (Fig. 2.5C). Mild to moderate hypopharyngeal overdistension also occurs, but seldom is it as marked as in croup. In addition, as opposed to croup, the subglottic portion of the trachea appears normal, on lateral view. On frontal view, however, some cases of epiglottitis demonstrate subglottic edema and

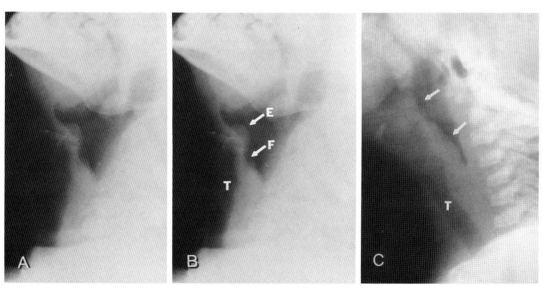

Figure 2.5. *Epiglottitis.* (**A and B**) Classic case demonstrating a swollen epiglottis (*E*), swollen aryepiglottic folds (*F*) and no narrowing of the subglottic trachea (*T*). There is moderate hypopharyngeal overdistension. The configuration of the epiglottis constitutes the so-called "thumb" sign. Evaluation of the aryepiglottic folds should be made at their midpoint, or just behind the epiglottis, and not at their base, where they normally appear thick (20). (**C**) A more pronounced case has resulted in the epiglottis and aryepiglottic folds fusing so as to present as a large supraglottic mass (*arrows*). Note that the subglottic portion of the trachea (*T*) is of normal diameter.

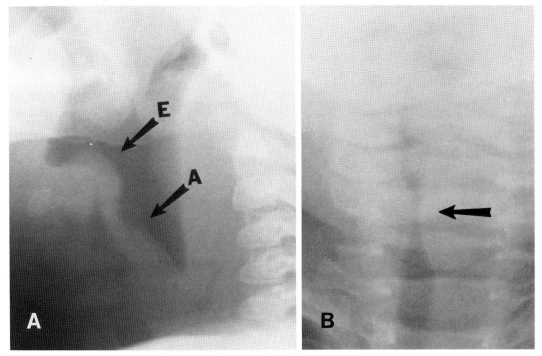

Figure 2.6. *Epiglottitis with subglottic edema.* (*A*) Note typical findings of epiglottitis on lateral view. Note, however, that the subglottic portion of the trachea is of normal diameter. Thickened epiglottis (*E*) and aryepiglottic folds (*A*). (*B*) Frontal view shows a funnel-shaped glottic and subglottic region (*arrow*) due to glottic edema. The findings, on this view, mimic those of croup.

a funnel-shaped glottic area indistinguishable from that seen in croup (Fig. 2.6). In these cases, although the primary problem still is supra- and glottic edema, enough edema extends into the subglottic portion of the trachea to produce the funnel deformity (40). In terms of therapy of epiglottitis, while it was once advocated that tracheostomy need be performed in almost all patients (30), currently most centers suggest nasotracheal intubation (28, 33, 38, 45).

It is most important to note that the aryepiglottic folds in epiglottitis become thickened, for with croup and other causes of stridor the aryepiglottic folds are thin and normal (20). However, one must evaluate fold thickening at the proper level. In this regard, it has been noted that the folds should be evaluated at their midpoint, or just behind the epiglottis, and not at their

base (20). At the base, as they drape over the arytenoid cartilage, they normally are thick, and overlap with abnormal thickening is too great to be of value. This does not occur at the other two levels (20).

In addition, in epiglottis, it is important to note whether the posterior wall of the midportion of the epiglottis is still visible. In most cases of epiglottitis, because the epiglottis swells, the posterior wall becomes invisible (see Fig. 2.5). Unfortunately, in mild cases of epiglottitis the posterior wall of the epiglottis may still be visible and the aryepiglottic folds only minimally thickened (Fig. 2.7). This, however, is the exception more than the rule, for in most cases of epiglottitis the posterior wall of the body of the epiglottis is obliterated (20). All of these points are important in the evaluation of these patients, and if one is not certain of the findings,

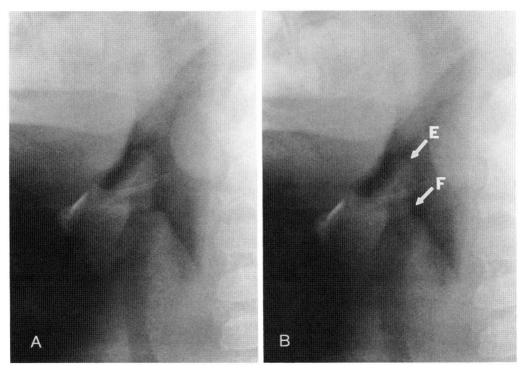

Figure 2.7. *Mild epiglottitis—evaluation of aryepiglottic folds.* (*A* and *B*) In this patient note that the epiglottis (*E*) is swollen. The posterior wall of the midportion of the epiglottis is barely visible. The aryepiglottic folds (*F*) themselves are indistinct but mildly thickened.

then a repeat film should be obtained. Finally, clinical correlation with endoscopy, if deemed necessary, should follow.

It is also important not to misinterpret the normal, so-called "omega" epiglottis for a thickened epiglottitis. In these patients, stridor may be due to croup or some other cause, but the epiglottis may appear a little thickened. This impression is erroneous, for it is merely a floppy epiglottis with prominent downward-curving lateral flaps (19). This results in an inverted "U" or omega-shaped epiglottis that appears thickened on lateral view (Fig. 2.8). However, in these cases no thickening of the aryepiglottic folds will be seen, and this should strongly rule against epiglottitis (19). *If one is not able to make this distinction on a lateral neck roentgenogram, it usually is because the inspiratory effort is not deep enough, and thus, the study should be repeated. One must be abso-*

lutely sure about the diagnosis of epiglottitis.

Croup. Most cases of croup are of viral origin (9), but bacterial croup, often severe and refractory, can occur. It carries terms such as membranous croup, pseudomembranous croup, membranous tracheitis, bacterial croup, or refractory croup (6, 13, 14, 22, 29, 35). In these cases, symptoms often are more severe, subglottic narrowing more pronounced, and response to usual treatment refractory. Indeed, intubation often is required.

Croup also has been demonstrated to be more common in allergic children (48), and this also has been our experience. Indeed, in older children, croup can occur on a purely allergic basis. In these cases, it is not associated with any type of infection at all, and can be very abrupt and severe in onset.

Classically, in croup, stridor primarily is

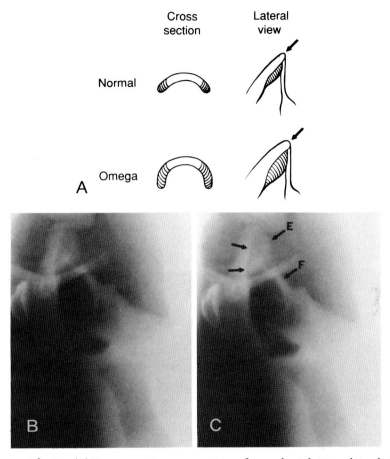

Figure 2.8. *Omega epiglottis.* (**A**) Diagrammatic representation of normal epiglottis on lateral view. Note that the normal epiglottis (*arrows*) is thin and the lateral walls (*shaded area*) are not prominent. With an omega epiglottis, the lateral walls (*shaded areas*) are more prominent and on lateral view can cause the epiglottis to appear thickened. (**B and C**) Note pseudothickening of the epiglottis (*E*) due to an omega epiglottis. The aryepiglottic folds (*F*) are normal. Also note that the posterior wall (*arrows*) of the body of the epiglottis still is clearly visible. This usually does not occur with epiglotittis. Part A reprinted with permission from S.D. John and L.E. Swischuk: Stridor and upper airway obstruction in infants and children. RadioGraphics 12: 625–643, 1992.

inspiratory, and the entire picture, including the barking cough, is rather typical. Characteristically, the disease is one of infants and young children, with the peak age incidence being between 6 months and 3 years (7, 43). Many of these children also have a full-blown viral lower respiratory tract infection, and in the evening, croup develops. Overall, *the clinical findings are so typical that there is question as to why roentgenograms should be obtained in these children.* Nonetheless, the study seems to be quite popular mostly because

it can easily differentiate croup from epiglottitis (3, 5, 8, 9, 13, 14, 16, 32, 34, 43).

Roentgenographically, with croup, there is marked hypopharyngeal overdistension during inspiration, but the epiglottis and aryepiglottic folds are normal. The vocal cords, however, usually appear thickened and fuzzy, and the subglottic portion of the trachea narrowed (Fig. 2.9*A*). This narrowing is primarily paradoxical and represents tracheal collapse secondary to negative intraluminal pressures that develop in this area during in-

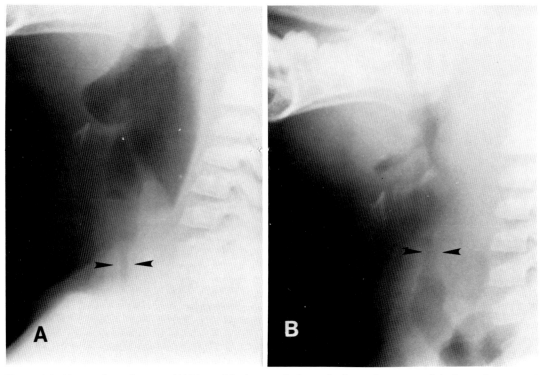

Figure 2.9. *Croup—lateral view.* (A) Typical findings include marked overdistension of the hypopharynx and paradoxical narrowing of the subglottic portion of the trachea (*arrows*). The epiglottis and aryepiglottic folds are normal. (B) Expiratory film demonstrating that the subglottic narrowing is not fixed, for on this view the subglottic area appears much wider (*arrows*). In most cases, the narrowing disappears entirely. Also note overdistension of the subglottic trachea.

spiration (17, 32, 43). This is a nonspecific response that occurs with any glottic obstruction, but in childhood it is most commonly seen with croup and is an important feature of this condition (Fig. 2.10). On expiration, it should be noted that such narrowing is not as fixed as it first appears (Fig. 2.9B). Indeed, it usually diminishes or completely disappears and thus, further attests to the fact that in typical viral, or spasmodic, allergic croup, such narrowing is not due to fixed edematous, subglottic tracheal narrowing (Fig. 2.10). In more severe cases, however, and these usually are cases of bacterial croup, inflammation may extend into the subglottic trachea and render the narrowing more pronounced and persistent. Indeed, it may not completely disappear on expiration. In addition, actual

membranes in the trachea may be seen in some of these cases (Fig. 2.11).

On frontal view, in croup, the vocal cords appear thickened and funnel-like in configuration (Fig. 2.12A). They appear this way because they are edematous and in spasm. Normally, on inspiration, the vocal cords should fall away and reveal a wide-open airway (Fig. 2.12B), while with crying or forced expiration (i.e., Valsalva maneuver), the inferior aspect of the vocal cord should appear shoulder-like or squared-off (Fig. 2.12C). With croup, there is little change in the appearance of the cords between inspiration and expiration, and thus the funnel-shaped configuration is almost always present and, interestingly enough, usually best seen on standard frontal chest roentgenograms.

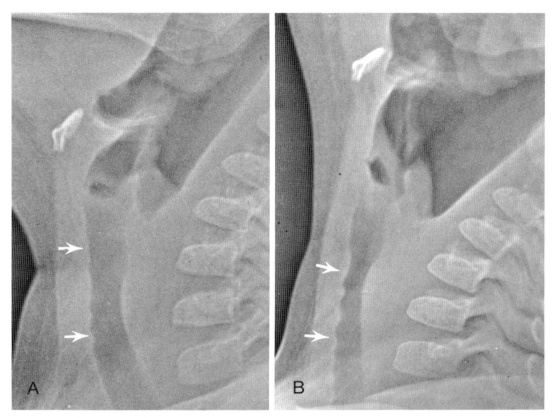

Figure 2.10. *Croup—paradoxical subglottic tracheal narrowing.* (*A*) Moderate inspiration. Note that the diameter of the subglottic trachea (*arrows*) is normal. (*B*) With deep inspiration, the hypopharynx shows gross overdistension and the subglottic portion of the trachea (*arrows*) now shows paradoxical narrowing. Also note that with marked overdistension of the hypopharynx the aryepiglottic folds appear thin and normal but with the lesser degree of hypopharyngeal distension noted in *A* the folds erroneously appear thickened. This study is a xeroradiogram, which is not currently used or advised. However, it does demonstrate the tracheal dynamics to greater advantage. (Reproduced with permission from S.D. John and L.E. Swischuk: Stridor and upper airway obstruction in infants and children. RadioGraphics 12: 625–643, 1992.)

Unfortunately, not all children display as classic a picture of croup as that just outlined, for if obstruction is less marked, and/or the inspiratory effort not as deep, less hypopharyngeal overdistension and paradoxical subglottic tracheal narrowing occur (29). In these patients, the only finding may be thickening or fuzziness of the vocal cords (Fig. 2.13). However, this configuration is just as suggestive of croup as is the classic one illustrated in Figure 2.9. In such instances, with a deeper inspiratory effort the findings become more classic. To be sure, the degree of roentgenographic abnormality in croup is more dependent on the degree of inspiration than on the severity of disease (34).

There are one or two other lesions that might present with croupy symptoms and initially might be misdiagnosed as croup. These include *congenital subglottic stenosis* (3, 4, 9, 43), and *subglottic hemangioma* (42, 47). In congenital subglottic stenosis, the findings are remarkably similar to those of croup, for there is hypopharyngeal overdistension and narrowing of the subglottic portion of the trachea (Fig. 2.14A). However, as compared with most cases of croup, the degree of narrowing does not diminish during expiration, for it is truly fixed and stenotic. With subglottic hemangioma, the characteristic finding is an eccentric posterior or lateral mass projecting into the subglottic portion of the trachea (Fig. 2.14B). These tumors most often are posterior or lateral, but occasionally can be anterior. Hemangiomas may be present elsewhere in the body or on the skin and, under such circumstances, make the diagnosis even more binding. Both congenital subglottic stenosis and subglottic hemangioma are mentioned at this point because, during episodes of viral res-

piratory tract infection, they may become more symptomatic and lead to a clinical picture suggestive of acute croup.

Another lesion that may mimic the roentgenographic findings of croup is a laryngeal web, and this is the one lesion that is almost impossible to demonstrate roentgenographically. Generally the findings mimic croup, and consequently, endoscopy usually is required for diagnosis. Vocal cord paralysis also can produce findings similar to croup on frontal and lateral views, but, of course, hoarseness, or apho-

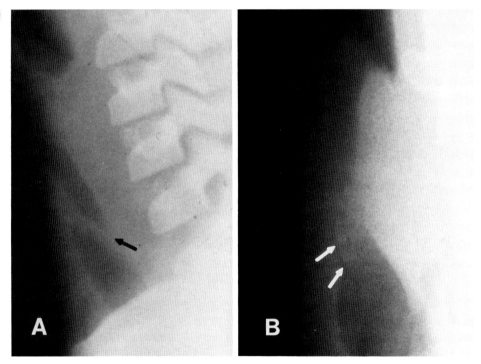

Figure 2.11. *Membranous croup or bacterial tracheitis.* (*A*) Note the membrane (*arrow*) in the trachea of this patient with severe respiratory stridor. (*B*) Another patient with severe stenosis of the trachea (*arrows*) and an indistinct, subglottic membrane. (Part *A* courtesy of Robin Gaup, M.D.)

Figure 2.12. *Croup—frontal view.* (*A*) Typical funnel-shaped glottic and subglottic narrowing in infant with croup (*arrows*). Edema and spasm of the glottis and, to a lesser extent, edema of the subglottic portion of the trachea lead to this typical funnel-shaped upper airway narrowing. (*B*) Normal child, inspiratory film for comparative purposes, showing how normal vocal cords open during inspiration to leave a wide airway (*arrows*). (*C*) Normal child, expiratory film (forced Valsalva maneuver) for comparative purposes, showing the normal right angle configuration of the inferior aspect of the closed vocal cords (*arrows*).

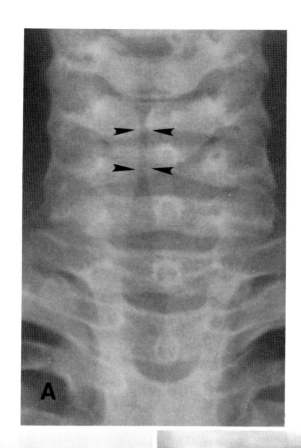

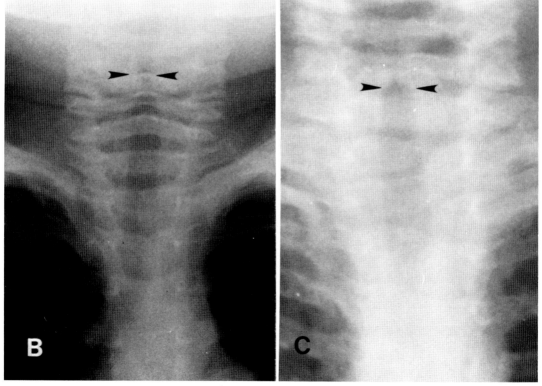

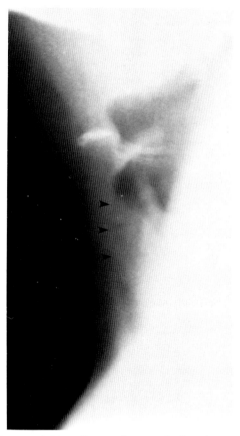

Figure 2.13. *Croup—fuzzy, thickened vocal cords.* Lateral view showing moderate hypopharyngeal overdistension and a normal epiglottis and aryepiglottic folds. However, the region of the vocal cords is fuzzy and thickened (*arrows*). This configuration is just as typical for croup as is the one demonstrated in Figure 2.9, and if the inspiratory effort were deeper, one would be able to see paradoxical collapse of the subglottic trachea.

nia, also usually is present. Finally, it might be noted that other infections of the larynx such as *Candida* (18) and herpes (27) can lead to croup or epiglottitis and stridor, and that upper airway obstruction in general has been shown to cause pulmonary edema (17, 24, 34, 39) and systemic hypertension (43). Although of unknown etiology, hypoxia is suspected as the basic trigger for these complications.

Uvulitis. Uvulitis as a part of pharyngitis (25) or in association with epiglottitis

(39) also can cause airway obstruction. In such cases, however, the uvula becomes quite large and swollen and may be a cause of inspiratory stridor or even dysphagia. Radiographically, the enlarged uvula is readily demonstrable (Fig. 2.15).

REFERENCES

1. Balsam, D., Sorrano, D., and Barax, Ch.: *Candida* epiglottitis presenting as stridor in a child with HIV infection. Pediatr. Radiol. 22: 235en?236, 1992.
2. Brilli, R.G., Benzing, G., III, and Cotcamp, D.H.: Epiglottitis in infants less than two years of age. Pediatr. Emerg. Care 5: 16–21, 1989.
3. Capitanio, M.A., and Kirkpatrick, J.A., Jr.: Upper respiratory tract obstruction in infants and children. Radiol. Clin. North Am. 6: 265–277, 1968.
4. Cuncy, R.L., and Bergstrom, L.B.: Congenital subglottic stenosis. J. Pediatr. 82: 282–284, 1973.
5. Currarino, G., and Williams, B.: Lateral inspiration and expiration radiographs of the neck in children with laryngotracheitis (croup). Radiology 145: 365–366, 1982.
6. Denneny, J.C., III, and Handler, S.D.: Membranous laryngotracheobronchitis. Pediatrics 70: 705–707, 1982.
7. Denny, F.W., Murphy, T.F., Clyde, W.A., Jr., Collier, A.M., and Henderson, F.W.: Croup: An 11-year study in a pediatric practice. Pediatrics 71: 871–876, 1983.
8. Dunbar, J.S.: Epiglottitis and croup. J. Can. Assoc. Radiol. 12: 95–97, 1961.
9. Dunbar, J.S.: Upper respiratory tract obstruction in infants and children. A.J.R. 109: 225–247, 1970.
10. Gershan, W.M., Gillman, K., Baxter, M., Manoukian, J., and Gordon, J.: Acute airway obstruction in a seven-month-old infant with epiglottitis. Pediatr. Emerg. Care 4: 197–199, 1988.
11. Goldhagen, J.L.: Supraglottitis in three young infants. Pediatr. Emerg. Care 5: 175–177, 1989.
12. Grattan-Smith, T., Forer, M., Kilham, H.L., and Gillis, J.: Viral supraglottitis. J. Pediatr. 110: 434–435, 1987.
13. Green, R., and Stark, P.: Trauma of the larynx and trachea. Radiol. Clin. North Am. 16: 309–320, 1978.
14. Henry, R.L., Mellis, C.M., and Benjamin, B.: Pseudomembranous croup. Arch. Dis. Child. 58: 180–183, 1983.
15. Herman, T.E., and McAlister, W.H.: Epiglottic enlargement: Two unusual causes. Pediatr. Radiol. 21: 139–140, 1991.
16. Howard, J.B., McCracken, G.H., Jr., and Luby,

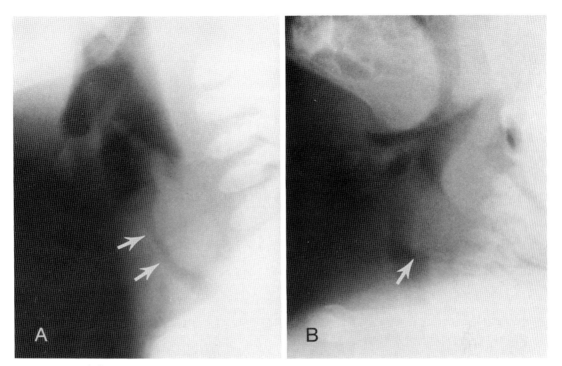

Figure 2.14. *Subglottic stenosis.*   (*A*) Note narrowing of the subglottic portion of the trachea (*arrows*). On expiration, such narrowing does not disappear. (*B*) Subglottic hemangioma. Note characteristic posterior wall subglottic mass (*arrow*). In other cases, the mass may come off the lateral wall of the subglottic portion of the trachea.

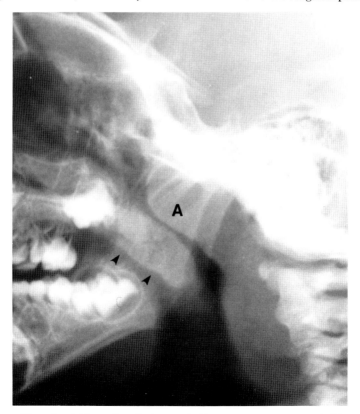

Figure 2.15. *Uvulitis.*   Note the thickened uvula (*arrows*). Also note prominent, probably inflamed, adenoids (A) and retropharyngeal lymphoid tissue.

J.P.: Influenza A2 virus as a cause of croup requiring tracheostomy. J. Pediatr. 81: 1148–1150, 1972.

17. Hurley, R.M. and Kearns, J.R.: Pulmonary edema and croup. Pediatrics 65: 860, 1980.

18. Jacobs, R.F., Yasuda, K., Smith, A.L., and Benjamin, D.R.: Laryngeal candidiasis presenting as inspiratory stridor. Pediatrics 69: 234–236, 1982.

19. John, S.D., and Swischuk, L.E.: Stridor and upper airway obstruction in infants and children. RadioGraphics 12: 625–643, 1992.

20. John, S.D., Swischuk, L.E., and Hayden, C.K., Jr.: Aryepiglottitis fold width in epiglottitis: Where should measurements be obtained? Radiology in press, 1993.

21. Jones, H.M.: Acute epiglottitis and supraglottitis. J. Laryngol. 72: 932–939, 1958.

22. Jones, R., Santos, J.I., and Overall, J.C.: Bacterial tracheitis. J.A.M.A. 242: 721–726, 1979.

23. Joseph, P.M., Berdon, W.E., Baker, D.H., et al.: Upper airway obstruction in infants and small children: Improved radiographic diagnosis by combining filtration, high kilovoltage, and magnification. Radiology 121: 143, 1976.

24. Kanter, R.K., and Watchko, J.F.: Pulmonary edema associated with upper airway obstruction. Am. J. Dis. Child. 138: 356–358, 1984.

25. Kotloff, K.R., and Wald, E.R.: Uvulitis in children. Pediatr. Infect. Dis. 2: 392–393, 1983.

26. Kulick, R.M., Selbst, S.M., Baker, M.D., and Woodward, G.A.: Thermal epiglottitis after swallowing hot beverages. Pediatrics 81: 441–444, 1988.

27. Lallemand, D., Huault, G., Laboureau, J.P., and Sauvegrain, J.: Lesions of the larynx and esophagus in herpes simplex infection. Ann. Radiol. 17: 317–325, 1974.

28. Lewis, J.R., Gartner, J.C., and Galvis, A.G.: A protocol for management of acute epiglottitis: Successful experiences with 27 consecutive instances treated by nasotracheal intubation. Clin. Pediatr. 17: 494–496, 1978.

29. Liston, S.L., Gehrz, R.C., Siegel, L.G., and Tilelli, J.: Bacterial tracheitis. Am. J. Dis. Child. 137: 764–767, 1983.

30. Margolis, C.Z., Colletti, R.B., and Grundy, G.: Haemophilus influenzae type B: The etiologic agent in epiglottitis. J. Pediatr. 87: 322–323, 1975.

31. Mauro, R.D., Poole, S.R., and Lockhart, C.H.: Differentiation of epiglottitis from laryngotracheitis in the child with stridor. Am. J. Dis. Child. 142: 679–682, 1988.

32. Meine, F.J., Lorenzo, R.L., Lynch, P.F., Capitanio, M.A., and Kirkpatrick, J.A.: Pharyngeal distension associated with upper airway obstruc-

tion. Experimental observations in dogs. Radiology 111: 395–398, 1974.

33. Milko, D.A., Marshak, G., and Striker, T.W.: Nasotracheal intubation in the treatment of acute epiglottitis. Pediatrics 53: 674–677, 1974.

34. Mills, J.L., Spackman, T.J., Borns, P., Mandell, G.A., and Schwartz, M.W.: The usefulness of lateral neck roentgenograms in laryngotracheobronchitis. Am. J. Dis. Child. 133: 1140–1142, 1979.

35. Phelan, P., and Hey, E.: Progressive inflammatory subglottic narrowing responsive to steroids. Arch. Dis. Child. 58: 228–230, 1983.

36. Poole, C.A., and Altman, D.H.: Acute epiglottitis in children. Radiology 80: 798–805, 1963.

37. Rapkin, R.H.: Diagnosis of epiglottitis: Simplicity and reliability of radiographs of neck in differential diagnosis of croup syndrome. J. Pediatr. 80: 96–98, 1972.

38. Rapkin, R.H.: Simultaneous uvulitis and epiglottitis. J.A.M.A. 243: 1843, 1980.

39. Rivera M., Hadlock, F.P., and O'Meara, M.E.: Pulmonary edema secondary to acute epiglottitis. A.J.R. 132: 991–992, 1979.

40. Shackelford, G.D., Siegel, M.J., and McAlister, W.H.: Subglottic edema in acute epiglottitis in children. A.J.R. 131: 603–605, 1978.

41. Stankiewicz, J.A., and Bowes, A.K.: Croup and epiglottitis: A radiologic study. Laryngoscope 95: 1159–1160, 1985.

42. Sutton, T.J., and Nogrady, M.B.: Radiologic diagnosis of subglottic hemangioma in infants. Pediatr. Radiol. 1: 211–216, 1973.

43. Swischuk, L.E., Smith, P.C., and Fagan, C.J.: Abnormalities of the pharynx and larynx in childhood. Semin. Roentgenol. 9: 283–300, 1974.

44. Travis, K.W., Todres, I.D., and Shannon, D.C.: Pulmonary edema associated with croup and epiglottitis. Pediatrics 59: 695–698, 1977.

45. Watts, F.B., Jr., and Slovis, T.L.: The enlarged epiglottis. Pediatr. Radiol. 5: 133–136, 1977.

46. Weber, M.L., Desjardins, R., Perreault, G., Rivard, G., and Turmel, Y.: Acute epiglottitis in children: Treatment with nasotracheal intubation: Report of 14 consecutive cases. Pediatrics 57: 152–155, 1976.

47. Williams, H.E., Phelan, P.D., Stocks, J.G., et al.: Hemangiomas of the larynx in infants: Diagnosis, respiratory mechanics and management. Aust. Paediatr. J. 5: 149–154, 1968.

48. Zach, M., Erben, A., and Olinsky, A.: Croup, recurrent croup, allergy and airways hyper-reactivity. Arch. Dis. Child. 56: 336–341, 1981.

Chest Film in Airway Obstruction.

Obstruction of the airway below the glottis

manifests itself primarily as an expiratory problem, and although there may be both inspiratory and expiratory breathing difficulty, it is the expiratory air trapping that predominates roentgenographically. Because of this, the chest tends to be over-aerated, and classic examples of lesions leading to such overaeration include obstructing vascular rings and mediastinal masses and cysts. With obstruction in and around the glottis, however, air cannot enter the chest in adequate amounts, and thus, the chest often appears underaerated (1). Furthermore, there is a paradoxical increase in heart size during inspiration (1, 3). The reason for this is that, with glottic or supraglottic obstruction, inspiratory intrathoracic pressures become negative and, in so doing, cause the cardiac silhouette to become larger and more prominent. Normally, of course, it would become smaller during inspiration.

Pulmonary edema also occurs in some cases of airway obstruction (2, 5–7). It can occur during or after the obstruction but occurs most often after the obstruction has been relieved. The exact cause of the pulmonary edema is not known, but most likely it lies in the realm of increased permeability of the capillaries secondary to hypoxia (4). The phenomenon is similar to that seen with postatelectic pulmonary edema.

REFERENCES

1. Capitanio, M.A., and Kirkpatrick, J.A.: Obstructions of the upper airway in children as reflected on the chest radiograph. Radiology 107: 159–161, 1973.
2. Galvis, A.G.: Pulmonary edema complicating relief of upper airway obstruction. Am. J. Emerg. Med. 5: 294–297, 1987.
3. Grunebaum M., Adler, S., and Varsano, I.: The paradoxical movement of the mediastinum. A diagnostic sign of foreign-body aspiration during childhood. Pediatr. Radiol. 8: 213–218, 1979.
4. Izsak, E.: Pulmonary edema due to acute upper airway obstruction for aspirated foreign body. Pediatr. Emerg. Care 2: 235–237, 1986.
5. Kanter, R.K., and Watchko, J.F.: Pulmonary edema associated with upper airway obstruction. Am. J. Dis. Child. 138: 356–358. 1984.
6. Rivera, M., Hadlock, F.P., and O'Meara, M.E.: Pulmonary edema secondary to acute epiglottitis. A.J.R. 132: 991–992, 1979.
7. Travis, K.W., Todres, I.D., and Shannon, D.C.: Pulmonary edema associated with croup and epiglottitis. Pediatrics 59: 695–698, 1977.

Foreign Bodies in the Upper Airway and Hypopharynx. With hypopharyngeal foreign bodies, after the initial coughing episode the foreign body can remain surprisingly silent. Roentgenographically, lateral neck films are invaluable (2), and if such foreign bodies are opaque, they are readily identified (Fig. 2.16A). If, however, they are radiolucent (i.e., aluminum, wood, plastic, etc.) they are almost impossible to detect (Fig. 2.16D). If perforation occurs, a retropharyngeal abscess may result (Fig. 2.16B). With other perforations, only free air is seen (Fig. 2.17).

Hypopharyngeal foreign bodies, unless they totally occlude the hypopharynx, seldom result in acute respiratory catastrophes. Laryngeal foreign bodies, on the other hand, commonly present with severe respiratory distress, stridor, and even apnea (Fig. 2.16C). Indeed, the problem often is so acute that there is not time for roentgenograms to be obtained (4, 5).

Foreign bodies that lodge in the vocal cords usually are slender and either flat or long. The classic such foreign body is an eggshell fragment (3), but eggshell aspiration is not as common as it was in former days. However, if it should occur, the eggshell may be seen on end, located between the vocal cords. In this position, it appears as a thin, opaque, vertical stripe. Occasionally, other opaque foreign bodies such as chicken and turkey bones can be visualized in the same position (Fig. 2.16C). Fish bones, however, almost always elude detection (1), for only those that are large and heavily calcified can be detected.

The problem of confusing a foreign body with normally calcified laryngeal car-

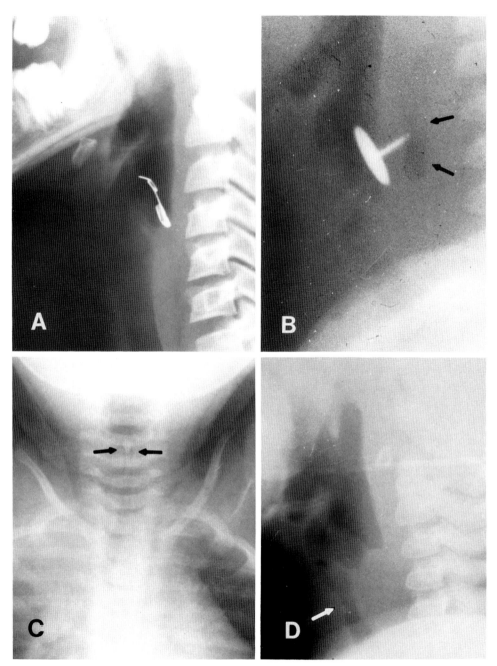

Figure 2.16. *Upper airway foreign bodies.* (*A*) Foreign body in hypopharynx. Note safety pin in this young infant. (*B*) Another infant with a thumbtack in the hypopharynx. Note that the retropharyngeal space is markedly thickened and that there are air bubbles in it (*arrows*). These findings represent a retropharyngeal abscess secondary to perforation of the posterior pharyngeal wall. (*C*) *Opaque laryngeal foreign body.* A chicken bone is present in the larynx just at the level of the glottis (*arrows*). (*D*) *Radiolucent upper airway foreign body—indirect findings only.* This patient had an acute episode of coughing and hemoptysis, and then persistent stridor for 3 weeks. The only roentgenographic finding was a persistent soft tissue mass bulging from the anterior tracheal wall, just below the glottis (*arrow*). On subsequent endoscopy, a small piece of aluminum foil was found embedded just below the glottic region.

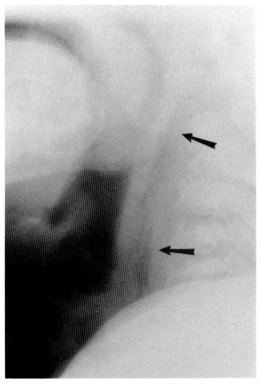

Figure 2.17. *Perforation of the hypopharynx.* Note streaks of free air (*arrows*) in the retropharyngeal soft tissues secondary to hypopharyngeal perforation due to a swallowed chicken bone.

tilage is not as great in childhood as it is in adulthood. These calcifications are discussed with upper esophageal foreign bodies in Chapter 3.

REFERENCES

1. Campbell, D.R., Brown, S.J., and Manchester, J.S.: An evaluation of the radio-opacity of various ingested foreign bodies in the pharynx and esophagus. J. Can. Assoc. Radiol. 19: 183–186, 1968.
2. Gay, B.B. Jr., Atkinson, G.O., Vanderzalm, T., Harmon, J.D., and Porubsky, E.S.: Subglottic foreign bodies in pediatric patients. Am. J. Dis. Child. 140: 165–168, 1986.
3. Naveh, Y., Friedman, A., and Altmann, M.: Eggshell aspiration. Am. J. Dis. Child. 129: 498–499, 1975.
4. Steichen, F.M., Fellini, A., and Einhorn, A.H.: Acute foreign body laryngotracheal obstruction: A cause of sudden and unexplained death in children. Pediatrics 48: 281–285, 1971.
5. Weston, J.T.: Airway foreign body fatalities in children. Ann. Otol. Rhinol. Laryngol. 74: 1144–1148, 1965.

Other Causes of Upper Airway Obstruction. Edema of the larynx and paraglottic structures can be seen with caustic burns secondary to lye ingestion (Fig. 2.18A), laryngeal trauma (Fig. 2.18B), and, in some cases, hot air or smoke inhalation. In such cases, hypopharyngeal overdistension and enlargement or obliteration of the glottic and paraglottic structures is seen. With *trauma to the larynx,* associated fractures of the hyoid bone and laryngeal cartilage also can be seen. In this regard, it is important not to confuse the separate ossification centers of the normal body and wings of the hyoid bone for a fracture (Fig. 2.18B). CT scanning is very valuable in further documenting laryngeal fractures.

Acute stridor occasionally is seen with *angioneurotic (allergic) edema of the epiglottis* or uvula (5). In some of these cases, symptoms may be profound, since nearly total airway occlusion may occur. Roentgenographically, the swollen, enlarged epiglottis (Fig. 2.18C) or uvula is readily demonstrable. In other cases, a chronically lodged *foreign body in the upper esophagus may lead to tracheal compression* and acute stridor (1–4). These patients often do not present with a history of dysphagia, and roentgenograms may demonstrate compression of the trachea only (see Fig. 3.151).

Vascular rings or other vascular anomalies usually present with chronic airway obstructive problems, but if a superimposed respiratory tract infection is present, acute stridor or wheezing may occur. In such cases, it is most important to identify the presence of a right-sided aortic arch, for this is almost always present with a vascular ring (Fig. 2.19). Of course, tracheal compression may be seen on plain films, but, generally speaking, the workup of stridor secondary to a vascular ring is not an emergency room procedure. A similar statement can be made regarding mediastinal masses and cysts that might present with airway obstruction.

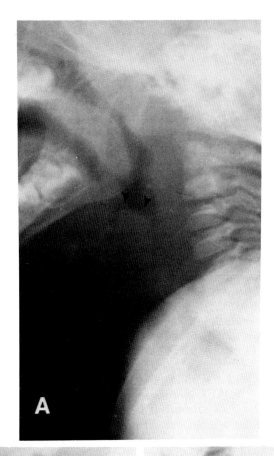

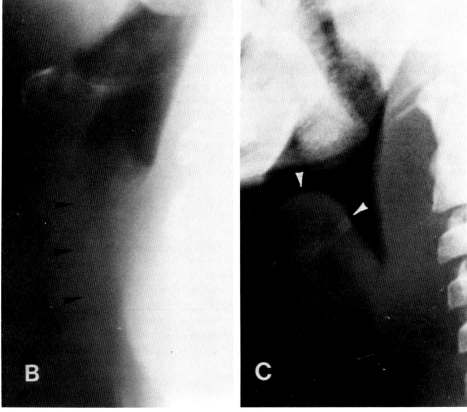

REFERENCES

1. Lallemand, D., Roussel, B., and Sauvegrain, J.: Narrowing of the cervical trachea following foreign body aspiration. Ann. Radiol. 18: 413–418, 1975.
2. Schidlow, D.V., Palmer, J., Balsara, R.K., Turtz, M.G., and Williams, J.L.: Chronic stridor and anterior cervical "mass" secondary to an esophageal foreign body. Am. J. Dis. Child. 135: 869–870, 1981.
3. Smith, P.C., Swischuk, L.E., and Fagan, C.J.: An elusive and often unsuspected cause of stridor or pneumonia (the esophageal foreign body). 122: 80–89, 1974.
4. Tauscher, J.W.: Esophageal foreign body: An uncommon cause of stridor. Pediatrics 61: 657–658, 1978.
5. Watts, F.B., Jr., and Slovis, T.L.: The enlarged epiglottis. Pediatr. Radiol. 5: 133–136, 1977.

RETROPHARYNGEAL ABSCESS

Retropharyngeal abscess usually presents with fever, neck pain and stiffness, and dysphagia (1–4). Stridor can be seen in these patients, but usually is not a predominant feature. Adenopathy usually is present in the neck and, in some cases, may be striking. In most instances, the retropharyngeal abscess results from suppuration of lymphoid tissue in the retropharyngeal space, but occasionally can result from perforation of the hypopharynx by a foreign body.

Roentgenographically, the findings consist of thickening of the retropharyngeal soft tissues and forward, bulging displacement of the airway (Fig. 2.20). If gas is present in the abscess, the diagnosis is more readily established (see Fig. 2.16B). In those cases where findings are minimal and one is in doubt, a barium swallow is helpful. This study will show the abnormal forward position of the esophagus and more clearly demonstrate the presence of soft tissue swelling in the retropharyngeal space.

The cervical spine usually is straight or flexed in cases of retropharyngeal abscess and often there is some degree of anterior offsetting of C_2 on C_3. This latter finding results from the intense muscle spasm present and does not represent true dislocation. By the same token, C_1 may be displaced forward on C_2, and as a result the space between the anterior arch of C_1 and the dens will become widened. It has been stated that this finding is due to inflammation-induced laxity of the ligaments in the area, and this may be true. However, it should be remembered that normal hypermobility of the upper cervical spine in infants is common.

It is important to differentiate normal tracheal buckling and prominent lymphoid tissue from true thickening of the retropharyngeal soft tissues. In this regard, with true thickening there is loss of the normal step-off from the posterior pharyngeal wall to the posterior wall of the trachea (Fig. 2.20). With normal retropharyngeal soft tissues, this does not occur and the step-off generally is preserved (Fig. 2.21). However, if uncertainty persists, a barium swallow can determine whether true thickening is present. Currently in most cases of retropharyngeal inflammation, either ultrasound, CT, or magnetic resonance imaging (MRI) now are utilized to determine whether an actual abscess is present (Figs. 2.22–2.23).

Figure 2.18. *Miscellaneous causes of upper airway obstruction.* (*A*) Lye burns to larynx. Note the edematous cords (*arrows*) in this patient who sustained lye burns to the esophagus, hypopharynx, and vocal cords. (*B*) Trauma to larynx. This boy was hit in the anterior neck by a fist and became hoarse. Note the edematous, indistinct vocal cords (*arrows*). Note the separately ossified body and wings of the hyoid bone. These should not be misinterpreted for a fracture. (*C*) Angioneurotic edema of the epiglottis. Note the markedly thickened epiglottis, aryepiglottic folds (*arrows*), and retropharynx in this patient presenting with acute respiratory distress. (Part *C* reprinted with permission from F.B. Watts, Jr., and T.L. Slovis: The enlarged epiglottis. Pediatr. Radiol. 5: 133–316, 1977.)

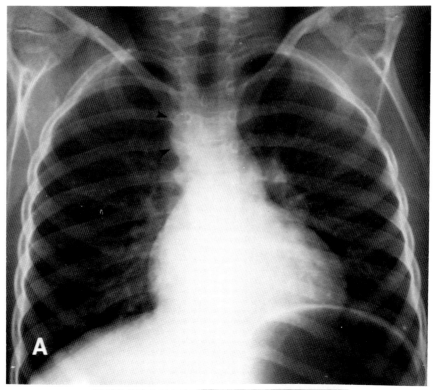

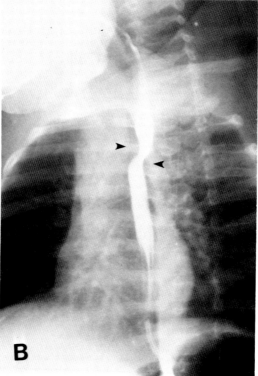

Figure 2.19. *Vascular ring causing stridor.* (**A**) Note the right-sided aortic (*arrow*) in this patient with a vascular ring (double aortic arch). The trachea is displaced to the left and indented on the right by the right-sided aortic arch. On lateral view in these patients, one occasionally can see anterior displacement of the trachea. (**B**) Barium swallow demonstrating characteristic reverse "S," double indentation of the esophagus (*arrows*).

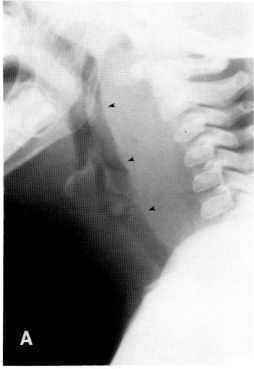

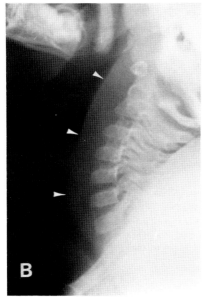

REFERENCES

1. Capitanio, M.A., and Kirkpatrick, J.A., Jr.: Upper respiratory tract obstruction in infants and children. Radiol. Clin. North Am. 6: 265–277, 1968.
2. Dunbar, J.S.: Upper respiratory tract obstruction in infants and children. A.J.R. 109: 225–246, 1970.
3. John, S.D., Swischuk, L.E.: Stridor and upper airway obstruction in infants and children. Radio-Graphics 12: 625–643, 1992.

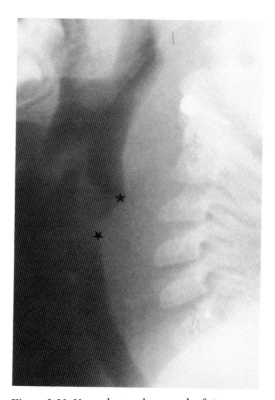

Figure 2.21. *Normal retropharyngeal soft tissue prominence.* In this patient, normal retropharyngeal lymphoid tissue causes indentation of the posterior wall of the hypopharynx. However, note that the posterior walls of the trachea and hypopharynx (°) remain offset. Therefore, even though a retropharyngeal disease process might be suggested, the smooth, curving deformity of the combined posterior hypopharyngeal and tracheal walls as demonstrated in Figure 2.20 are absent.

Figure 2.20. *Retropharyngeal abscess.* (*A*) Large retropharyngeal abscess causing thickening of the retropharyngeal space and smooth anterior displacement of the airway (*arrows*). The spine shows mild kyphosis secondary to intense muscle spasm. (*B*) Less striking case showing less thickening of the retropharyngeal tissues (*arrows*). Note, also, that the neck is in its normal extended position. Nonetheless, the pre-

vertebral soft tissues are thickened and the airway displaced anteriorly in a smooth, curving fashion. In addition, the normal step-off of the airway at the level of the larynx is lost.

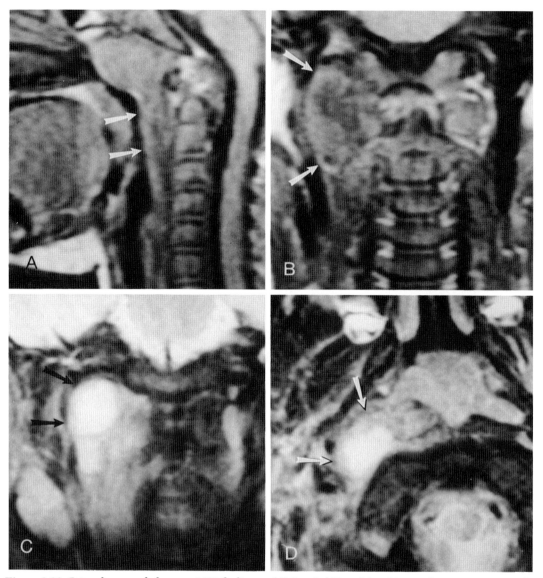

Figure 2.22. *Retropharyngeal abscess—MRI findings.* (*A*) Saggital T_1 weighted image demonstrates retropharyngeal soft tissue thickening (*arrows*). (*B*) Coronal section demonstrates an inflammatory mass on the right (*arrows*) with a mixed signal. (*C*) T_2 weighted image demonstrates the high signal abscess cavity and surrounding edema (*arrows*). (*D*) Similar findings on the axial view (*arrows*). (Courtesy of Phillip F. Tirman, M.D., Santa Barbara, California).

4. Swischuk, L.E., Smith, P.C., and Fagan, C.J.: Abnormalities of the pharynx and larynx in childhood. Semin. Roentgenol. 9: 283–300, 1974.

SINUSITIS, MASTOIDITIS, AND NASAL PASSAGE ABNORMALITIES

Sinusitis. Sinusitis is common in infants and children, and those who suggest that roentgenographic examination of the sinuses in this age group is of limited value (12) do these patients an injustice. This is not to say, however, that dealing with sinusitis in infants and children is easy, but, still, it must be dealt with. Sinusitis comes in varying degrees of severity and may be allergic or inflammatory, and frequently is

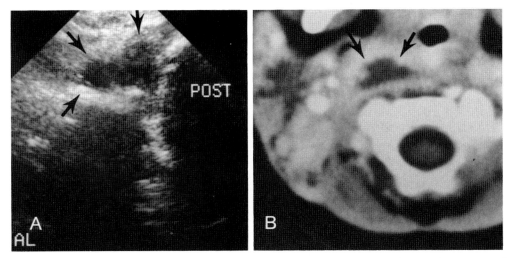

Figure 2.23. *Retropharyngeal abscess—ultrasound and CT findings.* (A) Ultrasound. Note the irregular, basically hypoechoic abscess (*arrows*). (B) Axial CT more precisely demonstrates the location and the extent of the abscess (*arrows*). (Reprinted from John, S.D., and Swischuk, L.E.: Stridor and upper airway obstruction in infants and children. RadioGraphics 12: 625–643, 1992. Courtesy of Joanna J. Seibert, M.D., Arkansas Children's Hospital, Little Rock.)

subacute (13). In addition, it is variably symptomatic and, when all of these factors are considered, it becomes a difficult entity to deal with.

Part of the problem of recognizing sinus disease in children, especially in young infants, arises from the fact that it was, and to a large extent still is, generally held that sinuses are not developed in infants. This is untrue, for the maxillary and ethmoid sinuses often are present at birth and can become infected at ages as young as 3–6 months (13). The problem, however, is that roentgenographic examination of the sinuses in infants less than 1 year of age is difficult and interpretation of the findings is even more difficult (1, 3, 5, 8). Consequently, it is easier to say that the sinuses have not as yet developed than to try to find them and interpret the findings. In such cases, it is only when the sinus cavities clear with treatment that one realizes that they were present all the time (Fig. 2.24). Similarly, proof that sinus cavities exist in young infants is present when disease is unilateral (Fig. 2.24C).

Another problem is that accomplishing a satisfactory roentgenographic examination is difficult in infants. Most often, the Waters' view, the single most important view in evaluating sinusitis in children, is obtained with too steep an angle (Fig. 2.25). While this most common problem is not always completely circumvented in very young infants, one's awareness of it can prompt repeat studies and, thus, proper interpretation.

In addition to these considerations, it seems doubtful that, as previously proposed, crying can cause enough mucosal edema and sinus obliteration to mimic disease (2–5, 8, 13). By the same token, mucosal redundancy, suggested as a normal phenomenon of young infants causing opacification of sinuses in the very young, also seems a doubtful concept. One only has to ask why, of all the mucosal surfaces in a young infant, would the mucosa in the paranasal sinuses selectively be redundant. Consequently, we have come, more and more, to the conclusion that the only normal sinus cavity is the one completely clear. However, when a sinus cavity is opacified, one cannot predict severity of

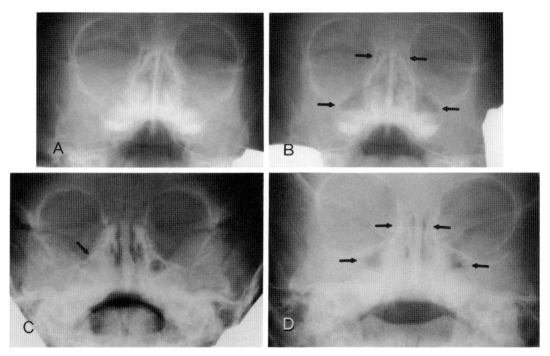

Figure 2.24. *Sinusitis in infancy.* (**A**) Note that the maxillary sinuses are difficult to see in this 11-month-old infant. The reason is that they are completely obliterated by inflammatory changes. However, one might be tempted to erroneously conclude that the maxillary sinuses are not yet developed. (**B**) After treatment, just 3 weeks later, one can see the normally aerated maxillary (*lower arrows*) and ethmoid (*upper arrows*) sinuses. (**C**) Another patient with unilateral maxillary sinus opacification on the right (*arrow*). One could see how easy it would be to say that the sinuses were not developed if the left maxillary sinus also were obliterated. This patient was 5 months old. (**D**) Note bilateral mucosal thickening of the maxillary sinuses (*lower arrows*) and obliteration of the ethmoid sinuses (*upper arrows*). Mucosal thickening in the maxillary sinuses might at first be missed and the maxillary sinuses erroneously believed to be clear.

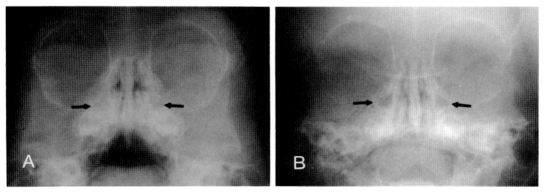

Figure 2.25. *Faulty Waters' view.* (**A**) This Waters' view was obtained too steeply and the maxillary sinuses (*arrows*) appear obliterated. (**B**) With proper angulation (less steep than in adults), the sinuses are seen to be clear (*arrows*).

the problem; the exception being the presence of air-fluid levels that signify acute, purulent, bacterial sinusitis. Viral infection seldom produces air-fluid levels. Mucosal thickening is common in allergic sinusitis, a frequently seen problem in children with asthma (2, 9, 13). It also is seen with viral and bacterial infection. Complete opacification, of course, can be seen with all three of the foregoing types of "sinusitis."

The fact that the roentgenograms, for the most part, cannot yield data regarding severity of sinusitis can explain why various studies have shown that patients with no complaints show opacified sinuses (7, 12). Indeed, most likely, if a random population were examined, a fair number of individuals would have opacified sinuses and yet not be overly complaintive of them. Sinusitis is a disease with a wide clinical spectrum and many individuals, including children, can tolerate certain degrees of sinusitis. This does not mean, however, that the sinuses are normal, only that the disease is not very severe. *Overall, then, the roentgenogram is quite sensitive in detecting sinus opacification and hence disease,* and we have come to utilize it quite regularly in cases of suspected sinusitis. Furthermore, because it is difficult to differentiate purulent rhinitis from purulent sinusitis on a clinical basis alone, the sinus films have become even more valuable, for with rhinitis alone, the sinus cavities are clear.

In terms of which views to obtain, it is the Waters' view that is most beneficial, but we also obtain the lateral view for evaluation of the sinuses and nasopharynx. The reason the Water's view is so valuable is that it is designed to visualize the maxillary and ethmoid sinus cavities, and, in infants and young children, these are the cavities most often involved. The maxillary sinus cavities, however, are more readily evaluated than the ethmoid and sphenoid sinus cavities. In terms of sinus development, the ethmoid and maxillary sphenoid sinus

cavities are present at least by 6 months, the sphenoid sinus cavities, at least by 2 years, but the frontal sinuses are usually not present until 7–10 years of age. Therefore frontal sinusitis does not exist in infants and young children.

Before embarking on a discussion of the roentgenographic findings of sinusitis, it is probably worthwhile to try to understand the pathophysiology of sinusitis. Normal sinus cavities are well aerated, for drainage is normal, but when drainage becomes impaired, the sinus cavities become occluded, and then superimposed bacterial infection becomes a high risk. The question is, how do the sinus cavities become occluded in the first place, and the most common causes are viral upper respiratory tract infection or allergy. In these cases, the mucosa of the sinuses becomes congested, occludes the orifices of the sinus cavities, and leads to impaired drainage. Once this occurs, the possibility of superimposed bacterial infection increases.

In terms of clinical significance, it has been shown that opacified paranasal sinuses in children are bacterially infected in 70% of cases (1). Of further interest is the fact that the vast majority of these patients did not have symptoms that would have prompted the initial physician to consider sinus disease. This phenomenon has been correlated by others (5) and, certainly, this has been our experience. Once one accepts these aspects of sinus disease in infants and children, one can begin to accept the premise that the only normal sinus cavity is the one that is completely aerated.

The roentgenographic manifestations of sinusitis include total opacification of the sinuses, variable thickness of the mucosa, and air-fluid levels (Figs. 2.24 and 2.26). Mucosal thickening is most common and, in this regard, as correlated with clinical and MRI findings in patients examined for reasons other than sinus disease, thickening of the mucosa in the maxillary sinuses of 4 mm or greater proved significant in

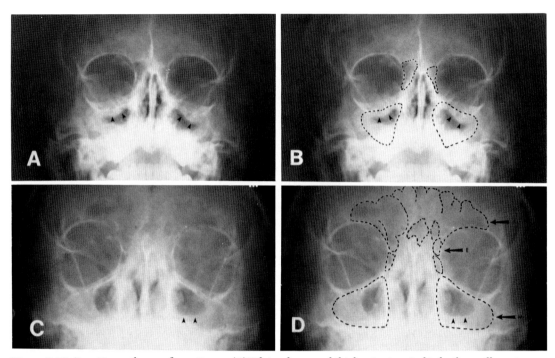

Figure 2.26. *Sinusitis—other configurations.* (*A*) Bilateral mucosal thickening is noted in both maxillary sinuses (*arrows*). This configuration frequently is seen in allergic children. In addition, the ethmoid sinuses, located just along the medial aspect of the orbital rims, also are partially obliterated and involved by inflammatory change. (*B*) For comparative purposes, the bony cortex of the maxillary and ethmoid sinuses in this patient have been delineated by *dotted lines.* (*C*) Another patient with an air-fluid level in the left maxillary sinus (*arrows*). The right maxillary sinus is almost completely obliterated by inflammatory change (exudate and mucosal thickening) and the ethmoid and frontal sinuses also are involved. Air-fluid levels most often are seen with acute sinusitis of bacterial origin. (*D*) *Dotted lines* once again outline the sinus cavities for comparative purposes. Maxillary sinus (*M*), ethmoid sinus (*E*), frontal sinus (*F*).

terms of associated symptomatology consistent with sinusitis (10).

When interpreting mucosal thickening, it is important not to misinterpret the findings as merely being representative of small sinus cavities (Fig. 2.27). This is a common mistake in the assessment of paranasal sinus disease in the pediatric age group, especially in infants and young children where the bony walls of the sinus cavities are thin (Fig. 2.27C). Air-fluid levels in any sinus cavity suggest acute bacterial sinusitis and, for their demonstration, upright views are necessary. Totally opacified sinuses, as noted earlier, are seen with all types of sinusitis but often escape notice until treatment and clearing of the sinus cavities occurs (see Fig. 2.24).

Symptoms of sinusitis in childhood often are not like those in adults (2, 4, 7, 9, 11, 13), and while pain and redness can occur over an acutely infected sinus cavity in a child, more often sinusitis is a chronic problem presenting with a persistent cough (due to a postnasal drip and often worse at night) and recurrent bouts of otitis media (4, 5, 13). Headache is not nearly as common a symptom as it is in adults and, indeed, a poor heralding finding of sinusitis in children. In other children with maxillary and ethmoid sinusitis, proptosis due to orbital edema may be the presenting problem and actually is quite common. In such cases, CT studies are invaluable and indeed mandatory. They clearly will show whether the pathologic process is due to

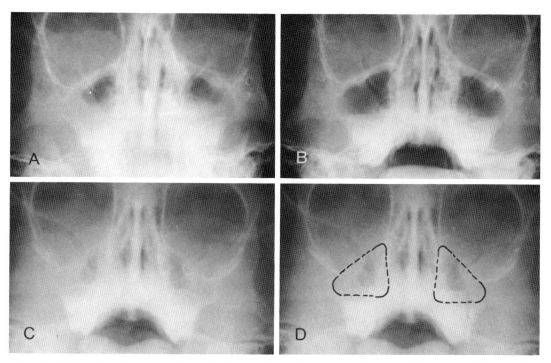

Figure 2.27. *Pseudosmall sinus pitfall.* (**A**) Note moderately pronounced mucosal thickening of the maxillary sinuses, which might erroneously suggest that the sinuses are clear but small. (**B**) With treatment the sinuses now are clear. (**C**) Extensive mucosal thickening of the maxillary sinuses in an infant, which, again, might at first erroneously suggest that the maxillary sinuses are clear but small. The bony walls are difficult to see. (**D**) *Dotted lines* outline the true sinus cavities.

preseptal cellulitis or intraorbital inflammation, even to the point of abscess formation. Preseptal cellulitis manifests in soft tissue swelling of the tissues anterior to the globe (Fig. 2.28A). When inflammation extends into the retro-orbital space, it most often occurs medially and displaces the medial rectus muscle (Fig. 2.28B and C). Abscess formation can occur anywhere (Fig. 2.28D). CT studies are invaluable in these patients and should be performed for any patient with inflammatory proptosis. In addition, computerized tomography is essential for preoperative assessment of sinus disease (6), and overall is gaining in popularity in all patients. It is much more informative than plain films, especially for disease in the ethmoid and splenoid sinuses.

Finally, in terms of the clinical diagnosis of sinusitis, a problem arises in distinguishing acute viral upper respiratory tract infections with coryza, from sinusitis. Our experience has been that in cases of acute viral upper respiratory tract infection, even though the patient may feel congested and look congested, the paranasal sinuses are clear. It is not until later when enough mucosal thickening and edema have occurred that the sinuses become abnormal. Furthermore, we have noted that patients with rhinitis have normal paranasal sinuses.

Before finally leaving the topic of sinusitis, two pitfalls in the interpretation of paranasal sinuses should be discussed in more detail. The first deals with the fact that the maxillary sinuses are not cuboid but rather triangular. As a result, either the superior or lateral orbital wall can be so

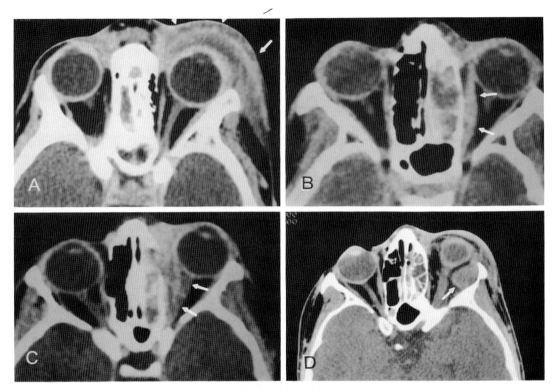

Figure 2.28. *Maxillary and ethmoid sinusitis with orbital complications.* (*A*) Preseptal cellulitis. Note extensive swelling of the preseptal soft tissues (*arrows*). There is no edema extending into the retro-orbital space and the medial rectus muscle is normal. (*B*) Another patient with thickening of the medial rectus muscle and adjacent soft tissues (*arrows*). Note adjacent sinusitis in the ethmoid cells. (*C*) Still another patient with more extensive edema along the medial retro-orbital space (*arrows*). Adjacent sinusitis is present but a frank abscess is not suggested. (*D*) Another patient with an abscess in the retro-orbital region (*arrow*).

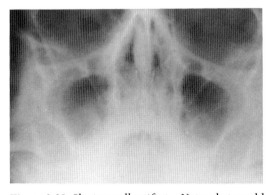

Figure 2.29. *Sloping wall artifact.* Note what would appear to be mucosal thickening along the roof and lateral walls of both maxillary sinuses. However, the thickening is not as pronounced laterally and certainly is not present medially or along the floor of the sinus cavities. This would be unusual if mucosal thickening were the problem. The findings are due to normal sloping of the roof and lateral wall of the maxillary sinuses, which erroneously suggest mucosal thickening on these slightly steep films.

slanted that pseudothickening of the mucosa is erroneously suggested (Fig. 2.29). The other pitfall lies in the fact that with just the right Waters' projection the floor of the maxillary sinuses appears extremely horizontal, suggesting an air-fluid level.

Ultrasound also has been utilized to determine the degree of aeration of the sinus cavities, but we have not done so. The procedure is not in widespread use.

Rhinitis. Rhinitis is a common problem in the pediatric age group. As with sinusitis, it can be allergic, viral, or bacterial in origin. It is not a radiographic diagnosis. *It becomes important only when it must be differentiated from sinusitis. In this regard, we have found that patients with rhinitis usually have normal paranasal sinuses.*

Acute mastoiditis, in terms of plain films

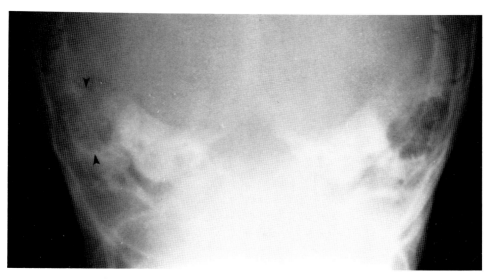

Figure 2.30. *Acute mastoiditis.* Note the hazy, obliterated right mastoid air cells (*arrows*). The mastoid air cells on the left are normal and well aerated. In such cases, often it is difficult to determine whether one is dealing with extensive acute inflammatory disease or early destruction secondary to an abscess.

is best demonstrated on Towne's projection of the skull. In these cases, one has both mastoid areas to compare and acute mastoiditis will be reflected by haziness or obliteration of the mastoid air cells (Fig. 2.30) and, in more acute cases, actual destruction of the bone with abscess formation. Obliteration of the mastoid air cells also occurs with bleeding associated with calvarial trauma and bone destruction as seen with histiocytosis X, leukemia, and lymphoma.

Aeration of the mastoid antra is present at birth and mastoid air cell development occurs rapidly thereafter. Consequently, mastoid air cell aeration usually is present in infants as young as 3 months of age and thus the diagnosis of acute mastoiditis with obliteration of the air cells can be made roentgenographically at this age. In those patients who suffer chronic repeated bouts of otitis media, overall air cell development is impaired, and bony sclerosis supervenes (14). Overall, in these patients, there are fewer aerated air cells, and dense or white appearing petrous bones. Currently, CT scanning more clearly delineates all of these acute and chronic problems (Fig. 2.31).

REFERENCES

1. Arruda, L.K., Mimica, I.M., Sole, D., et al: Abnormal maxillary sinus radiographs in children: Do they represent bacterial infection? Pediatrics 85: 553–558, 1990.
2. Furukawa, C.T., Shapiro, G.G., and Rachelefsky, G.S.: Children with sinusitis. Pediatrics 71: 133–134, 1983.
3. Glasier, C.M., Mallory, G.B., Jr., and Steele, R.W.: Significance of opacification of the maxillary and ethmoid sinuses in infants. J. Pediatr. 114:45–50, 1989.
4. Kogutt, M.S., and Swischuk, L.E.: Diagnosis of sinusitis in infants and children. Pediatrics 52: 121–124, 1973.
5. Kovatch, A.L., Wald, E.R., Ledesma-Medina, J., Chiponis, D.M., and Bedingfield, B.: Maxillary sinus radiographs in children with nonrespiratory complaints. Pediatrics 73: 306–308, 1984.
6. McAlister, W.H., Lusk, R., and Muntz, H.R.: Comparison of plain radiographs and coronal CT scans in infants and children with recurrent sinusitis. A.J.R. 153: 1259–1264, 1989.
7. McLain, D.C.: Sinusitis in children: Lessons from 25 patients. Clin. Pediatr. 9: 342, 1970.
8. Odita, J.C., Akamaguna, A.I., Ogisi, F.O., Amu, O.D., Ugbodaga, C.I.: Pneumatisation of the maxillary sinus in normal and symptomatic children. Pediatr. Radiol. 16: 365–367, 1986.
9. Rachelefsky, G.S., and Shapiro, G.G.: Diseases of the paranasal sinuses in children. In Bierman C.W., and Pearlman, D.S. (eds.): *Allergic Diseases of Infancy, Childhood and Adolescence,* pp. 526–624. W.B. Saunders, Philadelphia, 1980.

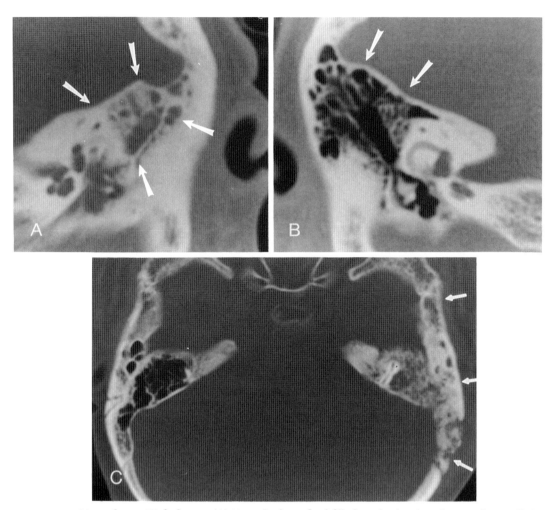

Figure 2.31. *Mastoiditis—CT findings.* (**A**) Note the hazy fluid-filled, underdeveloped mastoid air cells (*arrows*). (**B**) Normal side for comparison. Note the normal-appearing air-filled mastoid air cells (*arrows*). (**C**) Another patient with chronic mastoiditis and extensive destruction of the adjacent calvarium due to osteomyelitis (*arrows*).

10. Rak, K.M., Newell, J.D.II, Yakes, W.F., Damiano, M.A., and Luethke, J.M.: Paranasal sinuses on MR images of the brain: Significance of mucosal thickening. A.J.R. 156: 381–384, 1991.

11. Rulon, J.T.: Sinusitis in children. Postgrad. Med. 48: 107, 1970.

12. Shopfner, C.E., and Rossi, J.O.: Roentgen evaluation of the paranasal sinuses in children. A.J.R. 118: 176–186, 1973.

13. Swischuk, L.E., Hayden, C.K., Jr., and Dillard R.A.: Sinusitis in children. Radiographics 2: 241–252, 1982.

14. Tos, M., Strangerup, S.-E., Hvid, G.: Mastoid pneumatization. Evidence of the environmental theory. Arch. Otolaryngol. 110: 502–507, 1984.

EPISTAXIS

Epistaxis is a common problem in childhood. Most often it results from a simple nosebleed, and no roentgenograms are obtained. However, one should be aware of the fact that juvenile angiofibromas often present with epistaxis and sinusitis (1, 2). These angiofibromas occur most commonly in adolescent boys and, on the lateral roentgenogram of the paranasal sinuses, present as a mass in the nasopharynx (Fig. 2.32). This mass should not be con-

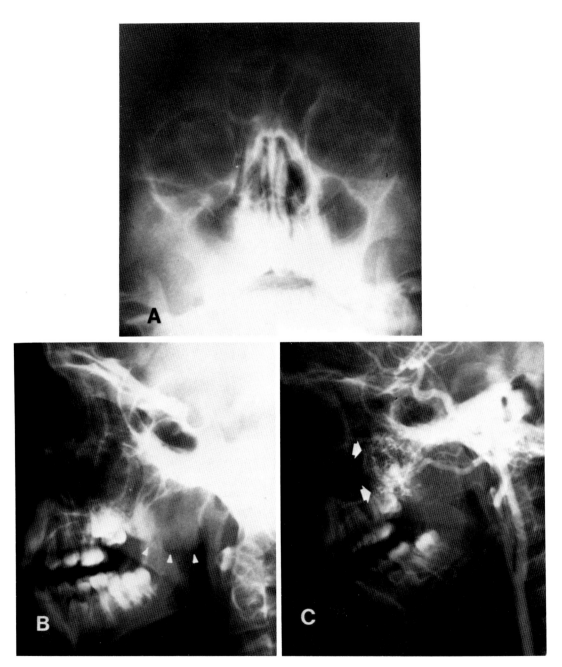

Figure 2.32. *Juvenile angiofibroma of nasopharynx presenting with epistaxis.*   (*A*) Note the partially obliterated right maxillary sinus in this patient with epistaxis. (*B*) Lateral view showing large nasopharyngeal mass (*arrows*), which might be mistaken for large adenoids. (*C*) Subsequent arteriogram demonstrates extensive tumor vascularity (*arrows*) characteristic of this lesion. It is being supplied by the external maxillary artery.

fused with normal adenoidal tissue, which often is very abundant in normal children. Nasopharyngeal angiofibromas are now best defined with magnetic resonance imaging, where high signal, on second echo, T_2-weighted images is characteristic. Nonetheless, angiography still is necessary prior to therapy, which now includes pre-operative embolization.

Epistaxis also may result from an acute or chronic foreign body in the nose, and if such a foreign body is radiolucent, it may remain undetected for extended periods of time. Of course, the most common cause of epistaxis is idiopathic or trauma to the face and nose.

REFERENCES

1. Fitzpatrick, P.J.: The nasopharyngeal angiofibroma. Clin. Radiol. 18: 62–68, 1967.
2. Holman, C.B., and Miller, W.E.: Juvenile nasopharyngeal fibroma: Roentgenologic characteristics. A.J.R. 94: 292–298, 1965.

CHAPTER 3
The Abdomen

Analyzing the abdominal roentgenogram is more difficult and often less rewarding than analyzing the chest roentgenogram, but yet it is an important study. In the chest, symmetry of structures and densities from side to side is of paramount importance, but in the abdomen symmetry is a minor consideration. In the abdomen, it is a matter of becoming familiar with the appearance of relatively fixed organs seen through changing intestinal gas patterns. No one normal configuration looks exactly like another, and the overall "normal" picture comes only through examining many roentgenograms over many years.

In beginning one's assessment of the abdominal roentgenogram, it is worthwhile to localize the stomach, rectum, and both the hepatic and splenic flexures of the colon. These areas of the gastrointestinal tract are relatively fixed, usually contain gas, and look much the same from one patient to another. After this, one should attempt to define the solid abdominal viscera, and of these the easiest to visualize are the liver, spleen, kidneys, psoas muscles, and urinary bladder, if filled (Fig. 3.1). After the abdominal viscera are examined, one should cast an eye over the diaphragmatic leaflets and bony structures such as the vertebrae, ribs, and pelvis. This is especially important in abdominal trauma.

All of the foregoing points are most pertinent to plain films which, of course, will continue to be obtained for the evaluation of acute abdominal problems in children. However, ultrasonography, even more than CT (CT), has come to play a significant role in the evaluation of the acute abdomen in children (1–5). In trauma, however, CT excels over ultrasound. With ultrasonography, almost invariably the first organs to be imaged are the right kidney and liver (Fig. 3.2). Thereafter, the spleen and left kidney are identified and then, primarily in cross-section, one can assess the retroperitoneal structures (Fig. 3.2). The lower abdomen and pelvic regions also can be assessed in longitudinal and cross-section, but to do so, the urinary bladder must be distended, either with urine or with saline introduced by the examiner.

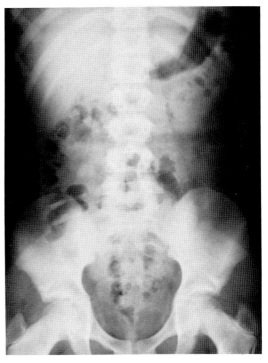

Figure 3.1. *Normal abdomen.* The distribution and volume of gastrointestinal gas is about average. The renal silhouettes are clearly visible and the psoas shadows are seen as broad triangular structures on either side of the spine. A distended urinary bladder is seen in the pelvis.

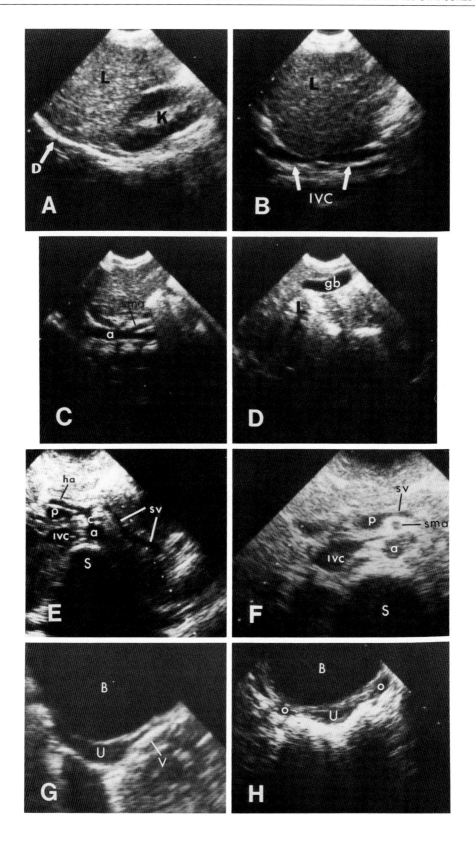

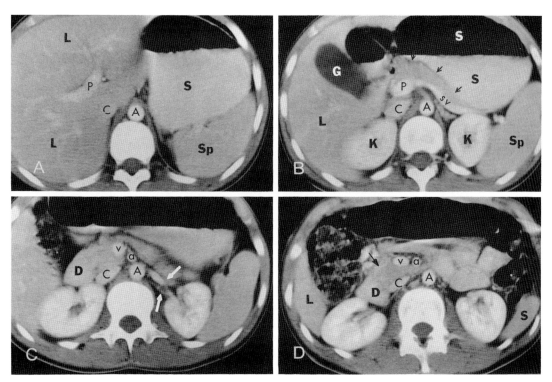

Figure 3.3. *Normal abdomen: CT findings.*   (A) Axial cut through the upper abdomen demonstrates the liver (L), the spleen (Sp), the stomach (S), the aorta (A), the inferior vena cava (C) and the intrahepatic portal vein (P). (B) Slightly lower cut demonstrates many of the same structures, but, in addition, note the gallbladder (G), kidneys (K), the portal vein (p), and the body and tail of the pancreas (*arrows*) lying just anterior to the splenic vein (*sv*). (C) Lower cut demonstrates the duodenum (D), the aorta (A), the inferior vena cava (C), the left renal artery and vein (*arrows*), the superior mesenteric artery (a), and the superior mesenteric vein (v). (D) Many of the previously noted structures are again demonstrated, but specifically note the relationship of the superior mesenteric artery (a) and the superior mesenteric vein (v). Duodenum (D), head of the pancreas (*arrow*). *Continued on next page.*

Figure 3.2. *Normal abdomen: ultrasound.*   (A) Longitudinal scan, *on the right* demonstrates the diaphragm (D), right kidney (K), and liver (L). (B) Longitudinal scan somewhat more medial demonstrates the inferior vena cava (IVC) and liver (L). (C) Longitudinal scan over the aorta demonstrates the aorta (a) and the superior mesenteric artery (sma) branching from it. (D) Another longitudinal scan demonstrates the liver (L) and gallbladder (gb). (E) Transverse scan demonstrates the spine (S), the aorta (a), the celiac artery (c), and the hepatic artery (ha). In addition, note the inferior vena cava (ivc), portal vein confluence (p), and the splenic vein (sv). (F) Another transverse cut demonstrating the spine (S), the aorta (a), and the superior mesenteric artery (sma). Characteristically, the superior mesenteric artery is surrounded by a collar of echogenicity. Also note the portal vein confluence (p), the inferior vena cava (ivc), and the splenic vein (sv). (F) Another transverse cut demonstrating the spine (S), the aorta (a), and the superior mesenteric artery (sma). Characteristically, the superior mesenteric artery is surrounded by a collar of echogenicity. Also note the portal vein confluence (p), the inferior vena cava (ivc), and the splenic vein (sv). The thin sonolucent steak heading medially from the inferior vena cava is the left renal vein. The pancreas lies above the splenic vein but is not clearly delineated here. (G) Longitudinal scan in the pelvis demonstrates the bladder (B), the uterus (U), and the vagina (V). The thin, sonolucent channel in the vagina is the vaginal lumen. (H) Transverse scan in the pelvis demonstrates the urinary bladder (B), the uterus (U), and both ovaries (o).

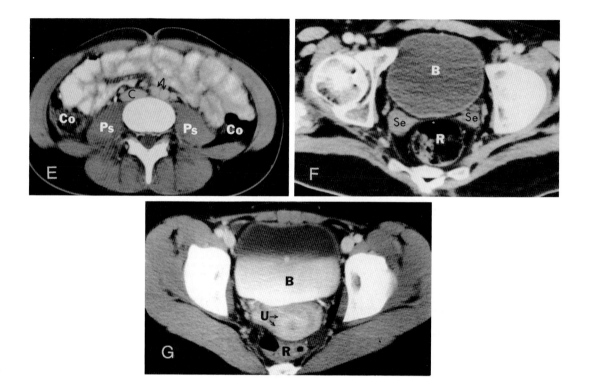

Figure 3.3 *Normal abdomen: CT findings—continued.* (*E*) Axial cut just above the iliac wings demonstrates the inferior vena cava (*C*), the iliac arteries (*arrows*), the ascending and descending colon (*Co*), and the psoas muscles (*Ps*). (*F*) Pelvis in male. Note the bladder (*B*), rectum (*R*), and the prominent seminal vesicles (*Se*). (*G*) Axial pelvic cut in female demonstrates the bladder (*B*), rectum (*R*), and uterus (*U*).

Computerized tomography yields cross-sectional anatomical data and, while it is quite useful in adults, it is less useful in infants and young children because usually there is less fat present. Because of this, separation of the various intra-abdominal structures from one another is not as rewarding as in adults. Nonetheless, it still is a very important imaging modality and one should be familiar with the anatomy, as demonstrated with CT (Fig. 3.3).

REFERENCES

1. Mendelson, R.M., and Lindsell, D.R.M.: Ultrasound examination of the paediatric "acute abdomen": preliminary findings. Br. J. Radiol. 60: 414–416, 1987.
2. See, C.C., Glassman, M., Berezin, S., Inamdar S., and Newman, L.J.: Emergency ultrasound in the evaluation of acute-onset abdominal pain in children. Pediatr. Emerg. Care 4: 169–171, 1988.
3. Seibert, J.J., Williamson, S.L., Golladay, E.S., Mollitt, D.L., Seibert, R.W., and Sutterfield, S.L.: The distended gasless abdomen: A fertile field for ultrasound. J. Ultrasound Med. 5: 301–308, 1986.
4. Shanon, A., Martin, D.J., and Feldman, W.: Ultrasonographic studies in the management of recurrent abdominal pain. Pediatrics 86: 35–38, 1990.
5. Simeone, J.F., Noveline, R.A., and Ferrucci, J.T., Jr.: Comparison of sonography and plain films in evaluation of the acute abdomen. A.J.R. 144: 49–52, 1985.

ACUTE ABDOMINAL PROBLEMS

Examination of the acute abdomen, regardless of cause, *requires supine and upright views of the abdomen, and both postero-anterior and lateral views of the chest.* This combined examination should never be cut short, and if the patient's condition is such that upright films are impossible to obtain, *cross-table lateral or decubitus views should be substituted. There is no room for a compromise, and he who cuts the examination short will regret it sooner or later.* The concept of a lesser examination (1) has no place in the evaluation of the acute abdomen in infants and children. After evaluation of these plain films, one's best imaging tool is ultrasound where a negative study is as important as a positive study. Negative studies are helpful when clinical findings are equivocal, for they add support to the final impression that not much of significance is going on.

REFERENCE

1. Mirvis, S.E., Young, J.W.R., Keramati, B., McCrea, E.S., and Tarr, R.: Plain film evaluation of patients with abdominal pain: Are three radiographs necessary? A.J.R. 147: 501–503, 1986.

ABNORMAL INTRALUMINAL GAS PATTERNS

Airless Abdomen. An airless abdomen usually is abnormal, and most often results from excessive vomiting and/or diarrhea (Fig. 3.4). Many times this occurs with gastroenteritis (1, 2, 4, 8), but an airless abdomen also can be seen in the early stages of acute appendicitis. It is also a feature of the adrenogenital syndrome in young infants (14) and of Addison's disease. Less

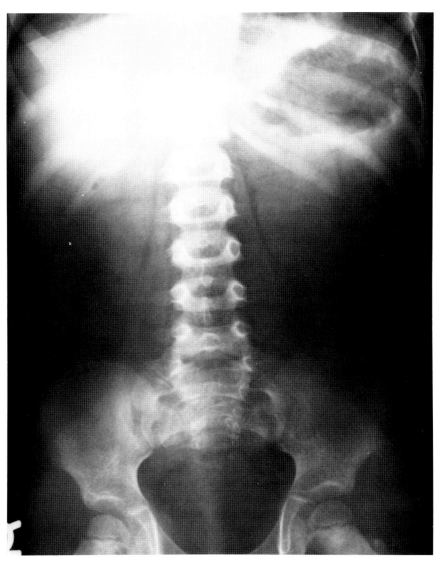

Figure 3.4. *Airless abdomen.* Gas is present in the stomach only (*left upper quadrant*). Most often, an airless abdomen is seen with gastroenteritis or acute appendicitis; this patient had gastroenteritis.

commonly, a relatively airless abdomen is seen in patients with such a degree of cerebral depression that swallowing is markedly impaired (2).

Paralytic Ileus. Generalized paralytic ileus can be seen with gastroenteritis, intestinal ischemia, neurogenic spinal shock, and conditions such as sepsis and hypokalemia (11). Paralytic ileus differs from mechanical ileus (mechanical obstruction) in that there is no differential distension of the gastrointestinal tract. In other words, all portions of the gastrointestinal tract dilate in proportion to each other, and in the classic case the colon remains larger than the small bowel (Fig. 3.5). Furthermore, the picture of dilated intestinal loops is much less orderly than in mechanical obstruction, for, generally speaking, many more loops are dilated. Indeed, in many

cases, dilated, disorganized, sluggish, intestinal loops seem to be present from top to bottom and side to side. On upright view, numerous air-fluid levels are seen, but the majority appear rather "inactive" and tend to extend over long lengths of bowel. In this regard, they are quite different from the short fluid levels seen in the acute, inverted, hairpin loops of the distended bowel seen with classic mechanical obstruction (Fig. 3.6).

The preceding description of the roentgenographic appearance of generalized paralytic ileus is more or less classic, but by no means the only one seen. Indeed, paralytic ileus can be quite variable and, in some cases, so localized that obstruction is suggested. Most often, this occurs with gastroenteritis (see Fig. 3.11B), and in such cases close clinical-roentgenographic

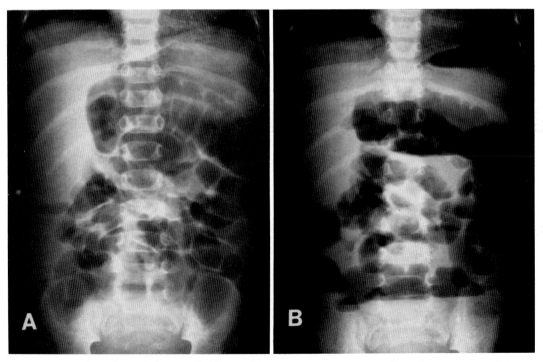

Figure 3.5. *Paralytic ileus.* (*A*) Distended loops of intestine are present everywhere, but proportional distension persists and the transverse colon (uppermost loop of distended intestine) remains larger than the numerous loops of distended small bowel. (*B*) Upright view showing numerous sluggish, long air-fluid levels scattered throughout the abdomen. Compare this adynamic appearance with the dynamic appearance of mechanical obstruction seen in Figure 3.6.

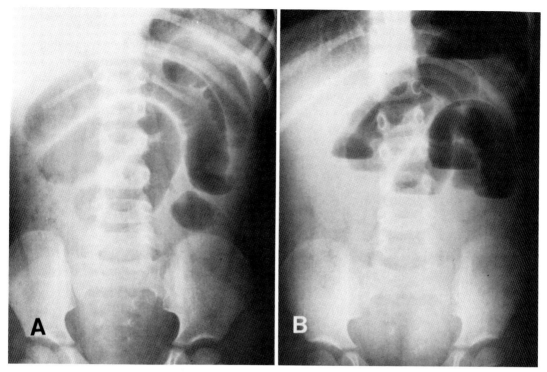

Figure 3.6. *Mechanical ileus.* (*A*) Note the well-organized loops of distended small bowel in the upper abdomen. No gas is seen distal to these loops which are arranged in the so-called "stepladder" configuration. (*B*) Upright view showing persistence of the orderly pattern with acute inverted "U" or "hairpin" loops characteristic of mechanically obstructed intestine. Also note that the air-fluid levels within any given loop are at different heights.

correlation is mandatory, for otherwise, roentgenographic misinterpretations will be common.

Mechanical Ileus. As compared with paralytic ileus, the pattern of distended intestinal loops in mechanical obstruction is much more orderly, especially when one is dealing with small bowel obstruction (6, 7, 13). With low colonic obstruction, if ileocecal valve incompetence is present, there may be less orderliness and more difficulty in differentiating the findings from those of paralytic ileus, but in the classic case of small bowel obstruction, the findings are rather typical (Fig. 3.6). The number of dilated loops visualized depends on the level of obstruction, but, in any case, the loops are discretely visualized and rather orderly in appearance. If, as often occurs on

the supine view, the loops are stacked one over the other, the term "stepladder" is applied to the configuration. In those cases where obstruction has existed for a long enough period of time, no gas will be seen distal to the obstruction, but if the duration of obstruction is short, or if the obstruction is incomplete, some gas may be seen in loops of intestine distal to the site of obstruction. Of course, these latter intestinal loops will not be distended, or at least not as distended as the more proximal obstructed loops.

On upright view, the loops of intestine form acute, hairpin loops with short air-fluid levels visible in both limbs of any given loop (Fig. 3.6). In addition, these fluid levels usually are at different heights in the two limbs of any given loop of intestine. This clearly demonstrates that mechanical obstruction is an active or dynamic process. In other words, in their effort to overcome the obstruction, the loops show hyperperistalsis, and as the intestinal contents churn back and forth, the air-fluid levels are captured at different heights in each limb of a loop.

The classic case of well-developed intestinal obstruction is not difficult to recognize and, indeed, the radiologist's real job is to detect obstructions before they reach this stage. This represents a true challenge, for in such cases signs of obstruction are much more subtle. Indeed, in some cases the loop, or loops, are quite inconspicuous, and unless the roentgenogram is closely scrutinized they will be missed (Fig. 3.7). Such loops can be considered sentinel loops (see p. 194), and their presence may be confirmed with upright films (Fig. 3.7). In those children too ill to be placed in the upright position, decubitus or cross-table views can be helpful.

One other point regarding obstructed loops of intestine is in order. In some cases, very little air is present in the distended intestinal loops, for they are filled with fluid. The loops of intestine may be seen as vague opaque sausage-like structures in the abdomen. On upright views, as the small amount of gas becomes trapped between the valvulae conniventes, a "string-of-beads" sign results (Fig. 3.8). On ultraso-

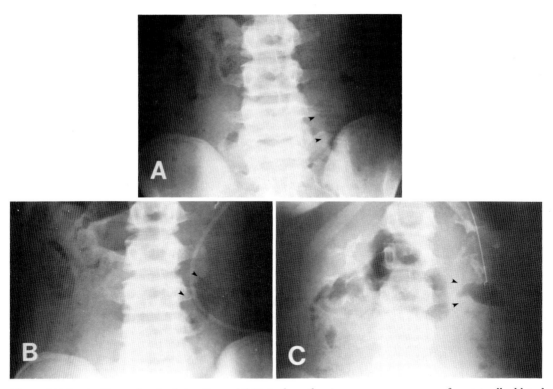

Figure 3.7. *Sentinel loop of early obstruction.* (*A*) Note the rather innocuous appearance of a minimally dilated loop of small intestine, just to the left of the lumbar spine (*arrows*). Transverse opaque lines representing the valvulae conniventes identify the loop as being dilated jejunum. On any one film, this loop probably would be dismissed as an incidental finding. (*B*) However, later in the day the same loop is visible in the same general location (*arrows*). (*C*) The next day on an upright view obtained during an intravenous pyelogram, note that the isolated loop is present again (*arrows*). The presence of this one loop of distended jejunum on three separate, well-spaced occasions is very significant; this patient had a small bowel obstruction secondary to adhesions from a previous laparotomy.

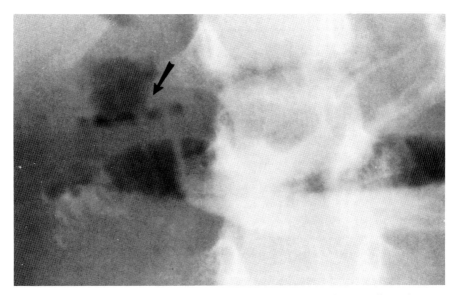

Figure 3.8. *"String-of-beads" sign.* On this upright view, note the string-of-beads effect of air trapped in between the valvulae conniventes (*arrow*).

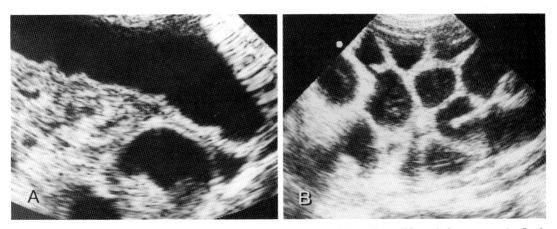

Figure 3.9. *Dilated small bowel: ultrasonographic demonstration.* (*A*) With small bowel obstruction, the fluid-filled loops are large and show considerable peristalsis. (*B*) With paralytic ileus, the fluid-filled loops are more numerous, of more uniform size, and show far less in the way of peristalsis.

nography, such fluid-filled loops may be seen as markedly dilated, anechoic circular or sausage-like hyperperistaltic structures (Fig. 3.9A). With paralytic ileus, more uniform, circular, and less dilated loops are seen, and peristalsis is diminished (Fig. 3.9B).

After determining that an intestinal obstruction is present, the second job for the roentgenologist is to determine its level.

This is relatively easily accomplished with gastric and duodenal obstructions, but with small bowel and colonic obstructions it may be more difficult. Generally speaking, however, the number of loops visualized in these cases is the best clue to the level of obstruction: i.e., the lower the obstruction, the more loops will one see. In those cases of low small bowel obstruction where differentiation from colonic obstruction is difficult, one should not waste time in trying to make the decision from plain films alone. A contrast study of the colon is most helpful in these cases and should be performed on an emergent basis. With such a study, one clearly can identify problems such as sigmoid volvulus, intussusception, Hirschsprung's disease, etc. Later one might even employ a barium meal and/or enterolysis for detecting poorly defined or elusive small bowel obstructions (3, 10).

Mixed Paralytic and Mechanical Ileus. In some patients with a mechanical obstruction there is some supervening systemic illness such as sepsis or peritonitis, which may then predispose the patient to a mixed picture of paralytic and mechanical ileus. In these cases, the abdominal film findings may be difficult to interpret, and close clinical correlation is required.

Closed Loop Obstruction. When a loop of intestine is obstructed at both ends, it is termed a closed loop obstruction. In many of these cases, the intestinal loop becomes strangulated and gangrenous before the obstruction is diagnosed. Consequently, a closed loop obstruction is one of the most serious forms of mechanical obstruction of the intestinal tract, and the condition must be recognized early. Closed loop obstructions can occur with colonic or small bowel volvulus, internal hernias, or when loops of intestine twist around congenital peritoneal bands or postoperative adhesions.

Roentgenographically, the hallmark of closed loop obstruction is the presence of a fixed, dilated loop of bowel, frequently assuming the configuration of the letter "U" or a "coffee bean" (9, 12). If such a loop is all that is visualized the diagnosis is relatively easy (Fig. 3.10), but if a more classic small bowel obstruction begins to develop behind the strangulated loop, the loop itself may be more difficult to isolate. In other cases, the loop is full of fluid, and although it still may occasionally retain its "coffee bean" configuration, more often it

produces a less specific mass on the abdominal roentgenograms. A similar mass-like configuration results if the loop of intestine becomes ischemic and extremely edematous.

Sentinel Loop. The sentinel loop usually refers to a segment of intestine that becomes paralyzed and dilated as it lies next to an inflamed intra-abdominal organ (15). It represents short segment paralytic ileus, and because it alerts one to the presence of an adjacent inflammatory process, it has been termed the "sentinel" loop. In the *right upper quadrant,* the sentinel loop can be seen with cholecystitis, pyelonephritis, and hepatic inflammatory or traumatic disease, while in the *left upper quadrant,* it is usually seen with pancreatitis, pyelonephritis, or splenic injury. In the *right lower quadrant,* the sentinel loop classically occurs with appendicitis, Meckel's diverticulitis, and regional enteritis. Sentinel loops in the *left lower quadrant* are much less common, but in the lower abdomen in female patients, genital problems such as salpingitis and hemorrhagic or torsed ovarian cysts or tumors also can produce a sentinel loop. In the **upper midabdomen**, most sentinel loops are seen with pancreatitis or trauma to the duodenum.

Roentgenographically, sentinel loops are visualized as isolated loops of distended intestine (Fig. 3.11A). However, it is most important that when a sentinel loop is suspected it be demonstrated to remain in one general position from film to film, for although the loops of distended intestine in these cases are not absolutely fixed, they should remain in the same general vicinity on repeated views. This is most important, for it is not unusual to see isolated loops of dilated intestine fortuitously present on a single film of some patients (Fig. 3.11B). Such loops can appear in perfectly normal individuals or in patients with gastroenteritis, and thus it is only when a sentinel loop persists that it is significant. Because of this, the sentinel loop must be assessed with caution and clinical correla-

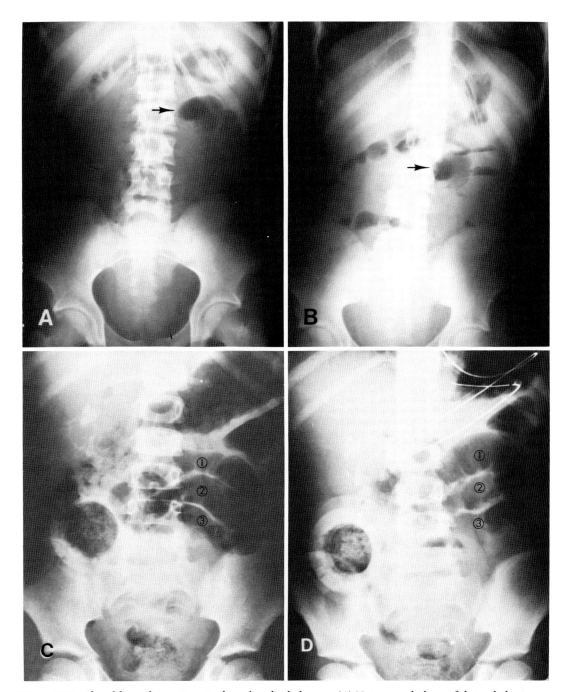

Figure 3.10. *Closed loop obstruction: single and multiple loops.* (*A*) Note a single loop of distended jejunum (*arrow*) in this child with a closed loop obstruction. A nasogastric tube is present in the stomach. (*B*) On upright view, note that the loop does not change position or configuration (*arrow*) and that its tapered end suggests a twisted or volved loop. One or two other loops of distended intestine with air-fluid levels are visualized, but it is the unchanging loop identified by the *arrows* that is most significant in indicating the presence of a closed loop obstruction. (*C*) Another patient with postoperative adhesions leading to a closed loop obstruction. Note the 1-2-3 arrangement of the distended loops of small bowel. (*D*) On upright view, this arrangement is essentially the same (i.e., fixed loops). Also note the colostomy bag and calculi in the right kidney.

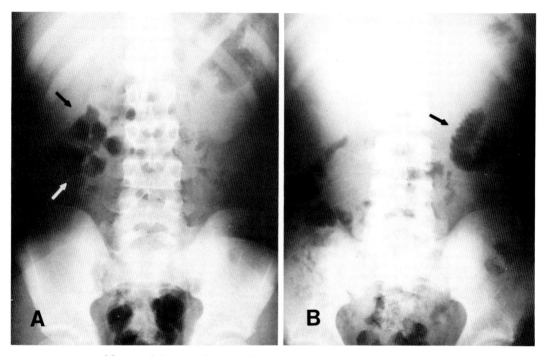

Figure 3.11. *Sentinel loops.* (*A*) Sentinel loops adjacent to intra-abdominal inflammation. In this patient with suspected appendicitis, note the presence of a number of dilated loops of intestine in the right flank (*arrows*). These are sentinel loops lying adjacent to an inflamed retrocecal appendix. (*B*) *Pseudosentinel loop*—fortuitous demonstration of an isolated loop of distended intestine. Note the single loop of distended jejunum on the left side of the abdomen (*arrow*) of this patient with gastroenteritis. Such fortuitous demonstration of a transiently dilated loop (or loops) of small bowel is not uncommon in gastroenteritis.

tion, for on as many occasions as it is helpful, on an equal number it can be misleading.

A special form of the sentinel loop occurs as the so-called *colon "cutoff" sign.* Most often this sign has been said to occur in the left transverse colon with pancreatitis, but it also can be seen on the right side with perforated appendicitis (see Fig. 3.50).

A sentinel loop also can be seen in early intestinal obstruction. In such cases, the visualized loop is the leading (sentinel) loop of an early intestinal obstruction and as such is quite valuable. However, often it is overlooked, for it may be difficult to detect (see Fig. 3.7).

Acute Gastric Dilatation. Acute gastric dilatation can be seen in extremely sick individuals and reflects a profound degree of localized paralytic ileus. It can be a lethal condition, for it induces a vagal re-

sponse that may result in cardiorespiratory arrest. Consequently, prompt treatment with nasogastric tube decompression is in order. Not all cases of a grossly dilated stomach represent acute gastric dilatation, however. Indeed, dilatation of the stomach is commonly seen in gastroenteritis (see Fig. 3.41), some normal infants, and in infants and children with respiratory distress. In these latter cases, the finding results from excessive air swallowing. In addition, it has been noted that acute gastric dilatation can occur in neglected children (14). In these cases, gastric dilatation usually occurs after the first full meal (14). Evidently the stomach is not able to handle this unusually large load, perhaps because there is some atrophy of the gastric muscle in these children (14). Once they get over the acute episode, they usually do not have further problems.

REFERENCES

1. Benson, H.H., and Jacobson, G.: Deficiency of small intestinal gas simulating obstruction. A.J.R. 82: 450–454, 1952.

2. Burko, H.: Toxic depression of the newborn causing deficient intestinal gas pattern. A.J.R. 88: 575–578, 1962.

3. Eklof, O., and Ringertz, H.: The value of barium enema in establishing nature and level of intestinal obstruction. Pediatr. Radiol. 3: 6–11, 1975.

4. Feinberg, S.B., et al.: Dehydration and deficiency of intestinal gas in infants. A.J.R. 76: 551–554, 1956.

5. Franken, E.A., Jr., Fox, M., Smith, J.A., and Smith, W.L.: Acute gastric dilatation in neglected children. A.J.R. 130: 297–299, 1978.

6. Hodges, P.C., and Miller, R.E.: Intestinal obstruction. A.J.R. 74: 1015–1025, 1955.

7. Levin, B.: Mechanical small bowel obstruction. Semin. Roentgenol. 8: 281–297, 1973.

8. Margulis, A., et al.: Deficiency of intestinal gas in infants with diarrhea. Radiology 66: 93–96, 1956.

9. Mellins, H.Z., and Rigler, L.G.: The roentgen signs in strangulating obstructions of the small intestine. A.J.R. 71: 404–415, 1954.

10. Nelson, S.W., and Christoforidis, A.J.: The use of barium sulfate suspensions in the study of suspected mechanical obstruction of the small intestine. A.J.R. 101: 367–378, 1967.

11. Preeyasombat, C., Pitchayayothin, N., and Viravekin, A.: Hypokalemic crisis simulating intestinal obstruction in a 4-year old girl. Am. J. Dis. Child. 130: 1143–1145, 1976.

12. Rigler, L.: Roentgen diagnosis of acute abdominal conditions. Bull. Univ. Minn. Hosp. 16: 120, 1944.

13. Schwartz, S.S.: The differential diagnosis of intestinal obstruction. Semin. Roentgenol. 8: 323–338, 1973.

14. Weens, H.S., and Golden, A.: Adrenal cortical insufficiency in infants simulating high intestinal obstruction. A.J.R. 74: 213–219, 1955.

15. Young, B.R.: Significance of regional or reflex ileus in roentgen diagnosis of cholecystitis, perforated ulcer, pancreatitis and appendiceal abscess, as determined by survey examination of acute abdomen. A.J.R. 78: 581–586, 1957.

ABNORMAL EXTRALUMINAL GAS PATTERNS

Extraluminal air may lie in the intestinal wall itself (intramural) or, more often, completely outside the intestine. In the latter cases, such air may be seen in the peritoneal cavity or retroperitoneal space and as such signifies the presence of a gastrointestinal perforation. Extraluminal, intramural air (pneumatosis cystoides intestinalis) usually is associated with a loss of intestinal mucosal integrity secondary to intestinal ischemia or severe inflammation with resulting necrotizing enterocolitis. However, pneumatosis cystoides intestinalis also is seen in the absence of these problems and as such is termed "benign pneumatosis."

Portal vein gas most often occurs in association with intestinal infarction or necrotizing enterocolitis, while biliary tree air usually is seen with intestinal obstructions around the duodenum, distal to the ampulla of Vater.

Pneumoperitoneum (Free Peritoneal Air). Pneumoperitoneum usually signifies the presence of gastrointestinal tract perforation but also occasionally can be seen secondary to pneumomediastinum. Gastrointestinal perforations usually occur with peptic ulcer disease, inflammatory disease such as Meckel's diverticulitis and appendicitis, foreign body ingestion, and abdominal trauma. Roentgenographically, the findings are virtually the same as in adults, but, in general, perforations resulting from nontraumatic causes are not nearly as common in children as in adults (33).

In the *supine position*, it is surprising to see how large a collection of free air may remain undetected. Such large collections are most likely to occur in neonates and very young infants with gastric or colonic perforation, but the problem also can occur with small intestinal perforation associated with obstruction. In any of these cases, one may note an extremely sharp, almost diagrammatic appearance to a generally hyperlucent abdomen (Fig. 3.12). In addition, the falciform ligament (30), urachus (15), or as an inverted "v," the inferior epigastric arteries or lateral umbilical ligaments (3, 37) can be outlined by air. Air also can collect in the fossa for the ligamentum teres as a vertical stripe of air over the liver (6). The overall configuration of massive pneumoperitoneum, as it appears on

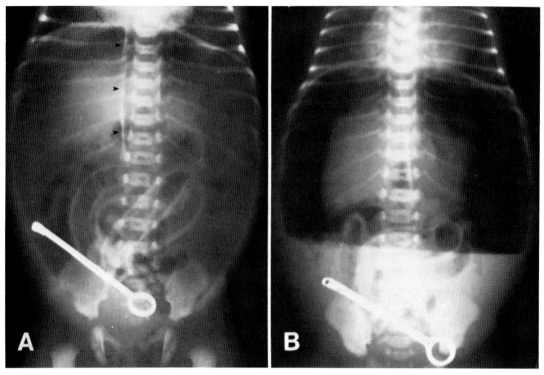

Figure 3.12. *Massive pneumoperitoneum: supine film findings.* (*A*) Note the hyperlucent appearance of the entire abdomen. Both aspects of the walls of the loops of intestine clustered in the center of the abdomen are well visualized. Because of this they appear as discrete linear and curvilinear white stripes. A similar phenomenon is seen along the falciform ligament (*arrows*). This aesthetically pleasing, almost diagrammatic appearance of the roentgenogram is characteristic of massive pneumoperitoneum, but is overlooked with surprising regularity. (*B*) Upright view confirms the presence of a massive volume of free air in the peritoneal cavity. Note how the liver, spleen, and stomach have been compressed centrally.

the supine roentgenogram of these infants, often receives one or other of the following descriptive terms: "saddlebag" or "football" sign (24).

In addition to the findings just noted, one usually will see loops of intestine with their walls outlined by air on both sides (28): that is, both their serosal and mucosal surfaces (Fig. 3.12A). Indeed, it is this latter finding that becomes most useful in the older child with lesser volumes of free air who is examined in the supine position, but before proceeding to this problem, one or two more points regarding massive pneumoperitoneum in the young infant are in order. In some of these infants, air may extend into the scrotum or groin, for the processus vaginalis is patent in male infants of this age, and in other infants, the abdominal viscera, especially the liver and spleen, become compressed toward the center of the abdomen. This latter finding often is more readily appreciated on upright or cross-table lateral views (Fig. 3.12B).

In the older child with lesser volumes of free air in the peritoneal cavity, the most useful finding on the supine film is visualization of both the outer and inner aspects of a dilated loop of intestine (Fig. 3.13). However, a word of caution is in order regarding this sign, for it also can be present in the absence of pneumoperitoneum in children with grossly distended intestines. In such cases, one loop is visualized through another (8), and because these loops contain so much air, segments of the bowel wall appear to be outlined by air on both sides (Fig. 3.14). In other cases of

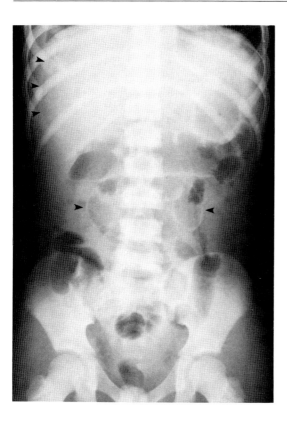

Figure 3.13. *Small volume pneumoperitoneum: supine film findings.* Note the *fine white line* representing intestinal wall (*lower arrows*) visualized in this manner because air is present both inside the lumen of the intestine and along its outer surface in the peritoneal cavity. Also note the presence of free air overlying the liver anteriorly (*upper arrows*). A similar parahepatic collection of air can be seen in Figure 3.16A. There also is a pleural effusion in the right costophrenic angle of this patient.

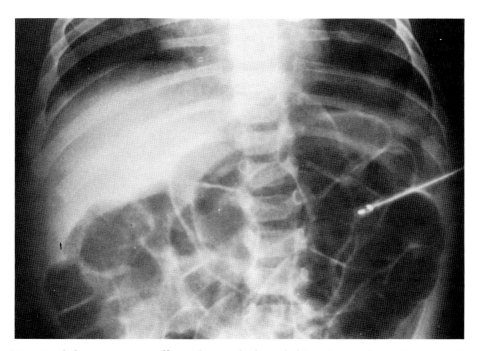

Figure 3.14. *Pseudofree air on supine film.* The grossly distended intestines in this patient cause the walls of each loop to be projected through other loops. This being the case, the walls appear to be outlined by air on both sides. However, no free air is present, but the finding is misleading and often misinterpreted as free air.

pneumoperitoneum, air will be seen to collect over the anterior surface, or along the inferior aspect, of the liver (21), and as such will appear as a variety of formless or linear parahepatic collections of air (Figs. 3.13, 3.15, and 3.16A).

On *upright view*, of course, free air characteristically collects beneath the diaphragmatic leaflets (Fig. 3.16), but if upright positioning is impossible to accomplish because of the patient's condition, *cross-table lateral or decubitus views* will demonstrate the same findings (Fig. 3.17). Indeed, with proper upright or decubitus positioning, it is said that as little as 1 cc of free air can be detected. Of course, the patient must remain in one of these positions for more than just a few seconds, for otherwise the air will not trickle up to the uppermost portion of the abdomen.

Small volume collections of air beneath the diaphragmatic leaflet (Fig. 3.18A) must be differentiated from certain normal, almost artifactual findings. One of these occurs when a diaphragmatic leaflet is visualized just over the lower edge of a rib (Fig. 3.18B), while the other occurs when the gastric bubble is visualized under the left diaphragmatic leaflet (Fig. 3.18C). In differentiating the stomach bubble from pneumoperitoneum, it should be noted that the combined thickness of the distended stomach and diaphragm usually is thicker than that of the diaphragm alone (Fig. 3.18C).

Most cases of pneumoperitoneum eventually are associated with peritonitis, for they result from perforation of the gastrointestinal tract, but occasionally one can encounter pneumoperitoneum without

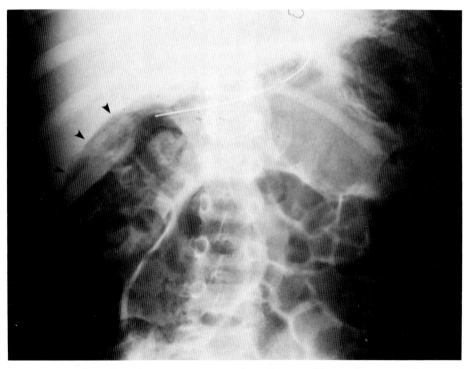

Figure 3.15. *Free air under inferior liver margin.*   Note the collection of free air lying just inferior to the lower aspect of the liver (*arrows*). Also note the presence of pneumatosis cystoides intestinalis in this patient. It is visualized best as curvilinear and bubbly collections of intramural gas in the splenic flexure. This patient was severely burned and demonstrated so-called "benign" pneumatosis cystoides intestinalis secondary to profound distension of the intestines. The free air was a complication of the pneumatosis.

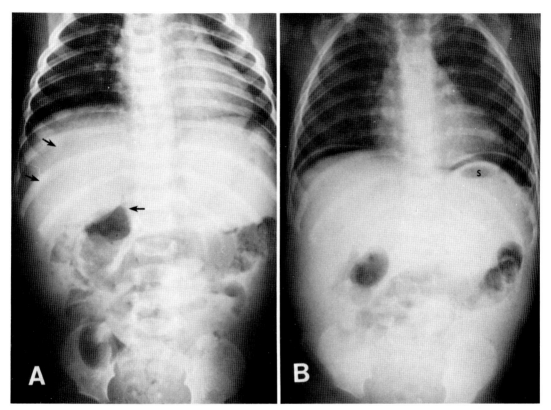

Figure 3.16. *Free peritoneal air: utilizing the upright view.* (*A*) On this supine view, it may be difficult to detect that free air is present. However, some is present over the anterior aspect of the liver (*upper arrows*), and some can be seen under the liver along its inferior medial aspect (*lower arrow*). Actually, the air probably outlines the gallbladder. (*B*) Upright positioning clearly identifies the presence of free air as it accumulates in characteristic fashion under both diaphragmatic leaflets. Stomach air bubble (*S*).

peritonitis. This can occur with pneumatosis cystoides intestinalis, pneumomediastinum, and after laparotomy. With regard to pneumatosis cystoides intestinalis, it is not the intestine that perforates, but merely the outer serosal surface, and thus free air may escape into the peritoneal cavity but no intestinal content escapes.

The mechanism of pneumoperitoneum in cases of pneumomediastinum is poorly understood, but it has been suggested that air may track into the abdomen along the aorta and abdominal vessels, or that there may actually be a congenital pleural-peritoneal communication present. At any rate, whatever the precise etiology, massive amounts of peritoneal air can accumulate this way, and it is remarkable that both the pneumomediastinum and pneumoperitoneum so incurred can remain rather silent. In addition, in some of these cases the presence of the initial lesion, that is, pneumomediastinum, may be difficult to detect, and only the pneumoperitoneum will be seen.

Retroperitoneal Free Air. Free air in the retroperitoneal space is much less commonly encountered than is free intraperitoneal air. Often such air layers itself against the psoas muscles or kidneys (Fig. 3.19), and in the more subtle cases can be missed even by the experienced observer. Retroperitoneal free air can be seen with perforation of the duodenum, retrocecal

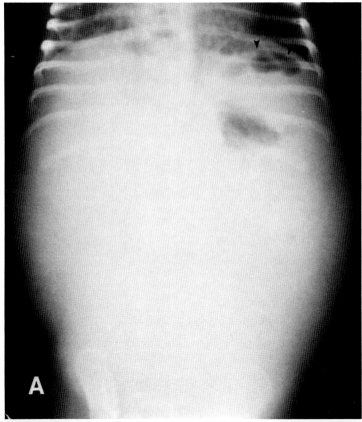

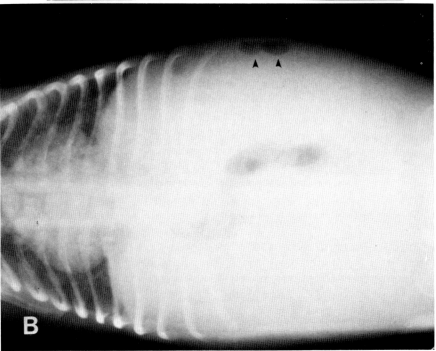

Figure 3.17. *Free peritoneal air: value of decubitus views.* (*A*) In this patient with intestinal perforation and peritonitis, the presence of free air in the abdominal cavity may be difficult to detect. However, the air demarcated by the *arrows* will turn out to be free air on the decubitus view. (*B*) Decubitus view demonstrating how the collection of free air has shifted in position and come to lie just below the abdominal wall (*arrows*).

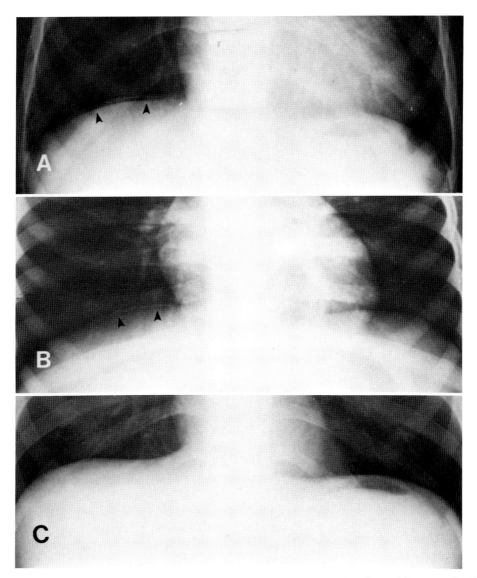

Figure 3.18. *Small volume pneumoperitoneum versus artifact.* (*A*) Note the thin sliver of free air under the right diaphragmatic leaflet (*arrows*). Note how thin the diaphragmatic leaflet appears. (*B*) Pseudo-free air resulting from superimposition of the top of the right diaphragmatic leaflet over the lower aspect of the underlying rib (*arrows*). (*C*) Pseudopneumoperitoneum produced by gas in the stomach. Note that the white line (*arrows*) above the collection of gas in the stomach is thicker than that seen in (*A*). It is thicker because it represents both gastric wall and diaphragmatic leaflet. The bolus of food present in the stomach further adds to the illusion that free air is present under the diaphragmatic leaflet.

appendicitis, or perforation of the rectum (Fig. 3.19*B*). It also can be seen with pneumomediastinum (Fig. 3.19*A*).

On supine view, when retroperitoneal air collects beneath the diaphragmatic leaflet, the leaflet itself is outlined (Fig. 3.19*A*). In addition, in some cases one can see oblique striations crossing over the liver area, representing air between the muscle bundles of the diaphragm (7). One also may visualize the inferior aspect of the heart border as a clear, distinct line (19).

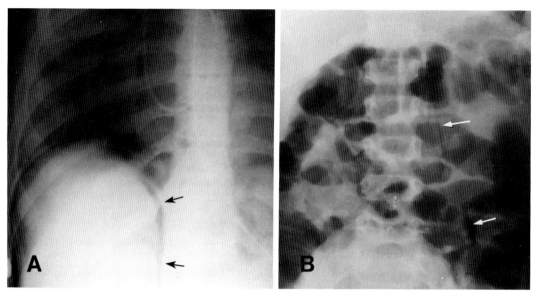

Figure 3.19. *Retroperitoneal air.* (*A*) Note air outlining the liver, right diaphragmatic leaflet, and right kidney (*arrow*). This air tracked from a pneumomediastinum resulting from ventilator therapy in a patient with a closed head injury. (*B*) Another patient with retroperitoneal air along the left psoas muscle (*arrows*). This resulted from a rectal perforation in a battered child.

Intramural Air (Pneumatosis Cystoides Intestinalis). "Pneumatosis cystoides intestinalis" is a term utilized to designate the presence of intramural gas. Most frequently such gas is seen with loss of mucosal integrity as incurred by extensive inflammatory or ischemic disease of the intestine, and classically it is a feature of necrotizing enterocolitis of the newborn infant (27, 29, 31, 32, 36). In these latter cases, intramural air is believed to represent gas formed by an overgrowth of bacteria in the bowel wall, and often such air first appears in the terminal ileum and ascending colon. Pneumatosis cystoides intestinalis secondary to enterocolitis also is seen in some infants with Hirschsprung's disease, and is a feature of ischemia induced by mechanical catastrophes such as closed loop strangulation or intestinal volvulus.

Pneumatosis intestinalis also can be seen in older infants and children (38) in association with intestinal obstruction (29), collagen vascular diseases (10, 11, 23, 25, 26), cystic fibrosis (11, 38, 39, 42), leuke-mia, steroid or other immunosuppressive therapy (2, 11, 14, 16, 20), gastroenteritis (5), and occasionally with perforated duodenal ulcer or jejunal diverticula (4). With intestinal obstruction, simple overdistension is believed to lead to mucosal tears and leakage of intraluminal gas into the bowel wall. Most often, this is seen with chronic small bowel obstructions. Dilatation with loss of integrity of the mucosa also is believed to lead to pneumatosis cystoides intestinalis in children with collagen vascular diseases, but it should be noted that some of these patients also may develop pneumatosis cystoides intestinalis secondary to intestinal ischemia and necrotizing enterocolitis (10, 19).

Pneumatosis cystoides intestinalis in cystic fibrosis and in children on steroids or other immunosuppressive therapy is of unknown etiology. With immunosuppressive therapy, it has been suggested that atrophy of submucosal lymphoid tissue may render the mucosa prone to tear more easily with overdistension. Pneumatosis cystoides intestinalis secondary to pneumomediasti-

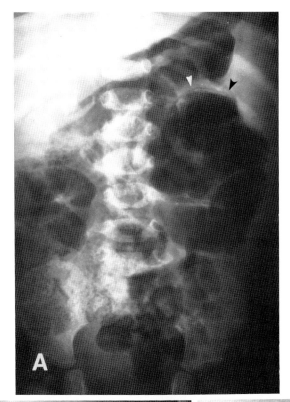

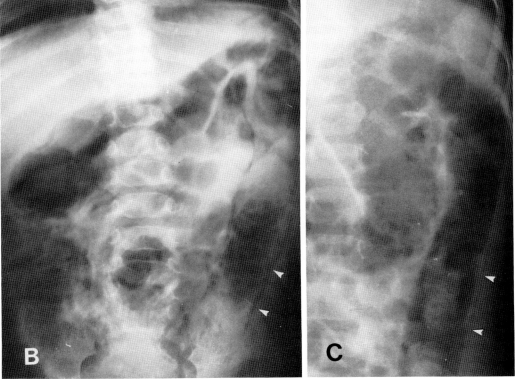

Figure 3.20. *Pneumatosis cystoides intestinalis (intramural air).* (**A**) Note classic curvilinear collections of air within distended loops of intestine (*arrows*). The bubbly pattern over the remainder of the abdomen often is misinterpreted as feces mixed with air, but actually represents another configuration of pneumatosis cystoides intestinalis. (**B**) Typical curvilinear collections of free air are seen in the ascending colon, while linear collections of air are noted in the descending colon (*arrows*). (**C**) *Normal properitoneal fat line* mimicking pneumatosis cystoides intestinalis. In this normal infant, the properitoneal fat line (*arrows*) might be misinterpreted for pneumatosis cystoides intestinalis.

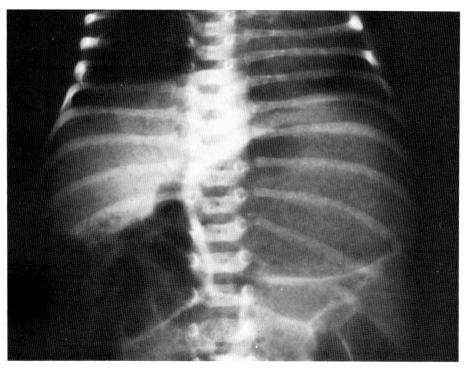

Figure 3.21. *Portal vein gas.*   Note the linear collections of gas in the portal vein radicles of the liver. Characteristically, they radiate toward the porta hepatis. This patient had necrotizing enterocolitis.

num, with or without obstructive emphysema, is uncommonly seen in children. Because pneumatosis in many of these children is not related to intestinal ischemia, it is a relatively benign finding (see Fig. 3.15).

The classic roentgenographic appearance of pneumatosis cystoides intestinalis consists of linear or curvilinear collections of gas within the bowel wall (Fig. 3.20). Unfortunately, not all patients present with this configuration, and in others the collection of gas appears so bubbly that it is difficult to differentiate it from food in the stomach, fecal material in the colon, or an intra-abdominal abscess (Fig. 3.20). Linear air collections must be differentiated from the normal properitoneal fat stripe (Fig. 3.20C).

Pneumatosis cystoides intestinalis occasionally can be limited to the stomach (12, 13, 22, 34), and while in most of these cases it merely is a part of more generalized, widespread enterocolitis, in others it truly is an isolated phenomenon. In these latter cases, it is believed to result from chronic overdistension of the stomach, such as is seen with infantile pyloric stenosis.

Portal Vein and Biliary Tract Gas.
Portal vein gas is a common finding in necrotizing enterocolitis of infancy (1, 34, 36, 40, 41), but can be seen with small bowel necrosis due to any number of causes. For this reason, it usually is seen hand in hand with pneumatosis cystoides intestinalis. Presumably, in these cases, gas enters the portal circulation from the intestinal wall, either through the veins or lymphatics, and then passes into the liver (Fig. 3.21). Biliary tract gas is quite uncommon and usually is seen with duodenal obstructions distal to the entrance of the common bile duct (9, 17).

REFERENCES

1. Arnon, R.G., and Fishbein, J.F.: Portal venous gas in pediatric age group: Review of the literature and report of 12 new cases. J. Pediatr. 79: 255–259, 1971.
2. Bornes, P.F., and Johnston, T.A.: Indolent pneumatosis of the bowel wall associated with immune suppressive therapy. Ann. Radiol. 16: 163–166, 1973.
3. Bray, J.F.: The "inverted V" sign of pneumoperitoneum. Radiology 151: 45–46, 1984.
4. Bryk, D.: Unusual causes of small bowel pneumatosis: Perforated duodenal ulcer and perforated jejunal diverticula. Radiology 106: 299–302, 1973.
5. Capitanio, M.A., and Greenberg, S.B.: Pneumatosis intestinalis in two infants with rotovirus gastroenteritis. Pediatr. Radiol. 21: 361–362, 1991.
6. Cho, K.C., and Baker, S.R.: Air in the fissure for the ligamentum teres: New sign of intraperitoneal air on plain radiographs. Radiology 178: 489–492, 1991.
7. Christensen, E.E., and Landay, M.J.: Visible muscle of the diaphragm: Sign of extraperitoneal air. A.J.R. 135: 521–523, 1980.
8. De Lacey, G., Bloomberg, T., and Wignall, B.K.: Pneumoperitoneum: The misleading double wall sign. Clin. Radiol. 28: 445–448, 1977.
9. Frates, R.E.: Incompetence of sphincter of Oddi in newborn. Radiology 85: 875–879, 1965.
10. Fischer, T.J., Cipel, L., and Stiehm, E.R.: Pneumatosis intestinalis associated with fatal childhood dermatomyositis. Pediatrics 61: 127–129, 1978.
11. Gupta, A.: Pneumatosis intestinalis in children. Br. J. Radiol. 51: 589–595, 1978.
12. Henry, G.W.: Emphysematous gastritis. A.J.R. 68: 15–18, 1952.
13. Holgersen, L.O., Bornes, P.F., and Srouji, M.N.: Isolated gastric pneumatosis. J. Pediatr. Surg. 9: 813–816 1974.
14. Jaffe, N., Carlson, D.H., and Vawter, F.G.: Pneumatosis cystoides intestinalis in acute leukemia. Cancer 30: 239–243, 1973.
15. Jelasco, D.V., and Schultz, E.H., Jr.: The urachus—an aid to the diagnosis of pneumoperitoneum. Radiology 92: 295–296, 1969.
16. Keats, T.E., and Smith, T.H.: Benign pneumatosis intestinalis in childhood leukemia. A.J.R. 122: 150–152, 1974.
17. Kirks, D.R., and Baden, M.: Incompetence of the sphincter of Oddi associated with duodenal stenosis. J. Pediatr. 83: 838–843 1973.
18. Klein, D.L.: Visibility of the inferior heart border in pneumoperitoneum. A.J.R. 137: 622–623, 1981.
19. Kleinman, P., Meyers, M.A., Abbott, G., and Kazam, E.: Necrotizing enterocolitis with pneumatosis intestinalis in systemic lupus erythematosus and polyarteritis. Radiology 121: 595–598 1976.
20. Kleinman, P.K., Brill, P.W., and Winchester, P.: Pneumatosis intestinalis: Its occurrence in the immunologically compromised child. Am. J. Dis. Child. 134: 1149–1151, 1980.
21. Menuck, L., and Siemers, P.T.: Pneumoperitoneum: Importance of right upper quadrant features. A.J.R. 127: 753–756, 1976.
22. Meyes, H.I., and Parker, J.J.: Emphysematous gastritis. Radiology 89: 426–431, 1967.
23. Miercort, R.D., and Merrill, F.G.: Pneumatosis and pseudo-obstruction in scleroderma. Radiology 92: 359–362, 1969.
24. Miller, R.E.: Perforated viscus in infants. A new roentgen sign. Radiology 74: 65–67, 1960.
25. Mueller, C.F., Morehead, R., Alter, A.J., and Michener, W.: Pneumatosis intestinalis in collagen disorders. A.J.R. 115: 300–305, 1972.
26. Oliveros, M.A., Herbst, J.J., Lester, P.D., and Ziter, F.A.: Pneumatosis intestinalis in childhood dermatomyositis. Pediatrics 52: 711–712, 1973.
27. Richmond, J.A., and Mikity, V.: Benign form of necrotizing enterocolitis. A.J.R. 123: 301–306, 1975.
28. Rigler, L.G.: Spontaneous pneumoperitoneum: A roentgenologic sign found in the supine position. Radiology 37: 604–607, 1941.
29. Robinson, A.E., Grossman, H., and Brumley, G.W.: Pneumatosis intestinalis in the neonate. A.J.R. 120: 333–341, 1974.
30. Schultz, E.H., Jr.: An aid to the diagnosis of pneumoperitoneum from supine abdominal films. Radiology 70: 728–731, 1958.
31. Seaman, W.B., Fleming, R.J., and Baker, D.H.: Pneumatosis intestinalis of the small bowel. Semin. Roentgenol. 1: 234, 1966.
32. Touloukian, R.J., Posch, J.N., and Spencer, R.: The pathogenesis of ischemic gastroenterocolitis of the neonate: Selective gut mucosal ischemia in asphyxiated neonatal piglets. J. Pediatr. Surg. 7: 194–205, 1972.
33. Tucker, A.S., Soine, L., and Izant, R.J., Jr.: Gastrointestinal perforations in infancy: Anatomic and etiologic gamuts. A.J.R. 123: 755–763, 1975.
34. Vaughan, B.R.: Emphysema of the stomach with portal vein gas. Australas. Radiol. 16: 377–378, 1972.
35. Vicki, G.F., Maggini, M., Moggi, P., Gori, F., and Paoli, F.: Pneumatosis intestinalis in infants: Clinical, radiological and anatomo-pathological study on eighteen patients. Ann. Radiol. 16: 153–161, 1973.
36. Vollman, J.H., Smith, W.L., and Tsang, R.C.:

Necrotizing enterocolitis with recurrent hepatic portal vein gas. J. Pediatr. 88: 486–487, 1976.

37. Weiner, C.I., Diaconis, J.N., and Dennis, J.M.: The "inverted V": A new sign of pneumoperitoneum. Radiology 197: 47–48, 1973.

38. West, K.W., Rescorla, F.J., Grosfeld, J.L., and Vane, D.W.: Pneumatosis intestinalis in children beyond the neonatal period. J. Pediatr. Surg. 24: 818–822, 1989.

39. White, H., and Rowley, W.F.: Cystic fibrosis of the pancreas: Clinical and roentgenographic manifestations. Radiol. Clin. North Am. 1: 539–556, 1963.

40. Wiot, J.F., and Felson, B.: Gas in the portal venous system. A.J.R. 86: 920, 1961.

41. Wolfe, J.N., and Evans, W.A.: Gas in the portal veins of liver in infant. A.J.R. 74: 186, 1955.

42. Wood, R.E., Herman, C.J., Johnson, K.W., and di Sant Agnese, P.A.: Pneumatosis coli in cystic fibrosis. Am. J. Dis. Child. 129: 246–248, 1975.

THICKENED AND PSEUDOTHICKENED BOWEL WALLS

True thickening of the intestinal wall can be seen with any type of inflammatory disease of the intestine, chronic intestinal obstruction, and intestinal ischemia or infarction (Fig. 3.22). Pseudothickening of the bowel wall is seen with ascites or peritonitis, or when loops of distended intestine contain more fluid than air (1, 2). In the first instance, as the loops of air-filled bowel float in the peritoneal fluid, they become separated to such a degree that bowel wall thickening is suggested (Fig. 3.23A). In the second case, bowel wall thickening is suggested when small amounts of gas collect at the top of a primarily fluid-filled loop of intestine. The cap of free air in each such loop is so small that an optical illusion suggesting thickened bowel wall is suggested (Fig. 3.23B and C). All of these findings are summarized in the diagram illustrated in Figure 3.24, but it should be noted that if true bowel wall thickening is present it tends to persist on upright view (see Fig. 3.22).

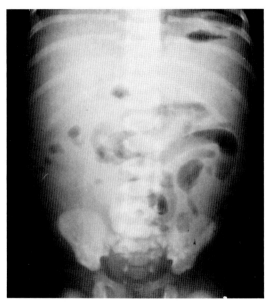

Figure 3.22. *True thickening of intestinal wall.* Note that on this upright view, the space between the air-filled loops of intestine is increased. This type of thickening would not persist on the upright view if it were pseudothickening. This infant had necrotizing enterocolitis and the intestine was thickened.

Figure 3.23. *True versus pseudothickening of bowel walls.* (*A*) In this infant, ascites is causing separation of the distended loops of intestine so as to mimic bowel wall thickening. (*B*) In this infant with low small bowel obstruction, the presence of large volumes of fluid within the dilated loops erroneously suggests bowel wall thickening. However, on upright view (*C*), note that the bowel walls are not thickened (*arrows*), but that the intestinal loops contain large volumes of fluid. In these cases, the relatively small amount of air in the intestinal loops is so small that on supine view, as it floats to the top of each loop, the fluid under it causes the space between any two given air collections to be widened. In this manner, bowel wall thickening is suggested, but actually is not present (see Fig. 3.24A for diagrammatic depiction of this phenomenon).

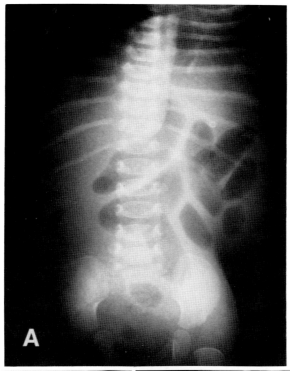

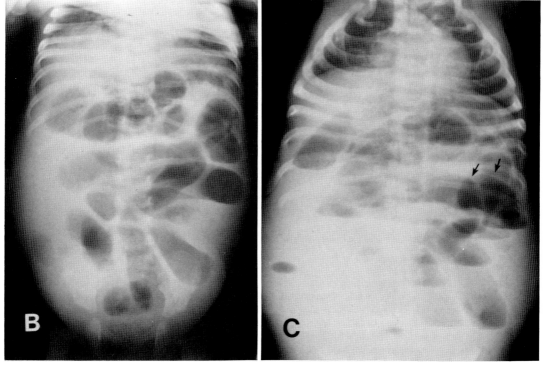

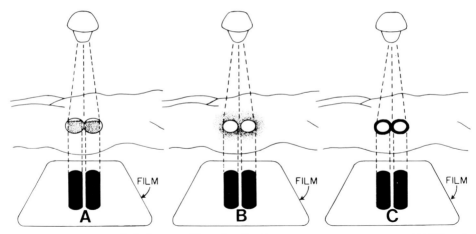

Figure 3.24. *True versus pseudothickening of bowel walls: diagrammatic representation.* (*A*) When large volumes of fluid are present in intestinal loops and only small amounts of gas float on top of this fluid, the resultant roentgenographic image is such that the space between the loops of intestine appears widened and bowel wall thickening is suggested. The bowel wall, however, is not thickened. (*B*) With ascitic fluid between the bowel loops, the loops themselves are separated, and since the space between them is widened, bowel wall thickening is once again erroneously suggested. (*C*) True thickening of the bowel wall. The widened space between the loops of air-filled intestine truly represents thick intestinal walls. (Reprinted with permission from R. B. Hoffman et al.: Pseudoseparation of bowel loops: A fallacious sign of intraperitoneal fluid. Radiology 87: 845–847, 1966.)

REFERENCES

1. Hoffman, R.B., Wankmuller, R., and Rigler, L.G.: Pseudoseparation of bowel loops: A fallacious sign of intraperitoneal fluid. Radiology 87: 845–847, 1966.
2. Nelson, S.W., and Eggleston, W.: Findings on plain roentgenograms of the abdomen associated with mesenteric vascular occlusion with a possible new sign of mesenteric venous thrombosis. A.J.R. 83: 886–894, 1960.

ABDOMINAL FLUID COLLECTIONS (ASCITES, PERITONITIS, HEMOPERITONEUM)

The roentgenographic findings of fluid in the abdomen are much the same from case to case, and depend primarily on the volume, not the type, of fluid present (5, 11). *Types of fluid that might be encountered include serous effusions, chyle, urine, bile, blood and pus.* With massive fluid collections the diagnosis is relatively easy, for the abdomen becomes distended and opaque, and the normally visible liver edge and retroperitoneal structures become obscured (Fig. 3.25A). If distended loops of intestine also are present, they tend to float toward the center of the abdomen (Fig. 3.25B) and in so doing result in the clinically percussable "tympanic cap." In addition to these findings, in many cases one will be able to delineate the edge of the medially displaced liver (Fig. 3.25B). This

Figure 3.25. *Massive ascites.* (*A*) Massive ascites in a young infant produces marked distension and opacity of the abdomen, obliteration of the inferior liver edge, and obliteration of all the retroperitoneal structures. In the right upper quadrant, one can see a slight difference in density between the medially displaced liver and the adjacent ascitic fluid. (*B*) With more penetration of the abdomen, the interface between the liver and ascitic fluid is more clearly visualized (*arrows*). In addition, note that some air is now present in the intestines and that the air-filled loops of intestine cluster and float in the center of the abdomen. (*C*) Enhanced visualization of the liver after injection of contrast material for an intravenous pyelogram. The increased density of the liver is secondary to the circulating contrast material and is useful in substantiating that the findings in Parts *A* and *B* actually were due to the ascitic fluid-liver interface.

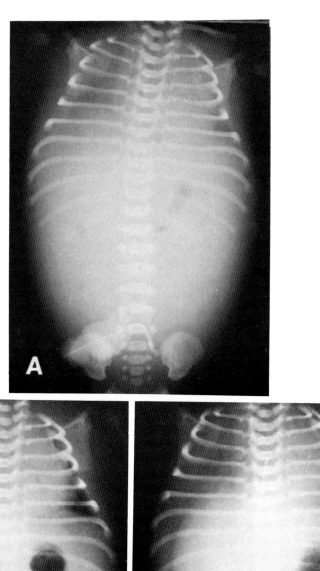

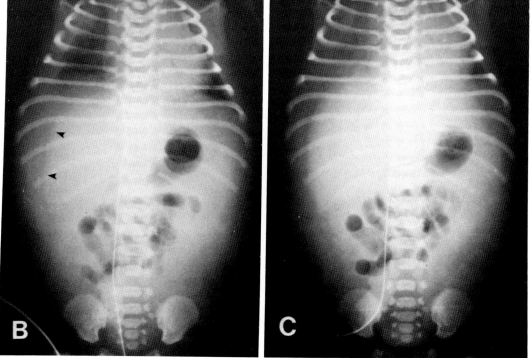

subtle finding is present more often than generally appreciated and results from the fact that the densities of the liver and adjacent fluid are just different enough that a roentgenographically perceptible interface between them develops (13, 19). This phenomenon is even more dramatically portrayed with CT scanning.

With lesser volumes of fluid, the findings on supine views of the abdomen often are subtle, and in this regard it should be noted that fluid first accumulates in the pelvis in the peritoneal cul-de-sac (Fig. 3.26A). When enough fluid accumulates here the cul-de-sac bulges laterally and the term "dog ears" has been assigned to this finding (Fig. 3.27A). However, it is not an easy finding to detect and in young infants it is almost impossible to detect. However, this is no longer a problem, for ultrasonography and CT are far superior in the detection of peritoneal fluid in its various nooks and crannies.

With larger fluid collections, fluid accumulations tend to pass upward between the abdominal wall and both the ascending

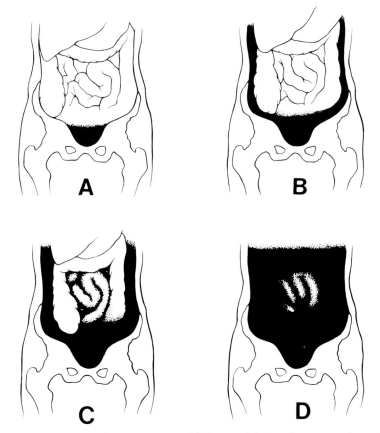

Figure 3.26. *Peritoneal fluid accumulation: sequence of findings.* (**A**) In early cases, in the supine position, fluid accumulates in the cul-de-sac. (**B**) With larger volumes, fluid begins to track upward and accumulates primarily between the abdominal wall and the ascending colon on the right, and the abdominal wall and descending colon on the left. (**C**) With even greater volumes of fluid, displacement of the ascending and descending colon medially becomes more pronounced, and fluid begins to accumulate beneath and around the liver. (**D**) With massive peritoneal fluid accumulations, the entire abdomen becomes filled with fluid, gas is forced out of the ascending and descending colon, and the few remaining air-filled loops of small bowel cluster and float in the center of the abdomen.

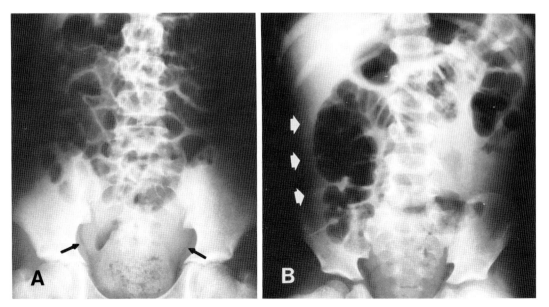

Figure 3.27. (A) Fluid in peritoneal cul-de-sac—the so-called "dog ears" sign. Fluid first accumulates in the peritoneal cul-de-sac, and when the cul-de-sac bulges laterally, a dog ear-like configuration is suggested (*arrows*). (B) Fluid collecting between ascending colon and abdominal wall. This patient was in an automobile accident and had hemoperitoneum. The best evidence for the presence of peritoneal blood (fluid) lies in the increased distance between the right abdominal wall and the ascending colon (*arrows*).

and descending portions of the colon (Figs. 3.26B and 3.27B). Eventually fluid reaches the liver, and as it collects along the inferior aspect of this organ, the liver angle (14) and its entire inferior edge become invisible (Figs. 3.25 and 3.26C). At the same time, fluid accumulates between the abdominal wall and liver and causes medial displacement of the liver (Figs. 3.25 and 3.26). Meanwhile, the accumulating fluid also tends to gather in between and separate the centrally floating loops of intestine (see Fig. 3.25).

Currently, ultrasonography is the best tool for detecting the presence of peritoneal fluid of any volume. It is especially useful in detecting small volume fluid collections in and around the liver, in the lesser sack, and in the peritoneal cul-de-sac. Various configurations of such free abdominal fluid are presented in Figures 3.28 and 3.29. CT also vividly displays these fluid collections (Fig. 3.30), but a problem can be encountered with fluid over the liver and its differentiation from

pleural fluid (Fig. 3.31). This does not occur with ultrasound, for in the sagittal plane fluid is clearly defined to be either above or below the diaphragm (see Fig. 1.60).

Serous ascitic effusions in children can be seen with many conditions including: (a) renal disease, (b) liver disease with portal hypertension, (c) portal vein obstruction, (d) hypoproteinemia, (e) protein-losing enteropathy, (f) congestive heart failure, and (g) pancreatitis (5, 21). Chylous ascites usually occurs on a congenital basis and results from congenital defects or obstructions of the thoracic duct (2, 3, 5, 9, 16), but it also can occur on a spontaneous basis, secondary to abdominal trauma (22), and with intestinal lymphangiectasia. In any of these cases, if fat content is high enough, the chylous fluid may appear more radiolucent than the adjacent liver, both on plain films and CT.

Urine ascites is another cause of peritoneal fluid accumulation, and most com-

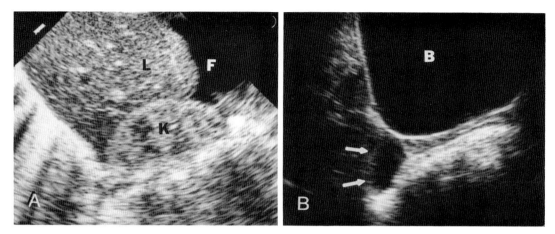

Figure 3.28. *Abdominal fluid: ultrasonographic findings.* (*A*) Note fluid (*arrows*) anterior to the liver (*L*) and kidney (*K*) in this young infant. (*B*) Adolescent girl with ruptured ovarian cyst, demonstrating fluid in the cul-de-sac (*arrows*). Bladder (*B*).

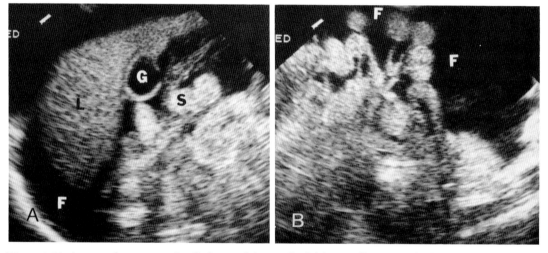

Figure 3.29. *Ascites: ultrasonographic findings.* (*A*) Free fluid (*F*) virtually surrounds the liver (*L*). There also is fluid between the gallbladder (*G*) and the echogenic small intestine (*S*). (*B*) Another view through the mid-abdomen demonstrates massive ascitic fluid (*F*) with the mesentery and loops of bowel floating in the fluid.

monly occurs with urinary tract obstruction (5, 7), but, of course, also can be seen with renal or urinary bladder injuries secondary to abdominal trauma. When peritoneal fluid accumulation is due to rupture of the urinary tract with urinary tract obstruction, it is believed that there is extravasation of urine into the perirenal space and then, through normal congenital defects, into the peritoneal cavity. Bile asci-

tes can occur on a congenital basis from obstruction, tears, or defects of the bile ducts (4, 10, 17, 21), but it also can result from bile duct injuries secondary to abdominal trauma.

Peritonitis in childhood may occur secondary to gastrointestinal perforations or as a primary infection (1, 6, 8, 12, 15). In these latter cases, the causative organism often, but not always, is *Streptococcus*

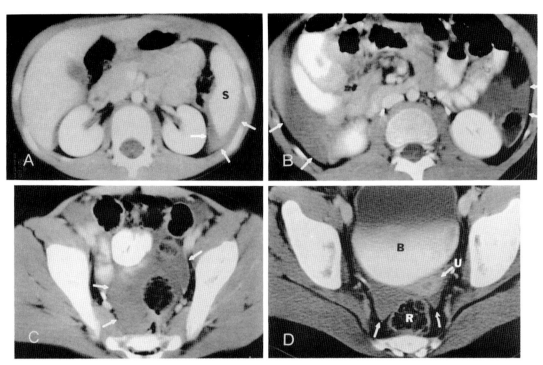

Figure 3.30. *Abdominal fluid: CT demonstration.* (*A*) Note hypodense fluid (*arrows*) around the spleen (*S*). There also is a little fluid between the liver and the kidney on the other side. (*B*) Large volume of paracolic fluid on both sides. (*C*) Same patient demonstrating a large collection of fluid (*arrows*) in the pelvis separating the various contrast and air-filled loops of intestine. (*D*) Classic fluid in the cul-de-sac (*arrows*) between the bladder (*B*) and rectum (*R*). The uterus (*U*) lies just off midline.

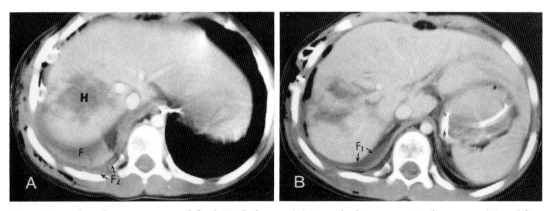

Figure 3.31. *Pleural versus peritoneal fluid: CT findings.* (*A*) Note the liver contusion-hematoma (*H*) and free abdominal fluid (*F*) between the liver and diaphragm. Also note pleural fluid (*F2*) above the diaphragm and some periportal tracking of blood along the portal vein branches. (*B*) Lower cut again demonstrates the liver contusion. In addition, note fluid (*F1*) between the diaphragmatic leaflet and liver.

pneumoniae, and these primary infections are especially prone to develop in children with the nephrotic syndrome (21). Tuberculous peritonitis is uncommonly seen in childhood, but when it occurs it tends to produce a more adhesive peritoneal reaction; consequently, the loops of bowel, instead of floating freely in the fluid, tend to remain more fixed from view to view. Peritonitis secondary to ascaris infection (18, 20) is uncommon in this country, and meconium peritonitis, of course, is a problem of neonates. In these patients, peritoneal calcification frequently is present.

Hemoperitoneum is most often seen secondary to abdominal trauma with splenic or liver injury. However, it also can be seen with injuries to the mesenteric vessels and aorta. The clinical setting, of course, is what alerts one to the diagnosis, for the roentgenographic findings are similar to those of any other abdominal fluid collection.

Very few conditions can mimic the presence of free peritoneal fluid, but in some patients with voluminous collections of fluid in the bowel, the findings at first might suggest free peritoneal fluid. This can occur with severe viral gastroenteritis, *Shigella* infection, or small bowel obstruction, and ultrasonography is excellent in demonstrating the fluid-filled intestinal loops (see Fig. 3.9).

In addition to these situations, it should be mentioned that in some patients with large, extremely thin-walled, mesenteric, or lymphangiectatic cysts, the cysts may be so fluctuant that peritoneal fluid is mimicked both clinically and roentgenographically (5). Indeed, even paracentesis, the final tool in the investigation of any abdominal fluid collection, may not solve the problem. This occurs because as the cyst is drained it becomes so flaccid that no residual "mass" remains, and one believes that ascites was the problem. Of course, such fluid almost always recurs, and it may require numerous paracenteses before one realizes that the real problem is a

thin-walled lymphangiectatic mesenteric cyst.

REFERENCES

1. Bose, B., Keir, W.R., and Godberson, C.V.: Primary pneumococcic peritonitis. Can. Med. Assoc. J. 110: 305–307, 1974.
2. Boysen, Bette E.: Chylous ascites. Am. J. Dis. Child. 129: 1338–1339, 1975.
3. Craven, C.E., Goldman, A.S., Larson, D.L., Patterson, M., and Hendrick, C.K.: Congenital chylous ascites: Lymphangiographic demonstration of obstruction of the cisterna chyli and chylous reflux into the peritoneal space and small intestine. J. Pediatr. 70: 340–345, 1967.
4. Esposito, G.: Biliary peritonitis in a child due to spontaneous perforation of the bile duct. Ann. Chir. Inf. 13: 339–346, 1972.
5. Franken, E.A.: Ascites in infants and children. Roentgen diagnosis. Radiology 102: 393–398, 1972.
6. Freji, B.J., Votteler, T.P., and McCracken, G.H., Jr.: Primary peritonitis in previously healthy children. Am. J. Dis. Child. 138: 1058–1061, 1984.
7. Friedland, G.W., Tune, B., and Mears, E.M.: Ascites due to spontaneous rupture of the renal pelvis in an 11-month-old infant with uretero-pelvic junctional obstruction. Pediatr. Radiol. 2: 263–264, 1974.
8. Geley, L., and Brandesky, G.: Pneumococcic peritonitis in childhood. Z. Kinderchir. 11: 42–49, 1972.
9. Gribetz, D., and Ganog, A.: Chylous ascites in infancy. Pediatrics 7: 632–639, 1951.
10. Hansen, R.C., Wasnich, R.D., Devries, P.A., and Sunshine, P.: Bile ascites in infancy: diagnosis with 133-rose bengal. Pediatrics 84: 719–721, 1974.
11. Keefe, E.J., Gagliardi, R.A., and Pfister, R.C.: The roentgenographic evaluation of ascites. A.J.R. 101: 388–396, 1967.
12. Khan, A.J., Evans, H.E., Macabuhay, M.R., Lee, Y., and Werner, R.: Primary peritonitis due to group G streptococcus: A case report. Pediatrics 56: 1078–1079, 1975.
13. Love, L., Demos, T.C., Reynes, C.J., Williams, V., Shkoinik, A., Gandhi, V., and Zerofos, N.: Visualization of the lateral edge of the liver in ascites. Radiology 122: 619–622, 1977.
14. Margulies, M., and Stoane, L.: Hepatic angle in roentgen evaluation of peritoneal fluid. Radiology 88: 51, 1967.
15. McDougal, W., Izant, R., and Zollinger, R.: Primary peritonitis in infancy and childhood. Ann. Surg. 181: 310–313, 1975.
16. McKendry, J.B.J., Lindsay, W.K., and Gerstein,

M.C.: Congenital defects of the lymphatics in infancy. Pediatrics 19: 21–35, 1957.

17. Moore, T.C.: Massive bile peritonitis in infancy due to spontaneous bile duct perforation with portal vein occlusion. J. Pediatr. Surg. 10: 537–538, 1975.

18. Parashar, S.K., Nadkarni, S.V., and Varma, R.A.: Primary roundworm peritonitis. Indian J. Surg. 36: 200–201, 1974.

19. Porto, A.V., and Lane, E.J.: Visualization of differences in soft-tissue densities. The liver in ascites. Radiology 121: 19–23, 1976.

20. Rao, P.L.N.G., Satyanarayana G., and Venkatesh A.: Intraperitoneal ascariasis. J. Pediatr. Surg. 23: 936–938, 1988.

21. Rubin, M., Blau, E.B., and Michaels, R.H.: Hemophilus and pneumococcal peritonitis in children with the nephrotic syndrome. Pediatrics 56: 598–601, 1975.

22. Vollman, R.W., Keenan, W.J., and Eraklis, A.J.: Post-traumatic chylous ascites in infancy. N. Engl. J. Med. 275: 875–877, 1966.

ABDOMINAL ABSCESS

Most abdominal abscesses are not visible on plain films. In the classic case an abdominal abscess has a bubbly, amorphous pattern, but in other instances only a mass displacing adjacent intestines is seen (Fig. 3.32). The granular appearance must be differentiated from a somewhat similar appearance seen in normal patients when gas is mixed with: (a) fecal material in the colon, (b) food in the stomach, and (c) a bezoar in the gastrointestinal tract. Abscesses in the right lower quadrant usually result from perforation of the appendix or a Meckel's diverticulum and are dealt with in the section on appendicitis. In the right upper quadrant, an abscess may be subhepatic or intrahepatic. Intrahepatic abscesses may be bacterial or amebic in origin, and currently are best imaged with ultrasound or CT. On plain films, one may be presented with a large liver, elevated right diaphragmatic leaflet, and associated changes in the right lung base (Fig. 3.33A). Pyogenic abscesses may be encountered in totally normal children, but it also should be noted that one of the classic presentations of children with chronic granuloma-

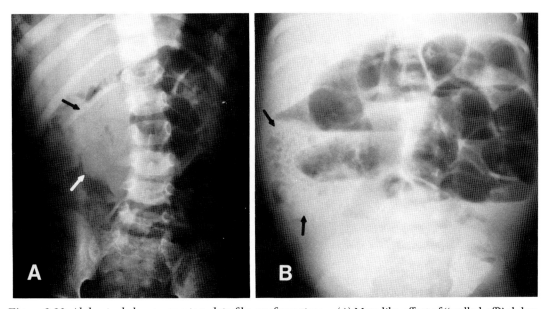

Figure 3.32. *Abdominal abscess: varying plain film configurations.* (**A**) Mass-like effect of "walled-off" abdominal abscess (*arrows*) secondary to perforated appendicitis. Note pronounced ipsilateral scoliosis secondary to spasm of the psoas muscle. (**B**) Typical granular appearance of an abscess (*arrows*) in the right lower quadrant secondary to intestinal perforation in a young infant.

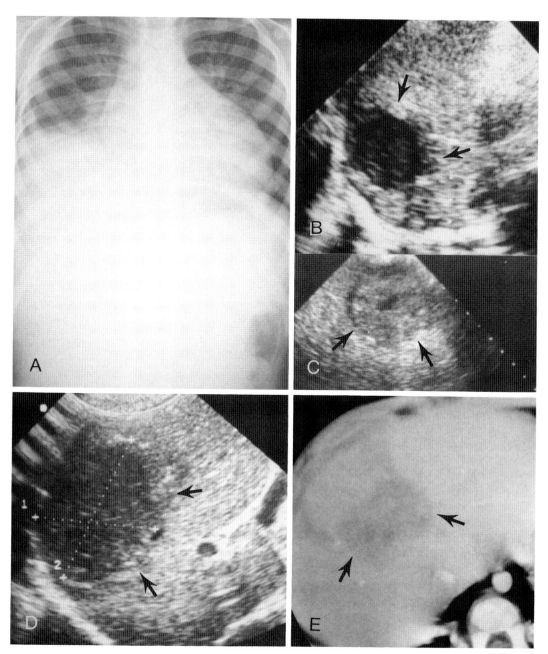

Figure 3.33. *Hepatic abscess.* (*A*) Plain film findings. Note the elevated right diaphragmatic leaflet and enlargement of the liver. Also note secondary changes in the right lung base. (*B*) Ultrasonogram in a patient with a liver abscess demonstrating a relatively hypoechoic amebic abscess (*arrows*). (*C*) Another patient with an almost solid, highly echogenic staphylococcal abscess (*arrows*). (*D*) Still another patient with a large liver abscess (*arrows*) of mixed echoes. (*E*) CT study in this patient demonstrates the hypodense abscess (*arrows*).

tous disease of childhood (neutrophil dysfunction) is liver abscess (23, 27). Amebic liver abscess also can be seen in children, but liver abscess secondary to ascaris infection is uncommon (22). Subhepatic abscesses can develop after perforation of a retrocecal appendix, a duodenal ulcer, or the gallbladder.

Abscesses in the upper midabdomen usually are located in the lesser sac or in, and around, the pancreas. Lesser sac abscesses may result from perforation of duodenal ulcers (4), while pancreatic abscesses result from more fulminant forms of pancreatitis (1). Abscesses in the pelvis usually result from appendiceal perforation, but also can be seen with salpingitis or bladder perforations.

A subphrenic abscess often will elevate the diaphragmatic leaflet and be associated with pulmonary changes such as atelectasis and pleural effusion (Fig. 3.34). On the right, such an abscess often displaces the liver downward, while on the left it displaces the stomach and splenic flexure medially and/or downwardly (8, 18, 21). Perinephric abscesses produce mass-like configurations in the retroperitoneal area, obliteration of the retroperitoneal soft tissues, and, on intravenous pyelography, decreased function and/or displacement of the kidney (2, 5, 13–16). They are, however, relatively uncommon in children (26, 29), as are intrarenal abscesses (19). Perinephric abscesses and renal infections, in general, are dealt with in a later section. Abscesses along or in the psoas muscle may be tuberculous or nontuberculous in origin (7, 9, 21), and are best demonstrated with CT (Fig. 3.35).

Ultrasonography, as the screening imaging modality in the investigation of abdominal abscess, is virtually indispensable. Characteristically, with ultrasound, abscesses present with a sonolucent center and an irregular or well-defined wall but more solid figurations also occur (Fig. 3.36). CT also is excellent in delineating

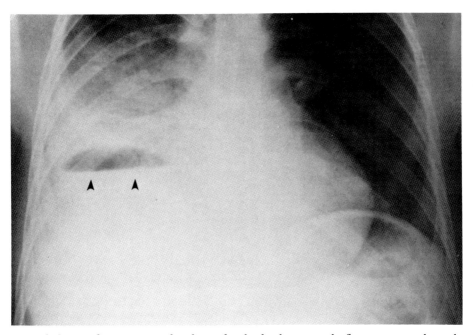

Figure 3.34. *Subphrenic abscess.* Note the elevated right diaphragmatic leaflet, gas accumulation beneath it (*arrows*), and associated changes in the right lung base. This patient had a right subphrenic abscess secondary to a perforated retrocecal appendix.

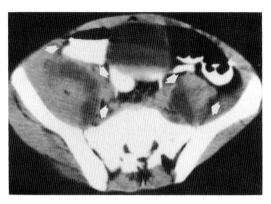

Figure 3.35. *Psoas abscess.* Bilateral psoas abscesses (*arrows*). The right is much larger than the left. Loculated fluid is seen within the abscesses.

abscesses and usually is more informative than ultrasound as far as precise abscess localization is concerned (Fig. 3.36).

Liver abscesses may be pyogenic or amebic in origin (3, 6, 10–12, 17, 20, 24, 25, 28–30) and amebic abscesses, more than pyogenic liver abscesses, tend to be strikingly anechoic (10). Amebic abscesses also may erode the diaphragm and extend into the chest or even the pericardial cavity (Fig. 3.37). Demonstration of these complications is extremely important, and when such an abscess is demonstrated to be near the diaphragmatic leaflet or the pericardium, impending penetration

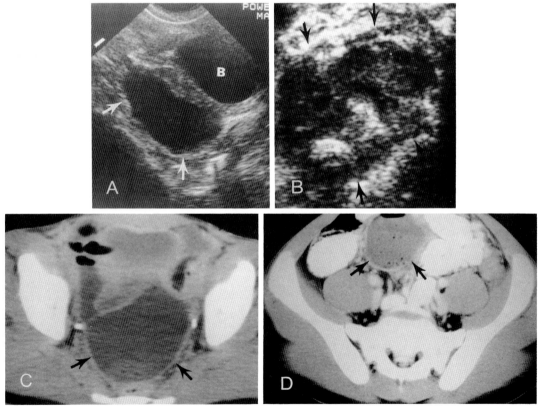

Figure 3.36. *Abdominal abscess: ultrasonographic and CT configurations.* (*A*) Patient with basically sonolucent pelvic abscess (*arrows*). Urinary bladder (*B*). (*B*) Another patient with an abscess (*arrows*) demonstrating heterogeneous echogenicity. (*C*) CT demonstration of another pelvic abscess (*arrow*) posterior to the bladder. (*D*) Another patient with an abscess demonstrating gas bubbles scattered throughout its substance and a bubble of air at the top of the abscess (*arrows*).

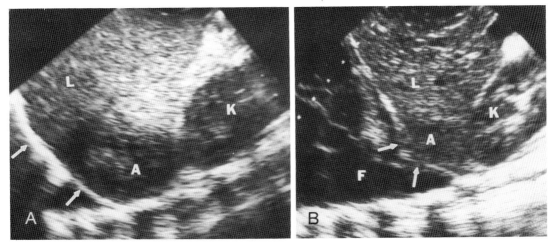

Figure 3.37. *Amebic abscess penetrating into the pleural space.* (*A*) Note the sonolucent liver abscess (*A*). Liver (*L*), kidney (*K*), diaphragmatic leaflet (*arrows*). (*B*) Later, with penetration through the diaphragm, note accumulation of fluid (*F*) in the pleural space and a defect in the diaphragmatic leaflet (*arrows*). The abscess (*A*) now is much smaller.

should be considered a real possibility. For this reason, the abscess should be drained immediately.

REFERENCES

1. Agnos, J., and Holmes, R.: Gas in the pancreas as a sign of abscess. A.J.R. 80: 60, 1958.
2. Bliznak, J., and Ramsey, J.: Emphysematous pyelonephritis. Clin. Radiol. 23: 61–64, 1972.
3. Boultbee, J.E., Sinjee, A.E., Rooknooden, F., and Engelbrecht, H.E.: Experiences with gray scale ultrasonography in hepatic amoebiasis. Clin. Radiol. 30: 683–689, 1979.
4. Boyce, M.J., Burwood, J.R., Johnson, M., and Wood, C.B.S.: Chronic duodenal ulcer in infancy complicated by hemorrhage, perforation, and cyst formation in the lesser sac. J. Pediatr. Surg. 8: 323–324, 1973.
5. Evans, J.A., Meyers, M.A., and Bosniak, M.A.: Acute renal and perirenal infections. Semin. Roentgenol. 61: 274–291, 1971.
6. Foster, S.C., Schneider, B., and Seaman, W.B.: Gas-containing pyogenic intrahepatic abscesses. Radiology 94: 613–618, 1970.
7. Graves, V.B., and Schreiber, M.H.: Tuberculous psoas muscle abscess. J. Can. Assoc. Radiol. 24: 268–271, 1973.
8. Gwinn, J.L., and Lee, F.A.: Radiological case of the month (subphrenic abscess). Am. J. Dis. Child. 129: 1333, 1975.
9. Hardcastle, J.D.: Acute non-tuberculous psoas abscess. Br. J. Surg. 57: 10, 1970.
10. Hayden, C.K., Jr., Toups, M., Swischuk, L.E., and Amparo, E.G.: Sonographic features of hepatic amebiasis in childhood. J. Can. Assoc. Radiol. 35: 279–282, 1984.
11. Isaac, F.: Roentgen findings in amebic disease of liver. Radiology 45: 581–587, 1945.
12. Kuligowska, E., Conners, S.K., and Shapiro, J.H.: Liver abscess: Sonography in diagnosis and treatment. A.J.R. 138: 253–257, 1982.
13. Langston, C.S., and Pfister, R.C.: Renal emphysema: A case report and review of the literature. A.J.R. 110: 778–786, 1970.
14. Levy, A.H., and Schwinger, H.N.: Gas-containing perinephric abscess. Radiology 60: 720–723, 1953.
15. Lipsett, P.J.: Roentgen ray observations in acute perinephritic abscess. J.A.M.A. 111: 1374–1376, 1928.
16. Love, L., Baker, D., and Ramsey, R.: Gas-producing perinephric abscess. A.J.R. 119: 783–792, 1973.
17. McCarty, E., Pathmanand, C., Sunakorn, P., and Scherz, R.G.: Amebic liver abscess in childhood: A case study of a 21-month-old Thai child and a literature review. Am. J. Dis. Child 126: 67–70, 1973.
18. Miller, W.T., and Talman, E.A.: Subphrenic abscess. A.J.R. 101: 961–969, 1967.
19. Moenne-Locloz, J.P., Bomsel, F., Gatti, J.M., and Prot, D.: Renal abscess in children: A rare but important radiological diagnosis. Pediatr. Radiol. 7: 150–154, 1978.
20. Newlin, N., Silder, T.M., Stuck, K.J., and San-

dler, M.A.: Ultrasonic features of pyogenic liver abscess. Radiology 139: 155–159, 1981.

21. Parbhoo, A., and Govendel, S.: Acute pyogenic psoas abscess in children. J. Pediatr. Orthop. 12: 663–666, 1992.

22. Parodi-Hueck, L.E., Wenger, F., and Montiel-Villasmil, D.: Ascaris hepatic abscess in children. J. Pediatr. Surg. 7: 69, 1972.

23. Preimesberger, K.F., and Goldberg, M.E.: Acute liver abscess in chronic granulomatous disease of childhood. Radiology 110: 147–150, 1974.

24. Rab, S.M., Alam, N., Hoda, A.N., and Yee, A.: Amoebic liver abscess: Some unique presentations. Am. J. Med. 43: 811–816, 1967.

25. Ralls, P.W., Colletti, P.M., Quinn, M.F., and Halls, J.: Sonographic findings in a hepatic amebic abscess. Radiology 145: 123–126, 1982.

26. Rote, A.R., Bauer, S.B., and Retik, A.B.: Renal abscess in children. J. Urol. 119: 254–258, 1978.

27. Samuels, L.D.: Liver scans in chronic granulomatous disease of childhood. Pediatrics 48: 41–50, 1971.

28. Schmidt, A.G.: Plain film roentgen diagnosis of amebic hepatic abscess. A.J.R. 107: 47–50, 1969.

29. Sukow, R.J., Cohen, L.J., and Sample, W.F.: Sonography of hepatic amebic abscesses. A.J.R. 134: 911–915, 1980.

30. Vanni, L.A., Lopez, P.B., Porto, S.O., and Brazil, P.A.: Solitary pyogenic liver abscess in children. Am. Dis. Child. 132: 1142, 1978.

ACUTE INFLAMMATORY PROBLEMS

Pneumonia Causing Acute Abdomen. Pneumonia, usually pneumococcal in origin, is notorious for producing symptoms

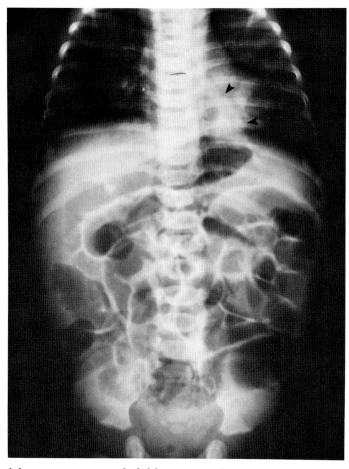

Figure 3.38. *Acute abdomen: pneumonia in the left base.* Note the extensive paralytic ileus in this patient with an acute abdomen. However, also note the area of increased density behind the left side of the heart (*arrows*) representing a pneumonia in the left lower lobe.

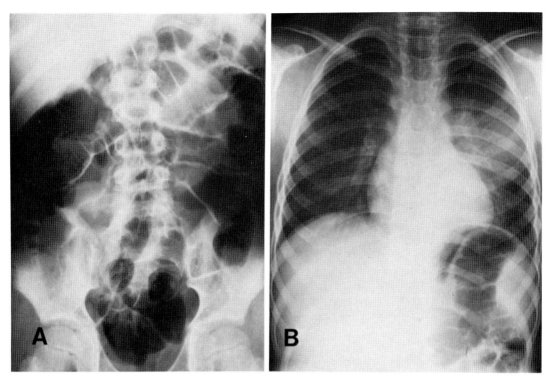

Figure 3.39. *Acute abdomen: value of chest film.* (*A*) Note extensive paralytic ileus in this patient presenting with an acute abdomen and suspected appendicitis. (*B*) Chest film demonstrates a large consolidating pneumonia in the left midlung.

suggesting an acute abdominal problem. Very often (1–3), but not always, the pneumonia is in the base of one of the lungs, and interestingly enough these pneumonias often are best seen on abdominal films (Fig. 3.38). The reason for this is that the higher kilovolt technique utilized for abdominal roentgenography tends to accentuate the density of the pneumonia, and, in addition, since many of these pneumonias are hidden behind the left or right side of the heart, a relatively overpenetrated roentgenographic technique actually is desirable. On the other hand, it should be remembered that not all such pneumonias are located in this area, and, indeed, *many are located higher in the lungs and surely will be missed if a chest roentgenogram is not obtained (Fig. 3.39).*

Most often when a pneumonia produces symptoms referable to the abdomen, a condition such as appendicitis is at first suspected, but as opposed to instances of appendicitis, roentgenographic examination of the abdomen usually is normal. On occasion, however, one will encounter both appendicitis and pneumonia in the same patient (1, 2). We have seen a few such cases, and it does require close clinical and roentgenographic correlation, maximal objectiveness, and diligence in analysis of the roentgenograms.

REFERENCES

1. Baechli, D., and Braun, P.: Concomitant pneumonia and acute appendicitis in a child. Z. Kinderchir. 23: 409–411, 1978.
2. Gongaware, R.D., Weil, R., III, and Santulli, T.V.: Right lower lobe pneumonia and acute appendicitis in childhood: A therapeutic disorder. J. Pediatr. Surg. 8: 33–35, 1973.
3. Jona, J.Z., and Belin, R.P.: Basilar pneumonia simulating acute appendicitis in children. Arch. Surg. 111: 552–553, 1976.

Acute Gastroenteritis. Gastroenteritis is the single most common abdominal inflammatory problem, and most often one is dealing with a viral infection. The clinical symptoms of vomiting and/or diarrhea are well known, and dehydration, especially in young infants, is a common and potentially serious complication. Roentgenographically, dehydration commonly is reflected on the chest films by the presence of markedly overaerated lungs, decreased pulmonary vascularity, and a small cardiac silhouette (see Fig. 1.150).

In the abdomen, the abnormal roentgenographic patterns are extremely variable and, to say the least, frequently very puzzling. However, the most common pattern is that of many loops of air-filled, distended intestine. Both large and small bowel are involved, but so gross are the findings that frequently it is difficult to differentiate one from the other. Indeed, one frequently first believes that mechanical obstruction is present (Fig. 3.40). In other cases of gastroenteritis, only a portion of the gastrointestinal tract may be dilated, and in such cases if: (a) the stomach shows predominant dilatation, a gastric outlet obstruction may be suggested (Fig. 3.41); (b) one or two loops of small bowel predominate, a small bowel obstruction may erroneously be diagnosed (Fig. 3.42A); and (c) the findings are confined to the colon, colon obstruction will be suggested (Fig. 3.42B). Finally, it should be noted that early in the course of gastroenteritis, when vomiting is the basic problem, one also may see a totally airless abdomen (see Fig. 3.4). In still other instances, a locally dilated loop of small intestine (pseudo-sen-

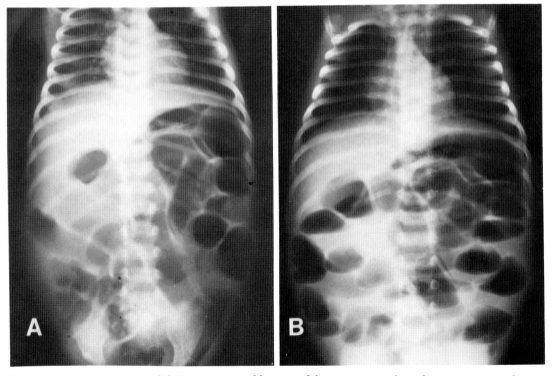

Figure 3.40. *Gastroenteritis.* (*A*) Note extensive dilatation of the intestines in this infant presenting with signs and symptoms of gastroenteritis. (*B*) Upright film demonstrates numerous air-fluid levels in the intestines. Although the characteristic dynamic, inverted "U," or hairpin, configuration of obstructed intestinal loops is absent, these findings still often are mistaken for intestinal obstruction.

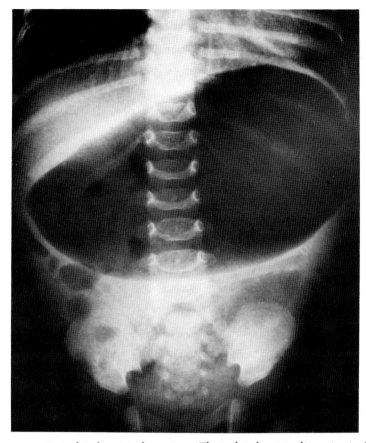

Figure 3.41. *Gastroenteritis: isolated gastric distension.* The isolated gastric distension in this infant with gastroenteritis could be misinterpreted as a gastric outlet obstruction.

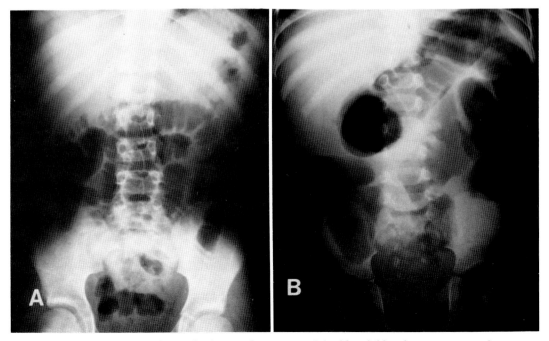

Figure 3.42. *Gastroenteritis: other misleading configurations.* (**A**) Older child with gastroenteritis demonstrating a picture suggesting jejunal obstruction. (**B**) Infant with gastroenteritis showing distension of the colon only.

tinel loop) may be encountered (see Fig. 3.11*B*). With ultrasound, gastroenteritis presents with dilated loops, hyperperistalsis, and, in some cases, muscosal thickening (Fig. 3.43).

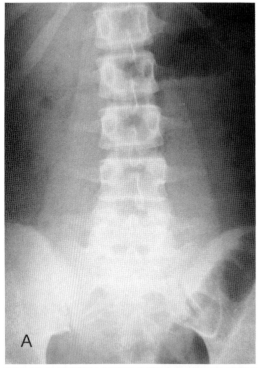

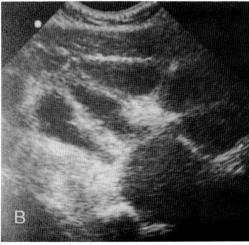

Figure 3.43. *Gastroenteritis: value of ultrasound.* (*A*) Note the virtually airless abdomen. (*B*) Ultrasonogram, however, demonstrates numerous loops of fluid-filled intestine.

Appendicitis. After gastroenteritis, *appendicitis is the most common acute abdominal inflammatory problem in childhood, and its accurate diagnosis remains as challenging as ever.* Indeed, many times the diagnosis is not secured until 24–48 hours have passed and by that time perforation has occurred. In this regard, it has been demonstrated that observation in a hospital environment can significantly remedy this problem and result in a greater yield of positive laparotomies (53). However, White and associates (53) underscore the fact that these patients must be observed in the hospital and not on an outpatient basis.

The classic clinical findings of appendicitis are well known but, of course, not all always are present in any one patient. In addition, there is the controversial problem of recurrent appendicitis (19), and because of this, the clinician may look for help. In this regard, the additional studies and tests most often obtained were: (a) the white blood cell (WBC) count and (b) the abdominal roentgenogram. For a short period of time, the barium enema gained popularity in the diagnosis of acute appendicitis, but currently if an additional imaging study is needed, ultrasonography is favored. In terms of the WBC count, it has been suggested that a count of <10,000 WBC/mm of blood is virtually incompatible with the diagnosis of acute appendicitis (26). By the same token, it can be stated that a count of >20,000 WBC/mm of blood also is unlikely to be due to appendicitis, but, of course, neither limit completely excludes the diagnosis.

As far as the abdominal roentgenogram is concerned, although there have been numerous dissertations on the subject (3, 14, 15, 18, 20, 22, 30, 32, 48, 50, 54), many still consider it valid only for the demonstration of a fecalith, free air, or some other complication of acute appendicitis. However, there is no question that the study is of far more value than this, but to be of such value the *relationship of the pathology of perforated and nonperforated appendicitis to the roentgenographic findings must be understood.*

In this regard, it should first be noted that *most children with acute nonperforated appendicitis show diminished air in the gastrointestinal tract.* Indeed, in some cases the abdomen is virtually airless (Fig. 3.44), while in others a few sentinel loops are seen on the right or, in the right lower quadrant (Fig. 3.45). In explaining the paucity of intestinal gas in these children, one must only recall that acute nonperforated appendicitis usually is associated with one or all of the following: (a) anorexia, (b) nausea, (c) vomiting, and (d) diarrhea. In any combination, these findings readily lead to a paucity of air in the gastrointestinal tract. Of course, in those cases where symptoms have not been present for a long enough period of time, usually under 12–18 hours, the airless gas pattern may not

have had enough time to develop and the roentgenograms will be normal, except, perhaps for the presence of scoliosis. On the other hand, seldom if ever is the gas pattern increased and, actually, if in a patient with suspected appendicitis intestinal gas is abundant and the bowel dilated, perforation should be suspected (Fig. 3.46).

The reasons for this change in the intestinal gas pattern with appendiceal perforation are multiple. First of all, just after perforation there is a relatively quiet clinical period, and as the acute anorexia and nausea settle down, more air is swallowed and retained in the gastrointestinal tract. At the same time peritonitis develops, and progressive paralytic ileus in the intestines is induced. Because of this, the swallowed air becomes trapped in the paralyzed intestine, and in many cases the degree of intestinal dilatation and gas accumulation is startling (Fig. 3.46). In such cases, if the

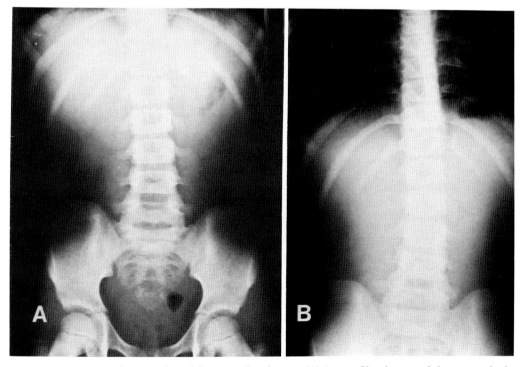

Figure 3.44. *Acute appendicitis: airless abdomen and scoliosis.* (*A*) Supine film showing abdomen in which gas is virtually absent. There is a minimal degree of scoliosis present. (*B*) On the upright film, however, note how much more pronounced the degree of scoliosis has become. Only a little gas is seen in the stomach.

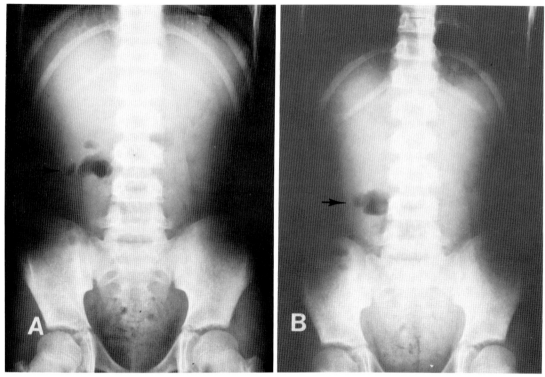

Figure 3.45. *Acute appendicitis: localized right-sided gas collections and indistinct right psoas shadow.* (**A**) Supine film showing a few isolated loops of distended intestine in the right flank (*arrow*). The right psoas shadow is less distinct than the left. (**B**) On upright view air-fluid levels are seen in the isolated loops of distended intestine (*arrow*). Indistinctness of the right psoas muscle is more apparent. No real scoliosis is present.

findings are considered in the absence of clinical correlation, confusion with gastroenteritis can occur (i.e., compare Fig. 3.46 with Fig. 3.40).

Other roentgenographic signs of acute appendicitis consist of the following: (a) lumbar or lumbosacral scoliosis with concavity to the right, (b) absence or indistinctness of the right psoas margin, (c) localized loops of dilated intestine in the right lower quadrant or flank, (d) air in the appendix, and (e) the presence of a calcified fecalith in the appendix.

Scoliosis with concavity to the right results from splinting of the paraspinal and psoas muscles, and the curve produced usually involves the lumbar spine or the lumbosacral junction. Scoliosis should be assessed on both the supine and upright views, for minimal degrees of scoliosis

often become more apparent on upright views (Fig. 3.44). Absence or indistinctness of the right psoas muscle margin also is a common finding in acute appendicitis and in the past has been explained in terms of obliteration due to adjacent edema. However, another, more likely explanation is distortion of the muscle edge due to spasm of the muscle (56). With spasm, the psoas muscle changes its cross-sectional shape and the normal, sharp outer edge is lost (Fig. 3.47). Localized right lower quadrant loops of distended intestine are sentinel loops and result from paralytic ileus of the terminal ileum and cecum secondary to the adjacent inflammatory process in the appendix (18, 29, 33, 54).

Air in the appendix is a relatively rare finding in acute appendicitis (Fig. 3.48), but generally is believed to be suggestive

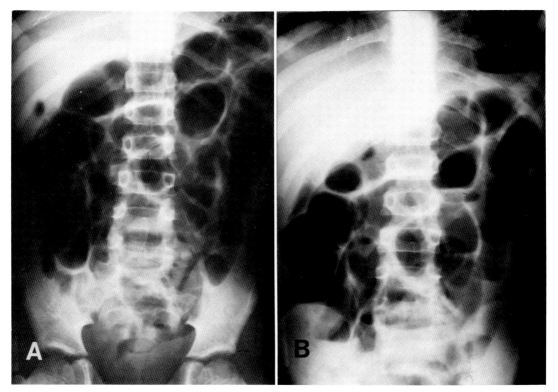

Figure 3.46. *Perforated appendicitis: large volumes of gas in the intestine.* (*A*) Note large volumes of gas present in both the large and small bowel in this patient with perforated appendicitis. The findings are distinctly different from those seen with nonperforated acute appendicitis as demonstrated in Figures 3.44 and 3.45. (*B*) Upright view showing numerous air-fluid levels scattered throughout both the large and small intestine. On the supine view, there is a small fecalith visualized just to the right of the midsacral spine, and there may be some suggestion of fluid displacing the cecum medially from the right abdominal wall, but otherwise the findings easily could be misinterpreted as those of gastroenteritis.

Effect of Psoas Angle on Radiographic Visualization

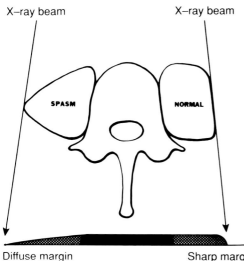

Figure 3.47. *Explanation of lack of psoas margin visualization.* Spasm of the psoas muscle distorts its contour and makes its outer edge appear more angled. As a result, the flat outer surface of the muscle is lost and the incidental x-ray beam (*arrows*), as it passes through the muscle and along the angled edge, does not produce a sharp margin. (From S.M. Williams, R.K. Harned, S.A. Hultman, and M.A. Qualfe: The psoas sign: A reevaluation. RadioGraphics 5: 525–536, 1985.)

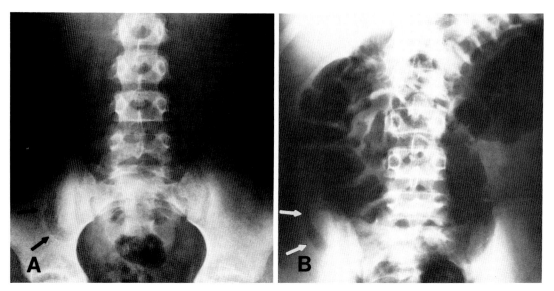

Figure 3.48. *Air in the appendix: acute appendicitis.* (*A*) Note air in an irregular and overdistended appendix (*arrows*). In addition, note absence of the right psoas shadow and a virtually airless abdomen. (*B*) Another patient with a distended, air-filled appendix (*arrows*), with an irregular lumen. There is proximal narrowing and distal distension. Also note the soft tissue mass effect around the appendix.

of the condition (13, 24, 43). On the other hand, it has been pointed out that air may be present in the appendix of patients with profound paralytic ileus or other inflammatory bowel disease (28). Nevertheless, in a case of suspected acute appendicitis, the persistent presence of air in the appendix should be taken as a positive finding. This is especially true if the abdomen is airless and the appendix overdistended or its lumen irregular in diameter (Fig. 3.48*A* and *B*). If these additional criteria are absent, one should be cautious about one's interpretation of air in the appendix. In acute appendicitis, gas accumulates in the appendix because it is occluded and because gas-producing organisms grow within it. Occlusion can be secondary to a fecalith (calcified or uncalcified), inspissated feces, or, rarely, inflammatory lymphadenopathy.

A calcified fecalith in the right lower quadrant, in the pelvis, or on the right side of the abdomen (Fig. 3.49) should virtually assure the diagnosis of acute appendicitis (4, 10, 11, 14, 15, 48, 54, 55). This is not to say, however, that calcified fecaliths are seen only in patients with acute appendicitis, for occasionally one encounters a calcified fecalith in a totally asymptomatic child. However, since it is generally held that over 50% of cases of perforated appendicitis are accompanied by fecaliths, the presence of this finding certainly does place even the asymptomatic patient in a higher risk category. To be sure, there is continued debate as to whether prophylactic appendectomy is warranted in such cases, for there is the strong likelihood that acute appendicitis will develop in these individuals sooner or later.

Roentgenographic signs of perforated appendicitis may consist of any of the following: (a) right side colon cutoff sign, (b) small bowel obstruction with or without a paucity of gas in the right lower quadrant, (c) inflammatory mass or abscess in the right lower quadrant or pelvis, (d) positive flank stripe sign, (e) obliteration of the properitoneal fat line on the right, and (f) free

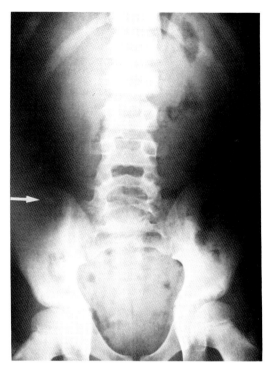

Figure 3.49. *Acute appendicitis with calcified fecalith.* Note that the abdomen shows virtual absence of intestinal gas. In addition, however, note the presence of a calcified fecalith in the right lower quadrant (*arrow*).

intraperitoneal air. Many times, more than one of the findings are present in any one patient, but free air is relatively rare (31, 50).

The right colon cutoff sign (23, 49) often is the first roentgenographic sign of perforation (49). It results from a combination of spasm of the cecum and ascending colon induced by the adjacent inflammatory process, and reflex paralytic ileus of the transverse, or remaining, ascending colon. As a result, the two areas of the colon are demarcated by a sharp cutoff of gas in the right upper quadrant. This finding is best assessed on the supine view, for on upright view shifting gas and fecal material in the colon can totally obscure its presence (Fig. 3.50). It is most important that, when the colon cutoff sign is present, it be deter-

mined that right side colon gas is diminished because of spasm and not because the cecum and ascending colon are full of feces. If gas is present in the transverse colon and absent in the ascending colon because it is full of fecal material, the colon cutoff sign is invalid (Fig. 3.51). In any such case, if there is doubt about the validity of the sign, a decubitus film, with right side up, can be employed. If one is dealing with a false cutoff sign, then the ascending colon should fill on the decubitus view (Fig. 3.52).

The right colon cutoff sign, of course, is not seen in all cases of perforated appendicitis and, actually, more commonly one will encounter a picture suggestive of low small bowel obstruction (Figs. 3.53 and 3.54). This type of obstruction has been termed "functional obstruction," for it probably represents a combination of mechanical and paralytic ileus (30, 32, 39). The mechanical component results from the obstructive effects of the progressive inflammatory process developing in the right lower quadrant, while the paralytic aspect represents reflex paralysis of the small bowel (39). Together these factors lead to varying degrees of obstruction, and in some cases the picture of obstruction is so distracting that, unless one is cognizant of the phenomenon, one will not consider perforated appendicitis as the primary diagnosis. Other findings associated with perforated appendicitis include signs of peritonitis, a positive flank stripe sign, and obliteration of the properitoneal fat line.

Signs of peritonitis are those of fluid in the abdomen (Fig. 3.55), while a positive flank stripe sign consists of an increase in the soft tissue distance between the abdominal wall and air-filled descending colon or cecum. The soft tissue space is widened by inflammatory edema or frank abscess formation (7). There is no question that when the finding is present it is very useful, but most often so many other findings of perforated appendicitis also are

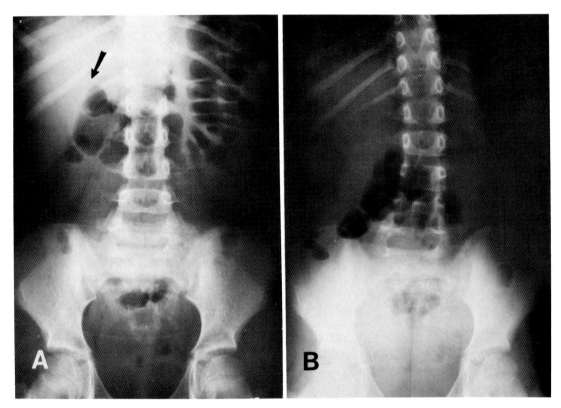

Figure 3.50. *Acute appendicitis: colon cutoff sign.* (*A*) Note gas in the transverse colon. The transverse colon is not unduly dilated, but gas terminates abruptly in the region of the hepatic flexure (*arrow*). This is the colon cutoff sign. The ascending colon and cecum are virtually empty but there are one or two locally distended sentinel loops of intestine in the right lower quadrant. (*B*) Upright view demonstrating the development of significant scoliosis, loss of the colon cutoff sign, and confirmation of the presence of locally distended loops of dilated intestine in the right lower quadrant.

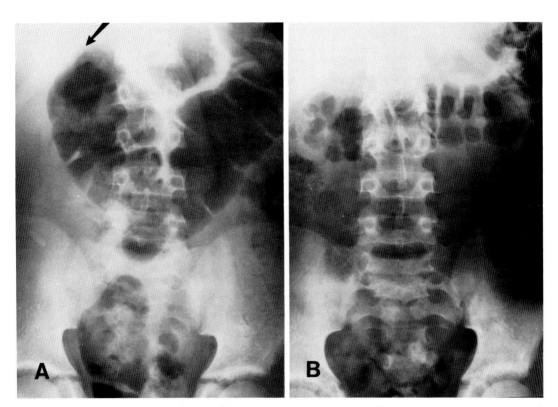

Figure 3.51. *Acute appendicitis: colon cutoff sign.* (*A*) Note the colon cutoff sign (*arrow*) and the presence of a fecalith. (*B*) Two years earlier the patient had symptoms suggestive of appendicitis; the fecalith was present and a colon cutoff sign was suggested. However, note feces in the ascending colon and lack of dilatation of the transverse colon. This negates the colon cutoff sign, but a decubitus film was not obtained. The patient was not operated upon at this time, but returned 2 years later with perforated appendicitis as demonstrated in (*A*).

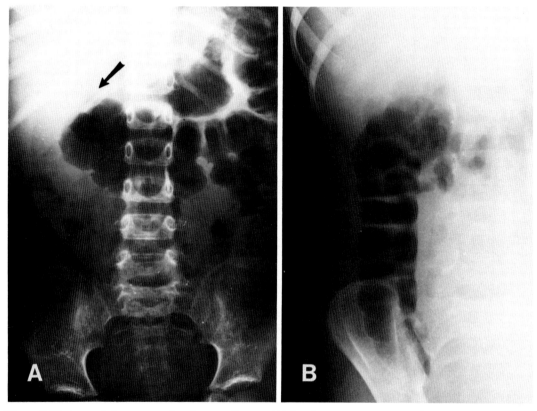

Figure 3.52. *Acute abdomen: pseudocolon cutoff sign.*   (**A**) On this supine view, note that a colon cutoff sign is suggested (*arrow*). (**B**) Decubitus film shows the ascending colon to readily fill with air. This negates the original suggestion of a colon cutoff sign.

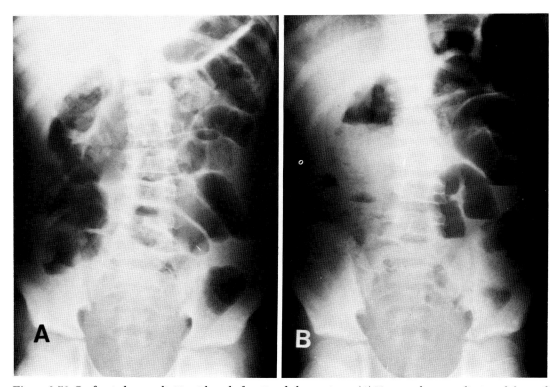

Figure 3.53. *Perforated appendicitis with early functional obstruction.* (*A*) Note moderate scoliosis and three of four loops of distended small bowel just to the left of the spine. (*B*) Upright view showing the same loops, but this time with air-fluid levels. These findings represent early functional obstruction secondary to perforated appendicitis.

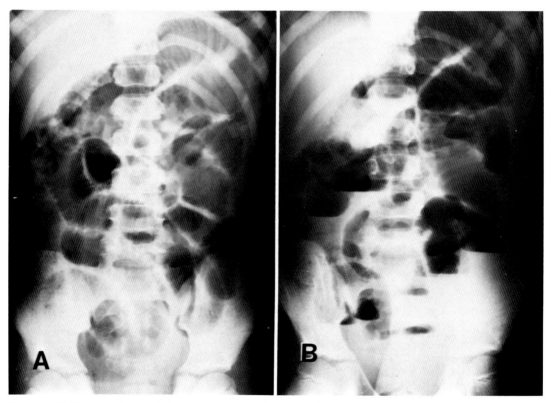

Figure 3.54. *Perforated appendicitis with pronounced functional obstruction.* (*A*) Supine view demonstrating numerous loops of distended intestine. However, note that the loops of jejunum are disproportionately distended when compared with gas in the colon. (*B*) The findings are visualized with greater clarity on the upright view where numerous, acute-appearing air-fluid levels are noted within the distended loops of jejunum. These findings represent pronounced functional obstruction secondary to perforation of the appendix.

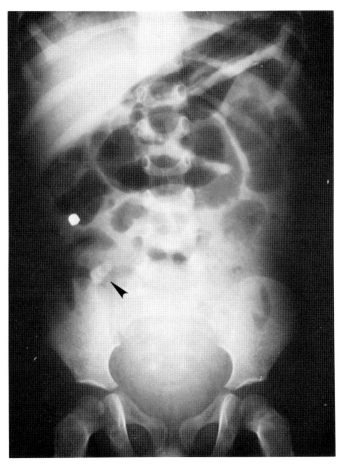

Figure 3.55. *Perforated appendicitis with abscess, fecalith, and peritonitis.*   First note that there are numerous loops of distended intestine in the abdomen (i.e., functional obstruction). However, note that the space between the individual loops is thickened. This indicates the presence of intraperitoneal fluid (pus) and, hence, the presence of peritonitis. Also note the calcified fecalith (*arrow*) and surrounding inflammatory mass (abscess). Increased density and whiteness of the lower abdomen and pelvic regions are due to the presence of intraperitoneal pus. An incidental colonic foreign body is seen above the calcified fecalith.

present that its practical value is diminished (Fig. 3.56). Absence of the right properitoneal fat line also is seen in advanced cases of appendiceal perforation, but as with the positive flank stripe sign, absence of the properitoneal fat line often is a superfluous finding, for other findings of perforation usually are present (Fig. 3.56). The presence of free air is the least common finding in perforated appendicitis and, when present, usually is of small volume and more difficult to detect.

An abscess clearly reflects an underlying perforation, and while in some cases the abscess may appear classically granular or dense and well defined, more often it is less well organized (Figs. 3.55 and 3.56). In still other instances, fixed, formless air bubbles are present within the generalized opacity of the abscess (Fig. 3.57), and, finally, in some cases massive accumulations of air are seen in abscess cavity (Fig. 3.58).

Ultrasonography now commonly is used for the evaluation of acute appendicitis but much as the physical examination is not perfect (1, 8, 16, 21, 25, 36, 40, 45, 46, 51,

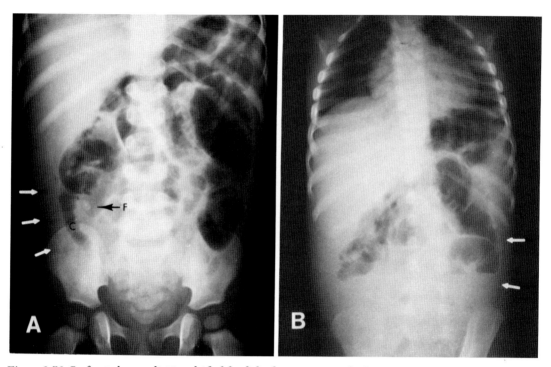

Figure 3.56. *Perforated appendicitis-calcified fecalith, abscess, positive flank stripe sign, and absent properitoneal fat stripe.* (*A*) Supine view demonstrating abundant gas within dilated intestines, a calcified fecalith (*F*), and medial displacement of the contracted cecum (*C*). The cecum is displaced medially because of the presence of fluid and edema between it and the abdominal wall. This constitutes a positive flank stripe sign (*arrows*). (*B*) Upright view showing the presence of a few distended loops of jejunum with air-fluid levels, but in addition clear-cut evidence that the properitoneal fat stripe on the right is absent. The properitoneal fat stripe on the left (*arrows*) is present. In addition, note that the gas-filled intestine on the right continues to be displaced medially from the abdominal wall (i.e., positive flank stripe sign).

57). Generally, the criteria utilized for the diagnosis of acute appendicitis include focal tenderness over the inflamed appendix, lack of compressibility of the appendix, fluid in the appendiceal lumen, and a transverse diameter of 6 mm or more (36). The normal appendix, not uncommonly identified, is not distended or tender (Fig. 3.59).

Once an inflamed appendix is identified, a variety of configurations can be seen, but the appendix will be distended and visible in almost all cases (38). In some cases, the distending intraluminal fluid is relatively sonolucent, while in others it is more echogenic due to debris. The mucosa is variably intact and in some cases is virtually de-

stroyed. Of course, a fecalith frequently is identified and such fecaliths may not be calcified; thus more fecaliths are identified with ultrasound than on plain films. Fluid may be seen around the appendix but does not necessarily indicate perforation (16), and in many cases localized adenopathy is also present (16). All of these findings are demonstrated in Figures 3.60 and 3.61.

Recently, color flow Doppler has been shown to demonstrate increased flow to the wall of the inflamed appendix (37). This finding has proved additionally useful for us (Fig. 3.61) and overall there is no question that ultrasonography has made a significant impact on the investigation of

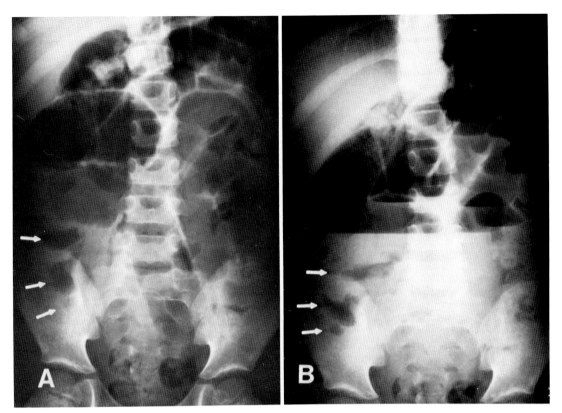

Figure 3.57. *Perforated appendicitis with abscess: fixed bubbles.* (**A**) Supine view demonstrating numerous loops of distended small bowel in the abdomen and two or three formless loops of gas in the right lower quadrant. In addition, a soft tissue inflammatory mass around these latter air collections is suggested (*arrows*). (**B**) Upright view shows the development of numerous air-fluid levels in the distended loops of small bowel. A functional obstruction is present. However, note that the formless collections of gas in the *right lower quadrant* (*arrows*) have not changed significantly in configuration or position. This lack of change in the appearance of the bubbles from supine to upright view can be taken as presumptive evidence for the presence of an abscess (which was surgically confirmed).

acute appendicitis, but it is unlikely that it will replace the physical examination. On the other hand, it is very complementary and, indeed, most useful in confusing and minimally symptomatic cases (46). In this regard, ultrasound also has the capability of documenting aborted cases of appendicitis, where the clinical and ultrasonographic findings never reach their full-blown stage before they spontaneously dissipate.

With perforated appendicitis, ultrasound may demonstrate the presence of free peritoneal fluid, a fluid collection in juxtaposition to the appendix, periappendiceal fat echogenicity, or actual abscess formation. It has also been demonstrated that there is loss of the echogenic submucosal layer (38), but one of the most important and problematic features, in our experience, has been that the appendix itself collapses and becomes more difficult to identify (Fig. 3.62). This has been noted by others (38). Color flow Doppler, with its ability to show increased blood flow to the inflamed appendiceal wall, may prove useful in such cases. Overall, however, imaging the perforated appendix is more diffi-

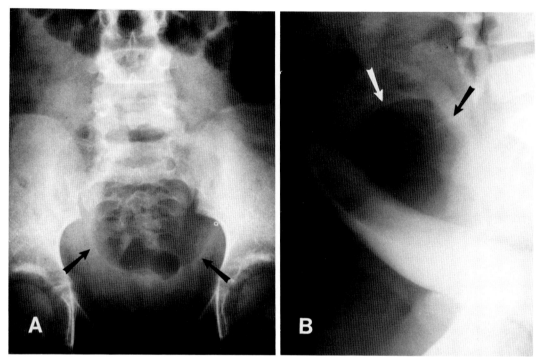

Figure 3.58. *Appendiceal abscess.* (**A**) Note the large gas-filled abscess (*arrows*). (**B**) Lateral view showing the same abscess (*arrows*) behind the contrast-filled bladder.

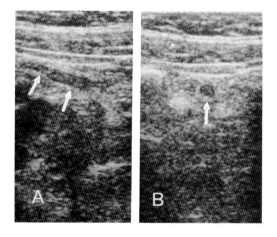

Figure 3.59. *Normal appendix.* (**A**) Longitudinal view demonstrating the normal appendix (*arrows*). (**B**) Cross-sectional view showing the appendix (*arrow*).

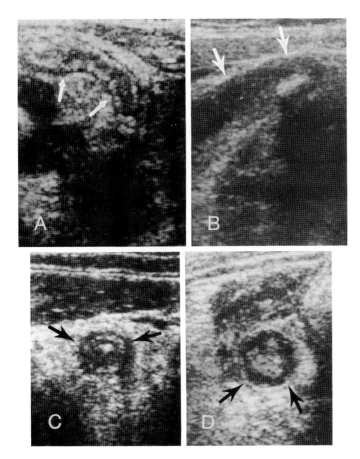

Figure 3.60. *Acute appendicitis: ultra-sonographic features.* (**A**) Note the distended, fluid-filled appendix (*arrows*). The echogenic mucosa is still intact. (**B**) Another patient with a distended appendix (*arrows*), but with the mucosa less intact. There is an echogenic fecalith in the tip of the appendix. (**C**) Cross-sectional view in another patient of a swollen, distended appendix (*arrows*). Note the concentric ring configuration. An echogenic, but nonshadowing fecalith is present in the center. (**D**) Another patient with a markedly distended appendix (*arrows*) with a sonolucent rim and a great deal of echogenic debris within its lumen.

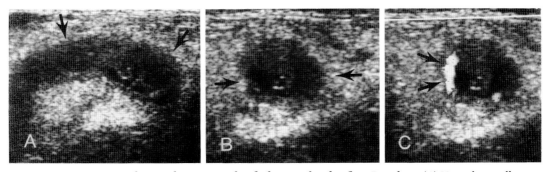

Figure 3.61. *Acute appendicitis: ultrasonographic findings with color flow Doppler.* (**A**) Note the swollen appendix (*arrows*) on longitudinal view. There is very little residual echogenic mucosa. (**B**) Cross-sectional view shows the distended appendix (*arrows*). (**C**) Color flow Doppler demonstrates excessive flow to the appendiceal wall (*arrows*).

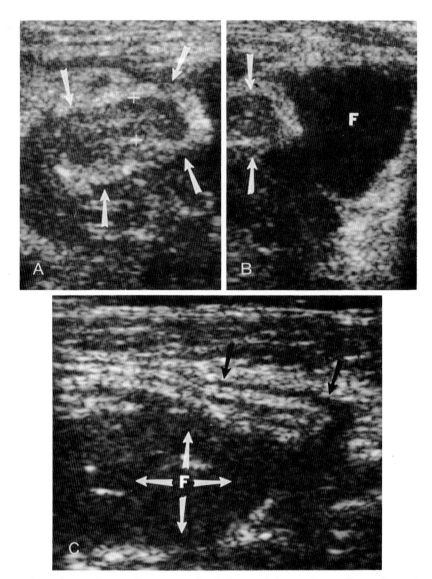

Figure 3.62. *Perforated appendicitis: ultrasonographic findings.* (*A*) Note the swollen, collapsed appendix surrounded by echogenic, thickened fat (*arrows*). (*B*) The appendix (*arrows*) is seen in cross-section. A large fluid collection (*F*) is seen adjacent to the appendix. (*C*) Another patient with a collapsed appendix (*arrows*) with an adjacent fluid collection (*F*). Note that the tip of the appendix is indistinct suggesting that this is where the perforation occurred.

cult than imaging the nonperforated appendix (16, 38).

Abscesses after perforation can be located in a variety of places and have a number of configurations ranging from oval to round to lobulated. They may have a sonolucent center, contain debris, be virtually solid, or show a hyperechoic rim (Fig.

3.63). CT, of course, is also very useful in the detection of postperforation abscesses (Fig. 3.64), and, in addition, can clearly identify the presence of free fluid in the abdomen, especially in the cul-de-sac. An important clinical feature of completely walled-off abscesses is that they do not present with acute findings. The patient

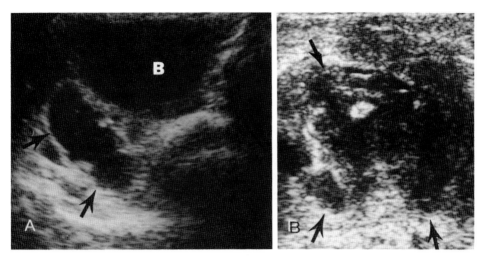

Figure 3.63. *Perforated appendicitis with abscess; ultrasound findings.* (**A**) Note the sonolucent irregular abscess (*arrows*) behind the urinary bladder (**B**). (**B**) Another abscess (*arrows*) basically sonolucent but with echogenic debris and a central fecalith.

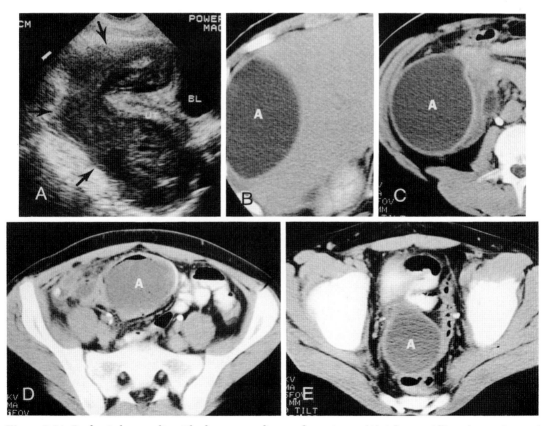

Figure 3.64. *Perforated appendix with abscess; peculiar configurations.* (**A**) A large midline abscess (*arrows*) surrounding the uterus. Bladder (*bl*). (**B**) Another patient 3 weeks after perforation demonstrates a well-circumscribed abscess (**A**) adjacent to the liver. The abscess appears intrahepatic but was extrahepatic. (**C**) A little lower in the abdomen one can see the well-defined abscess (**A**) with a slightly hyperintense rim. (**D**) Low in the pelvis another abscess (**A**) is demonstrated. Some air is present in this abscess. There is also adjacent soft tissue edema on the right. (**E**) Lower, this same abscess (**A**) extends in front of the rectum. These abscesses were drained percutaneously.

usually is obviously not completely healthy, but yet not seriously ill. In such cases, the abscesses responsible may appear unusually benign and/or bizarre (Fig. 3.64).

The diagnosis of *retrocecal appendicitis* is more difficult than the diagnosis of appendicitis in its usual location, and in such cases the clinical findings may mimic those of cholecystitis, pancreatitis, hepatitis, or kidney disease. Consequently, a delay in

diagnosis is common, and because of this, perforation occurs more often (19, 33, 50). Roentgenographically, in these cases, the findings may be very subtle and may differ from the usual case of appendicitis in the following ways: (a) scoliosis may be located in the upper lumbar or thoracolumbar spine, (b) sentinel loops may lie more in the right upper quadrant, and (c) a fecalith may lie higher than expected.

The *barium enema examination* once

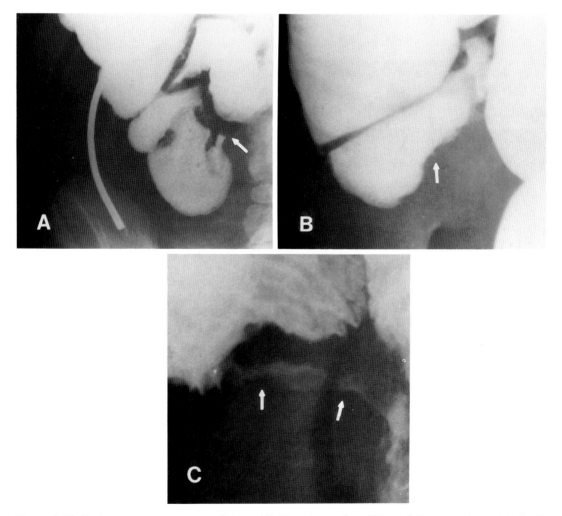

Figure 3.65. *Barium enema: acute appendicitis.* (**A**) Note incomplete filling of the appendix and lack of a rounded bulbous end (*arrow*). (**B**) Nonfilling of the appendix with a barium-filled pointed beak at its base (*arrow*). Also note minimal associated cecal indentation. (**C**) Incomplete filling of the appendix with mucosal edema causing gross cobblestoning (*arrows*).

was becoming popular for the diagnosis of acute, nonperforated appendicitis (12, 27, 44). It was a safe and valuable procedure, but as ultrasound arrived on the scene, its role virtually has been relegated to confusing cases of perforated appendicitis. Basically, in acute appendicitis, one was looking for filling or nonfilling of the appendix. One of the problems was that 10–15% of normal appendices do not fill on barium enema examination (42). On the other hand, positive findings included complete or partial lack of filling of the appendix, a pointed beak of barium at the base of the nonfilled appendix, cobblestoning and other signs of mucosal edema and spasm,

and irregularity or deformity of the adjacent cecum (Fig. 3.65).

With perforated appendicitis, many cases are confusing clinically, and in others it may be difficult to clearly identify an abscess with ultrasound. Of course, one might proceed to CT in these cases, but if a barium enema is obtained, it will demonstrate the presence of an adjacent inflammatory process (35) that should be presumed secondary to perforated appendicitis until proven otherwise (Figs. 3.66 and 3.67). In these cases, the adjacent intestine, be it colon or small bowel, will be displaced by the inflammatory process, and at the same time, these and other loops

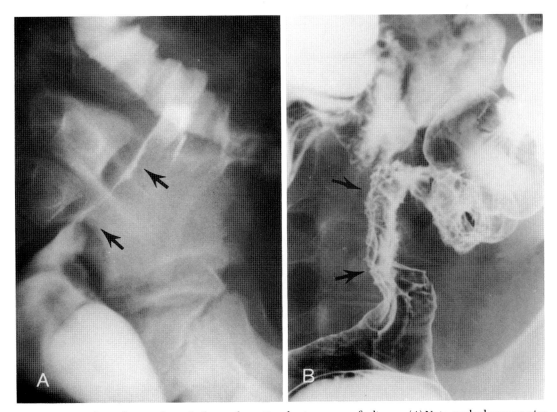

Figure 3.66. *Perforated appendix with abscess formation: barium enema findings.* (A) Note marked compression and narrowing of the rectum (*arrows*) just in front of the spine. A large abscess was present anteriorly. (B) Another patient demonstrating entrapment of a segment of the rectum (*arrows*) by a surrounding abscess. Note spiculation and tethering of the intestine.

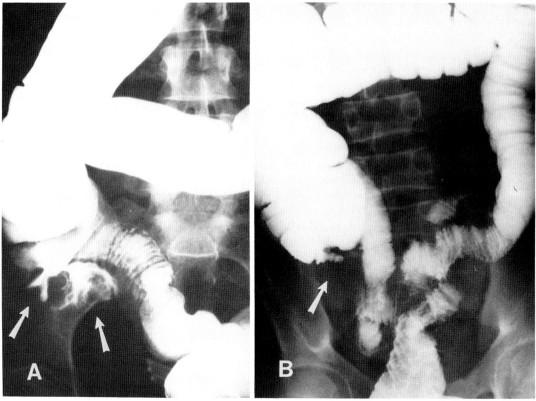

Figure 3.67. *Perforated appendicitis: barium enema findings.* (*A*) Note the contracted, deformed cecum (*arrows*) and absence of filling of the appendix even though the terminal ileum is well filled. (*B*) Another patient demonstrating similar findings but a less deformed cecum (*arrow*). Also note changes in the sigmoid colon suggesting pericolonic inflammation. The colon contour is irregular and edema and deformity of the wall are suggested.

of bowel will appear plastered to the inflammatory mass (Fig. 3.66 and 3.67).

Other interesting features of acute appendicitis include the following: (a) appendiceal foreign bodies can lead to appendiceal inflammation (6), (b) urinary tract disease can present as appendicitis or vice versa, (c) a genitourinary fistula may result (17, 41), and (d) an inflamed or perforated appendix can lie in an inguinal or femoral hernia, or in the scrotum of a young male infant (2, 5, 52). In these latter cases, the infant may present with an acute abdomen, intestinal obstruction, or a mass in the inguinal region or scrotum. With urinary tract involvement, symptoms such as pyuria, hematuria, right flank pain, etc., may render the problem virtually indistinguishable from that of true urinary tract infection. Indeed, if an intravenous pyelogram is performed, paralytic ileus of the ureter with apparent ureteral obstruction of the ureter may further add to one's erroneous initial impressions (9, 34). Liver abscess also can be seen as a complication of perforated appendicitis (47).

REFERENCES

1. Abu-Yousef, M.M., Bleicher, J.J., Maher, J.W., Urdaneta, L.F., Franken, E.A., Jr., and Metcalf, A.M.: High resolution sonography of acute appendicitis. A.J.R. 149: 53–58, 1987.
2. Alvear, D.T., and Rayfield, M.M.: Acute appendicitis presenting as a scrotal mass. J. Pediatr. Surg. 11: 91–92, 1976.

3. Bakhda, R.K., and McNair, M.M.: Useful radiological signs in acute appendicitis in children. Clin. Radiol. 28: 193–196, 1977.

4. Brady, B., and Carroll, D.: The significance of the calcified appendiceal enterolith. Radiology 68: 648, 1957.

5. Carey, L.C.: Acute appendicitis occurring in hernias: A report of 10 cases. Surgery 61: 236, 1967.

6. Carey, L.S.: Lead shot appendicitis in northern native people. J. Can. Assoc. Radiol. 28: 171–174, 1977.

7. Casper, R.B.: Fluid in the right flank as a roentgenographic sign of acute appendicitis. A.J.R. 110: 352–354, 1970.

8. Ceres, L., Alonso, I., Lopez, P., Parra, G., and Echeverry, J.: Ultrasound study of acute appendicitis in children with emphasis for the diagnosis of retrocecal appendicitis. Pediatr. Radiol. 20: 258–261, 1990.

9. Chiu, R., and Gambach, R.: Radiographic ureteral changes with appendicitis. J. Can. Assoc. Radiol. 25: 154–160, 1974.

10. Faegenburg, D.: Fecalith of the appendix: Incidence and significance. A.J.R. 89: 752–759, 1963.

11. Felson, B., and Bernhard, C.M.: The roentgenologic diagnosis of appendiceal calculi. Radiology 49: 178–191, 1947.

12. Figiel, L.S., and Figiel, S.J.: Barium examination of cecum in appendicitis. Acta Radiol. 57: 469–480, 1962.

13. Fisher, M.S.: A roentgen sign of gangrenous appendicitis. A.J.R. 81: 637–639, 1959.

14. Graham, A.D., and Johnson, H.F.: The incidence of radiographic findings in acute appendicitis compared to 200 normal abdomens. Milit. Med. 131: 272–276, 1966.

15. Hatten, L.E., Miller, R.C., Hester, C.L., Jr., and Moynihan, P.C.: Appendicitis and the abdominal roentgenogram in children. South. Med. J. 66: 803–806, 1973.

16. Hayden, C.K., Jr., Kuchelmeister, J., and Lipscomb, T.S.: Sonography of acute appendicitis in childhood: Perforation vs. nonperforation. J. Ultrasound Med. 11: 209–216, 1992.

17. Hoffer, F.A., Ablow, R.C., Gryboski, J.D., and Seashore, J.H.: Primary appendicitis with an appendio-tuboovarian fistula. A.J.R. 138: 742–743, 1982.

18. Holgerson, L.O., and Stanley-Brown, E.G.: Acute appendicitis with perforation. Am. J. Dis. Child. 122: 288–293, 1971.

19. Homer, M.J., and Braver, J.M.: Recurrent appendicitis: reexamination of controversial disease. Gastrointest. Radiol. 4: 295–301, 1979.

20. Isdale, J.M.: The radiological signs of acute appendicitis in infancy and childhood. S. Afr. Med. J. 53: 363–364, 1978.

21. Jeffrey, R.B., Jr., Laing, F.C., and Townsend, R.R.: Acute appendicitis: Sonographic criteria based on 250 cases. Radiology 167: 327–329, 1988.

22. Joffe, N.: Some uncommon roentgenologic findings associated with acute perforative appendicitis. Radiology 110: 301–305, 1974.

23. Johnson, J.F., Pickett, W.J., and Enzenauer, R.W.: Contrast enema demonstration of a colon cut-off sign in a baby with perforated appendicitis. Pediatr. Radiol. 12: 150–151, 1982.

24. Killen, D.A., and Brooks, D.W., Jr.: Gas-filled appendix: A roentgenographic sign of acute appendicitis. Ann. Surg. 161: 474–478, 1965.

25. Larson, J.M., Pierce, J.C., Ellinger, D.M., Parish, G.H., Hammond, D.C., Ferguson, C.F., Verde, F.J., and Vander Kolk, H.L.: The validity and utility of sonography in the diagnosis of appendicitis in the community setting. A.J.R. 153: 687–691, 1989.

26. Lee, P.W.R.: The leukocyte count in acute appendicitis. Br. J. Surg. 60: 618, 1973.

27. Lewin, G.A., Mikity, V., and Wingert, W.A.: Barium enema: An outpatient procedure in the early diagnosis of acute appendicitis. J. Pediatr. 92: 451–453, 1978.

28. Lim, M.S.: Gas-filled appendix: Lack of diagnostic specificity. A.J.R. 128: 209–210, 1977.

29. May, L.M., O'Neill, F.E., and Allen, S.W.: Cecal ileus: An undescribed and helpful sign in acute appendicitis. Tex. J. Med. 54: 92, 1958.

30. Mayson, P.B., Jr., and Rosenthal, S.J.: Roentgen findings in delayed diagnosis of appendicitis. A.J.R. 103: 347–350, 1968.

31. McCort, J.J.: Extra-alimentary gas in perforated appendicitis. A.J.R. 84: 1087–1092, 1960.

32. Melamed, M., Melamed, J.L., and Rabushka, S.E.: Appendicitis: "Functional" bowel obstruction associated with perforation of the appendix. A.J.R. 99: 112–117, 1967.

33. Meyers, M.A., and Oliphant, M.: Ascending retrocecal appendicitis. Radiology 110: 295–299, 1974.

34. Moncada, R., Raffensperger, J., Wasserman, D., and Freeark, R.: Hydronephrosis secondary to acute appendicitis in children. Pediatr. Radiol. 2: 121–124, 1974.

35. Picus, D., and Shackelford, G.D.: Perforated appendix presenting with severe diarrhea: Findings on barium enema examination. Radiology 149: 141–143, 1983.

36. Puylaert, J.B.C.M., Rutgers, P.H., Lalisang, R.I., deVries, B.C., van der Werf, S.D.J., Dorr, J.P.J., and Blok, R.A.P.R.: A prospective study of ultrasonography in the diagnosis of appendicitis. N. Engl. J. Med. 317: 666–669, 1987.

37. Quillin, S.P., and Siegel, M.J.: Appendicitis in

children: Color Doppler sonography. Radiol. 184: 745–747, 1992.

38. Quillin, S.P., Siegel, M.J., and Coffin, C.M.: Acute appendicitis in children: Value of sonography in detecting perforation. A.J.R. 159: 1265–1268, 1992.

39. Riggs, W., and Parvey, L.S.: Perforated appendix presenting with disproportionate jejunal distention. Pediatr. Radiol. 5: 47–49, 1976.

40. Rioux, M.: Sonographic detection of the normal and abnormal appendix. A.J.R. 158: 773–778, 1992.

41. Rizen, B.K., Itzig, C., and Quinn, P.J.: Case report, appendicovesical fistula in childhood. Am. J. Dis. Child. 130: 530–531, 1976.

42. Sakover, R.P., and DelFava, R.L.: Frequency of visualization of the normal appendix with the barium enema examination. A.J.R. 121: 312–317, 1974.

43. Samuel, E.: The gas-filled appendix. Br. J. Radiol. 30: 27–30, 1957.

44. Schey, W.L.: Use of barium in the diagnosis of appendicitis in children. A.J.R. 118: 95–103, 1973.

45. Sivit, C.J., Newman, K.D., Boenning, D.A., Nussbaum-Blask, A.R., Bulas, D.I., Bond, S.J., Attorri, R., Rebolo, L.C., Brown-Jones, C., and Garin, D.B.: Appendicitis: Usefulness of US in diagnosis in a pediatric population. Radiology 185: 549–552, 1992.

46. Skaane, P., Amland, P.R., Nordshus, T., and Solheim, K.: Ultrasonography in patients with suspected acute appendicitis: A prospective study. Br. J. Radiol. 63: 787–793, 1990.

47. Slovis, T.L., Haller, J.O., Cohen, H.L., Berdon, W.E., and Watts, F.B., Jr.: Complicated appendiceal inflammatory disease in children: Pylephlebitis and liver abscess. Radiology 171: 823–825, 1989.

48. Soteropoulos, C., and Gilmore, J.H.: Roentgen diagnosis of acute appendicitis. Radiology 71: 246–257, 1958.

49. Swischuk, L.E., and Hayden, C.K., Jr.: Appendicitis with perforation: The dilated transverse colon sign. A.J.R. 135: 687–689, 1980.

50. Vaudagna, J.S., and McCort, J.J.: Plain film diagnosis of retrocecal appendicitis. Radiology 117: 533–536, 1975.

51. Vignault, F., Filiatrault, D., Brandt, M.L., Garel, L., Grignon, A., and Ouimet, A.: Acute appendicitis in children: Evaluation with US. Radiology 176: 501–504, 1990.

52. Voitk, A.J., MacFarlane, J.K., and Estrada, R.L.: Ruptured appendicitis in femoral hernias. Ann. Surg. 179: 24, 1974.

53. White, J.J., Santillana, M., and Haller, J.A., Jr.: Intensive in-hospital observation: A safe way to decrease unnecessary appendectomy. Ann. Surg. 41: 793–798, 1975.

54. Wilkinson, R.H., Bartlet, R.H., and Eraklis, A.J.: Diagnosis of appendicitis in infancy: Value of abdominal radiograph. Am. J. Dis. Child. 118: 687–690, 1969.

55. Williams, H.H.: Coproliths in children: Recognition and significance. Pediatrics 34: 372–377, 1964.

56. Williams, S.M., Harned, R.K., Hultman, S., A., and Qualfe, M.A.: The psoas sign: A reevaluation. RadioGraphics 5: 525–536, 1985.

57. Worrell, J.A., Drolshagen, L.F., Kelly, T.C., Hunton, D.W., Durmon, G.R., and Fleischer, A.C.: Graded compression ultrasound in the diagnosis of appendicitis: A comparison of diagnostic criteria. J. Ultrasound Med. 9: 145–150, 1990.

Conditions Mimicking Acute Appendicitis. The most common right lower quadrant conditions mimicking the clinical and roentgenographic findings of acute appendicitis are: (a) mesenteric adenitis, (b) *Yersinia* ileocolitis, (c) Crohn's disease or regional enteritis, (d) Meckel's diverticulitis, (e) the so-called ileocecal syndrome or typhlitis in children with leukemia, and (f) the occasional case of infarction of the appendices epiploicae. In addition, some cases of urinary tract disease, pelvic inflammatory disease, and noninflammatory adnexal disease also can mimic appendicitis. All of these latter conditions are discussed at later points in this chapter.

Mesenteric adenitis often is diagnosed by exclusion, but more recently ultrasonographically documented adenopathy in these patients has become possible (Fig. 3.68A). Unfortunately, however, adenopathy also can be seen with acute appendicitis, but in the absence of findings suggesting the latter condition, mesenteric adenitis can be suggested as the diagnosis.

So-called "suppurative mesenteric lymphadenitis" (3) is a much more severe illness and laparotomy is difficult to avoid. In these cases, lymph node infection probably is of bacterial origin and as such closely parallels the findings of acute appendicitis. A variety of enteric organisms have been found to cause the problem, including *Yersinia* (2, 3, 5, 11, 17). In-

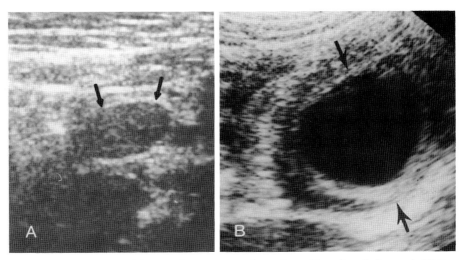

Figure 3.68. *Mesenteric adenitis.* (*A*) Typical appearance of an enlarged lymph node (*arrows*). (*B*) Suppurative adenitis. Note the large lymph node (*arrows*) with a sonolucent center.

deed, *Yersinia* ileocolitis is being recognized more and more as a cause of abdominal symptoms mimicking acute appendicitis. If barium enemas are performed in these patients, one may see extensive edema and nodularity of the ileocecal region (Fig. 3.69) and nonspecific mucosal irregularities. In some cases, the findings might be confused with those of postperforation appendiceal abscess. Ultrasonographically, the suppurated lymph nodes may be detected as sonolucent, cyst-like structures (Fig. 3.68B).

Crohn's disease or regional enteritis is notorious for first presenting with findings suggestive of acute appendicitis (7, 13, 14, 16, 23). There is no real way to get around this dilemma, except to remember that such patients are going to be seen in the emergency room from time to time. Even then, they might still be operated upon for acute appendicitis. Ultrasonographically, regional enteritis presents with edematous thick bowel which then is confirmed with barium studies (Fig. 3.70).

Meckel's diverticulitis also can mimic acute appendicitis, but to spend a great deal of time on the plain film findings of this condition would not be fruitful. Indeed, in many cases the plain film findings

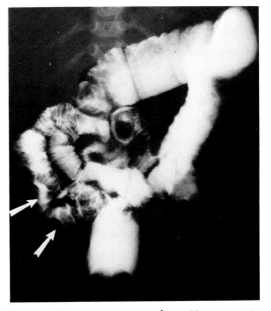

Figure 3.69. *Yersinia enterocolitis.* Note extensive edema and thumbprinting of the cecum and ascending colon (*arrows*). In other cases similar changes are seen in the terminal ileum. (Courtesy of B. Barlow, R. Gandhi, and L.W. Young: Radiological case of the month. Am. J. Dis. Child. 135: 171–172, 1981.)

are normal, and even barium studies of the gastrointestinal tract are seldom helpful (19). If inflammation is more pronounced, right lower quadrant findings similar to those seen in acute appendicitis may de-

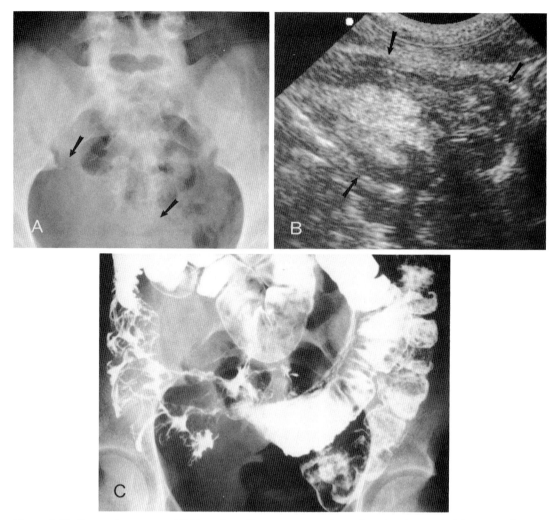

Figure 3.70. *Regional enteritis.* (*A*) Note the soft tissue mass in the right pelvis (*arrows*). (*B*) Longitudinal ultrasonographic scan through the mass demonstrates a large, oval-shaped heterogeneous soft tissue mass (*arrows*). (*C*) Upper GI series with follow-through demonstrates the extensive inflammatory mass due to regional enteritis. There are extensive mural thickening and sinus formation.

velop, and if perforation occurs, those associated with perforated appendicitis will be seen (4, 6, 10, 12, 18, 25). Other manifestations of Meckel's diverticulitis include a right lower quadrant or lower abdominal air or fluid-filled mass (with larger diverticula) and stone formation (4, 15). Occasionally the inflamed diverticulum can be identified with ultrasound and may resemble an inflamed appendix.

Typhlitis or the so-called ileocecal syndrome is an affliction of patients with leukemia (1, 2, 9, 21, 22, 24). It is characterized by a profound necrotizing inflammation of the terminal ileum, appendix, and cecum, and usually is a terminal event. However, just why it occurs is not known. The clinical findings mimic those of acute appendicitis, and the key to proper diagnosis is knowledge that the patient is suffering from leukemia. Ultrasonographically, the large, swollen cecum can be seen as an echogenic but disorganized segment of thickened bowel (Fig. 3.71).

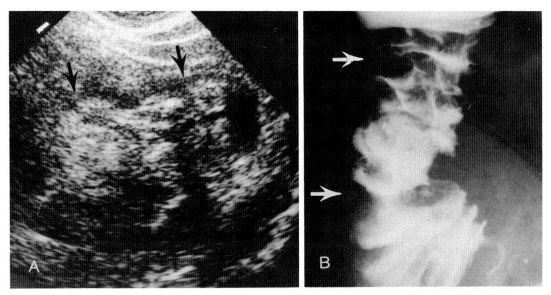

Figure 3.71. *Typhlitis.* (*A*) Sonogram demonstrates an oval, heterogeneous mass (*arrows*). (*B*) Barium enema demonstrating the cecal involvement consisting of spasm and intramural thickening with considerable thumb-printing (*arrows*).

Idiopathic infarction or torsion of the appendices epiploicae (8, 20) is not particularly common in childhood, but in some cases can mimic the findings of acute appendicitis.

REFERENCES

1. Alexander, J.E., Williamson, S.L., Seibert J.J., Golladay, E.S., and Jimenez, J.F.: The ultrasonographic diagnosis of typhlitis (neutropenic colitis). Pediatr. Radiol. 18: 200–204, 1988.
2. Abramson, S.J., Berdon, W.E., and Baker, D.H.: Childhood typhlitis: Its increasing association with myelogenous leukemia: Report of five cases. Radiology 146: 61–64, 1983.
3. Alvear, D.T., and Kain, T.M.: Suppurative mesenteric lymphadenitis, a forgotten clinical entity. J. Pediatr. Surg. 10: 969–970, 1975.
4. Baldero, J.: Calculi in a Meckel's diverticulum. J. Fac. Radiol. 9: 157–160, 1958.
5. Barlow, B., Tandhi, R., and Young, L.W.: Radiological case of the month—suppurative mesenteric adenitis: *Yersinia enterocolitica.* Am. J. Dis. Child. 135: 171–172, 1981.
6. Canty, T., Meguid, M.M., and Eraklis, A.J.: Perforation of Meckel's diverticulum in infancy. J. Pediatr. Surg. 10: 189–193, 1975.
7. Cohen, W.N., and Denbesten, L.: Crohn's disease with predominant involvement of the appendix. A.J.R. 113: 361–363, 1970.
8. Coultre, C. Le, and Braum, P.: Idiopathic infarction of appendices epiploica in children: Report of two cases. Ann. Chir. Inf. 17: 61–64, 1976.
9. Cronin, T.G., Jr., Calandra, J.D., and DelFava, R.L.: Typhlitis presenting as toxic cecitis. Radiology 138: 29–30, 1981.
10. Dalinka, M.K., and Wunder, J.F.: Meckel's diverticulum and its complications, with emphasis on roentgenologic demonstration. Radiology 106: 295–298, 1973.
11. Ekberg, O., Sjøstrom, B., and Brahme, F.: Radiological findings in *Yersinia* ileitis. Radiology 123: 15–19, 1977.
12. Enge, I., and Frimann-Dahl, J.: Radiology in acute abdominal disorders due to Meckel's diverticulum. Br. J. Radiol. 37: 775–780, 1964.
13. Ewen, S.W.B., Anderson, J., Galloway, J.M.D., et al.: Crohn's disease initially confined to the appendix. Gastroenterology 60: 853–857, 1971.
14. Hall, J.H., and Hellier, M.D.: Crohn's disease of the appendix presenting as acute appendicitis. Br. J. Surg. 56: 390–392, 1969.
15. Hirschy, J.C., Thorpe, J.J., and Cortese, A.F.: Meckel's stones: A case report. Radiology 119: 19–20, 1976.
16. Hollings, R.M.: Crohn's disease of the appendix. Med. J. Aust. 1: 639–641, 1964.
17. Martin, H.C.O., and Goon, H.K.: Salmonella ileocecal lymphadenitis masquerading as appendicitis. J. Pediatr. Surg. 21: 377–378, 1986.
18. Meguid, M., Canty, T., and Eraklis, A.: Compli-

cations of Meckel's diverticulum in infants. Surg. Gynecol. Obstet. 139: 541–544, 1974.

19. Meguid, M.M., Wilkinson, R.H., Canty, T., Eraklis, A.J., and Treves, S.: Futility of barium sulfate in diagnosis of bleeding Meckel's diverticulum. Arch. Surg. 108: 361–362, 1974.

20. Schikler, K.N., Nagaraj, H.S., and Hodge, K.M.: Torsion of appendix epiploica in systemic lupus erythematosus. Am. J. Dis. Child. 136: 748–749, 1982.

21. Sherman, N.J., and Woolley, M.W.: Ileocecal syndrome in acute childhood leukemia. Arch. Surg. 107: 39–42, 1973.

22. Teefey, S.A., Montana, M.A., Goldfogel, G.A., and Shuman, W.P.: Sonographic diagnosis of neutropenic typhlitis. A.J.R. 149: 731–733, 1987.

23. Threatt, B., and Appelman, H.: Crohn's disease of the appendix presenting as acute appendicitis: Report of 3 cases with a review of the literature. Radiology 110: 313–317, 1974.

24. Wagner, M.L., Harberg, F.J., and Kumbar, A.P.: Typhlitis a complication of leukemia in childhood. A.J.R. 109: 341–450, 1970.

25. White, A.F., Oh, K.S., Weber, A.L., and James, A.E., Jr.: Radiological manifestations of Meckel's diverticulum. A.J.R. 118: 86–94, 1973.

Other Intra-abdominal Inflammations or Infections.

These include pancreatitis, hepatitis, cholecystitis, cholelithiasis, renal infections, salpingitis, and a variety of colon inflammations. *Pancreatitis* is not a particularly common problem in childhood (3, 14) but is seen with cholecystitis (1), viral infections such as mumps and infectious mononucleosis, and after blunt abdominal trauma. The latter is especially common in the battered child syndrome (3, 14, 29). In addition, pancreatitis has been noted with cystic fibrosis (26) juvenile diabetes mellitus (17), hyperparathyroidism, refeeding in malnourished children (12), drug (especially steroid) therapy (3, 14), and on a hereditary basis in certain families (5, 15, 34).

Abdominal roentgenograms in acute pancreatitis most often are entirely normal, but in other instances one may see socalled sentinel loops of distended intestine overlying the inflamed pancreas (6). These loops may take the form of: (a) a dilated portion of the transverse colon (colon cutoff sign), (b) a dilated duodenum, or (c) dilated loops of small bowel in the upper midabdomen or left upper quadrant (2, 6, 11, 27). In all of these cases, the findings represent paralytic ileus of the loop of intestine lying next to the inflamed pancreas, and, in some cases, if inflammation is severe, there may be an increase in the soft tissue distance between the transverse colon and stomach (18). This latter finding represents the sequelae of edema extending into the adjacent soft tissues. In some cases, there may be actual necrosis of the transverse colon (32), *but overall all of these plain film findings are rare, and in most cases the plain films are normal.*

If pancreatic inflammation is so severe that pancreatic necrosis occurs, a gas abscess of the pancreas can develop (2, 7, 22). Such an abscess can assume the configuration of one large air and fluid-filled cavity or numerous small bubbles (Fig. 3.72). Very rarely, calcifications within the pancreas are seen.

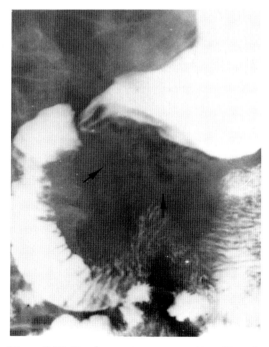

Figure 3.72. *Emphysematous pancreatitis.* Note the widened duodenal loop, elevated antrum of the stomach, and collection of bubbles in the region of the pancreas (*arrows*). These bubbles are gas collections in the pancreas.

In most cases, pancreatitis is suspected and diagnosed clinically. However, confirmation frequently is sought for with ultrasonography or CT, and while these studies usually are normal, when enlargement of the pancreas is seen, the diagnosis should be suspected (Figs. 3.73 and 3.74). On ultrasound, increased lucency of the pancreas may be seen (4, 8). In addition to these findings, one may see fluid around the pancreas (28), increased echogenicity in and around the kidney and liver due to lipolysis (31) of fat (Fig. 3.74C), and, of course, if a pseudocyst (25) is present, a large cystic cavity with or without debris is seen (Fig. 3.75). With ultrasonography now on the scene, seldom is a gastrointestinal series performed for acute pancreatitis, but if one should obtain such a study, one may see widening and compression of the duodenal loop, the so-called pad sign.

Traumatic pancreatitis in childhood can be seen with any type of blunt abdominal

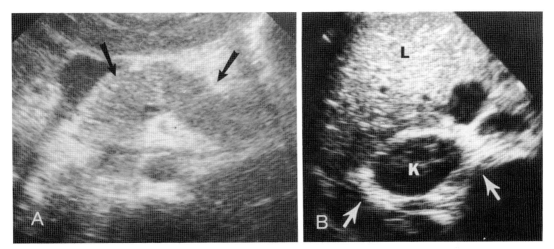

Figure 3.73. *Acute pancreatitis; ultrasound findings.* (*A*) Note the enlarged and slightly hypoechoic pancreas (*arrows*). (*B*) Another patient with an echogenic expanded fat compartment (*arrows*) around the kidney (*K*). Liver (*L*). This finding is due to lipolysis. Most often, however, the pancreas looks normal.

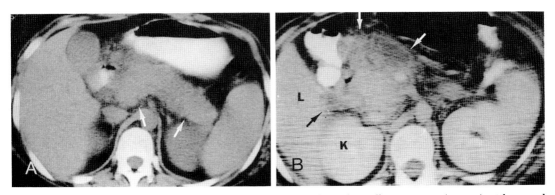

Figure 3.74. *Acute pancreatitis: CT findings.* (*A*) Note the enlarged, swollen pancreas (*arrows*) with ragged edges. There appears to be some fluid accumulating around the pancreatic head. (*B*) Slightly lower slice demonstrates the large, inflammatory fluid collection (*white arrows*). Some of the fluid has extended into the space (*black arrow*) between the liver (*L*) and kidney (*K*). Such an inflammatory reaction causes lipolysis of the fatty tissue, as seen in Figure 3.73*B*.

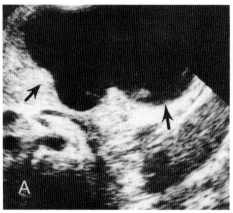
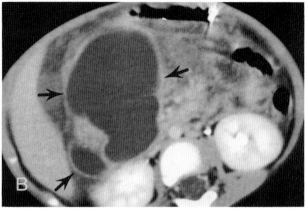

Figure 3.75. *Pancreatic pseudocyst.* (*A*) Ultrasonographic findings. Note the basically anechoic, lobulated pancreatic pseudocyst (*arrows*). (*B*) CT findings. Note the multilobulated pancreatic pseudocyst (*arrows*). With both ultrasound and CT, some cysts may contain more debris.

trauma, but is most common in the battered child syndrome. In these cases, the pancreas simply may be enlarged and edematous, but in other cases an actual fracture or laceration of the pancreas can be seen (see Fig. 3.127). These fractures can be identified with ultrasonography and CT. Initially the lesion may appear rather innocuous, although fluid around the fracture site can be seen. Eventually, however, pseudocyst formation is a very likely possibility.

It is important to realize that *although pancreatitis is an abdominal problem, many extra-abdominal clinical and roentgenographic manifestations also can be seen.* Indeed, these findings can distract one's attention from the main problem, and thus one must be aware of all findings. First, it should be noted that associated pleural effusions (Fig. 3.76) are very common (2, 19, 20, 22, 33) and that occasionally even pericardial effusions can be seen (20). In addition, when pancreatic enzymes are liberated into the bloodstream, pulmonary edema and profound respiratory insufficiency can result (9, 23). In other instances, hypocalcemia resulting from the binding of calcium to these same pancreatic enzymes can lead to electrocardiographic changes suggesting myocardial

ischemia (16). Hypocalcemia also can lead to neurologic manifestations.

Fat necrosis from the liberation of lipase into the bloodstream can produce subcutaneous nodules (24, 30), widespread necrosis of the fat of the mesentery (18), and in some cases fat necrosis-induced lytic lesions in the bones (10, 13, 16, 21, 29). These latter lesions can mimic osteomyelitis and usually are seen 2 or 3 weeks after the acute episode of pancreatitis.

Cholecystitis and cholelithiasis are more common in childhood than is generally appreciated (1, 3–7, 10–13, 17), and while it was generally believed that cholelithiasis most often was secondary to hemolytic blood disorders, it is becoming increasingly apparent that most cases, perhaps two-thirds or more, are due to other causes (4, 7, 14). Indeed, many are idiopathic and, just as in the adult, more cases occur in females than in males.

Clinical features are much the same as in adults, but in infancy the diagnosis may be difficult. Jaundice may be present, and in those cases of empyema or hydrops of the gallbladder (2, 3, 8, 9, 16), a mass may be palpable. Indeed, an enlarged gallbladder may be visible roentgenographically (Fig. 3.77). If calcified gallstones are present, they may be seen on plain films (Fig.

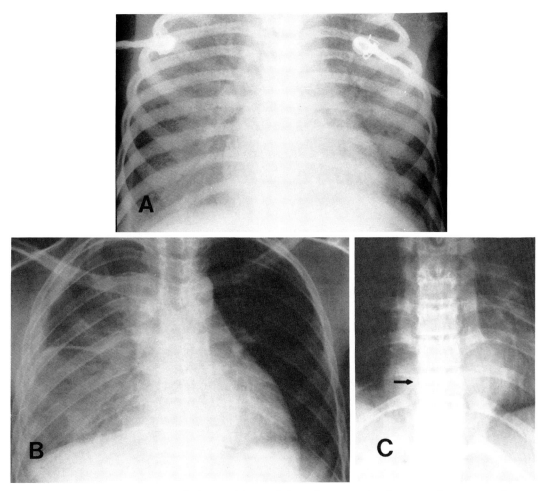

Figure 3.76. *Pancreatitis with chest findings.* (**A**) Note bilateral interstitial pulmonary edema causing haziness of the lungs in this patient with acute pancreatitis. (**B**) Another patient with a semi-opacified right hemithorax due to a pleural effusion secondary to pancreatitis. Pulmonary edema of the right lung also probably is present and a paraspinal mass is present on the left. (**C**) A week or two later this paraspinal mass was determined to be due to a compression fracture of a thoracic vertebra (*arrow*). The findings were believed to represent vertebral collapse secondary to osteolysis resulting from fat necrosis.

3.78*A*), and if gangrene or abscess formation develops in the gallbladder, one may see air in the gallbladder or within its wall (i.e., emphysematous cholecystitis). Otherwise, the diagnosis of most cases of cholecystitis and cholelithiasis is relegated to ultrasonography and, to some extent, nuclear scintigraphy.

Ultrasound can identify acute cholecystitis, the presence of gallstones, a hydropic gallbladder, and dilated intrahepatic ducts. Nuclear scintigraphy, utilizing one

or the other of the **IDA** isotopes, also can be utilized to identify acute cholecystitis, a hydropic gallbladder, or an obstructed biliary tract.

Gallstones, on ultrasound, are strongly echogenic with pronounced, distal acoustical shadowing (Fig. 3.78*B*). Shadowing, however, is not always present (Fig. 3.78*C*) and probably depends on the amount of calcium in the stone. Acute cholecystitis may show nothing more than a distended gallbladder, but edema of the

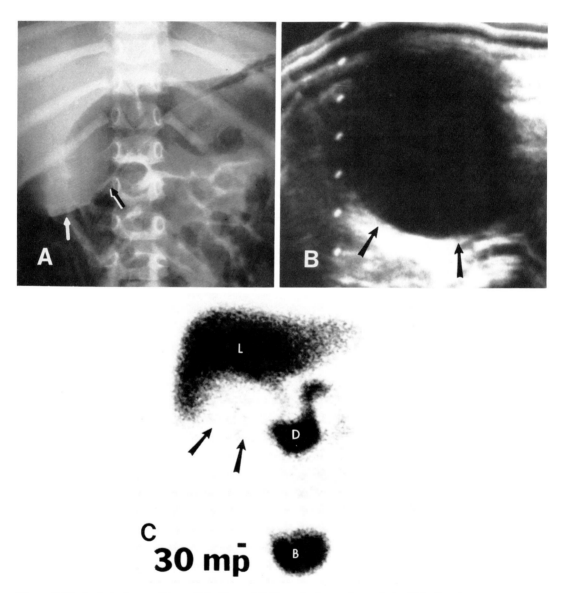

Figure 3.77. *Acute hydrops of the gallbladder.* (*A*) Note the large, distended gallbladder (*arrows*). (*B*) Ultrasound study demonstrating a hydropic gallbladder in another patient (*arrows*). (*C*) Isotope Tc-HIDA study demonstrates no isotope activity in the gallbladder (*arrows*). Isotope, however, has passed into the duodenum (*D*) and is being excreted into the urinary bladder (*B*).

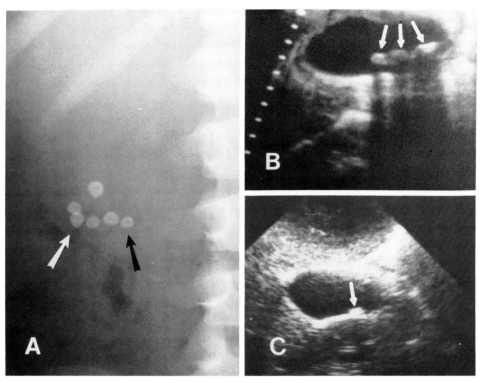

Figure 3.78. *Cholelithiasis.* (*A*) Note calcified gallstones (*arrows*) in this patient with sickle cell disease. (*B*) Ultrasonography demonstrates the gallbladder and numerous hyperechoic gallstones (*arrows*), with distal acoustical shadowing. (*C*) Another patient with a single gallstone (*arrow*).

wall also can be seen (Fig. 3.79*A*). Such edema is not present in every case and also is nonspecific (15, 18). In this regard, it can be seen with generalized anasarca and ascites. However, in most cases it is seen with inflammatory disease of the gallbladder and although it is a nonspecific finding is a valuable positive finding. Currently it is a common finding in patients with acquired immunodeficiency syndrome (**AIDS**).

If a hydropic gallbladder is present, it is easily identified as a large, cystic, anechoic structure (see Fig. 3.77*B*). In addition, one will not be able to identify a normal gallbladder. This is important, for with choledochal cysts, another condition presenting as a large cystic structure, the gallbladder usually is identified. Dilated intra- and extrahepatic bile ducts also can be identified with ultrasound (Fig. 3.80) as well as ob-

structing stones in the common bile duct (Fig. 3.80*D*).

Gallbladder sludge, ever since ultrasonography has come to be commonplace, is frequently identified in a variety of patients. For the most part, gallbladder sludge is secondary to stasis and such sludge can be a precursor of gallstone formation. Gallbladder sludge is a common finding in fasting patients and patients on hyperalimentation, but it also is seen in patients with acute cholecystitis and patients with obstructive pathology of the biliary tract (Figs. 3.79 and 3.80). In terms of nuclear scintigraphy, a technetium (Tc)-IDA study often is very useful. Normally there is progression of the isotope from the liver into the bile ducts, the gallbladder, and then the intestines. If obstruction is present, this sequence of events is interrupted.

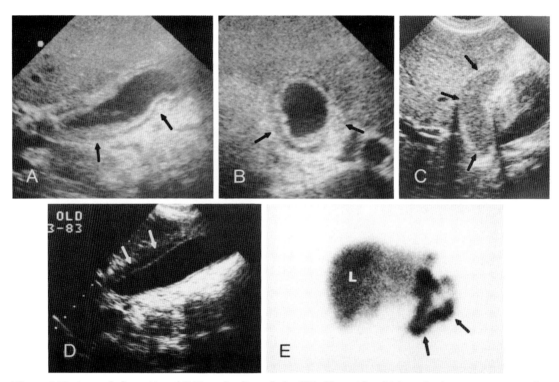

Figure 3.79. *Acute cholecystitis.* (*A*) Note the distended gallbladder with a thickened echogenic mucosa and a thickened hypoechoic muscular wall (*arrows*). (*B*) View in cross-section demonstrates the same findings (*arrows*). (*C*) Another patient with acalculus cholecystitis demonstrating a distended gallbladder full of sludge (*arrows*). (*D*) Another patient with a distended gallbladder and some fluid (*arrows*) around its wall. (*E*) Scintigram in the same patient demonstrates no accumulation of isotope material in the gallbladder. Isotope, however, is seen in the small bowel (*arrows*). Liver (*L*).

For example, with acute cholecystitis, because the cystic duct is obstructed, the gallbladder usually is not visualized (Fig. 3.79). Similarly, when hydrops of the gallbladder is present, the gallbladder does not accept any of the isotope. When the biliary tract is obstructed, accumulation of the isotope can be seen in the dilated biliary ducts (Fig. 3.80).

Acute *pyelonephritis and cystitis* are common in childhood, especially in girls. However, the plain film and ultrasound findings usually are normal. In a few cases, sentinel loops may be seen over the infected kidney or bladder, and if a unilateral problem such as a renal carbuncle or perinephric abscess exists, evidence of perirenal inflammation or an actual mass with

scoliosis to the ipsilateral side may be noted (Fig. 3.81). In these cases, pyelographic findings may demonstrate a displaced kidney with variably decreased renal function (Fig. 3.81*B*), but in acute pyelonephritis without these complications, except for mild to moderate calyceal dilatation and blunting in some cases, the pyelographic findings are normal. Similarly, with ultrasound the studies usually are normal. Occasionally, generalized renal enlargement and mild caliectasis can be seen, but unless a complication such as an abscess occurs, the findings usually are normal.

Renal or perirenal abscesses (3), in general, can be liquid or solid on ultrasonographic examination, and are readily de-

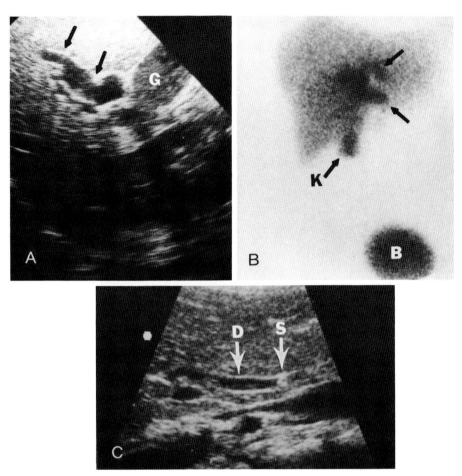

Figure 3.80. *Acute cholecystitis with obstruction.* (*A*) Note the distended gallbladder (*G*) containing some echogenic sludge. Also note the dilated hepatic duct (*arrows*). (*B*) Tc-IDA study demonstrates isotope in the dilated, obstructed bile ducts (*arrows*), but none in the gallbladder. In addition, none has passed into the GI tract. Some is being excreted, as would be expected, into the kidney (*K*) and the bladder (*B*). (*C*) Another patient with an obstructing stone (*S*) in a dilated (*D*) common bile duct.

monstrable with CT (Fig. 3.82). Many of these abscesses now are drained percutaneously. Lobar nephronia or focal nephritis also can be detected with ultrasound (2, 4). Generally, these inflamed areas present as a round or oval area in the kidney which is relatively hypoechoic. However, in other cases the lesion is echogenic, and it has been suggested that this is due to focal hemorrhage secondary to the vasculitis induced by the infection (4). These lesions also are readily demonstrable with cortical imaging agents such as 99mTc-DMSA or glucoheptonate (1, 5). Although uncommon, lobar nephronia usually presents with acute symptoms (Fig. 3.83).

Finally, a note regarding infection associated with hydronephrosis is in order. It is well known that obstructive uropathy predisposes one to urinary tract infection. In most such cases only the obstructed urinary tract is detected, but in other cases the entire tract may become filled with purulent material. This can occur both with bacterial and fungal infections and can lead to anuria. In these profound cases, ultra-

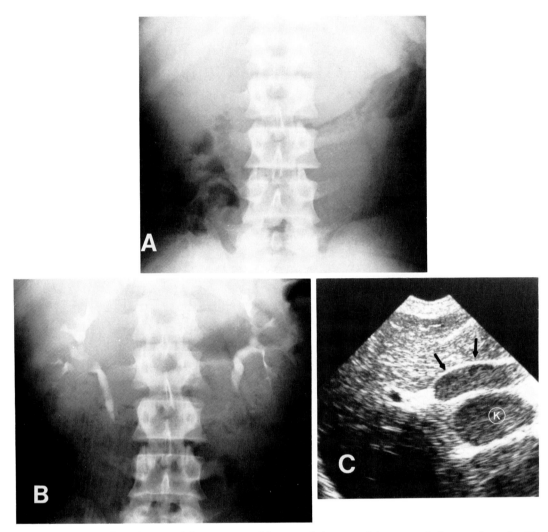

Figure 3.81. *Perinephric abscess.* (*A*) Note sentinel loops and absence of the psoas shadow on the right. The normal psoas shadow is visible on the left. Also note that the inferior edge of the liver is obliterated. (*B*) Intravenous pyelogram demonstrating poorly defined right renal margins and a right kidney that appears a little larger than the left. (*C*) Ultrasonographic findings in another patient demonstrate an echogenic abscess (*arrows*) just above the kidney (*K*).

sonography readily demonstrates the purulent material in the dilating collecting system (Fig. 3.84).

   Cystitis usually is seen in combination with pyelonephritis although it can occur as an isolated infection. Most often, it is of bacterial origin, but viral infections can occur (2, 3). In most cases of cystitis, one will note a spastic, irregular bladder, secondary to spasm and mucosal edema (Fig.

3.85). If blood clots are present, they may be seen as radiolucent filling defects in the bladder. Another form of cystitis in children is cyclophosphamide (Cytoxan) cystitis, but this problem is seen exclusively in patients with blood dyscrasias or other tumors requiring therapy with that agent (Fig. 3.85*C*).

   Generally, urinary bladder abnormalities are best demonstrated with the blad-

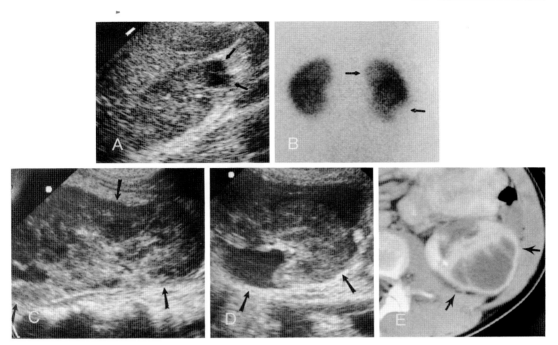

Figure 3.82. *Renal abscess.* (**A**) Note the small sonolucent abscess (*arrows*) in the inferior pole of the right kidney. (**B**) Tc-99m glucoheptenate study demonstrates the focal defect in the lower pole of the right kidney (*lower arrow*) but also demonstrates another suspicious defect in the upper pole (*upper arrow*). This second defect was not visible ultrasonographically. (**C**) Another patient with a markedly enlarged and completely distorted kidney (*arrows*) due to pyonephrosis. (**D**) Cross-sectional view demonstrates the distorted kidney and also two sonolucent subcapsular fluid (pus) collections (*arrows*). (**E**) CT study demonstrates the enlarged left kidney (*arrows*) demonstrating a complete loss of normal architecture and the two subcapsular fluid collections noted in (**D**).

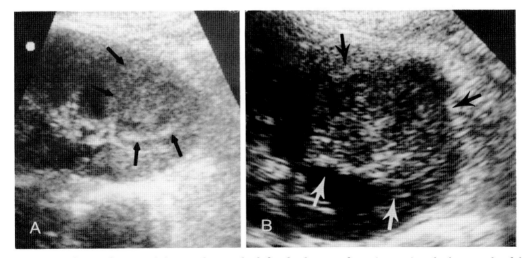

Figure 3.83. *Lobar nephronia.* (**A**) Note the poorly defined echogenic focus (*arrows*) in the lower pole of the kidney. (**B**) Another view demonstrates the echogenic focus to better advantage (*arrows*). On Tc-99m glucoheptenate studies these areas are photon deficient.

Figure 3.84. *Hydropyonephrosis.* Note the dilated calyces with numerous fluid debris levels (*arrows*).

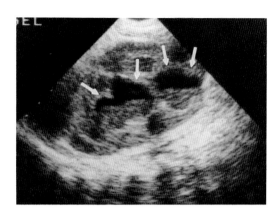

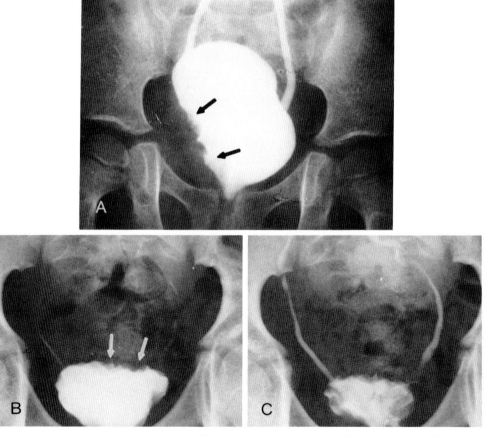

Figure 3.85. *Cystitis: various configurations.* (**A**) Note irregularity and mass-like indentation of the right side of the bladder (*arrows*) in this patient presenting with bleeding from the urinary tract. This patient had cytoxin cystitis. (**B**) Note irregularity over the top of the bladder (*arrows*) in this patient with symptoms of cystitis. (**C**) Postvoid film demonstrates marked mucosal irregularity and thickening of the bladder.

der fully distended, but often edema and irregularity of the mucosa are more clearly demonstrated on the postvoiding or partially filled study (Fig. 3.85C). In addition, now that ultrasonography is available, thickening of the bladder mucosa in cases of cystitis is readily detected with this modality (Fig. 3.86A). In some of these cases mucosal thickening can be profound and mimic the findings of a bladder tumor (1). Cystitis cystica is one such condition. Thickening of the bladder mucosa also is demonstrable with CT (Fig. 3.86B).

Salpingitis occurs in adolescent girls (2, 4) and has a real propensity to produce localizing, sentinel loops over the lower abdomen or profound paralytic ileus mimicking mechanical obstruction (Fig. 3.87). These findings result from the diffuse peritonitis induced by pus extruding into the peritoneal cavity from the fallopian tube. In other cases, mass-like configurations representing pus collections in the lower abdomen and pelvis can be seen. These pus collections can represent true pelvic abscesses, pyosalpinx, or tubo-ovarian abscesses. In any of these cases, the clinical findings may mimic acute appendicitis and,

to be sure, this also can be a problem with ultrasonography (3). However, ultrasound probably still is the best imaging modality for detecting all of these findings. Currently, transvaginal ultrasound tends to produce clearer and more definitive studies (1), but transabdominal ultrasound still is very satisfactory. Ultrasonographically, one may see a variety of findings including dilated, pus-filled fallopian tubes, a variety of configurations of tubo-ovarian abscess, fluid in the cul-de-sac, and fluid in the peritoneal cavity. Although all of these findings generally are nonspecific, in the proper clinical situation they are highly suggestive.

In terms of *inflammatory bowel disease,* more and more of these conditions are identified with ultrasound. The most common, of course, is simple viral gastroenteritis, but any number of inflammatory diseases can be identified. For the most part, two patterns exist. The most common is diffuse mucosal thickening due to mucosal disease and the second is transmural thickening due to diseases such as regional enteritis (Fig. 3.88). Overall, however, except for viral gastroenteritis, inflammatory

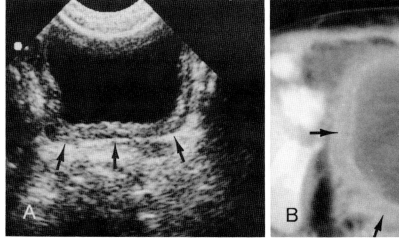
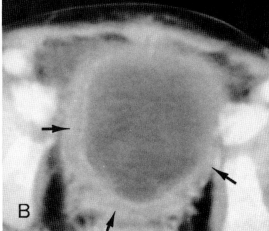

Figure 3.86. *Cystitis: ultrasonographic and CT findings.* (A) Note the markedly thickened echogenic mucosa *(arrows).* (B) CT study in another patient again demonstrates markedly thickened mucosa *(arrows).*

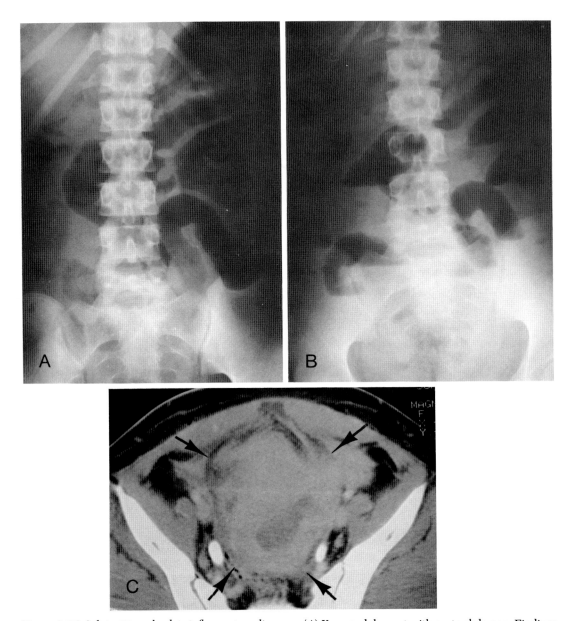

Figure 3.87. *Salpingitis and pelvic inflammatory disease.* (*A*) Young adolescent with acute abdomen. Findings suggest peritonitis and/or obstruction. (*B*) Upright film suggests intestinal obstruction. After antibiotic treatment, these findings disappeared in 24 hours.(*C*) Another patient whose CT study shows a large pelvic mass with mixed densities (*arrows*). The findings are nonspecific.

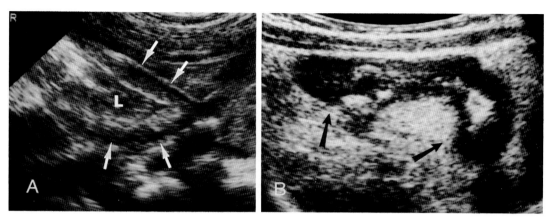

Figure 3.88. *Inflammatory bowel disease.* (*A*) Characteristic mucosal thickening (*arrows*) producing echogenic thickening of the mucosa. Intestinal lumen (*L*). (*B*) Transmural thickening due to late stage regional enteritis produces more uniform hypoechoic thickening of the intestinal wall (*arrow*).

problems of the gastrointestinal tract usually involve the colon (Fig. 3.89). On the other hand, focal mucosal thickening with obliteration of the normal soft tissue planes of the stomach also can be seen with acute gastritis and gastric ulcer disease (2).

Colitis, on an acute basis, can be seen with shigellosis (6), ulcerative colitis (Fig. 3.89*B* and *C*), pseudomembranous colitis (Fig. 3.89*A*), typhlitis, granulomatous colitis (Crohn's disease), amebiasis, food (milk) allergy in infants (3, 4, 14), and the hemolytic uremic syndrome (13). In the latter condition, changes can be so profound as to lead to colonic necrosis and perforation (7, 11). For the most part, plain film findings in colitis are lacking, except in those patients with toxic megacolon. Most often, this complication is seen with ulcerative colitis, and in such cases the colon (usually the transverse colon) is distended and paralyzed. It is void of haustral markings and its wall may be smooth, coarsely serrated, or thumbprinted (Fig. 3.90). The latter configurations result from extensive mucosal inflammation, edema, or pseudopolyp formation. As noted, toxic megacolon classically is seen with ulcerative colitis (2, 5, 9, 16), but it also can be seen with granulomatous colitis (8, 10) and amebic colitis (15, 17).

Necrotizing enterocolitis is primarily an affliction of premature infants, but also can be seen in older infants with any type of ischemic disease of the intestine (12). The findings consist of: (a) pronounced abdominal distension with severe paralytic ileus of the intestine, (b) pneumatosis cystoides intestinalis, (c) portal vein gas, (d) free air in the peritoneal cavity when perforation occurs, and (e) peritonitis. (See Figs. 3.20 and 3.21.)

Finally, a word regarding *shigellosis* is in order. This acute intestinal inflammation represents one of the most severe forms of gastroenteritis, and the volume of fluid loss through the colon is enormous. Indeed, the presence of massive volumes of fluid in the intestines can lead to a variety of plain film findings, some of which may suggest more serious problems such as ascites, peritonitis, or bowel obstruction (Fig. 3.91*A*). In other cases, the abdominal findings are not different from those seen with viral gastroenteritis. Every so often, one ends up performing a barium enema in patients with shigellosis, and the intense colonic spasm demonstrated can be striking (Fig. 3.91*B*).

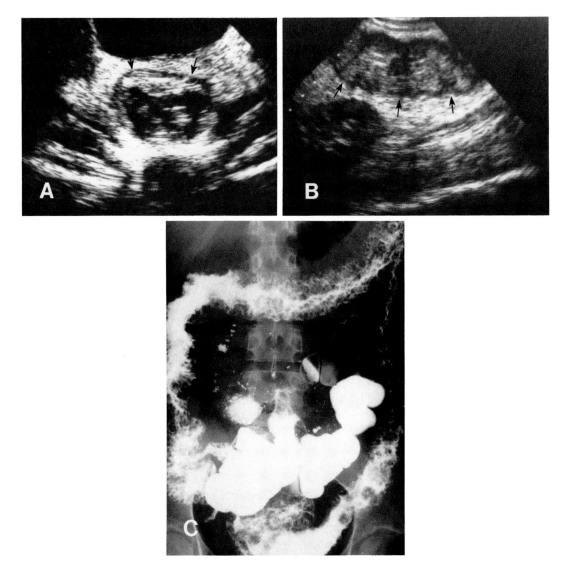

Figure 3.89. *Colitis: ultrasonographic findings.*   (**A**) Note the sonolucent rim of thickened rectal wall (*arrows*) in this patient with pseudomembranous colitis. Sonolucent fluid is present in the lumen and there are areas of echogenicity due to debris and thickened mucosa. (**B**) Another patient with ulcerative colitis. Note the sonolucent rim of thickened colon wall (*arrows*) and numerous echoes from the thickened mucosa within. (**C**) Barium enema in the same patient.

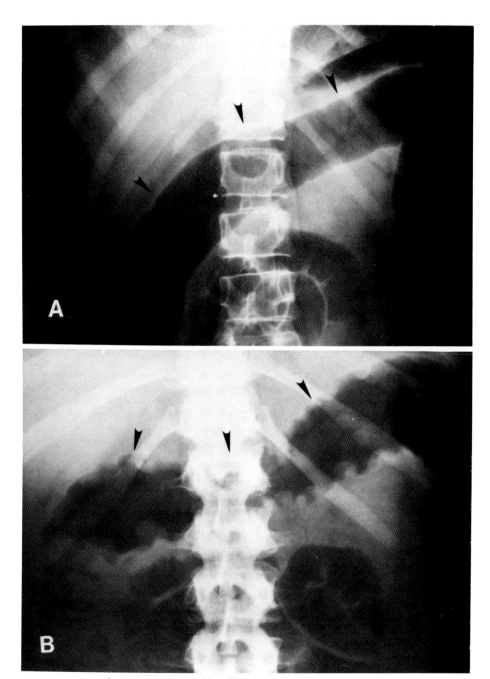

Figure 3.90. *Toxic megacolon.* (*A*) Note the dilated but smooth transverse colon with no haustral markings (*arrows*). (*B*) Another patient with a dilated colon, but in this case note the nodular projections into the lumen of the dilated colon (*arrows*). The findings represent thickening, edema, and pseudopolyp formation of the colon. (Part *B* courtesy of Virgil B. Graves, M.D.)

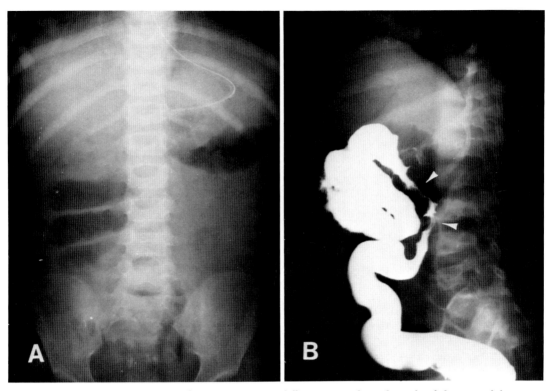

Figure 3.91. *Shigellosis.* (A) Supine film demonstrating diffuse opacity throughout the abdomen and three sentinel loops on the right. The findings could be misinterpreted as peritonitis, small bowel obstruction, or some other intra-abdominal problem. However, the patient had *Shigella* infection of the gastrointestinal tract. (B) Barium enema in another patient demonstrating extreme spasm with thumbprinting of the descending colon (*arrows*).

REFERENCES

Pancreatitis

1. Auldist, A.W.: Pancreatitis and choledocholithiasis in childhood. J. Pediatr. Surg. 7: 78, 1972.

2. Barry, W.F., Jr.: Roentgen examination of the abdomen in acute pancreatitis. A.J.R. 74: 220–225, 1955.

3. Buntain, W.L., Wood, J.B., and Woolley, M.M.: Pancreatitis in childhood. J. Pediatr. Surg. 13: 143–149, 1978.

4. Cox, K.L., Ament, M.E., Sample, W.F., Sarti, D.A., O'Donnell, M., and Byrne, W.J.: The ultrasonic and biochemical diagnosis of pancreatitis in children. J. Pediatr. 96: 407–411, 1980.

5. Crane, J.M., Amoury, R.A., and Hellerstein, S.: Hereditary pancreatitis: Report of a kindred. J. Pediatr. Surg. 8: 893–900, 1973.

6. Davis, S., Parbhoo, S.P., and Gibson, M.J.: The plain abdominal radiograph in acute pancreatitis. Clin. Radiol. 31: 87–93, 1980.

7. Felson, B.: Gas abscess of pancreas. J.A.M.A. 163: 637–641, 1957.

8. Fleischer, A.C., Parker, P., Kirchner, S.G., and James, A.E., Jr.: Sonographic findings of pancreatitis in children. Radiology 146: 151–155, 1983.

9. Goldberg, B.H., and Bergstein, J.M.: Acute respiratory distress in a child after steroid-induced pancreatitis. Pediatrics 61: 317–318, 1978.

10. Goluboff, N., Cram, R., Ramgotra, B., Singh, A., and Wilkinson, G.W.: Polyarthritis and bone lesions complicating traumatic pancreatitis in two children. Can. Med. Assoc. J. 118: 924–928, 1978.

11. Grollman, A.I., Goodman, S., and Fine, A.: Localized paralytic ileus: An early roentgen sign in acute pancreatitis. Surg. Gynecol. Obstet. 91: 65–70, 1950.

12. Gryboski, J., Hillemeier, C., Kocoshis, S., Anyan, W., and Seashore, J.S.: Refeeding pancreatitis in malnourished children. J. Pediatr. 97: 441–443, 1980.

13. Haller, J., Greenway, G., Resnick, D., Kindynis, P., Kang, H.S.: Intraosseous fat necrosis associated with acute pancreatitis: MR imaging. Radiology 173: 193–195, 1989.

14. Jordan, S.C., and Ament, M.E.: Pancreatitis in children and adolescents. J. Pediatr. 91: 211–216, 1977.

15. Kattwinkel, J., Lapey, A., di Sant'Agnese, P.A., Edwards, W.A., and Huffy, M.P.: Hereditary pancreatitis: Three new kindreds and a critical review of the literature. Pediatrics 51: 55–69, 1973.

16. Keating, J.P., Shackelford, G.D., Shackelford, P.G., and Ternberg, J.L.: Pancreatitis and osteolytic lesions. J. Pediatr. 81: 350–353, 1972.

17. Malone, J.I.: Juvenile diabetes and acute pancreatitis. J. Pediatr. 85: 825–827, 1974.

18. Meyers, M.A., and Evans, J.A.: Effects of pancreatitis on small bowel and colon: Spread along mesenteric planes. A.J.R. 119: 151–165, 1973.

19. Mitchell, C.E.: Relapsing pancreatitis with recurrent pericardial and pleural effusions: A case report and review of the literature. Ann. Intern. Med. 60: 1047–1053, 1964.

20. Morens, D.M., Hammar, S.L., and Heicher, D.A.: Idiopathic acute pancreatitis in children. Am. J. Dis. Child. 128: 401–404, 1974.

21. Neuer, F.S., Roberts, F.F., and McCarthy, V.: Osteolytic lesions following traumatic pancreatitis. Am. J. Dis. Child. 131: 738–740, 1977.

22. Poppel, M.H.: The roentgen manifestations of pancreatitis. Semin. Roentgenol. 3: 227–241, 1968.

23. Rovner, A.J., and Westcott, J.L.: Pulmonary edema and respiratory insufficiency in acute pancreatitis. Radiology 118: 513–520, 1976.

24. Schrier, R.W., Melmon, K.L., and Fenster, L.F.: Subcutaneous nodular fat necrosis in pancreatitis. Arch. Intern. Med. 116: 832–836, 1965.

25. Schulz, R.D., Stechele, V., Seitz, K.H., Rettenmaier, G., Weitzel, D., and Mildenberger, H.: Pancreatic pseudocyst in children: Echographic and angiographic demonstration. Ann. Radiol. 21: 173–178, 1978.

26. Schwachman, H., Lebenthal, E., and Khaw, K.: Recurrent acute pancreatitis in patients with cystic fibrosis with normal pancreatic enzymes. Pediatrics 55: 86–95, 1975.

27. Schwartz, S., and Nadelhaft, J.: Simulation of colonic obstruction at the splenic flexure by pancreatitis: Roentgen features. A.J.R. 78: 607–616, 1957.

28. Siegelman, S.S., Copeland, B.E., Saba, G.P., Cameron, J.L., Sanders, R.C., and Zerhouni, E.A.: CT of fluid collections associated with pancreatitis. A.J.R. 134: 1121–1132, 1980.

29. Slovis, T.L., Berdon, W.E., Haller, J.O., Baker, D.H., and Rosen, L.: Pancreatitis and the battered child syndrome: Report of two cases with skeletal involvement. A.J.R. 125: 456–461, 1975.

30. Swerdlow, A.B., Berman, M.E., Gibbel, M.I., et al.: Subcutaneous fat necrosis associated with acute pancreatitis. J.A.M.A. 173: 765–769, 1960.

31. Swischuk, L.E., and Hayden, C.K.: Pararenal space hyperechogenicity in childhood pancreatitis. A.J.R. 145: 1085–1086, 1985.

32. Thompson, W.M., Kelvin, F.M., and Rice, R.P.: Inflammation and necrosis of the transverse colon secondary to pancreatitis. A.J.R. 128: 943–948, 1977.

33. Weens, H.S., and Walker, L.A.: The radiologic diagnosis of acute cholecystitis and pancreatitis. Radiol. Clin. North Am. 2: 89–106, 1964.

34. Whitten, D.M., Feingold, M., and Iesenklam, E.J.: Hereditary pancreatitis. Am. J. Dis. Child. 116: 426–428, 1968.

Cholecystitis and Cholelithiasis

1. Bertin, P., Fortier-Beaulieu, M., Rymer, R., Patrois, R., and Pellerin, D.: Primary biliary lithiasis in children: 18 cases. Ann. Pediatr. 22: 203–212, 1975.

2. Bloom, R.A., and Swain, V.A.J.: Noncalculous distension of gallbladder and childhood. Arch. Dis. Child. 41: 503–508, 1966.

3. Chamberlain, J.W., and Hight, D.W.: Acute hydrops of the gallbladder in childhood. Surgery 68: 899–905, 1970.

4. Chrichlow, R.W., Seltzer, M.H., and Jannetta, P.J.: Cholecystitis in adolescents. Am. J. Dig. Dis. 17: 68–72, 1972.

5. Fortier-Beaulieu, M., and Rymer, R.: Radiological diagnosis of cholelithiasis in infancy and childhood (21 cases). Ann. Radiol. 16: 167–171, 1973.

6. Hanson, B.A., Mahour, G.H., and Woolley, M.M.: Disease of the gallbladder in infancy and childhood. J. Pediatr. Surg. 6: 277–283, 1971.

7. Harned, R.K., and Babbitt, D.P.: Cholelithiasis in children. Radiology 117: 391–393, 1975.

8. Jamieson, P.N., and Shaw, D.G.: Empyema of gallbladder in an infant. Arch. Dis. Child. 50: 482–484, 1975.

9. Kumari, S., Lee, W.J., and Baron, M.G.: Hydrops of the gallbladder in a child: Diagnosis by ultrasonography. Pediatrics 63: 295–297, 1979.

10. Lucus, C.E., and Walt, A.J.: Acute gangrenous acalculous cholecystitis in infancy: Report of a case. Surgery 64: 847–849, 1968.

11. Marks, C., Espinosa, J., and Hyman, L.J.: Acute acalculous cholecystitis in childhood. J. Pediatr. Surg. 3: 608–611, 1968.

12. Morales, L., Taboda, E., Toledo, L., and Radri-

gan, W.: Cholecystitis and cholelithiasis in children. J. Pediatr. Surg. 2: 565–568, 1967.
13. Natar, G.: Gallbladder disease in childhood. Aust. Paediatr. J. 8: 147–151, 1972.
14. Newman, D.E.: Gallstones in children. Pediatr. Radiol. 1: 100–104, 1973.
15. Patriquin, H.b., DePietro, M., and Barber, F.E.: Sonography of thickened gallbladder wall: Causes in children. A.J.R. 141: 57–60, 1983.
16. Scobie, W.G., and Bentley, J.F.R.: Hydrops of the gallbladder in a newborn infant. J. Pediatr. Surg. 4: 457–459, 1969.
17. Strauss, R.G.: Cholelithiasis in childhood. Am. J. Dis. Child. 117: 689–692, 1969.
18. Teefey, S.A., Baron, R.L., and Bigler, S.A.: Sonography of the gallbladder: Significance of striated (layered) thickening of the gallbladder wall. A.J.R. 156: 945–947, 1991.

Urinary Tract Infection

1. Bjørgvinsson, E., Majd, M., and Eggli, K.D.: Diagnosis of acute pyelonephritis in children: Comparison of sonography and 99mTc-DMSA scintigraphy. A.J.R. 157: 539–543, 1991.
2. Lee, J.K.T., McClennan, B.L., Melson, G.L., and Stanley, R.J.: Acute focal bacterial emphasis on gray scale sonography and computed tomography. Am. J. Roentgen. 135: 87–92, 1980.
3. Moenne-Locloz, J.P., Bomsel, F., Gatti, J.M., and Prot, D.: Renal abscess in children. A rare but important radiological diagnosis. Pediatr. Radiol. 7: 150–154, 1978.
4. Rigsby, C.M., Rosenfield, A.T., Glickman, M.G., and Hodson, J.: Hemorrhagic focal bacterial nephritis: Findings on gray-scale sonography and CT. A.J.R. 146: 1173–1177, 1986.
5. Traisman, E.S., Conway, J.J., Traisman, H.S., Yogev, R., Firlit, C., Skolnik, A., and Weiss, S.: Localization of urinary tract infection with 99mTc-glucoheptonate scintigraphy. Pediatr. Radiol. 16: 403–406, 1986.

Cystitis

1. Harris, V.J., Javapour, N., and Fizzotti, G.: Cystitis cystica masquerading as a bladder tumor. A.J.R. 120: 410–412, 1974.
2. Mufson, M.A., Zallar, L.M., Mankad, V.N., and Manalo, D.: Adenovirus infection in acute hemorrhagic cystitis. Am. J. Dis. Child. 121: 281–285, 1971.
3. Numazaki, Y., Shigeta, A., Kumasaka, K., Miyazawa, T., Yamanaka, M., Yano, N., Takai, S., and Ishida, N.: Acute hemorrhagic cystitis in children: Isolation of adenovirus II. N. Engl. J. Med. 278: 700–704, 1968.

Salpingitis

1. Bulas, D.I., Ahlstrom, P.A., Sivit, C.J., Nussbaum, A.R., and O'Donnell, R.M.: Pelvic inflammatory disease in the adolescent: Comparison of transabdominal and transvaginal sonographic evaluation. Radiology 183: 435–439, 1992.
2. Golden, N., Cohen, H., Gennari, Q., and Neuhobb, S.: The use of ultrasonography in the evaluation of adolescents with pelvic inflammatory disease. Am. J. Dis. Child. 141: 1235–1238, 1987.
3. Terry, J., and Forrest, T.: Sonographic demonstration of salpingitis: Potential confusion with appendicitis. J. Ultrasound Med. 8: 39–41, 1989.
4. Shafer, M.A.B., Irwin, C.E., and Sweet, R.L.: Acute salpingitis in the adolescent female. J. Pediatr. 100: 339–350, 1982.

Inflammatory Bowel Disease and Colitis

1. Bar-Ziv, J., Ayoub, J., and Fletcher, B.: Hemolytic uremic syndrome: Case presenting with acute colitis. Pediatr. Radiol. 2: 203–205, 1974.
2. Hayden, C.K., Jr., Swischuk, L.E., and Rytting, J.E.: Gastric ulcer disease in infants: US findings. Radiology 164: 131–134, 1987.
3. Hill, S.M., and Milla, P.J.: Colitis caused by food allergy in infants. Arch. Dis. Child. 65: 132–133, 1990.
4. Jenkins, H.R., Pincott, J.R., Soothill, J.F., Milla, P.J., and Harries, J.T.: Food allergy: The major cause of infantile colitis. Arch. Dis. Child. 59: 326–329, 1984.
5. Karjoo, M., and McCarthy, B.: Toxic megacolon of ulcerative colitis in infancy. Pediatrics 57: 962–965, 1976.
6. Kelber, M., and Ament, M.E.: Shigella dysenteriae; I. A forgotten cause of pseudomembranous colitis. Pediatrics 89: 595–696, 1976.
7. Liebhaber, M.I., Parker, B.R., Morton, J.A., and Tune, B.M.: Abdominal mass and colonic perforation in a case of the hemolytic-uremic syndrome. Am. J. Dis. Child. 131: 1168–1169, 1977.
8. Peterson, R.B., Meseroll, W.P., Shrago, G.G., et al.: Radiographic features of colitis associated with the hemolyticuremic syndrome. Radiology 118: 667–671, 1976.
9. Rice, R.P.: Plain abdominal film roentgenographic diagnosis of ulcerative diseases of the colon. A.J.R. 104: 544–550, 1968.
10. Schachter, H., Goldstein, M.J., and Kirsner, J.B.: Toxic dilatation complicating Crohn's disease of colon. Gastroenterology 53: 136–142, 1967.
11. Schwartz, D.L., Becker, J.M., So, H.B., and Schneider, K.M.: Segmental colonic gangrene: A

surgical emergency in the hemolytic-uremic syndrome. Pediatrics 62: 54–56, 1978.

12. Takayanagi, K., and Kapila, L.: Necrotizing enterocolitis in older infants. Arch. Dis. Child. 56: 468–471, 1981.

13. Tochen, M.L., and Campbell, J.R.: Colitis in children with the hemolytic-uremic syndrome. J. Pediatr. Surg. 12: 213–219, 1977.

14. Swischuk, L.E., and Hayden, C.K.: Barium enema findings (?segmental colitis) in four neonates with bloody diarrhea—possible cow's milk allergy. Pediatr. Radiol. 15: 34–37, 1985.

15. Vargas, M., and Pena, A.: Toxic amoebic colitis and amoebic colon perforation in children: An improved prognosis. J. Pediatr. Surg. 11: 223–225, 1976.

16. Wolf, B., and Marshak, R.: "Toxic" segmental dilatation of the colon during the course of fulminating ulcerative colitis: roentgen findings. A.J.R. 82: 985–995, 1959.

17. Wruble, L.A., Duckworth, J.K., Duke, D.D., and Rothschild, J.A.: Toxic dilatation of the colon in a case of amebiasis. N. Engl. J. Med. 275: 926–928, 1966.

MISCELLANEOUS ACUTE ABDOMINAL PROBLEMS

Systemic Conditions Presenting with an Acute Abdomen. An acute abdomen can be seen in patients with diabetes mellitus (1), sickle cell anemia, abdominal migraine, and pneumonia. For the most part, the abdominal roentgenograms in these patients are normal or merely show paralytic ileus. In diabetes mellitus the problem usually is ketoacidosis or electrolyte imbalance, while in sickle cell disease the problem is sludging of the blood and ischemia of the intestine. Abdominal migraine is a matter of vasospasm, while with pneumonia the problem is referred pain.

REFERENCE

1. Valerio, D.: Acute diabetic abdomen in childhood. Lancet 1: 66–67, 1977.

Peptic Ulcer Disease and Gastritis. A thorough, complete discussion of these entities is beyond the scope of this book, but it is worth noting that both conditions are more common in childhood than is generally appreciated (1–10). In some children, acute abdominal pain clearly suggestive of duodenal ulcer disease can be seen, but many children present with little in the way of abdominal pain, and vomiting is the predominant feature. In still other cases, bleeding may be the problem.

Roentgenographically, the actual ulcer may be seen (Fig. 3.92A), but most cases of peptic ulcer disease do not demonstrate an actual ulcer. More often, spasm of the antrum and duodenal bulb along with edema of the mucosa of these structures is seen. In addition, in some cases of gastritis, one may see a diffuse cobblestone appearance to the edematous mucosa (Fig. 3.92B). Ultrasound also can demonstrate the presence of gastritis (4). In these cases, the gastric wall is thickened and there is disruption of the normal layers of the wall (Fig. 3.92C). It is difficult to visualize an actual ulcer with ultrasound, but if the ulcer is large it may be seen.

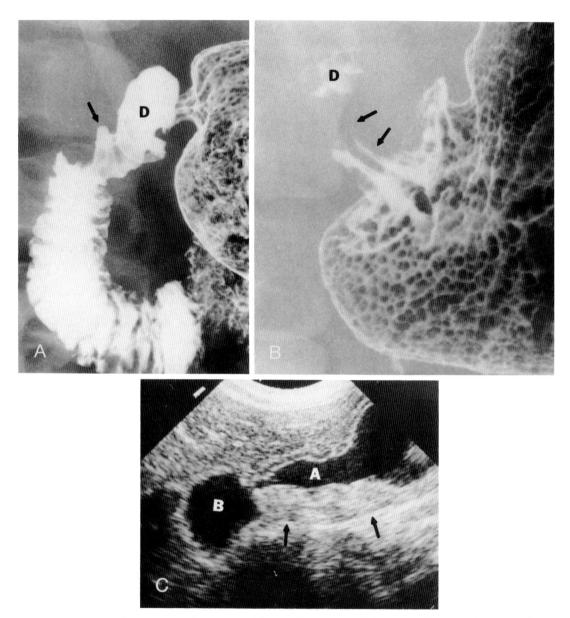

Figure 3.92. *Peptic ulcer disease and gastritis.*   (**A**) Note the postapical ulcer crater (*arrow*). There are edematous folds radiating from its base and marked spasm of the postapical portion of the duodenum. Duodenal bulb (*D*). (**B**) Gastritis. Note the diffuse mucosal nodularity throughout the stomach. In addition, note spasm of the antrum (*arrows*) and duodenal bulb (*D*). (**C**) Ultrasonogram demonstrating gastritis with marked thickening of the gastric wall (mucosa and submucosa) along the inferior curvature of the antrum (*arrows*). Note the normal layers on the opposite side. Duodenal bulb (*B*), antrum (*A*).

REFERENCES

1. Curci, M.R., Little, K., Sieber, W.K., and Kieswetter, W.B.: Peptic ulcer disease in childhood reexamined. J. Pediatr. Surg. 11: 329–335, 1976.
2. Deckelbaum, R.L., Roy, C.C., Lussier-Lazaroff, J., and Morin, C.L.: Peptic ulcer disease: A clinical study in 73 children. Can. Med. Assoc. J. 111: 225–228, 1974.
3. Habbick, B.F., Melrose, A.G., and Grant, J.C.: Duodenal ulcer in childhood. Arch. Dis. Child. 43: 23–27, 1968.
4. Hayden, C.K., Jr., Swischuk, L.E., and Rytting, J.E.: Gastric ulcer disease in infants: US findings. Radiology 164: 131–134, 1987.
5. Hsu, H.Y., Chang, M.H., and Want, T.H.: Acute duodenal ulcer. Arch. Dis. Child. 64: 774–779, 1989.
6. Murphy, M.S., Eastham, E.J., Jiminez, M., Nelson, and R. Jackson, R.H.: Duodenal ulceration: Review of 110 cases. Arch. Dis. Child. 62: 554–558, 1987.
7. Robb, J.D.A., Thomas, P.S., Orzulok, J., and Odling-Smee, G.W.: Duodenal ulcer in children. Arch. Dis. Child. 47: 688–696, 1972.
8. Rosenlund, M.L., and Koop, C.E.: Duodenal ulcer in childhood. Pediatrics 45: 283–286, 1970.
9. Singleton, E.B.: The radiologic incidence of peptic ulcer in infants and children. Radiology 84: 956–957, 1965.
10. Tsang, T.-M., Saing, H., and Yeung, C.-K.: Peptic ulcer in children. J. Pediatr. Surg. 25: 744–748, 1990.

Hiatus Hernia and Esophagitis. The symptoms of a hiatus hernia and gastroesophageal reflux are well known to all, and if one takes the time, a strongly suggestive history can be extracted from an older child if the problem is present. In younger infants the problem is more difficult, and vomiting may be the only symptom. Associated problems such as resistant asthma (2), sudden infant death syndrome (3, 4), and apnea (6) have been attributed to gastroesophageal reflux. While all of these problems do occur, they are not nearly as common as generally believed. Certainly our experience would suggest that gastroesophageal reflux is not a very common cause of refractory asthma or the sudden infant death syndrome.

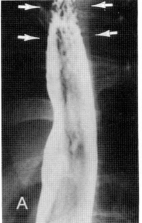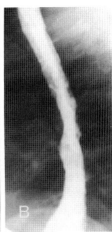

Figure 3.93. *Esophagitis.* (*A*) *Herpes.* Note the fine nodularity and mucosal fold thickening (*arrows*) in the upper esophagus. (*B*) *Monilia.* Note extensive spasm of the esophagus and irregularity of the mucosa of the esophagus.

Esophagitis secondary to the ingestion of corrosive materials is dealt with later in this chapter. Rarely, viral (herpes [1, 5]) or *Candida* esophagitis are encountered in childhood. These are seen more often now that human immunodeficiency virus (HIV)-infected patients have become commonplace. The findings usually involve the mucosa with diffuse edema, often manifesting in cobblestoning or edematous striation of the esophagus (Fig. 3.93). Of course, pronounced spasm is present, and with *Candida* esophagitis such spasm can be profound. Solitary ulcers are less common, for the problem usually is one of diffuse, superficial ulceration.

REFERENCES

1. Bastian, J.F., and Kaufman, I.A.: Herpes simplex esophagitis in a healthy 10-year-old boy. J. Pediatr. 100: 426–427, 1962.
2. Danus, O., Casar, C., Larrain, A., and Pope, C.E., II: Esophageal reflux: An unrecognized cause of recurrent obstructive bronchitis in children. J. Pediatr. 89: 220–224, 1976.
3. Herbst, J.J., Book, L.S., and Bray, P.F.: Gastroesophageal reflux in the "near miss" sudden infant death syndrome. J. Pediatr. 92: 73–75, 1978.
4. Leape, L.L., Holder, T.M., Franklin, J.D.,

Amoury, R.A., and Ashcraft, K.W.: Respiratory arrest in infants secondary to gastroesophageal reflux. Pediatrics 60: 924–928, 1977.

5. Meyers, C., Durkin, M.G., and Love, L.: Radiographic findings in herpetic esophagitis. Radiology 119: 21–22, 1976.

6. Walsh, J.K., Farrell, M.K., Kennan, W.J., Lucas, M., and Kramer, M.: Gastroesophageal reflux in infants: Relation to apnea. J. Pediatr. 99: 197–201, 1981.

Intestinal Infarction and Intramural Bleeding or Edema.

Intestinal infarction in children is uncommon except as seen with mechanical problems such as volvulus or intussusception, or after blunt abdominal trauma causing injury to the blood vessels of the gut. Plain films may show sentinel loops, generalized paralytic ileus, or edematous loops of infarcted intestine. Extremely edematous loops of the intestine may show so-called "thumbprinting" of the bowel wall, and with ultrasound, thickening of the intestinal wall is seen.

Bleeding into the intestinal wall can occur in hemophilia, Henoch-Schönlein purpura, and after trauma. Edema can occur with hypoproteinemia, portal hypertension, and with angioneurotic edema. Usually there is little to see on the plain films of these patients, but if the bleeding or edema is extensive, thumbprinting or a mass-like configuration of the intestine can be noted. Most often, these changes are demonstrated more clearly with barium studies of the upper gastrointestinal (GI) tract, but bowel thickening now is initially readily demonstrable with ultrasound.

Henoch-Schönlein purpura is not an uncommon cause of intestinal bleeding, and the findings of bleeding or an acute abdomen may precede the classic purpuric skin rash (6). The condition is believed to be a virus-induced hypersensitivity problem leading to small vessel thrombosis and subsequent bleeding. When the gastrointestinal tract is involved, the main clinical manifestation is abdominal pain (5, 9). The thickened hemorrhagic mucosa can be readily identified with ultrasound (1–4) (Fig. 3.94) and usually manifests as concentric thickening of the intestinal wall (6).

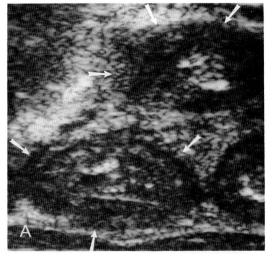

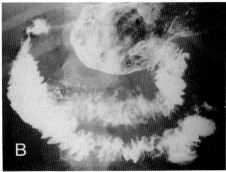

Figure 3.94. *Henoch Schönlein purpura.* (*A*) Note concentric thickening of the intestinal wall primarily due to echogenic mucosa (*arrows*). A number of loops of intestine are involved. (*B*) Another patient whose upper GI series demonstrates extensive edema and thickening of the intestinal wall producing marked spiculation and thumbprinting of the involved segments of the intestine.

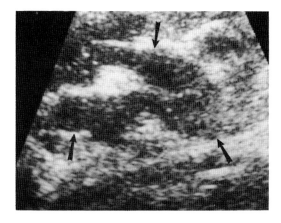

Figure 3.95. *Henoch Schönlein purpura: pseudo- intussusception.* Note the pseudokidney appearance of this liquified hematoma (*arrows*). The findings resemble those of intussusception. This patient was not obstructed and had a normal barium enema.

In other cases, it may be more eccentric (3). Free peritoneal fluid also can be seen in small amounts, and intussusception is a known complication of the condition (8, 9). The ultrasonographic appearance of the intussusception is no different than with other causes of intussusception, but we also have noted that a liquified hematoma can produce ultrasonographic findings similar to those seen with intussusception (Fig. 3.95). If a gastrointestinal barium study is performed (7, 10), the appearance of the thickened intestinal loops can be quite striking (Fig. 3.94).

REFERENCES

1. Agha, F.P., Nostrat, T.T., and Keren, D.F.: Leucocytoplastic vasculitis (hypersensitivity angiitis) of the small bowel presenting with severe gastrointestinal hemorrhage. Am. J. Gastroenterol. 81: 195–198, 1986.
2. Bomelburg, T., Claasen, U., and von Lengerke, H.J.: Intestinal ultrasonographic findings in Schönlein syndrome by high frequency ultrasound. European J. Pediatr. 150: 158–160, 1991.
3. Couture, A., Veyrac, C., Baud, C., Galifer, R.B., and Armelin, I.: Evaluation of abdominal pain in Henoch- Schönlein syndrome by high frequency ultrasound. Pediatr. Radiol. 22: 12–17, 1992.
4. Demirci, A., Cengiz, K., Baris, S., and Karagoz, F.: CT and ultrasound of abdominal hemorrhage in Henoch-Schönlein purpura. J. Comput. Assist. Tomogr. 15: 143–145, 1991.
5. Glasier, C.M., Siegel, M.J., MacAlister, W.H., and Schakelford, G.D.: Henoch-Schönlein syndrome in children: Gastrointestinal manifestations. A.J.R. 136: 1081–1085, 1981.
6. John, S.D., Swischuk, L.E., and Hayden, C.K., Jr.: Gastrointestinal sonographic findings in Henoch-Schönlein purpura. (In preparation)
7. Martinez-Frontanilla, L.A., Haase, G.M., Ernster, J.A., and Bailey, C.W.: Surgical complications in Henoch- Schönlein purpura. J. Pediatr. Surg. 19: 434–436, 1984.
8. Martinez-Frontanilla, L.a., Silverman, L., and Meagher, D.P., Jr.: Intussusception in Henoch-Schönlein purpura: Diagnosis with ultrasound. J. Pediatr. Surg. 23: 375–376, 1988.
9. Rodriquez-Erdman, F., and Levitan, R.: Gastrointestinal and roentgenological manifestations of Henoch-Schönlein purpura. Gastroenterology 54: 260–264, 1968.

Hepatitis. With hepatitis, as the liver enlarges it stretches its capsule, and abdominal pain can be the presenting problem. Hepatitis usually is viral in origin but also can be toxic in origin. There are few imaging findings with hepatitis. In most cases, ultrasonographically the liver merely is enlarged. However, in some cases of acute liver necrosis, edema of the liver can produce a sonolucent-appearing liver with marked periportal echogenicity (1, 2) (Fig. 3.96).

In addition, it has been noted in cat-scratch disease that multiple sonolucent granulomas may be seen in the liver and spleen (3–5). These also are demonstrable with CT (Fig. 3.96).

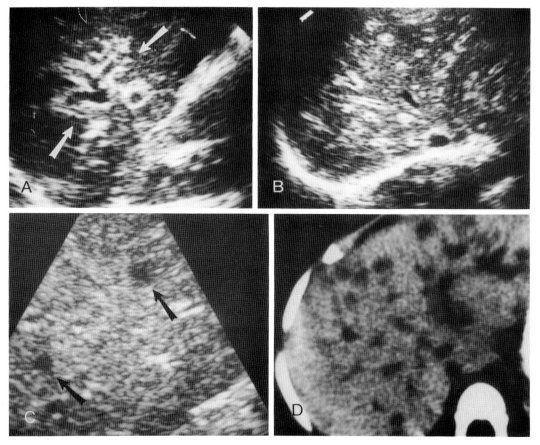

Figure 3.96. *Acute hepatic necrosis.* (*A*) Note the relatively hypoechoic lever parenchyma and marked periportal echogenicity (*arrows*). (*B*) Another view demonstrating similar findings. (*C*) *Cat-scratch disease granulomas.* Note the two hypoechoic areas in the liver (*arrows*). (*D*) CT scan demonstrates numerous low-density lesions scattered throughout the liver. (Parts *C* and *D* reproduced with permission from J.C. Leonidas et al.: Granulomatous hepatitis in cat-scratch disease. Pediatr. Radiol. 21: 598–599, 1991.)

REFERENCES

1. Blane, C.E., Jongeward, R.H., and Silver, T.M.: Sonographic features of hepatocellular disease in neonates and infants. A.J.R. 141: 1313–1316, 1983.
2. Kurtz, A.B., Rubin, C.S., Cooper, H.S., Nisenbaum, H.L., Cole-Beuglet, C., Medoff, J., and Goldberg, B.B.: Ultrasound findings in hepatitis. Radiology 136: 717–723, 1980.
3. Larsen, C.E., and Patrick, L.E.: Abdominal (liver, spleen) and bone manifestations of cat-scratch disease. Pediatr. Radiol. 22: 353–355, 1992.
4. Port, J., and Leonidas, J.C.: Granulomatous hepatitis in cat-scratch disease. Pediatr. Radiol. 21: 598–599, 1991.
5. Rappaport, D.C., Cumming, W.A., and Ros, P.R.: Case report. Disseminated hepatic and splenic lesions in cat-scratch disease: Imaging features. A.J.R. 156: 1227–1228, 1991.

Renal Colic. Renal colic is not as great a problem in children as it is in adults, but still it does occur. The clinical symptoms are exactly the same as in adults and imaging of these patients centers around plain films, ultrasonography, and intravenous pyelography. Plain films may reveal an enlarged renal silhouette and a calcified stone (Fig. 3.97*A*). Ultrasound can dem-

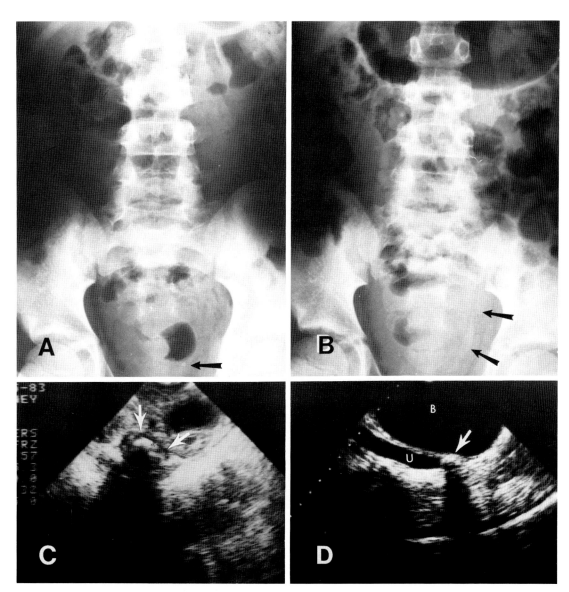

Figure 3.97. *Renal colic—calcified renal calculus.* (*A*) Note the small calcified renal calculus (*arrow*) in the pelvis of this patient who presented with renal colic. (*B*) Subsequent intravenous pyelogram demonstrates moderate dilatation of the distal ureter on the left (*arrows*). The small calcified calculus is visualized again. (*C*) Ultrasound delineation of renal calculi in another patient. Note multiple renal stones (*arrows*) with distal shadowing. (*D*) Note echoes, with distal shadowing, from stone impacted in distal ureter (*arrow*). Dilated ureter (*U*), bladder (*B*).

onstrate hydronephrosis, hydroureter, intrarenal stones (Fig. 3.97*C*) or the echogenic calculus in the ureter (Fig. 3.97*D*). Intravenous pyelography often still is used to diagnose renal colic, for it clearly demonstrates the level and the degree of obstruction of the kidney (Fig. 3.97*B*). With

acute obstruction, one sees a delayed nephrogram and diminished renal function of the involved kidney.

Adnexal Problems in Girls. The most common problem in this group of abnormalities is a simple ovarian cyst. Small follicular cysts 1 cm or less in diameter are commonly found in adolescent girls (Fig. 3.98A). If any of these cysts enlarge (Fig. 3.98B), they can cause lower abdominal and pelvic pain. Furthermore, bleeding into these cysts or into a corpus lutean cyst (Fig. 3.99) can produce considerable pain. Roentgenographically, simple cysts are anechoic, for they are fluid filled (Fig. 3.98B and C), but once hemorrhage occurs, the pattern becomes mixed (1, 2) (Fig. 3.98D). It is difficult to differentiate a hemorrhagic cyst from an ovarian tumor such as a teratoma or dermoid (Fig. 3.99).

With any of these pelvic problems, fluid often is present in the cul-de-sac. This fluid can be blood or simply reactive fluid. Normal fluid in the cul-de-sac is not as common in girls as it is in women, and thus in children it should be treated with more suspicion. Consequently, if a patient is encountered with pelvic pain, a few small cysts in the ovary, and fluid in the cul-de-sac, the clinician should become suspicious that one of these cysts may have hemorrhaged. These cysts do not have to be large to produce local hemorrhage. This is especially important when no other cause for the abdominal pain is detected. This is not to say that the findings are pathognomonic, but only that they are highly suggestive in the proper clinical setting.

Torsion of the normal adnexa also can

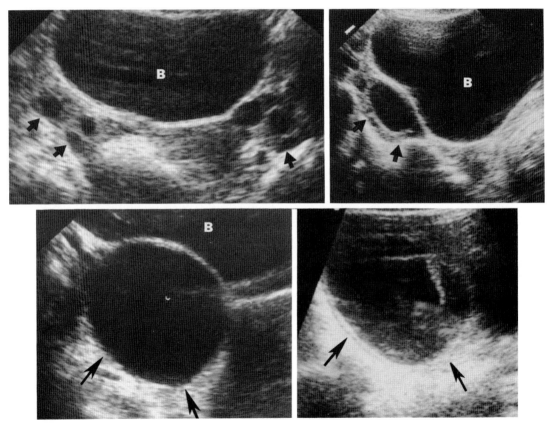

Figure 3.98. *Ovarian cysts.* (*A*) Note bilateral numerous small cysts in both ovaries (*arrows*) of this adolescent girl. Bladder (*B*). (*B*) Another patient whose sagittal view of one of the adnexal regions demonstrates one large cyst and numerous smaller cysts (*arrows*). Bladder (*B*). (*C*) Another patient with a large sonolucent cyst (*arrows*). Bladder (*B*). (*D*) Hemorrhage in this cyst produces echogenic debris and fibrin strands. Fibrin also layers the wall of the cyst producing an echogenic inner layer.

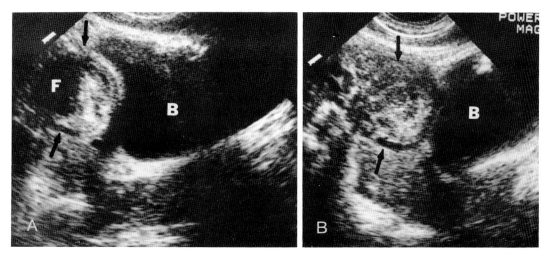

Figure 3.99. *Hemorrhagic corpus lutean cyst.* (*A*) Sagittal view demonstrates the large cyst (*arrows*) with a heterogeneous center. Fluid (*F*) in the cyst is suggestive, but not totally diagnostic of a hemorrhagic corpus lutean cyst. Bladder (*B*). (*B*) Cross-section through the hemorrhagic cyst (*arrows*) reveals the heterogeneous but virtually solid appearance of the cyst. Bladder (*B*). These findings are difficult to differentiate from torsion of normal ovaries or tumors of ovaries.

occur (3, 4, 6–8), and, in addition, torsion of an ovarian cyst (5) or a tumor such as a dermoid or teratoma can occur. Ultrasound is best for detecting all of these problems but, as mentioned earlier, differentiating one from another is difficult. For the most part, they each present as a round or oval mass with a mixed pattern of echogenicity and, frequently, fluid in the cul-de-sac. Calcification, of course, is the hallmark of a dermoid or teratoma.

ACUTE MECHANICAL PROBLEMS

Entities to be discussed in this section include intussusception, volvulus, hernia, and visceral torsion. Any of these conditions can present with acute, even catastrophic, clinical pictures, and the radiologist should be aware of them all and the pertinent plain film findings with which they might present.

Intussusception. The clinical findings of classic intussusception are well known and include: (a) crampy abdominal pain, (b) vomiting, (c) bloody (currant jelly) stools, and (d) either a palpable mass or palpable emptiness in the right flank or lower quadrant. However, not all of these findings need be present at the same time and, furthermore, in many patients they are intermittent. *Indeed, it is becoming more and more apparent that many cases of intussusception are atypical in their presentation.* For example, the classic triad of clinical findings in one series was noted to be present in only 20% of patients (45). Bleeding was present in only 36% of patients in another series (25), and some intussusceptions may be relatively painless (15, 17). In addition, a palpable abdominal mass has been shown to be present in only 50–60% of cases (25, 44, 45). Altered consciousness and apathy (3, 9, 11, 42) also have been documented as manifestations of intussusception, but it is not known why these phenomena occur. However, it is postulated that intestinal ischemia may lead to release of endotoxins which then could alter the blood brain barrier and lead to central nervous system depression (11). *Overall, then, one should realize that a good many cases of intussusception present with less than classic findings (3, 17)* *and, interestingly enough, it is here that ultrasound becomes very useful.*

Intussusception is most common between the ages of 6 months and 2 years, but, of course, can be seen in the older child or even the neonate. In most cases, the cause of intussusception is idiopathic, although mesenteric lymph node enlargement and/or redundant, edematous, intestinal mucosa (i.e., as part of a viral or other GI infection) probably account for the lead point in most cases. Indeed, now that ultrasound is available, adenopathy may be more frequently seen with intussusception. A more discrete leading lesion such as polyp, Meckel's diverticulum, duplication cyst, appendix, or hemangioma is found in <10% of cases and, in this regard, usually is found in older children or neonates (14, 16, 31, 61).

Most cases of intussusception are ileocolic (34), with ileo-ileo and ileo-ileocolic intussusceptions accounting for no more than 10–12% of cases (24, 35). Generally speaking, these latter intussusceptions are more difficult to diagnose and tend to be present for longer periods of time before definitive treatment is accomplished. Consequently, complications such as bowel necrosis and perforation are more common and, because of this, these intussusceptions generally are considered more serious. A very rare type of intussusception is back and forth, antegrade and retrograde telescoping of the bowel with multiple layers of intestine encountered within the intussusception. In addition, occasionally intussusceptions are chronic and after ultrasound, may be confirmed more expediently with an upper GI series and small bowel follow-through (24, 49).

Plain film roentgenographic findings of intussusception are useful, but variable, and depend primarily on the duration of the symptoms and the presence or absence of complications. In early cases, a normal gas pattern is usual, but the longer the intussusception is present, the more likely is one to see a pattern of typical small bowel

obstruction (Fig. 3.100A). In other cases, one can see the actual head of the intussusception on plain films (Fig. 3.100B and D), but this generally occurs in less than 50% of cases (44). Visualization of the head of the intussusception can be enhanced and increased to 60% by the use of decubitus views (64), but such views are not generally obtained. Perhaps more commonly than seeing the head of the intussusception, one sees lack of definition of the inferior aspect of the liver (26) and/or absence of gas in the right lower quadrant or flank (Fig. 3.100B). Absence of gas in the right lower quadrant or flank results from the fact that, as an intussusception develops, the air is squeezed out of the intestine, and failure of visualization of the liver edge occurs because, when right upper quadrant bowel gas is absent, the natural contrasting effect of liver against adjacent air-filled bowel is lost. Of course, if bowel necrosis and perforation ensue, the findings of peritonitis and free peritoneal air supervene. All of these points notwithstanding, however, it should be noted that *many cases still demonstrate normal or near-normal abdominal films, and this should not dissuade one from pursuing the diagnosis of intussusception if it is suspected clinically.* In this regard, although in some series the plain films are reportedly frequently highly suggestive of the diagnosis (64), our own experience has been less rewarding, and, consequently, we now perform ultrasonography in any case suggestive in any way of intussusception. Ultrasound is very effective in detecting intussusception and has increasingly become the next imaging modality after plain films (7, 23, 36, 38, 41, 54, 62). False negative studies are few, and although some suggest ultrasound should be used for clinically atypical cases only (5), it generally is in more widespread use. Ultrasound with color flow Doppler also may prove useful in detecting devitalized bowel that may be more susceptible to perforation (30).

In the earlier years of ultrasonography,

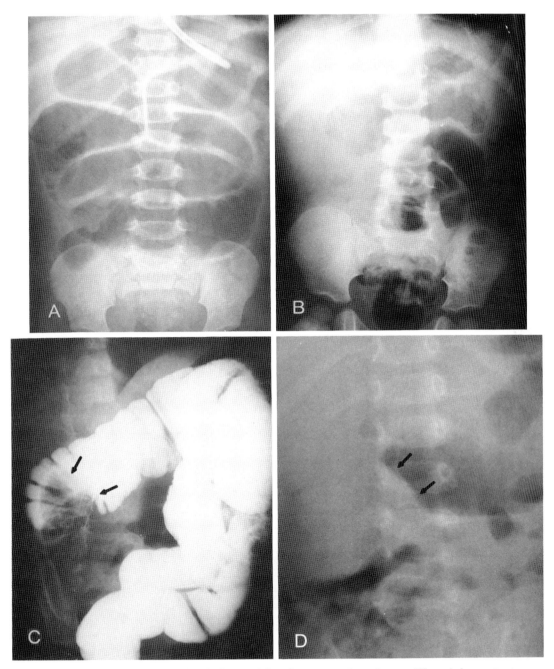

Figure 3.100. *Intussusception: plain film findings.*   (*A*) In this patient, classic low small bowel obstruction is present. (*B*) Classic configuration of intussusception consisting of paucity of gas in the right flank and two or three loops of distended (obstructed) small bowel just to the left of the lower lumbar spine. In addition, a vaguely apparent soft tissue defect is seen in the transverse colon just to the left of the hepatic flexure. Could this be the head of the intussusception? (*C*) Subsequent barium enema demonstrates the head of the intussusception (*arrows*) to correspond to its suspected location on the plain abdominal film seen in *B*. (*D*) Note, in another patient, a clear-cut mass (*arrows*) in the transverse colon. Otherwise the abdominal gas pattern is completely normal.

resolution of the various intestinal layers was not possible, and thus the intussusception appeared more sonolucent and lead to the sonolucent donut and pseudokidney signs (54). However, currently, with high-resolution linear transducers, visualization of the individual layers of the intussusceptions has become possible. As a result, the findings are now more those of a layered oval mass on longitudinal views and concentric rings on cross-section (Fig. 3.101). Indeed, depending on the number of mucosal layers seen, one concievably might even be able to distinguish ileocolic from ileo-ileocolic intussusceptions in some cases. The concentric ring pattern, when enough mesenteric fat is present, can be seen on plain films as the target sign (43, 44). However, this sign is very subtle.

In addition to the foregoing findings, a small amount of free peritoneal fluid (56) can be seen in some cases of intussusception (Fig. 3.102). This is important to note so as not to interpret the findings as being due to perforation or bowel necrosis. Free fluid in small amounts is not uncommonly seen at surgical exploration of these patients, and this should not be a surprising finding when seen with ultrasound. However, when fluid is more voluminous and especially when a fibrinous exudate is seen within the fluid, perforation, or impending perforation, should be considered (Fig. 3.103).

As far as contrast enema reduction of an intussusception is concerned, almost all patients with the disease should be afforded the study. Those patients to be excluded, for the most part, are those demonstrating signs of peritonitis and/or

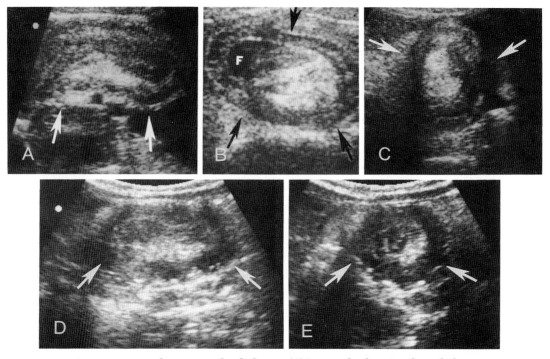

Figure 3.101. *Intussusception: ultrasonographic findings.* (**A**) Longitudinal section through the intussusception demonstrates an oval, somewhat layered mass with an echogenic center. (**B**) Slightly oblique view through the intussusception (*arrows*) demonstrates the various layers more clearly and also shows some fluid (*F*) in the lumen. (**C**) Cross-sectional view of the intussusception shows the echogenic center and the relatively hypoechoic rim. (**D**) Another patient with a more uniform sonolucent rim to the generally oval-shaped intussusception (*arrows*). (**E**) Cross-sectional view in the same patient demonstrates a sonolucent donut configuration (*arrows*).

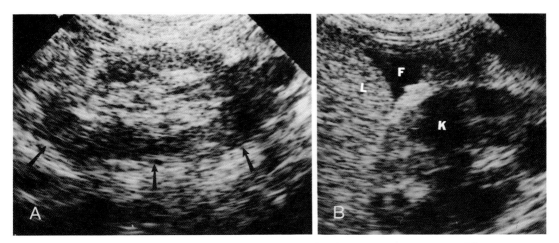

Figure 3.102. *Intussusception with peritoneal fluid.* (*A*) Note the characteristic appearance of the intussusception (*arrows*). (*B*) In another area, some free fluid (*F*) is seen between the liver (*L*) and the right kidney (*K*). (From L.E. Swischuk and S.D. Stansberry: Ultrasonographic detection of free peritoneal fluid in uncomplicated intussusception. Pediatr. Radiol. 21: 350–351, 1991.)

perforation (3, 30). The fact that the intussusception may have been present for 24 hours or more is no longer generally considered a contraindication to nonsurgical reduction (3, 6, 46, 52). In addition, the presence of the so-called "crescent sign" (contrast coating the head of the intussusception) is not considered a contraindication (3, 52).

In the past, barium was almost exclusively used for the nonsurgical reduction of intussusception, but currently there is a great wave of enthusiasm for reduction with air (4, 20, 27, 30, 39, 48, 50, 51, 58). Reduction with aqueous contrast material also can be utilized (3, 27, 33), but air is currently favored, and the end result is that barium eventually will cease to be used. In most general surveys, barium still tends to be used by less currently trained radiologists (10, 27, 33), but eventually it should pass off the scene (32, 53). Ultrasound guidance for the aqueous reduction of intussusception also has been used, and with good results (58, 63). However, it is a not a commonplace procedure.

Proponents of gas reduction list the following as the major advantages of utilizing either air or oxygen: higher reduction rates, no ionizing radiation, and a shorter study. All of this is true, but, in some studies, when reduction rates were compared with those obtained with barium, it became obvious that barium success rates of 40–50% simply reflected a problem with the method of reduction. A rate this low was not the common standard with barium reduction but certainly did add credence to the markedly improved reduction rates with the use of air. In the end, therefore, *when all of the data began to come in, it became apparent that the problem centered more around intracolonic pressures generated than around the contrast agent used.* The most important piece of information in this regard was provided by Kuta and Benator (29), who demonstrated that to generate the 120 mm Hg pressures obtained with air systems, one had to raise a barium column to 3½ feet and an aqueous material column to 5 feet. We have used the aqueous method for more than a decade and have had a success rate of around 80%. This compares favorably with success rates with gas, which generally range from 70–90% but are more around 80%. We have used gastrografin diluted 5:1 with normal saline to render it isotonic and have

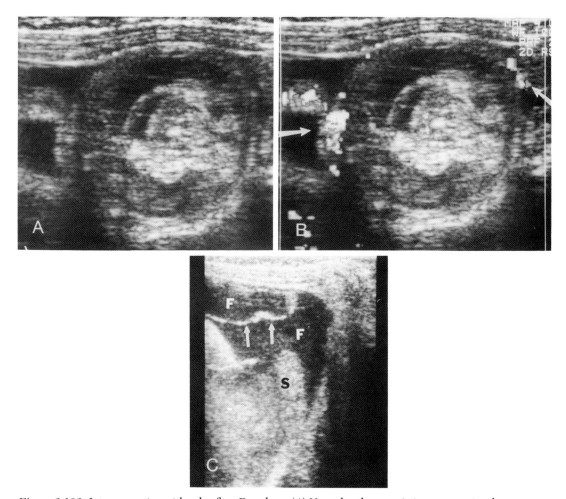

Figure 3.103. *Intussusception with color flow Doppler.* (*A*) Note the characteristic cross-sectional appearance of the intussusception. (*B*) On color flow Doppler, flow is seen around the periphery (*arrows*), but none is seen within the center. (*C*) Considerable fluid (*F*) is seen just around the tip of the spleen (*S*). Note the fibrinous strand within the fluid (*arrows*). At surgery, this patient showed areas of necrosis with impending perforation.

had no difficulty with visualization. We have not used other aqueous contrast agents but do not see why they would not see why they would not be effective.

In terms of air reduction, it has been demonstrated that pressures of 60 mm Hg are required to move an intussusception and 100 mm Hg to reduce it (51). Intramural pressures should not exceed 120 mm Hg for prolonged periods of time, for perforation becomes more likely. This aspect of the study must be monitored closely, and actually some form of safety valve to avoid going over this limit should

be included in one's system. All of this notwithstanding, however, what air has done is encourage a generally more aggressive approach to the reduction of intussusception (3, 6), for once barium is removed from the picture perforation is not such a devastating problem. Such an aggressive approach had been suggested in the past (34), and we have used it with gastrographin for over a decade.

Perforation rates with nonsurgical reduction generally run around 1–3% (3, 48), but in one general survey were noted to be *eight times more common with air reduction* (27).

The consequences of perforation still are incompletely answered with air reduction, but massive pneumoperitoneum can be a serious problem necessitating immediate needle decompression (48). In this regard, it is not as easy to visually detect air leaking into the peritoneal cavity as it is to detect positive contrast material leaking into the peritoneal cavity. On the other hand, with air, when perforation occurs there is an abrupt loss of pressure in the system being used. Once this occurs, the system should be shut down and decompressed immediately.

In the past, glucagon was advocated in stubborn cases, but it never really proved effective and now generally is not used. Sedation also has been popular (3, 34, 46) and seemed to help. Recently, however, air reduction proponents, now able to monitor pressures closely, suggest that without sedation the infant is able to generate, through straining, greater transient but beneficial pressures in the colon (27, 51). All of this is interesting, but over the years I have come to the conclusion that *in the end, most depends on just how well one seals off the anus. It must be totally occluded.*

Total occlusion of the anus usually is best accomplished by tight taping of the buttocks with abundant quantities of *good quality, cloth adhesive tape.* Transparent adhesive tape is no good for this job and this is important because inadequate taping will lead to repeat studies and lower reduction rates. In addition, *we utilize a Foley bulb in the rectum, and while not all will subscribe to this maneuver, we have found it indispensable in obtaining total occlusion.* We inflate it after the colon is filled and the intussusception identified. The balloon is inflated under fluoroscopic control to near the diameter of the contrast-filled rectum, and then it is pulled down as a plunger against the sealed anus. *We have found this to be the most important part of reduction, for if the anus is not totally occluded, reduction is impaired.*

The configuration of an intussusception, on any contrast study, generally is similar and typical. With positive contrast studies, however, the head of the intussusception in addition to appearing round and bulbous (Fig. 3.104A and B), could demonstrate the so-called "coiled spring" sign. With air, the latter two findings are difficult to see and the intussusception usually simply appears bulbous (Fig. 3.104C).

The retrograde progress of the head of the intussusception as it is pushed around the colon is easy to detect and document fluoroscopically. Often it tends to "hang up" at the splenic and hepatic flexures and also at the ileocecal valve. At any of these sites, if maximal pressures are reached and no progress is made, no matter which method one uses, it is best to decompress the system and try again. In this regard, with aqueous contrast agents one simply lowers the bag to the floor and drains the contents back into the bag. Thereafter, one raises the bag to the appropriate level (5 feet) and tries again. With air reduction, simple decompression by "leaking off" the system can be accomplished. With aqueous contrast material, we have repeated this decompressive maneuver up to five times, although in most cases three attempts suffice (3, 6). At any site, if no progress is made after 5 minutes with any contrast agent, it probably is wise to stop.

With final reduction at the ileocecal valve, the filling defect of the intussusception disappears and contrast material rushes into the dilated, obstructed small bowel. This is a most important observation, for otherwise one cannot say that reduction is complete. In addition, while contrast may enter the terminal ileum with ileo-ileocolic intussusceptions, it is only when the contrast material reaches the dilated small bowel proximal to the intussusception that one can say reduction is complete. In this regard, it is easier to see this latter phenomenon with aqueous contrast

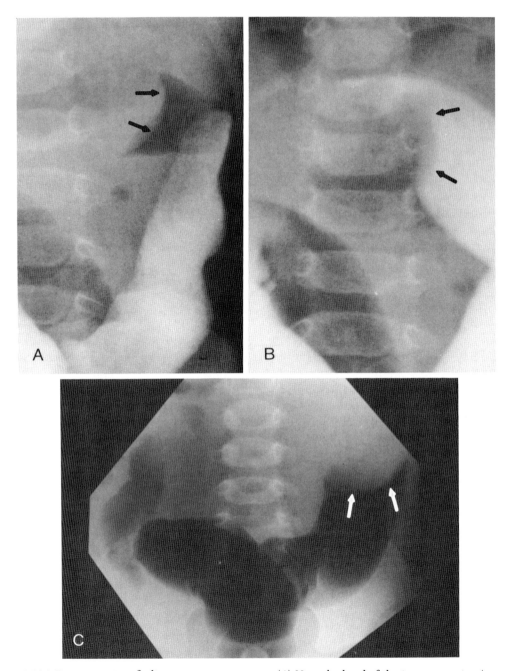

Figure 3.104. *Intussusception: findings on contrast enema.* (*A*) Note the head of the intussusception (*arrows*) and the advancing opaque gastrografin column introduced from below. (*B*) Later the gastrografin column meets the intussusception, which produces a characteristic radiolucent defect (*arrows*). (*C*) Air reduction of intussusception clearly demonstrates the head of the intussusception (*arrows*) in the descending colon.

agents than with air. In addition, it has been noted that air can rapidly gush into, and fill, the dilated small bowel before reduction actually occurs (21). This is not a problem with positive contrast agents, but at the same time these agents can unveil a variety of potentially confusing postreduction pseudotumoral, cecal and distal small bowel configurations (10, 11). These changes probably are multifactorial in origin, but most likely are due to inflammation and edema of the intestinal wall. They are not a cause for concern and eventually also may be seen, although perhaps not as clearly, with air reduction enemas.

A postevacuation film should be obtained after reduction is complete and a 24-hour follow-up film should be taken to determine whether the intussusception has remained reduced or has recurred. If the intussusception is not fully reduced, the small bowel obstruction will not disappear and the colon distal to the intussusception will remain spastic (13).

Recurrent rates after nonsurgical reduction range from 4–10% (3, 6, 27, 33), and the first recurrence should be treated with repeat contrast enema reduction. Recurrent intussusceptions occur more commonly in those cases where a definite leading point is seen and, by the same token, are more difficult to reduce in the first place (14). In addition, the longer the intussusception remains untreated or the lower it is in the colon, the more difficult will be the reduction.

Perforation rates, as mentioned earlier, hover at around 1–3%, but may become a little higher with the general trend toward more aggressive approaches to reduction. The actual perforation is not due so much to the reduction procedure as to the fact that the involved colon has become devitalized and more prone to perforation (8). However, now that barium is being used less and less, perforation is a more acceptable complication and, when it is detected, immediately converts the case to one which becomes surgical. Generally, as long as or aqueous agents are used, the perfo-

ration causes no real additional problems, but, at the same time, *nonsurgical reduction should not be attempted without prior notification of the surgical service.* With air reduction perforation may not be so benign, for massive pneumoperitoneum can lead to vasovagal complications.

Spontaneous reduction of intussusception is now more commonly encountered (55). The reason for this is that the phenomenon can be documented with ultrasound. It is not unusual to have a patient present with findings very suggestive of intussusception, demonstrate their presence with ultrasound, and yet not be able to find the intussusception with contrast studies. In such cases, one should be cognizant of the fact that the intussusception has spontaneously reduced (55).

In conclusion, it should be mentioned that intussusception can be a presenting feature of cystic fibrosis in older children (19, 22, 60). In these patients, fecal impactions (meconium ileus equivalent) and redundancy and thickening of the intestinal mucosa can predispose to intussusception. In addition, it should be noted that while the appendix can act as a lead point for intussusception, isolated intussusception of the appendix also can occur and may be seen in totally asymptomatic individuals (1, 2, 18).

REFERENCES

1. Atkinson, G.O., Gay, B.B., and Naffis, D.: Intussusception of the appendix in children. A.J.R. 126: 1164–1168, 1976.
2. Bachman, A.L., and Clemett, A.R.: Roentgen aspects of primary appendiceal intussusception. Radiology 101: 531–538, 1971.
3. Barr, L.L., Stansberry, S.D., and Swischuk, L.E.: Significance of age, duration, obstruction and the dissection sign. Pediatr. Radiol. 20: 454–456, 1990.
4. Beasley, S.W., and Glover, J.: Intussusception: Prediction of outcome of gas enema. J. Pediatr. Surg. 27: 474–475, 1992.
5. Bhisitkul, D.M., Listernick, R., Shkolnik, A., Donaldson, J.S., Henricks, B.D., Feinstein, K.A., and Fernbach, S.K.: Clinical application of ultrasonography in the diagnosis of intussusception. J. Pediatr. 121: 182–186, 1992.

6. Bissett, G.S., III, and Kirks, D.R.: Intussusception in infants and children: Diagnosis and therapy. Radiology 168:141–145, 1988.

7. Bowerman, R.A., Silver, T.M., and Jaffe, M.H.: Real-time ultrasound diagnosis of intussusception in children. Radiology 143: 527–529, 1982.

8. Bramson, R.T., and Blickman, J.G.: Perforation during hydrostatic reduction of intussusception: Proposed mechanism and review of the literature. J. Pediatr. Surg. 27: 589–591, 1992.

9. Braun, P., and Germann-Nicod, I.: Altered consciousness as a precocious manifestation of intussusception in infants. Z. Kinderchir. 33: 307–309, 1981.

10. Campbell, J.B.: Contrast media in intussusception. Pediatr. Radiol. 19: 293–296, 1989.

11. Conway, E.E., Jr.: Central nervous system findings and intussusception: How are they related? Pediatr. Emerg. Care 9:15–18, 1993.

12. Devred, P., Faure, F., and Padovani, J.: Pseudotumoral cecum after hydrostatic reduction of intussusception. Pediatr. Radiol. 14: 295–298, 1984.

13. Dklog, O., and Hugosson, C.: Post evacuation findings in barium enema-treated intussusceptions. Ann. Radiol. 19: 133–139, 1976.

14. Ein, S.H.: Leading points in childhood intussusception. J. Pediatr. Surg. 11: 209–211, 1976.

15. Ein, S.H., Stephens, C.A., and Minor, A.: Painless intussusception. J. Pediatr. Surg. 11: 563–564, 1976.

16. Eklof, O.A., Johanson, L., and Lohr, G.: Childhood intussusception: Hydrostatic reducibility and incidence of leading points in different age groups. Pediatr. Radiol. 10: 83–86, 1980.

17. Fanconi, S., Berger, D., and Rickham, P.P.: Acute intussusception: A classic clinical picture? Helv. Paediatr. Acta 37: 345–352, 1982.

18. Fink, V.H., Santos, A.L., and Goldberg, S.L.: Intussusception of the appendix: Case reports and reviews of the literature. Am. J. Gastroenterol. 42: 431–441, 1964.

19. Flux, M.: Intussusception in a patient with cystic fibrosis. South. Med. J. 60: 1184–1187, 1967.

20. Gu, L., Alton, D.J., Daneman, A., Stringer, D.A., Liu, P., Wilmot, D.M., and Reilly, B.J.: Intussusception reduction in children by rectal insufflation of air. A.J.R. 150: 1345–1348, 1988.

21. Hedlund, G.L., Johnson, J.F., and Strife, J.L.: Ileocolic intussusception: Extensive reflux of air preceding pneumatic reduction. Radiology 174: 187–189, 1990.

22. Holsclaw, D.S., Rocmans, C., and Schwachman, H.: Intussusception in patients with cystic fibrosis. Pediatrics 48: 51–58, 1971.

23. Holt, S., and Samuel, E.: Multiple concentric ring sign in the ultrasonographic diagnosis of intussusception. Gastrointest. Radiol. 3: 307–309, 1978.

24. Humphrey, A., Alton, D.J., and McKendry, J.B.J.: Atypical ileocolic intussusception diagnosed by barium follow through. Pediatr. Radiol. 12: 65–66, 1982.

25. Hutchinson, I.F., Olayiwola, B., and Young, D.G.: Intussusception in infancy and childhood. Br. J. Surg. 67: 209–212, 1980.

26. Jorulf, H.: Tip of the liver in intussusception of the bowel in infancy and childhood. Acta Radiol. [Diagn.] (Stockh.) 14: 26–32, 1974.

27. Katz, M.E., and Kolm, P.: Intussusception reduction 1991: An international survey of pediatric radiologists. Pediatr. Radiol. 22: 318–322, 1992.

28. Katz, H., Phelan, E., Carlin, J. B., and Beasley, S.W.: Gas enema for the reduction of intussusception: Relationship between clinical signs and symptoms and outcome. A.J.R. 160: 363–366, 1993.

29. Kuta, A.J., and Benator, R.M.: Intussusception: Hydrostatic pressure equivalents for barium and meglumine sodium diatrizoate. Radiology 175: 125–126, 1990.

30. Lam, A.H., and Firman, K.: Value of sonography including color Doppler in the diagnosis and management of long-standing intussusception. Pediatr. Radiol. 22: 112–114, 1992.

31. Macpherson, W.A., and Hays, D.M.: The malignant nature of pediatric intussusception secondary to specific etiologic lesions. Am. Surg. 29: 667, 1963.

32. Markowitz, R.I., and Meyer, J.S.: Pneumatic versus hydrostatic reduction of intussusception. Radiology 183:623–624, 1992.

33. Meyer, J.S.: The current radiologic management of intussusception: A survey and review. Pediatr. Radiol. 22: 323–325, 1992.

34. Minami, A., and Fujji, K.: Intussusception in children. Am. J. Dis. Child. 129: 346–348, 1975.

35. Mok, P.M., and Humphry, A.: Ileo-ileocolic intussusception: Radiological features and reducibility. Pediatr. Radiol. 12: 127–131, 1982.

36. Montali, G., Croce, F., DePra, L., and Solbiati, L.: Intussusception of the bowel: A new sonographic pattern. Br. J. Radiol. 56: 621–623, 1983.

37. Palder, S.B., Ein, S.H., Stringer, D.A., and Alton, D.: Intussusception: Barium or air? J. Pediatr. Surg. 26: 271–275, 1991.

38. Pariety, R.A., Lepreauy, J.F., and Gruson, G.: Sonographic and CT features of ileocolic intussusception. A.J.R. 136: 608–610, 1981.

39. Phelan, E., de Campo, J.F., and Malecky, G.: Comparison of oxygen and barium reduction of ileocolic intussusception. A.J.R. 150: 1349–1352, 1988.

40. Pokorny, W.J., Wagner, M.L., and Harberg, F.J.: Lateral wall cecal filling defects following successful hydrostatic reduction of cecalcolic intussusceptions. J. Pediatr. Surg. 15: 156–159, 1980.

41. Pracros, J.P., Tran-Minh, V.A., Morin DeFinfe, C.H., Desfrenne-Pracros, P., Louis, D., and Basset, T: Acute intestinal intussusception in children: Contribution of ultrasonography (145 cases). Ann. Radiol. 30: 525–530, 1987.

42. Rachmel, A., Rosenbach, Y., Amir, J., Dinari, G., Shoenfeld, T., and Nitzan, M.: Apathy as an early manifestation of intussusception. Am. J. Dis. Child. 137: 701–702, 1983.

43. Ratcliffe, J.F., Fong, S., Cheong, L., and O'Connell, P.: Plain film diagnosis of intussusception: Incidence of the target sign. A.J.R. 158: 619–621, 1991.

44. Ratcliffe, J.F., Fong, S., Cheong, L., and O'Connell, P.: The plain abdominal film in intussusception: The accuracy and incidence of radiographic signs. Pediatr. Radiol. 22: 110–111, 1992.

45. Raudkivi, P.J., and Smith, H.L.M.: Intussusception: Analysis of 98 cases. Br. J. Surg. 68: 645–648, 1981.

46. Rosenkrantz, J.G.,,Cox, J.A., Silverman, F.N., and Martin, L.W.: Intussusception in the 1970s: Indications for operation. J. Pediatr. Surg. 12: 367–373, 1977.

47. Smith, D.S., Bonadio, W.A., Losek, J.D., Walsh-Kelly, C.M., Hennes, H.M., Glaeser, P.W., Melzer-Lange, M., and Rimm, A.A.: The role of abdominal x-rays in the diagnosis and management of intussusception. Pediatr. Emerg. Care 8: 325–327, 1992.

48. Stein, M., Alton, D.J., and Daneman, A.: Pneumatic reduction of intussusception: 5-year experience. Radiology 183:681–684, 1992.

49. Stone, D.N., Kangarloo, H., Graviss, E.R., Danis, R.K., and Silberstein, M.J.: Jejunal intussusception in children. Pediatr. Radiol. 9: 65–68, 1980.

50. Sargent, M.A., and Wilson, B.P.M.: Are hydrostatic and pneumatic methods of intussusception reduction comparable? Pediatr. Radiol. 21: 346–349, 1991.

51. Shiels, W.E., II, Maves, C.K., Hedlund, G.L., and Kirks, D.R.: Air enema for diagnosis and reduction of intussusception: Clinical experience and pressure correlates. Radiology 181: 169–172, 1991.

52. Stephenson, C.A., Seibert, J.J., and Strain, J.D.: Intussusception: Clinical and radiographic factors influencing reducibility. Pediatr. Radiol. 20: 57–60, 1989.

53. Swischuk, L.E.: The current radiology management of intussusception: A survey and review. Pediatr. Radiol. 22: 317, 1992.

54. Swischuk, L.E., Hayden, C.K., and Boulden, T.: Intussusception: Indications for ultrasonography and an explanation of the donut and pseudo-kidney signs. Pediatr. Radiol. 15: 388–391, 1985.

55. Swischuk, L.E., John, S.D., and Swischuk, P.N.: Spontaneous reduction of intussusception: Ultrasonographic demonstration. (In preparation).

56. Swischuk, L.E., and Stansberry, S.D.: Ultrasonographic detection of free peritoneal fluid in uncomplicated intussusception. Pediatr. Radiol. 21: 350–351, 1991.

57. Tao, H., and Dunbar, J.S.: Intussusception of the appendix. J. Can. Assoc. Radiol. 22: 333–335, 1971.

58. Todani, T., Sato, Y., Watanabe, Y., Toki, A., Uemura, S., and Urushihara, N.: Air reduction for intussusception in infancy and childhood: Ultrasonographic diagnosis and management without x-ray exposure. Z. Kinderchir. 45: 222–226, 1990.

59. Tran-Minh, V.A., Pracros, J.P., Massard, P.E., Louis, D., and Pracros-Deffrenne, P.: Diagnosis of acute intestinal intussusception (AII) by real-time ultrasonography. Evaluation of 176 children with suspicion of AII. Pediatr. Radiol. 15: 267–268, 1985.

60. Tucker, A.S., Stern, R.C., Pittman, S.S., and Perrin, E.V.: Intussusception in older children: A complication of cystic fibrosis. Ann. Radiol. 16: 173–176, 1973.

61. Turner, D., Rickwood, A.M.K., and Brereton, R.J.: Intussusception in older children. Arch. Dis. Child. 55: 544–546, 1980.

62. Verschelden, P., Filiatrault, D., Garel, L., Grignon, A., Perreault, G., Boisvert, J., and Dubois, J.: Intussusception in children: Reliability of US in diagnosis: A prospective study. Radiology 184: 741–744, 1992.

63. Wang, G., Liu, S.: Enema reduction of intussusception by hydrostatic pressure under ultrasound guidance: A report of 377 cases. J. Pediatr. Surg. 23: 814–818, 1988.

64. White, S.J., and Blane, C.E.: Intussusception: Additional observations on the plain radiograph. A.J.R. 139: 511–513, 1982.

Volvulus. Conditions considered under the broad topic of volvulus include midgut volvulus, volvulus of the colon, gastric volvulus, and segmental small bowel volvulus. *Midgut volvulus* is associated with obstructing duodenal bands and intestinal malrotation. Usually it is a problem of the neonate, but it also can present in older infants and children. In such cases, the presentation often is atypical, both clinically and roentgenographically (6, 8, 10, 11, 13, 14, 16).

In the classic case of midgut volvulus in the neonate, there is acute onset of bilious vomiting, crampy abdominal pain, and varying degrees of abdominal distension. If vascular compromise is severe, signs of shock also will be evident and, as the bowel undergoes necrosis, perforation with peritonitis may supervene. Most such cases declare themselves in the first month of life, but in the older child, while symptoms occasionally are similar, more often they are atypical and confusing. Indeed, these children frequently first are considered to have chronic abdominal problems such as malabsorption ulcer disease, protein-losing enteropathy, or simply continue as cases of undiagnosed recurrent abdominal pain. It requires an astute physician to think of the diagnosis under these conditions. In this regard, Bonadio et al. (3) have shown that while bilious vomiting was seen in 97% of their patients, blood in the stool was present in only 16%. On physical examination, no abnormal abdominal findings were seen in 76% of their cases.

Roentgenographically, a wide spectrum of abnormality is seen in midgut volvulus, and, unfortunately, in some cases the abdominal roentgenograms can appear near normal. However, in those cases demonstrating abnormality, one of the most helpful findings is that of obstruction of the duodenum in its third and fourth portions (Fig. 3.105). In these cases, obstruction may be due to the associated duodenal bands only or to complicating midgut volvulus. With midgut volvulus, however, obstruction often is more pronounced. In those infants in whom the obstructed duodenum is full of fluid and a supine film only is obtained, air in the distended stomach erroneously will suggest a gastric outlet obstruction (Fig. 3.106).

Other patients with midgut volvulus may show evidence of a classic small bowel obstruction (Fig. 3.107) or a small bowel obstruction in association with a soft tissue

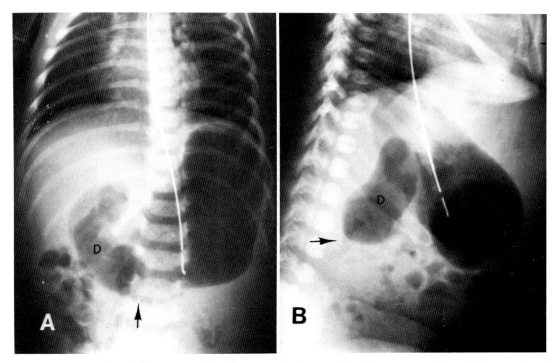

Figure 3.105. *Duodenal obstruction with malrotation.*   (A) Supine film demonstrating distended stomach and descending duodenum (*D*). The site of obstruction in the third and fourth portions of the duodenum is demarcated *by the arrow*. (B) Lateral view demonstrating site of obstruction (*arrow*) in the dilated descending duodenum (*D*) to better advantage. This level of obstruction is typical for the complex of malrotation, duodenal band, and midgut volvulus. (Reprinted from L.E. Swischuk: Radiology of the Newborn Infant and Young Child. Ed. 3. Williams & Wilkins, Baltimore, 1988.)

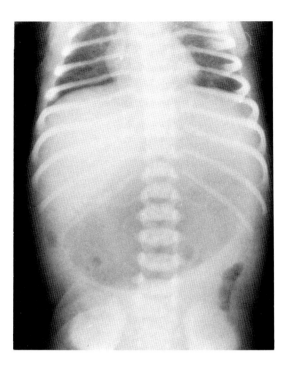

Figure 3.106. *Midgut volvulus appearing as a gastric outlet obstruction.* Note the distended stomach. There is no visible gas in the duodenum and very little is scattered throughout the remainder of the gastrointestinal tract. A gastric outlet obstruction might be suspected, but actually, this patient had midgut volvulus with descending duodenal obstruction. In the supine position, however, the duodenum is filled with fluid and thus is invisible roentgenographically. (Reprinted from L.E. Swischuk: Radiology of the Newborn Infant and Young Child. Ed. 3. Williams & Wilkins, Baltimore, 1988.)

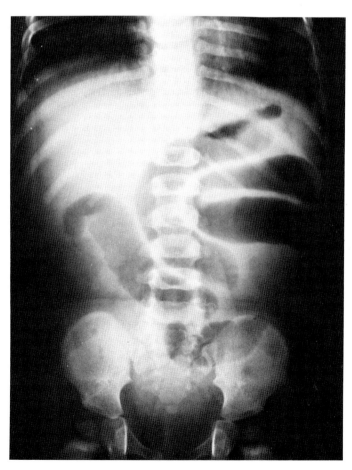

Figure 3.107. *Midgut volvulus—small bowel obstruction pattern.* Note the numerous loops of distended small intestine in this patient with midgut volvulus and obstruction.

mass (Fig. 3.108). In these latter cases, the mass represents fluid-filled, volved bowel, or, in other words, a form of closed-loop obstruction. The volved mass of intestine frequently is located in the right lower quadrant (12), but in fact can be seen anywhere in the abdomen.

Because of the high obstruction present in these patients, one would think that all of them would show deficient abdominal gas patterns. However, this is not so and some infants may show considerable volumes of gas in distended loops of intestine. The reason for this seeming paradox is that once venous compromise occurs, intestinal gas absorption is severely compromised (9). Consequently, the presence of numerous loops of distended intestine in patients with suspected midgut volvulus should be

considered an ominous sign. Of course, if bowel necrosis occurs, pneumatosis cystoides intestinalis may be seen, and if perforation occurs, signs of peritonitis and free air will develop.

Either the upper GI series or barium enema can be used to confirm the presence of midgut volvulus and should be performed immediately (2, 15). In our institution we prefer the upper GI series. With barium enema examinations, one can be totally certain that midgut volvulus is present only if the cecum is misplaced high into the midabdomen, behind the transverse colon (Fig. 3.109). In such cases, as the intestine volves, the cecum is drawn tightly behind the transverse colon and the findings are pathognomonic. However, if the cecum simply is out of place, that is, if it is

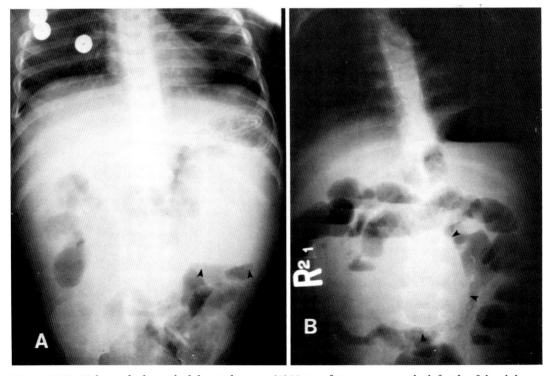

Figure 3.108. *Midgut volvulus with abdominal mass.* (*A*) Note soft tissue mass on the left side of the abdomen (*arrows*). (*B*) Upright view demonstrates that the mass has shifted to a new position (*arrows*). Note also that a small bowel obstruction is suggested. This patient was being investigated for malabsorption and one night developed severe crampy abdominal pain. At laparotomy, he had midgut volvulus. The soft tissue mass on the abdominal films represented fluid trapped in some of the volved loops.

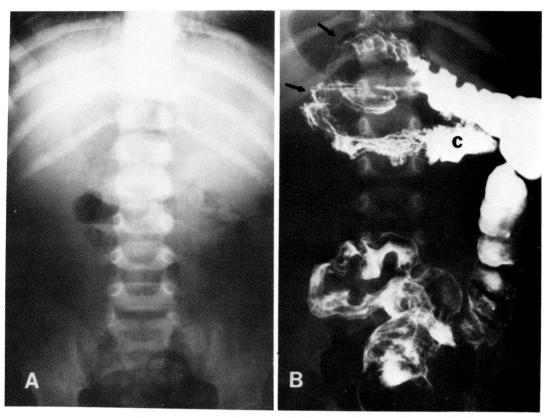

Figure 3.109. *Midgut volvulus, barium enema findings.* (*A*) Abdominal film revealing a misleadingly near-normal appearance. However, note that although some gas is present in the stomach, the remainder of the abdomen shows a paucity of gas. When these findings are considered with the fact that this patient had acute onset of bilious vomiting and crampy abdominal pain, one should think of some underlying acute mechanical problem. In this case, both midgut volvulus and intussusception were considered and because of this a barium enema was obtained. (*B*) Barium enema demonstrating the typical, totally abnormal position of the volved cecum (*C*) and the twisted colon (*arrows*).

medial in position and not in its normal right lower quadrant location (18), then one cannot assume that midgut volvulus is present. Furthermore, a normally placed cecum does not exclude underlying malrotation and hence the possibility that midgut volvulus could develop. Because of all these points, the upper GI series has gained popularity as the initial investigative procedure in patients with suspected midgut volvulus.

In midgut volvulus, the upper GI series will show either (a) obstruction of the third portion of the duodenum or (b) obstruction of the duodenum and associated, pa-

thognomonic spiraling of the small intestine around the superior mesenteric artery (Fig. 3.110). In addition, the point of duodenal obstruction will lie over the spine or just to the right of it. The small bowel after this point passes on to an abnormal midabdominal or right-side position. All of this reflects the presence of malrotation and poor intestinal fixation, including absence of the ligament of Treitz which normally fixes the bowel to the left of the spine. If edema of the loops of intestine distal to the area of spiraling also is noted, vascular compromise can be assumed with certainty.

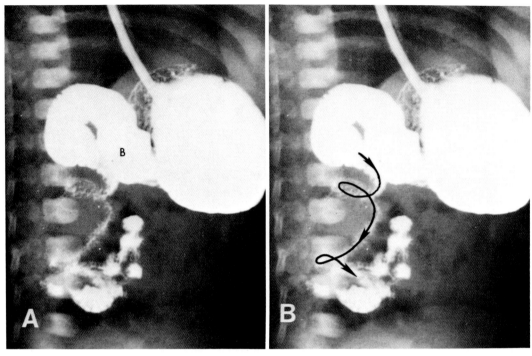

Figure 3.110. *Midgut volvulus: duodenal obstruction and spiraling of small bowel.* (**A**) Note the distended duodenal bulb (*B*) and descending duodenum. Also note spiraling of the small bowel distal to the site of obstruction of the duodenum. (**B**) Diagrammatic representation of spiraling of the small bowel.

Ultrasonography also can demonstrate findings of midgut volvulus, similar to those seen on an upper GI series (4, 5, 7). In addition, the twisted pedicle of the mesentery and reversal of the normal relationship of the superior mesenteric artery and vein can be seen (4, 7, 12, 19). The latter finding may not be so easy to demonstrate, but the obstructed duodenum basically is clearly identified (Fig. 3.111).

In older children, however, as mentioned earlier, clinical and roentgenographic findings usually are atypical. Indeed, considering that one may have apparently normal intestinal position with poor development of the mesentery (9) and incomplete rotation of the intestine with normal cecal position (17), one can easily understand why such atypia arises. Nonetheless, it is just this type of case that passes into older childhood, and then one must look for every possible clue on the

upper GI series, barium enema, or ultrasound study for proper diagnosis. In this regard, any bizarre configuration of the duodenum, small bowel, or the cecum should be treated with suspicion (1) (Fig. 3.112).

Segmental volvulus of the small bowel represents a classic cause of closed loop obstruction, and often is associated with anomalous peritoneal bands, congenital mesenteric defect, internal hernias, incomplete malrotation problems (14), or postoperative adhesions. As with all closed loop obstructions, diagnosis may be late in coming, but it has been noted that if a beaked configuration of the small bowel is seen on barium enema examination, volvulus should be considered the correct diagnosis (14). The beaking is similar to that seen with colon volvulus, a problem discussed in the next section.

Volvulus of the colon is not a common

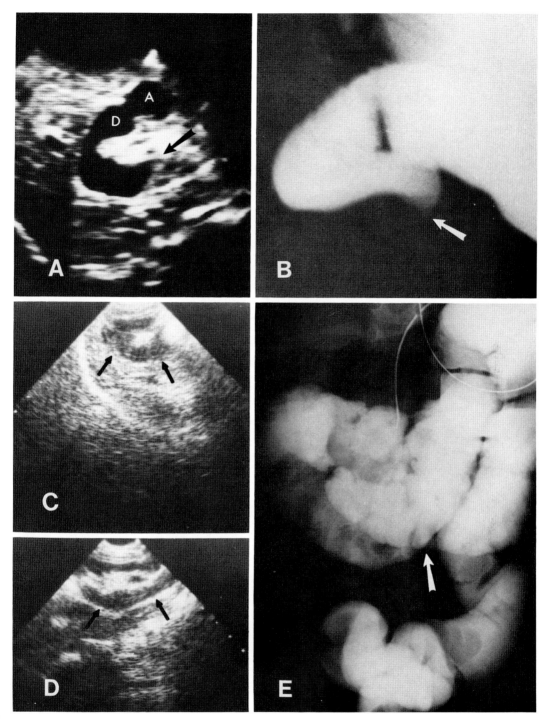

Figure 3.111. *Midgut volvulus: ultrasonographic findings.* (*A*) Note the distended antrum (*A*), duodenal bulb and loop (*D*), and beak (*arrow*). (*B*) Confirmatory upper GI series showing the same findings, including the beak (*arrow*). (*C*) Edematous intestine in midgut volvulus. Ultrasonographic cross-section demonstrates sonolucent donut due to edematous segment of intestine (*arrows*). (*D*) Longitudinal view demonstrates an oval mass-like configuration of the edematous intestine. (*E*) Barium enema in same patient, demonstrating the cecum to be in an abnormal position, behind the transverse colon. This was an older patient with midgut volvulus. (Part *A* from C.K. Hayden, Jr., T.F. Boulden, L.E. Swischuk, and T.E. Lobe: Sonographic demonstration of duodenal obstruction with midgut volvulus. A.J.R. 143: 9–10, 1984.)

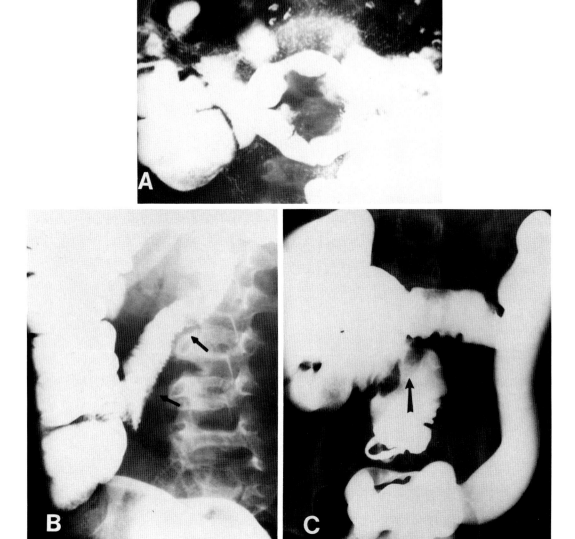

Figure 3.112. *Abnormal fixation of intestine.*   (*A*) In this patient with chronic intermittent abdominal pain, note the peculiarly spiraled and generally abnormal configuration of the upper small bowel. (*B*) Same patient shows unusual position of terminal ileum (*arrows*). (*C*) Another patient with abnormal positioning of the cecum and compression by a band (*arrow*). All of these configurations should make one suspect abnormal intestinal fixation. (Part *C* courtesy of the late Sue Jacobi, M.D., Austin, Texas.)

problem in childhood, but it does occur and does so most often in the sigmoid colon (1, 3–5, 7, 11, 13). In some of these cases, the U-shaped loop of the volved sigmoid colon appears typical, lying far to the right of the spine and having its apex pointing toward the liver (Fig. 3.113). However, this does not always occur and, overall, the findings of sigmoid volvulus in children are less specific than in adults. In addition, it should be noted that the normally redundant but nonvolved sigmoid colon can present with findings mimicking sigmoid volvulus (Fig. 3.114A). If, in such cases, the child is asymptomatic and volvulus is not suspected, the finding can be treated as being strictly fortuitous. In other cases, however, it may be difficult to discard the finding without barium enema verification (Fig. 3.114B). Cecal volvulus is less common than sigmoid volvulus (6), and the roentgenographic findings are different. With cecal volvulus, the dilated, volved cecum is located in the upper midabdomen or left upper quadrant (Fig. 3.115). Volvulus of the transverse colon is very rare (2, 10) but, when present, demonstrates the volved loop to be more central and in the upper abdomen. Volvulus of any type is more likely to occur in the bedridden

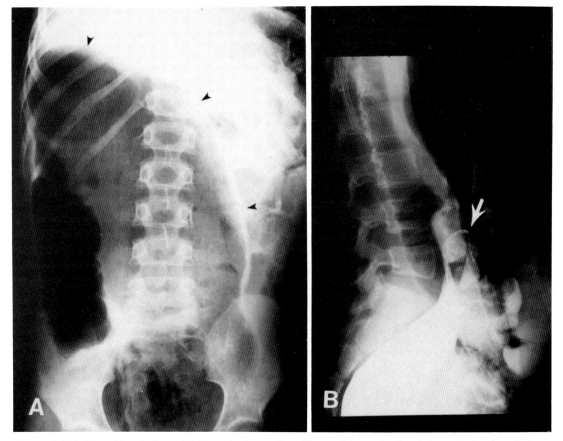

Figure 3.113. *Sigmoid volvulus.* (A) Note the large dilated loop of sigmoid colon in its typical right-sided position (*arrows*). (B) Barium enema showing narrowing at site of volvulus (*arrow*). (Reprinted with permission from J.R. Campbell and E. Blank: Sigmoid volvulus in children. Pediatrics 53: 702–705, 1974.)

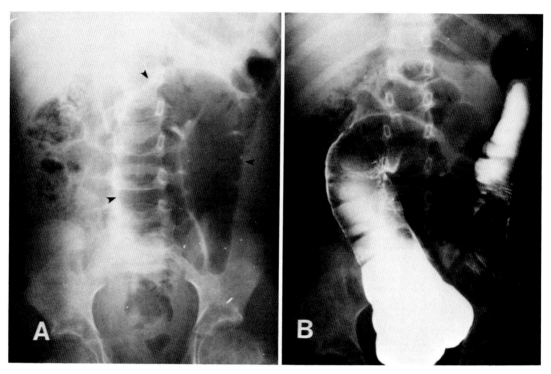

Figure 3.114. *Pseudovolvulus of sigmoid colon.* (*A*) Note the inverted "U" appearance of the sigmoid colon (*arrows*) which in this patient spuriously suggests sigmoid volvulus. However, this patient had no symptoms of obstruction and was being investigated for painless rectal bleeding. (*B*) Subsequent barium enema demonstrates normal, but very redundant, sigmoid colon. This, of course, is not to say that such a loop would not volve, for indeed it could.

child, and overall, this and normal redundancy of the sigmoid colon are the prime predisposing factors to the development of volvulus. A similar problem can occur with a chronically obstructed, redundant colon such as is seen in Hirschsprung's disease (9).

Once volvulus is suspected, a barium enema examination should be attempted, for not only will it demonstrate the typical beaking, narrowing, or twisting deformity of the volved segment of colon (Fig. 3.113*B*), but it also often is therapeutic. If the barium enema does not relieve the obstruction, proctoscopy with insertion of a decompressing tube should be attempted. After reduction, the colon may show persistent narrowing or thumbprinting as a result of residual edema and spasm (8). The

presence of such edema of the intestine also is demonstrable with ultrasound (Fig. 3.116).

Gastric volvulus is a true surgical emergency (1–6), and symptoms of vomiting and severe abdominal pain often have sudden onset. Shock may supervene, and chest and abdominal films will reveal a large, distended stomach causing the left diaphragmatic leaflet to be high in position (Fig. 3.117). In addition, one may note two air-fluid levels within the volved stomach (2). If barium is administered, it will either stop at the gastroesophageal junction or pass into the inverted, rotated stomach. If the barium stops at the gastroesophageal junction, it simply infers that volvulus is so tight that complete obstruction has occurred at this level. Volvulus of the stom-

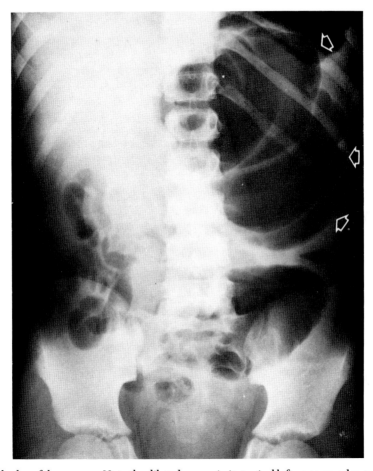

Figure 3.115. *Volvulus of the cecum.*   Note the dilated cecum in its typical left upper quadrant position (*arrows*).

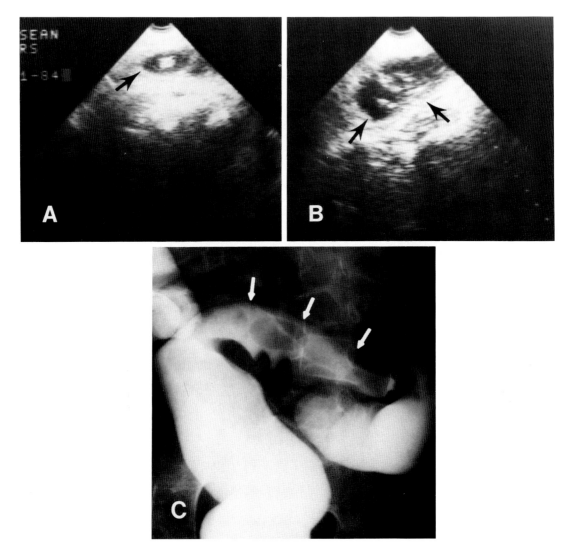

Figure 3.116. *Devolved sigmoid volvulus; ultrasonographic findings.* (*A*) Cross-section demonstrates a sonolucent donut (*arrow*). (*B*) Note an oval mass with a sonolucent rim (*arrows*). These findings represent edema of the intestinal wall. (*C*) Barium enema demonstrating thumbprinting of the involved segment of sigmoid colon (*arrows*).

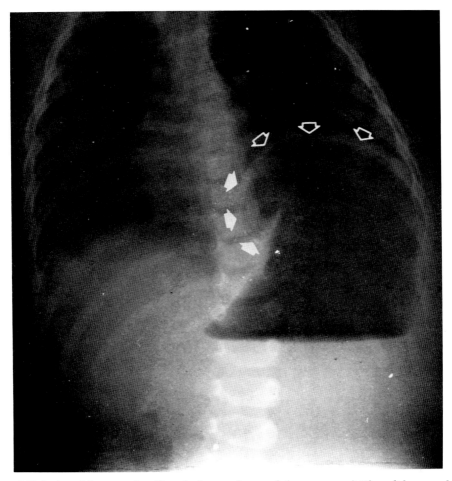

Figure 3.117. *Volvulus of the stomach.* Note the inverted stomach (*upper arrows*). The *solid arrows* demarcate the tapered tip of one end of the volved stomach. (Reprinted with permission from J.B. Campbell et al.: Acute mesentero-axial volvulus of the stomach. Radiology 103: 153–156, 1972.)

ach also can be seen with congenital diaphragmatic hernias, and in some cases may be a chronic, recurrent problem (1).

REFERENCES

Midgut Volvulus

1. Ablow, R.C., Hoffer, F.A., Seashore, J.H., and Touloukian R.J.: Z-shaped duodenojejunal loop: Sign of mesenteric fixation anomaly and congenital bands. A.J.R. 141: 461–464, 1983.

2. Berdon, W.E., Baker, D.H., Bull, S., and Santulli, T.V.: Midgut malrotation and volvulus: Which films are most helpful? Radiology 96: 375–383, 1970.

3. Bonadio, W.A., Clarkson, T., Naus, J.: The clinical features of children with malrotation of the intestine. Pediatr. Emerg. Care 7: 348–349, 1991.

4. Dufour, D., Delaet, M.H., Dassonville, M., Cadranel, S., and Perlmutter, N.: Midgut malrotation, the reliability of sonographic diagnosis. Pediatr. Radiol. 22: 21–23, 1992.

5. Hayden, C.K., Jr., Boulden, T.F., Swischuk, L.E., and Lobe, T.E.: Sonographic demonstration of duodenal obstruction with midgut volvulus. A.J.R. 143: 9–10, 1984.

6. Houston, C.S., and Wittenborg, M.H.: Roentgen evaluation of anomalies of rotation and fixation of the bowel in children. Radiology 84: 1–17, 1965.

7. Leonidas, J.C., Magid, N., Soberman, N., and Glass, T.S.: Midgut volvulus in infants: Diagnosis with US. Work in progress. Radiology 179: 491–493, 1991.

8. Janik, J.S., and Ein, S.H.: Normal intestinal rotation with non-fixation: A cause of chronic abdominal pain. J. Pediatr. Surg. 14: 670–674, 1979.

9. Kassner, E.G., and Kottmeier, P.K.: Absence and retention of small bowel gas in infants with midgut volvulus: Mechanisms and significance. Pediatr. Radiol. 4: 28–30, 1975.

10. Pochaczevski, R., Ratner, H., Leonidas, J.C., Naysan, P., and Feraru, F.: Unusual forms of volvulus after the neonatal period. A.J.R. 114: 390–393, 1972.

11. Powell, D.M., Othersen, H.B., and Smith, C.D.: Malrotation of the intestines in children: The effect of age on presentation and therapy. J. Pediatr. Surg. 24: 777–780, 1989.

12. Pracros, J.P., Sann, L., Genin, G., Tran-Minh, V.A., Morin, X.X., de Finfe, C.H., Foray, P., and Louis, D.: Ultrasound diagnosis of midgut volvulus: The "whirlpool" sign. Pediatr. Radiol. 22: 18–20, 1992.

13. Schaffer, I., and Ferris, I.: The mass sign in primary volvulus of small intestine in adults. A.J.R. 94: 374–378, 1965.

14. Siegel, M.J., Shackelford, G.D., and McAlister, W.H.: Small bowel volvulus in children: Its appearance on the barium enema examination. Pediatr. Radiol. 10: 91–93, 1980.

15. Simpson, A.J., Leonidis, J.C., Krasna, I.H., Becker, J.M., and Schneider, K.M.: Roentgen diagnosis of midgut malrotation: Value of upper gastrointestinal radiographic study. J. Pediatr. Surg. 7: 243–252, 1972.

16. Spigland, N., Brandt, M.L., and Yazbeck, S.: Malrotation presenting beyond the neonatal period. J. Pediatr. Surg. 25: 1139–1142, 1990.

17. Slovis, T.L., Klein, M.D., and Watts, F.B., Jr.: Incomplete rotation of the intestine with a normal cecal position. Surgery 87: 325–330, 1980.

18. Steiner, G.M.: The misplaced caecum and the root of the mesentery. Br. J. Radiol. 51: 406–413, 1978.

19. Zerin, J.M., and DiPietro, M.A.: Superior mesenteric vascular anatomy at US in patients with surgically proved malrotation of the midgut. Radiology 183: 693–694, 1992.

Volvulus of the Colon

1. Allen, R.P., and Nordstrom, J.E.: Volvulus of the sigmoid in children. A.J.R. 91: 690–693, 1964.

2. Asano, S., Konuma, K., Rikimaru, S., et al.: Volvulus of the transverse colon in a four-year-old boy. Z. Kinderchir. 35: 21–23, 1982.

3. Campbell, J.R., and Blank, E.: Sigmoid volvulus in children. Pediatrics 53: 702–705, 1974.

4. Carter, R., and Hinshaw, D.B.: Acute sigmoid volvulus in children. Am. J. Dis. Child. 101: 631–634, 1961.

5. Hunter, J.G., and Keats, T.E.: Sigmoid volvulus in children. A.J.R. 108: 621–623, 1970.

6. Kirks, D.R., Swischuk, L.E., Merten, D.F., and Filston, H.C.: Cecal volvulus in children. A.J.R. 136: 419–422, 1981.

7. Lillard, R.L., Allen, R.P., and Nordstrom, J.E.: Sigmoid volvulus in children. Case report. A.J.R. 97: 223–226, 1966.

8. Meyers, M.A., Ghahremani, G.G., and Govoni, A.F.: Ischemic colitis associated with sigmoid volvulus: New observations. A.J.R. 128: 591–595, 1977.

9. Neilson, I.R., and Youssef, S.: Delayed presentation of Hirschsprung's disease: Acute obstruction secondary to megacolon with transverse colonic volvulus. J. Pediatr. Surg. 25: 1177–1179, 1990.

10. Newton, N.A., and Reines, H.D.: Transverse colon volvulus: case reports and review. A.J.R. 128: 69–72, 1977.

11. Riddervold, H.O., Keats, T.E., and Son, K.S.: Sigmoid volvulus in children. A case report. J. Can. Assoc. Radiol. 22: 270–271, 1971.

12. van Buch, K., and Schumacher, W.: Torsion of the sigmoid in children. Z. Kinderchir. 15: 168–173, 1974.

13. Wilk, P.J., Ross, M., and Leonidas, J.: Sigmoid volvulus in an 11-year-old girl: Case report and literature review. Am. J. Dis. Child. 127: 400–402, 1974.

Gastric Volvulus

1. Ash, M.J., and Sheiman, N.J.: Gastric volvulus in children: report of two cases. J. Pediatr. Surg. 12: 1059–1062, 1977.

2. Campbell, J.B., Rappaport, L.N., and Skerker, L.B.: Acute mesentero-axial volvulus of the stomach. Radiology 103: 153–156, 1972.

3. Cole, B.C., and Dickinson, S.J.: Acute volvulus of the stomach in infants and children. Surgery 70: 707–717, 1971.

4. Honna, T., Kamii, Y., and Tsuchida, Y.: Idiopathic gastric volvulus in infancy and childhood. J. Pediatr. Surg. 25: 707–710, 1990.

5. Kilcoyne, R.F., Babbitt, D.P., and Sakaguchi, S.: Volvulus of the stomach. A case report. Radiology 103: 157–158, 1972.

6. Lorimer, A., and Penn, L.: Acute volvulus of the stomach. A.J.R. 77: 627, 1957.

Hernias. Internal hernias are difficult to diagnose. The clinical and roentgenographic findings usually are nonspecific and, at most, merely suggest an intestinal obstruction. These hernias often are par-

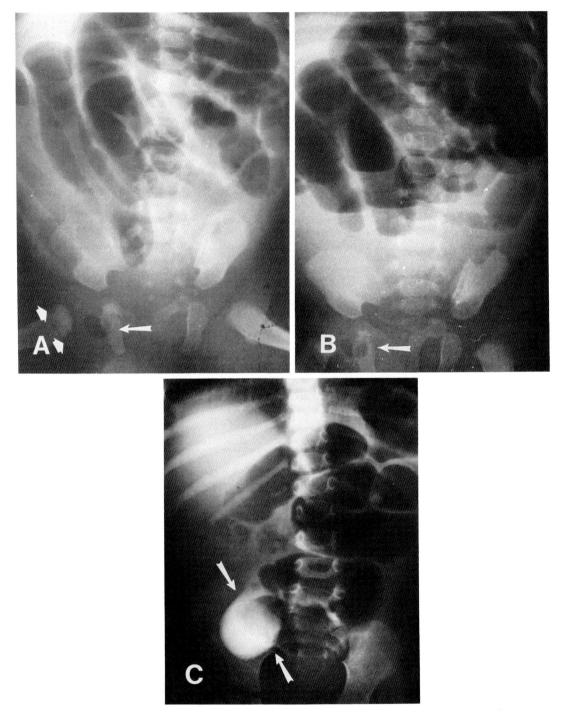

Figure 3.118. *Incarcerated inguinal hernia.* (**A**) Note numerous loops of distended small bowel suggesting a typical small bowel obstruction. In addition, however, note air within the incarcerated right inguinal hernia (*long arrow*). *Short arrows* delineate ipsilateral prominence of the inguinal soft tissue fold commonly seen with incarcerated inguinal hernias. (**B**) Upright view showing same findings. (**C**) Umbilical hernia with incarceration. Note obstructed loops of bowel and central umbilical hernia (*arrows*).

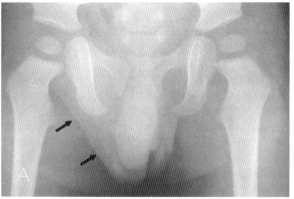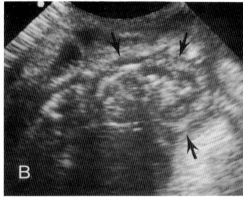

Figure 3.119. *Left incarcerated inguinal hernia; prominent inguinal soft tissue fold only.* (A) Note prominence of the right inguinal soft tissue fold (*arrows*). Compare with the normal appearance of the fold on the left. This patient had an incarcerated inguinal hernia on the right and presented with hip pain and restricted motion of the right leg. (B) Ultrasonographic findings in another patient. Note the layered appearance of incarcerated intestine (*arrows*).

aduodenal in location (4, 6) but, in fact, can be found anywhere along the mesentery or omentum (2, 7, 10). Hernias through the foramen of Winslow frequently involve the cecum, right colon, or terminal small bowel. In such cases, these structures herniate into the lesser sac behind the stomach (3, 5, 7–9, 11), and at first the plain film findings might suggest cecal volvulus. However, with lateral positioning, it will be seen that the dilated loop or loops of intestine are located behind the stomach and not in front as they would be with volvulus of the cecum.

Incarcerated **inguinal hernias** frequently are overlooked during physical examination of an infant with a distended abdomen secondary to the intestinal obstruction caused by the hernia. In such infants, in addition to the pattern of small bowel obstruction, one may see the incarcerated loops of air-filled intestine in the groin or scrotum (Fig. 3.118). If the loops of intestine do not contain air, one may see fullness of the cutaneous inguinal fold (1) on the involved side (Fig. 3.119A). In such cases, ultrasound is of value in demonstrating that the mass in the inguinal canal or scrotum is a hernia (Fig. 3.119B). In addition, color flow Doppler can be used to demonstrate the presence or absence of blood flow to the hernia. Incarcerated umbilical hernias with obstruction also occur but are less common (Fig. 3.118C).

REFERENCES

1. Currarino, G.: Incarcerated inguinal hernia in infants: Plain films and barium enema. Pediatr. Radiol. 2: 247–250, 1974.
2. Dalinka, M.K., Wunder, J.F., and Wolfe, R.D.: Internal hernia through the mesentery of a Meckel's diverticulum. Radiology 95: 39–40, 1970.
3. Henisz, A., Matesanz, J., and Westcott, J.: Cecal herniation through the foramen of Winslow. Radiology 112: 575–578, 1974.
4. McKail, R.A.: Hernia through the foramen of Winslow, hernia traversing the lesser sac, and allied conditions. Br. J. Radiol. 34: 611–618, 1961.
5. Meyers, M.A.: Paraduodenal hernias: Radiologic and arteriographic diagnosis. Radiology 95: 29–38, 1970.
6. Parsons, B.: Paraduodenal hernias. A.J.R. 69: 563–589, 1953.
7. Rubin, S.Z., Ayalon, A., and Berlatzky, Y.: The simultaneous occurrence of paraduodenal and paracecal herniae presenting with volvulus of the intervening bowel. J. Pediatr. Surg. 11: 205–208, 1976.
8. St. John, E.G.: Herniation through the foramen of Winslow. A.J.R. 72: 222–228, 1954.
9. Stankey, R.M.: Intestinal herniation through the foramen of Winslow. Radiology 89: 929–930, 1967.

10. Tovar, J., Bertin, P., and Bienayme. J.: Transmesenteric hernias. Ann. Chir. Inf. 17: 113–122, 1976.

11. Zer, M., and Dintsman, M.: Incarcerated "foramen of Winslow" hernia in a newborn. J. Pediatr. Surg. 8: 325, 1973.

Visceral Torsion. Visceral torsion usually involves the spleen or liver, but splenic torsion is more common (1–3, 5–8, 10–15). Torsion (volvulus) of the stomach and colon have been discussed in previous sections. An unusual cause of visceral torsion is torsion of the appendix causing symptoms similar to those of appendicitis (4).

In splenic and liver torsion, the predisposing factor usually is a hypermobile, poorly fixed organ. Clinical findings, with torsion of either the spleen or liver, usually consist of acute, crampy abdominal pain which may or may not refer itself to the expected upper quadrant of the abdomen. Symptoms also may be chronic and intermittent (1, 7, 10).

Abdominal roentgenograms in torsion of the spleen usually show absence of the normal splenic or liver silhouette and replacement of the space by gas-filled colon or small bowel. The organ itself may be seen as a soft tissue mass anywhere in the abdomen (10), but often the spleen lies on the left (Fig. 3.120). Small bowel obstruction also may occur. Ultrasonographically,

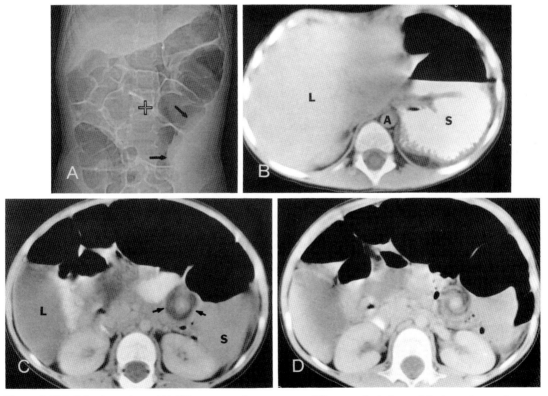

Figure 3.120. *Splenic torsion.* (*A*) CT topogram demonstrates diffuse paralytic ileus of the intestines and a mass (*arrows*) in the left lower quadrant. Note that the normal splenic silhouette is absent. (*B*) Scan through the upper abdomen demonstrates the liver (*L*), the aorta (*A*), and the stomach (*S*). There is no evidence of the spleen. The spleen should be visualized on this cut. (*C*) Lower cut demonstrates the liver (*L*), both kidneys to either side of the spine, and the spleen (*S*). Also note a peculiar round structure with a dense center (*arrows*). This represents the twisted pedicle of the spleen with some incorporated fat. (*D*) Slightly lower cut again demonstrates a whorl like appearance of the twisted pedicle. Reprinted with permission from L. E. Swischuk et al. (14).

clues to the diagnosis again consist of absence of the spleen in its normal location (9), but, in addition, color flow Doppler can show blood flow to the spleen and in the twisted pedicle to be diminished or absent. In more advanced cases, with splenic infarction, the spleen may show irregular sonolucent areas of hemorrhage (Fig. 3.120). CT also can identify the abnormal, torsed spleen (4) and twisted pedicle (14) (Fig. 3.120). Of course, if blood flow is seriously compromised the spleen will not enhance with contrast material.

Isotope spleen scans with 51Cr-labeled, heat-damaged, red blood cells show either totally absent uptake or partially absent uptake in the spleen (2, 7). In splenic torsion, blood smear findings show Howell-Jolly bodies, burr cells, a leukocytosis with shift to the left, and thrombocytosis (5).

REFERENCES

1. Bayer, H.P., Joppich, I., and Waag, K.L.: Chronic intermittent torsion of the spleen. Z. Kinderchir. 21: 386–391, 1977.
2. Broker, F.H.L., Khettry, J., Filler, R.M., and Traves, S.: Splenic torsion and accessory spleen: A scintigraphic demonstration. J. Pediatr. Surg. 10: 913–915, 1975.
3. Broker, F.H.L., Fellows, K., and Treves, S.: Wandering spleen in three children. Pediatr. Radiol. 6: 211–214, 1978.
4. Dewan, P.A., and Woodward, W.: Torsion of the vermiform appendix. J. Pediatr. Surg. 21: 379, 1986.
5. Dublin, A.B., and Rosenquist, C.F.: Diagnosis of splenic torsion: A combined radiographic approach. Case report. Br. J. Radiol. 49: 1045–1046, 1976.
6. Feins, N.R., and Borger, J.: Torsion of the right lobe of the liver with partial obstruction of the colon. J. Pediatr. Surg. 7: 724–725, 1972.
7. Gordon, D.H., Burrell, M.I., Levin, D.C., Mueller, C.F., and Becker, J.A.: Wandering spleen—the radiological and clinical spectrum. Radiology 125: 39–46, 1977.
8. Herman, T.E., and Siegel, M.J.: CT of acute splenic torsion in children with wandering spleen. Case report. A.J.R. 156: 151–153, 1991.
9. Hunter, T.B., and Haber, K.: Sonographic diagnosis of a wandering spleen. A.J.R. 129: 925–926, 1977.
10. Muckmel, E., Zer, M., and Dintsman, M.: Wandering spleen with torsion of pedicle in a child presenting as an intermittently appearing abdominal mass. J. Pediatr. Surg. 13: 127–128, 1978.
11. Sequeira, F.W., Weber, T.R., Smith, W.L., Caresky, J.M., and Cairo, M.S.: Budd-Chiari syndrome caused by hepatic torsion. A.J.R. 137: 393–394, 1981.
12. Shende, A., Lanzkowsky, P., and Becker, J.: Torsion of a visceroptosed spleen. Am. J. Dis. Child. 130: 88–91, 1976.
13. Smulewicz, J., and Clemett, A.: Torsion of the wandering spleen. Am. J. Dis. Child. 20: 274–279, 1975.
14. Swischuk, L.E., Williams, J.B., and John, S.D.: Torsion of wandering spleen: New CT finding. J. Pediatr. Radiol. 23:1993.
15. Thompson, J.S., Ross, R.J., and Pizzaro, S.T. The wandering spleen in infancy and childhood. Clin. Pediatr. 19: 221–224, 1980.

Omental Strangulation and Infarction.

These problems are quite rare, but do occur (1–3). They are very difficult to diagnose roentgenographically, but with the availability of ultrasound, one may be able to demonstrate an echogenic abdominal mass which then would mitigate toward surgical exploration of the abdomen.

REFERENCES

1. Holden, M.P.: Primary idiopathic segmental infarction of the greater omentum. J. Pediatr. Surg. 7: 77, 1972.
2. Iuchtman, M., Berant, M., and Assa, J.: Transomental strangulation. J. Pediatr. Surg. 13: 439–449, 1978.
3. Rich, R.H., and Filler, R.M.: Segmental infarction of the greater omentum: A cause of acute abdomen in childhood. Can. J. Surg. 26: 241–243, 1983.

ABDOMINAL TRAUMA

General Approach. In abdominal trauma, the abdominal roentgenogram now is used more as an initial screening examination than one for specific diagnosis. Ultrasound and even more so CT have supplanted its role in this regard. But the plain film still has some use and one should develop some type of general approach to its assessment.

In beginning one's assessment of the ab-

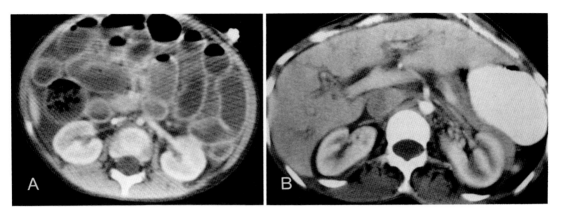

Figure 3.121. *(A) Hypovolemic shock; CT findings.* Note how hyperintense the kidneys appear and in addition note the hyperintense appearance of the intestinal walls. The intestines are dilated and filled with fluid and air. *(B) Periportal tracking.* Note extensive periportal tracking of fluid in this patient with intraperitoneal bleeding secondary to anticoagulant therapy.

domen, one should quickly scan the lung bases, diaphragmatic leaflets, larger abdominal viscera, and the overall gas pattern. Thereafter one should look at the pelvis, ribs, and vertebrae for fractures. One also should look at the spine for evidence of scoliosis, for scoliosis is very helpful in lateralizing abnormalities to one side or other. Thereafter, one should inspect the abdomen for evidence of free air, peritoneal fluid (blood, bile, etc.), focally distended loops of intestine (i.e., sentinel loops), and, as mentioned, fractures of the ribs, bony pelvis, or spine.

Both ultrasound and CT are now commonly utilized in the investigation of abdominal trauma. Although some suggest that plain films and ultrasound should suffice in cases of minor trauma (1, 6, 15), all agree that when intra-abdominal injury is seriously suspected, CT is much more informative and the preferred modality (1–4, 7, 8, 12, 15).

Intravenous pyelography is seldom used in the evaluation of blunt abdominal trauma, but the retrograde cystogram still is best for the evaluation of urinary bladder or urethral injury. Magnetic resonance imaging (MRI) is of minor, if any, value in the evaluation of abdominal trauma. Similarly, angiography is only occasionally required. It is utilized in select cases of vascular injury, if time allows.

Finally, one might note an interesting phenomenon occasionally visualized on CT scans with hypovolemia and shock (13, 14). In these cases, the organs become hyperintense and often this phenomenon is best visualized in the walls of the shocked, fluid-filled, and usually paralyzed, intestinal loops (Fig. 3.121A).

Another phenomenon often seen with abdominal trauma and especially hepatic trauma is so-called "periportal tracking of fluid" (9–11). Although originally believed to be due to blood tracking along the periportal space, there is now some question that the finding may be due to transudation of fluid into the periportal space from associated portal lymphatic obstruction (i.e., hematoma) or fluid overload from iatrogenic bolus intravenous fluid therapy (9–11). The latter may be the more common cause of the phenomenon but it may also be seen with underlying liver trauma (Fig. 3.121B).

REFERENCES

1. Akgur, F.M., Tanyel, F.C., Akhan, O., Buyuk-pamukdu, N., and Hicsonmez, A.: The place of ultrasonographic examination in the initial evaluation of children sustaining blunt abdominal trauma. J. Pediatr. Surg. 28: 78–81, 1993.

2. Babcock, D.S., and Kaufman, R.A.: Ultrasonography and computed tomography in the evaluation of the acutely ill pediatric patient. Radiol. Clin. North Am. 21: 527–550, 1983.

3. Berger, P.E., and Kuhn, J.P.: CT of blunt abdominal trauma in childhood. A.J.R. 13: 105–110, 1981.

4. Brody, A.S., Seidel, F.G., and Kuhn, J.P.: CT evaluation of blunt abdominal trauma in children: Comparison of ultrafast and conventional CT. A.J.R. 153: 803–806, 1989.

5. Bulas, D.I., Taylor, G.A., and Eichelberger, M.R.: The value of CT in detecting bowel perforation in children after blunt abdominal trauma. A.J.R. 153: 561–564, 1989.

6. Filiatrault, D., Longpre, D., Patriquin, H., Perreault, G., Grignon, A., Pronovost, J., and Bosvert, J.: Investigation of childhood blunt abdominal trauma: A practical approach using ultrasound as the initial diagnostic modality. Pediatr. Radiol. 17: 373–379, 1987.

7. Karp, M.P., Cooney, D.R., Berger, P.E., Khun, J.P., and Jewett, T.C., Jr.: The role of computed tomography in the evaluation of blunt abdominal trauma in children. J. Pediatr. Surg. 16: 316–323, 1981.

8. Kaufman, R.A., Towbin, R., Babcock, D.S., Gelfand, M.K., Guice, K.S., Oldham, K.T., and Noseworthy, J.: Upper abdominal trauma in children: Imaging evaluation. A.J.R. 142: 449–460, 1984.

9. Patrick, L.E., Ball, T.I., Atkinson, G.O., and Winn, K.J.: Pediatric blunt abdominal trauma: Periportal tracking at CT. Radiology 183: 689–691, 1992.

10. Siegel, M.J., and Herman, T.E.: Periportal low attenuation at CT in childhood. Radiology 183: 685–688, 1992.

11. Shanmuganathan, K., Mirvis, S.E., and Amoroso, M.: Periportal low density on CT in patients with blunt trauma: Association with elevated venous pressure. A.J.R. 160: 279–283, 1993.

12. Sivit, C.J., Taylor, G.A., Bulas, D.I., Bowman, L.M., and Eichelberger, M.R.: Blunt trauma in children: Significance of peritoneal fluid. Radiology 178: 185–188, 1991.

13. Sivit, C.J., Taylor, G.A., Bulas, D.I., Kushner, D.C., Potter, B.M., and Eichelberger, M.R.: Post-traumatic shock in children: CT findings associated with hemodynamic instability. Radiology 182: 723–726, 1992.

14. Taylor, G.A., Fallat, M.E., and Eichelberger, M.R.: Hypovolemic shock in children: Abdominal CT manifestations. Radiology 164: 479–481, 1987.

15. Zahran, M., Eklof, O., and Thomasson, B.: Blunt abdominal trauma and hollow viscus injury in children: The diagnostic value of plain radiography. Pediatr. Radiol. 14: 304–309, 1984.

Specific Organ Injury. One of the most commonly injured organs is the *spleen*. Clinically, upper abdominal, left upper quadrant, flank, or left shoulder (referred from the diaphragm) pain provides a clue to the diagnosis. The roentgenographic findings associated with splenic injury (2–4, 7) often are difficult to evaluate, but one or more of the following findings should be sought for: (a) medial displacement of the stomach, (b) downward and/or medial displacement of the splenic flexure, (c) elevation of the left diaphragmatic leaflet, (d) scoliosis of the spine with concavity to the left, (e) sentinel loops over the left upper quadrant, (f) pleural effusions or atelectasis in the left lung base, and, in a few cases, (g) associated rib fractures. Of course, not all these findings are present in any one patient, but being aware of all of them is most important (Fig. 3.122).

Splenic injuries are readily identified with CT scanning (5, 6). Ultrasonography, initially employed in the investigation of splenic injury (1), is not as productive, and we have found that splenic hematomas can be missed with ultrasound. Consequently, we seldom perform ultrasonography for suspected splenic injury, for CT scanning usually clearly identifies all forms of splenic injury (Fig. 3.123). In terms of the CT examination, one should be aware of the phenomenon of irregular contrast opacification of the spleen very early after the bolus contrast injection (Fig. 5.123*B*).

Liver injury with virtual exsanguinating hemorrhage is a true emergency, and often there is barely enough time to obtain abdominal roentgenograms. In such cases, emergency ligation or embolization of the hepatic artery frequently is performed (5, 6, 9). Intracapsular hematomas, a much more common problem, lead to enlargement of the liver, upward displacement of

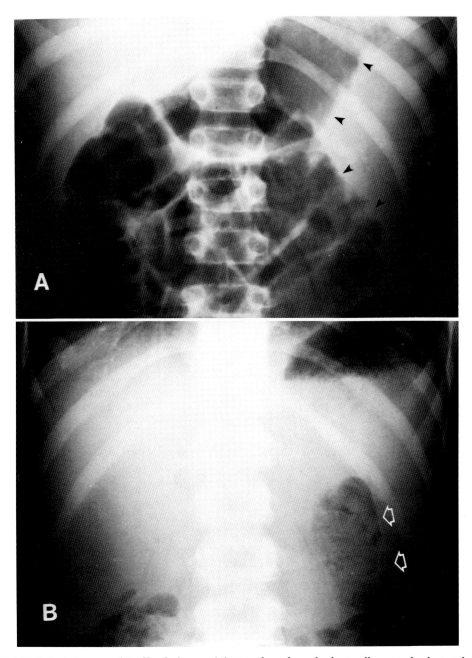

Figure 3.122. *Splenic trauma; plain film findings.* (*A*) Note the enlarged splenic silhouette displacing the stomach and intestines medially (*arrows*). (*B*) Another case showing a medially displaced splenic flexure (*arrows*). The spleen is difficult to identify as such, but the splenic space is increased in width.

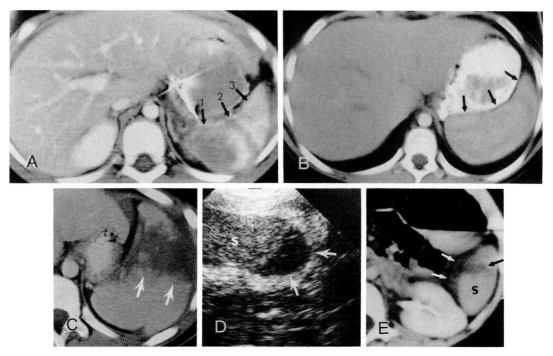

Figure 3.123. *Splenic trauma: CT findings.* (*A*) Note the completely abnormal spleen demonstrating a large hematoma (*1*), a central laceration (*2*), and residual, relatively normal splenic pulp (*3*). There is a little free fluid (blood) between the splenic pulp and the abdominal wall. (*B*) Normal irregular opacification of the spleen (*arrows*) due to imaging early during a bolus injection. This is an important artifact not to be misinterpreted for multiple splenic contusions. (*C*) Another patient with a splenic "fracture" (*arrows*). (*D*) Subcapsular splenic hematoma (*arrows*) visualized with ultrasound. Spleen (*S*). (*D*) CT findings in same patient demonstrate the spleen (*S*), a central laceration (*black arrow*), and the subcapsular collection of blood (*white arrows*).

the right diaphragmatic leaflet, medial displacement of the duodenum and stomach, downward displacement of the hepatic flexure, and, in some cases, downward displacement and compression of the right kidney (Fig. 3.124). Of course, atelectasis and pleural effusions in the right lung base also may be noted, along with right rib fractures. Intrahepatic air, probably forced into the liver from the intestinal tract, also has been described (1, 11). If blood escapes into the peritoneal cavity, the findings will be those of intraperitoneal fluid. Ultrasonography is more rewarding with liver injuries than with splenic injuries, but still CT scanning is the procedure of choice (8, 10)(Fig. 3.125). Arteriography usually is not utilized for diagnosis, but is necessary when selective artery embolization or ligation is contemplated.

Periportal tracking of blood also can be seen with liver injury (see Fig. 3.31).

Injury to the *bile ducts* or *gallbladder* often is difficult to diagnose and usually is accompanied by injury to other viscera in the area, mainly the liver. If the gallbladder or bile ducts are injured alone, however, bile peritonitis is the presenting feature (2–4, 7). In such cases, the peritonitis produced often is of a smoldering nature, and it is not until paracentesis is performed that the diagnosis is substantiated. In the past, direct cholangiography often was employed to detect these leaks, but currently less invasive radionuclide studies are considered just as rewarding. In such cases, a Tc-HIDA scan will demonstrate isotope activity outside the hepatobiliary system and gastrointestinal tract.

Pancreatic trauma in childhood is rela-

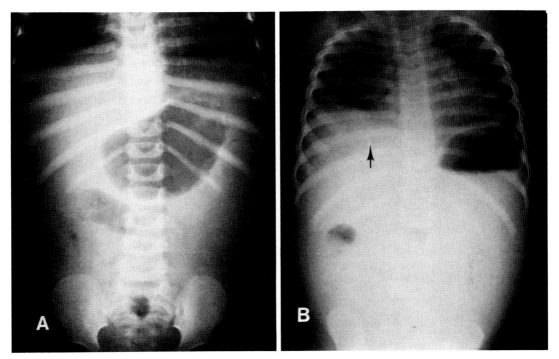

Figure 3.124. *Liver trauma.* Note the markedly enlarged liver (*arrows*) displacing the stomach far to the left and the intestines downwardly.

tively common (1–9) and can occur with surprisingly mild injury. Most often it is seen with automobile accidents, bicycle handlebar accidents, blows with the fist to the abdomen, falls on a blunt object, and seat belt injuries in older children. It is also commonly seen in the battered child syndrome.

The roentgenographic findings are variable, and actually most often the abdominal roentgenograms are normal. However, in other cases, one may see telltale sentinel loops of dilated intestine over the area of the pancreas. In any given case, these loops may be those of dilated small bowel, duodenum, or transverse colon (Fig. 3.126A). When the transverse colon is dilated, it results in the so-called "colon cutoff" sign (Fig. 3.126B). In addition to these findings, one may see widening of the soft tissue space between the stomach and transverse colon as a result of bleeding and/or edema in this area. However, all of

these findings either are rare or subtle, and thus suspected pancreatic injury is best assessed with ultrasound or CT scanning (4, 7).

In some cases the pancreas may be enlarged, and on ultrasound somewhat hypoechoic (edema). In other cases parapancreatic fluid collections are present and occasionally an actual laceration or "fracture" of the pancreas is seen (Fig. 3.127). These same findings are demonstrable with CT scanning (Fig. 3.127), and both ultrasound and CT can clearly document the presence of complicating post-traumatic pseudocysts (Fig. 3.75). Trauma to the *duodenum* often is seen in conjunction with pancreatic injury but, of course, can occur alone (4, 6, 8). It results from the same type of injury responsible for pancreatic trauma, and also is seen in the battered child syndrome. Trauma to the duodenum may manifest in actual duodenal rupture, intramural duodenal tears, or intramural

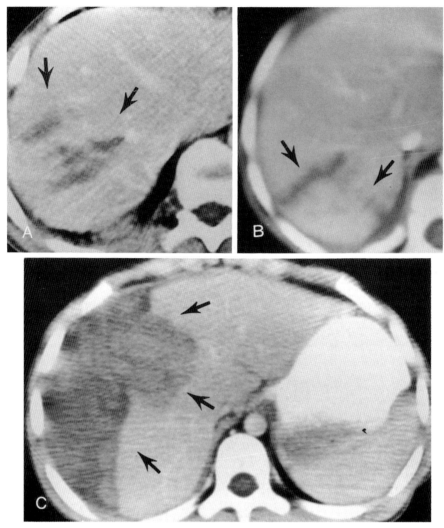

Figure 3.125. *Liver trauma: CT findings.* (*A*) Note numerous intrahepatic hypodense, irregular contusions (*arrows*). These areas represent small areas of hemorrhage. (*B*) Another patient with a laceration (fracture) through the right lobe of the liver (*arrows*). (*C*) Large subcapsular intrahepatic hematoma (*arrows*). Also see Figure 3.31.

hematoma formation (1–8). The latter injury, however, is most common. When duodenal rupture occurs, the usual site of perforation is along the posterior duodenal wall, and, subsequently, there is leakage of intestinal contents into the retroperitoneal space. Symptoms due to such leakage may not become apparent immediately, and, indeed, may take hours or days to develop. When they do develop, they consist of pain in the back or flank, and roentgenographi-

cally, if water-soluble contrast agents are administered to these patients, retroperitoneal extravasation can be demonstrated. The duodenum, of course, also will be deformed or even obstructed. Intraperitoneal rupture of the duodenum is rare.

With duodenal intramural hematoma formation, the plain films may show nothing abnormal, or they may show evidence of duodenal or gastric obstruction (Fig. 3.128A). Less commonly, the hematoma

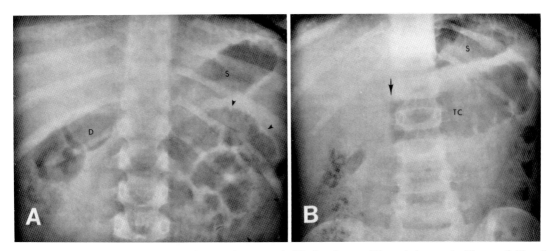

Figure 3.126. *Pancreatic trauma.* (*A*) Note the stomach (*S*), duodenum (*D*), and the sentinel loops of dilated small bowel in the left abdomen (*arrows*). The stomach is displaced upwardly, and the soft tissue space between the stomach and intestines is widened. The duodenal bulb is filled with air secondary to paralytic ileus. (*B*) Another case demonstrating the colon cutoff sign. Note the dilated transverse colon (*TC*) and the abrupt cutoff of gas just to the right of the spine (*arrow*). Also note that the soft tissue space between the stomach (*S*) and the transverse colon is increased. (Reprinted with permission from L.W. Young and J.T. Adams: Roentgenographic findings in localized trauma to the pancreas in children. A.J.R. 101: 639–648, 1967.)

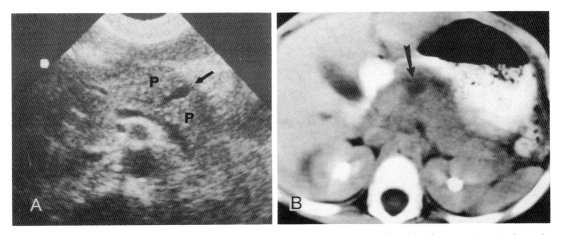

Figure 3.127. *Pancreatic fracture.* (*A*) Ultrasound study demonstrates a wedge-like fracture (*arrow*) through the pancreas (*P*). The pancreas is a little enlarged and there is some peripancreatic fluid present. (*B*) CT study in another patient demonstrates a similar wedge-like fracture (*arrow*). A little peripancreatic fluid also is present. In other cases, the findings in pancreatic trauma are no different than in other cases of pancreatitis from other causes (see Fig. 3.74).

itself may be seen as an abdominal mass. However, if duodenal injury is suspected, ultrasound or an upper GI series should be performed. The upper GI series will demonstrate the duodenal obstruction resulting from an intramural mass (Fig. 3.128*B*– *D*), and with intramural tears, barium will be seen to extravasate from the duodenum. Intramural hematomas eventually disappear, with the blood escaping into the bowel lumen and follow-up GI studies usually showing a complete return to normal.

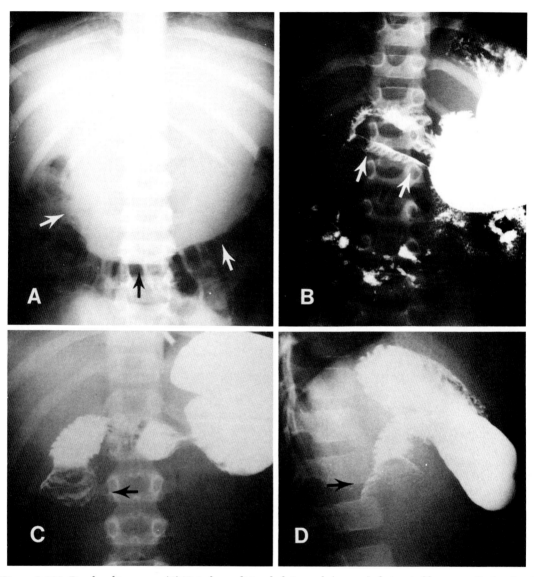

Figure 3.128. *Duodenal trauma.* (*A*) Note large distended stomach (*arrows*) obstructed because of a duodenal hematoma. (*B*) Typical appearance of the duodenal hematoma; an intramural lesion (*arrows*). (*C*) and (*D*) Another patient with classic findings of an intramural hematoma (*arrows*). (Parts *C* and *D* courtesy of Virgil Graves, M.D., Great Falls, Montana.)

Currently, duodenal hematomas are more likely to first be demonstrated with ultrasonography or CT scanning (4). CT findings are similar to those seen on upper GI series, in that there is a mass present due to the hematoma and associated displacement or deformity of the duodenum. With ultrasonography, the early hematoma ap-

pears as an echogenic mass (Fig. 3.129), but with maturation the hematoma liquifies and becomes anechoic (Fig. 3.130).

Small intestinal injury has become more common as seat belt injuries have become more common (3, 4), but, of course, any type of blunt trauma to the abdomen can cause small bowel injury. In terms of

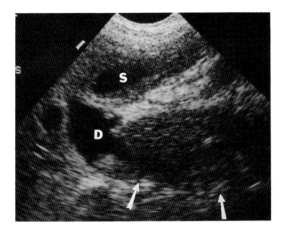

Figure 3.129. *Duodenal hematoma: ultrasonographic findings.* Note the echogenic, eccentric hematoma (*arrows*) located in the distal duodenum and producing some obstruction of the descending duodenum (*D*). Stomach (*S*).

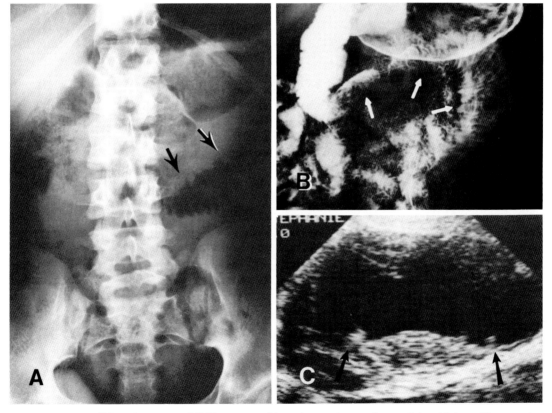

Figure 3.130. *Small bowel trauma.* (**A**) Note sentinel loop (*arrows*) secondary to jejunal injury. The next day the patient developed a classic small bowel obstruction. (**B**) Upper GI series demonstrating a large intramural jejunal hematoma (*arrows*). (**C**) Ultrasonogram demonstrates a large, sonolucent hematoma (*arrows*). (Parts (**B**) and (**C**) from R.A. Kaufman and D.S. Babcock: An approach to imaging the upper abdomen in the injured child. Semin. Roentgenol. 14: 308–320, 1984.)

the specific type of injury incurred, perforation and hematoma formation probably are most common (3–5, 8, 11, 12), and in either case, post-traumatic stenoses with obstruction of the intestine can result (2, 6, 7).

Protrusion of a loop of small bowel into an associated spinal fracture-dislocation is a rare phenomenon (9). In acute intestinal injury, however, abdominal roentgenograms frequently are normal, but in some cases, one or two sentinel loops of dilated, injured small bowel can be seen. If these loops appear thickened, intramural bleeding should be suspected, but often this is a difficult finding to appreciate on plain films and usually is best demonstrated with CT or upper gastrointestinal contrast studies. In some of these cases, the hematoma may be in the mesentery of omentum (1), but in either case, if large enough, the hematoma may present as an abdominal mass on plain films. However, in most cases ultrasonography or CT scanning are more productive in detecting these hematomas (Fig. 3.130).

In terms of seat belt injuries, ecchymotic changes across the lower abdomen should serve as a signal that internal or spinal injuries could be present (10). This is most important to appreciate, for in the rush of evaluating such patients these injuries may be overlooked.

Perforation of the stomach, small intestine, or colon may lead to free air being visualized in the abdomen (11, 12). With gastric or colonic perforations, such air usually is intraperitoneal and of such a volume that it is readily visualized. With small bowel perforations, however, little if any air is seen. Rectal perforations may lead to air accumulations in the pelvic soft tissues, and both rectal and duodenal perforations can lead to retroperitoneal air collections.

Esophageal perforation can present with widening of the mediastinum, air in the mediastinum, or a hydropneumothorax. Esophageal perforations can be confirmed with the administration of contrast material, and as far as etiology is concerned they usually result from acutely increased intraluminal pressures secondary to blunt trauma to the abdomen and lower chest. Perforation from foreign bodies is rare.

Injury to the *urinary tract* is one of the more common manifestations of abdominal trauma, and renal injury can range from simple renal parenchymal contusion to complete avulsion of the renal pedicle (3, 4, 6, 7, 9–15, 19, 22). A diagrammatic representation of these injuries is offered in Figure 3.131. Interestingly enough, however, most of these lesions can be treated conservatively, and it is only the massive injury to the kidney or its blood supply that requires immediate surgical intervention. In addition, initial studies, no matter what they consist of, usually are not useful in predicting future problems such as scarring and systemic hypertension. Therefore, over the years, the approach to renal trauma generally has become quite conservative. In this regard, it has been shown that, with renal trauma, if the patient is normotensive and red blood cells less than 50 per high-power field, no investigation is necessary (19).

In the past, one relied almost solely on the intravenous pyelogram for the evaluation of renal trauma and, although the study is still occasionally utilized, CT scanning has provided a more definitive method with which to document (17, 18, 21) and follow (21) renal injury. Ultrasonography also can be utilized, but there is no comparison with the information yielded with contrast-enhanced CT scanning. Indeed, small contusions and lacerations can be missed with ultrasound.

With simple *renal contusions or intrarenal hematomas* the renal silhouette is intact, but the kidney may be focally or generally enlarged. Intravenous pyelography usually demonstrates generalized or focal decreased renal function (Fig. 3.132), while ultrasound may show a focal echogenic lesion. CT, however, most clearly

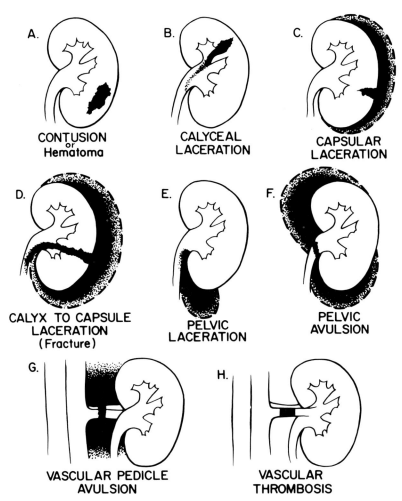

Figure 3.131. *Types of renal injury: diagrammatic representation.   Black areas* represent areas of blood accumulation, except in (*H*) where the *black area* represents the area of thrombosis. (Modified from R.I. Macpherson and A. Decter: Pediatric renal trauma. J. Can. Assoc. Radiol. 22: 10–21, 1971.)

identifies the non-contrast-enhancing contusion (Fig. 3.133). Renal lacerations, transected kidneys, crushed kidneys, and perirenal fluid collections (blood, urine) also are best demonstrated with CT (Fig. 3.133). If lacerations extend through the renal capsule, extravasation of contrast material into the perinephric space may be seen.

Injuries to the *renal pelvis* lead to extravasation of urine and contrast material around the kidney, and in some cases the urine collection may lead to the development of a so-called "urinoma" (7, 12). This collection of urine may be visualized as a soft tissue mass on plain abdominal roentgenograms, and on intravenous pyelography will eventually fill with contrast material (Fig. 3.134). Associated obstruction of the upper urinary tract is common in these cases, and the urine collections may extend into the thorax (2). These urine collections usually are readily demonstrable with ultrasonography, for they are sonolucent. They are also readily visualized with CT scanning.

Vascular injury to the renal pedicle may range from traumatic avulsion of both the

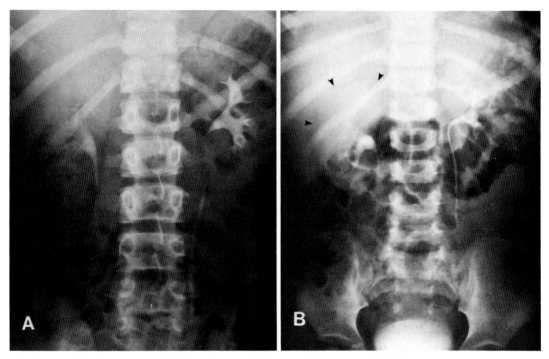

Figure 3.132. *Renal contusion.* (*A*) Note decreased function of the entire right kidney in this patient with a right renal contusion. (*B*) Another patient demonstrating decreased function and slight enlargement of the right upper renal pole only (*arrows*).

artery and vein to renal artery thrombosis (1, 15). With total avulsion of the renal pedicle, perinephric hematoma formation usually is profound, and, of course, no function of the involved kidney is seen. With traumatic renal artery thrombosis, the kidney usually is not enlarged and arteriography is required for demonstration of the obstructed artery.

Before leaving renal trauma, a note regarding *trauma to a previously unsuspected hydronephrotic kidney* is in order. In some of these cases, trauma seems to be relatively mild, but pain and hematuria cause the child to seek medical attention. Indeed, one often is surprised at just how large these hydronephrotic kidneys are, and how they remain silent until the time of injury (Fig. 3.135). In these cases, one most often is dealing with an underlying ureteropelvic junction obstruction, but ureteral stenosis at a lower level also can be encountered. When such a kidney is in-

jured, nothing more than hematuria may result, but in other instances, frank tears of the renal pelvis or calices lead to extravasation of urine, blood, and contrast material.

Injuries to the ureter are rare, but *bladder and urethral injury* is rather common, especially in the presence of pelvic fractures (4, 5, 14, 16). *Urethral injury* is most often seen in males, and as such usually involves the posterior urethra at its junction with the bladder neck. Tears of the nondistended bladder around the bladder neck and posterior urethra lead to extravasation of urine into the extraperitoneal pelvic soft tissues. In such instances, plain films frequently demonstrate the presence of an accompanying pelvic fracture and obliteration of the soft tissue planes of the pelvis. Intravenous urography or retrograde cystography will demonstrate extravasation of urine into the pelvic soft tissues. Ultrasonography and CT scanning, of course, also

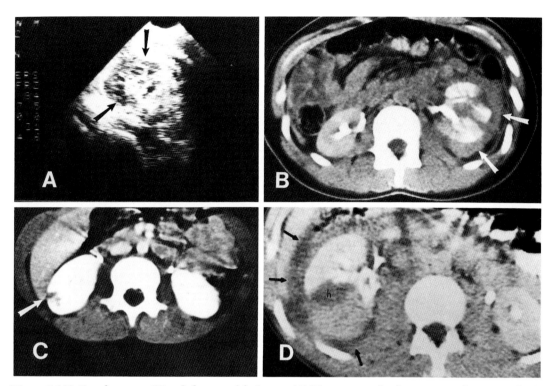

Figure 3.133. *Renal trauma: CT and ultrasound findings.* (*A*) Ultrasonography demonstrates disorganized echo activity in the poorly defined left kidney (*arrows*). (*B*) Contrast-enhanced CT study much more clearly demonstrates the fractured left kidney and blood around it (*arrows*). (*C*) Another patient demonstrating a small intrarenal hematoma or area of contusion (*arrow*). (*D*) Still another patient with a contrast-enhanced CT scan demonstrating a large intrarenal hematoma (*h*), some blood around the kidney (*arrows*), and a contusion over the lower pole. Note that the kidney also is displaced outward.

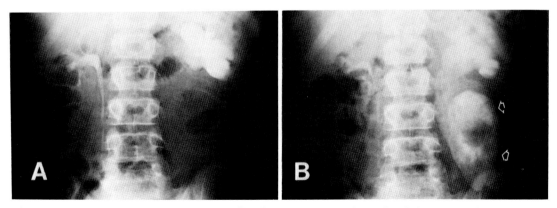

Figure 3.134. *Parapelvic urinoma.* (*A*) Early film demonstrating an elevated and obstructed left kidney. Note one or two curvilinear collections of contrast material below the left kidney. (*B*) Delayed films demonstrate filling of a large urinoma (*arrows*) which was obstructing the left kidney.

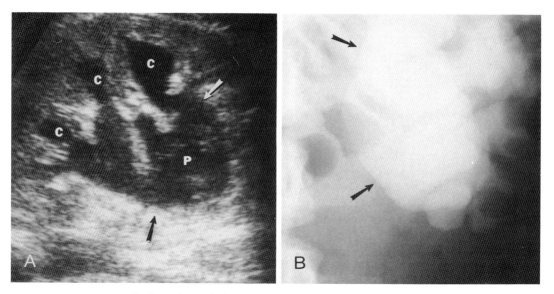

Figure 3.135. *Trauma to hydronephrotic kidney.* (*A*) This patient had abdominal trauma and subsequent hematuria. Abdominal ultrasound revealed a large hydronephrotic left kidney (*arrows*). Note the dilated renal pelvis (*P*) and calyces (*C*). (*B*) Subsequent intravenous pyelogram demonstrates the same findings with a markedly hydronephrotic renal pelvis and calyces (*arrows*). The patient had a ureteropelvic junction obstruction which was unsuspected until the time of trauma.

readily demonstrate these fluid collections.

In investigating a potential bladder or urethral injury, it is important to first perform a retrograde urethrogram. This will yield information as to the condition of the urethra (Fig. 3.136A) and, thereafter, if the urethra and bladder neck are normal a formal retrograde cystogram can be performed (Fig. 3.136B). However, if a Foley catheter is being utilized for this procedure, it should be placed in a position such that the inflated bulb does not occlude the bladder neck. This is important, for if the bulb occludes the bladder neck, it may also occlude a nearby perforation. In cases where a perforation is suspected but not demonstrated, oblique views of the bladder and bladder neck should be obtained, for these views often demonstrate smaller leaks.

Distended urinary bladders, when ruptured, often lead to urine extravasation into the peritoneal cavity. In such cases,

plain films will demonstrate the presence of abdominal fluid, and subsequent cystography will demonstrate the site and extent of the leak (Fig. 3.136C). Trauma to the bladder without perforation also can occur and is especially common with pelvic fractures. Such injury is difficult to document roentgenographically unless a pelvic hematoma surrounds the bladder. In these cases, the bladder may be minimally deformed or elevated, eccentrically deformed or elevated, or deformed in typical pear-shaped fashion (Fig. 3.137).

Ultrasonography (8) and CT scanning also can demonstrate these fluid collections around the bladder (Fig. 3.137A), but these studies have not replaced the cystogram. One of the reasons is that the cystogram is performed under fluoroscopic control and one can determine where the leak has occurred. However, with ultrasound, in some cases, an actual defect in the bladder wall can be seen (20). Most often, however, this does not occur.

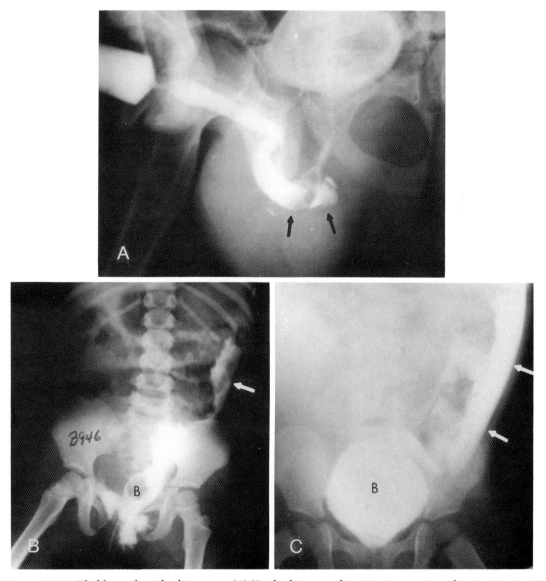

Figure 3.136. *Bladder and urethral trauma.* (**A**) Urethral tear resulting in extravasation of contrast material (*arrows*) on this retrograde urethrogram. (**B**) Patient with bladder trauma. Note the displaced urinary bladder (*B*). It is displaced to the left because of intrapelvic blood and urine accumulation. Below the bladder, note extravasation of contrast material into the pelvic soft tissues. Also note that there has been intraperitoneal leakage (*arrow*) of contrast material (*arrow*). (**C**) Intraperitoneal rupture (*arrows*) of the bladder (*B*) in a battered child. (Part *B* courtesy of Charles J. Fagan, M.D., and Part *C* courtesy of Theresa Stacy, M.D.)

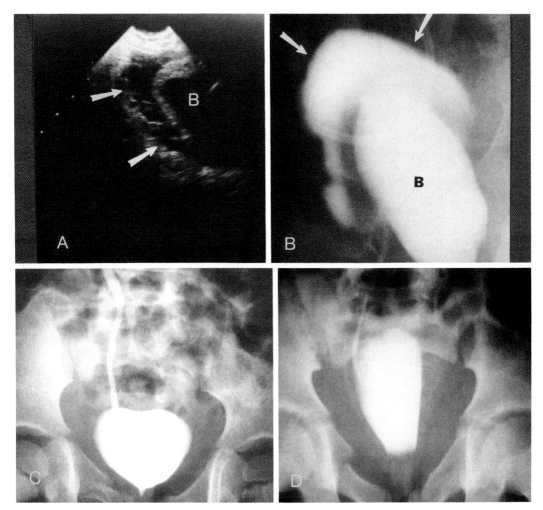

Figure 3.137. *Bladder trauma.*   (*A*) Sagittal sonogram demonstrating the urinary bladder (*B*) and fluid with echogenic strands within it, surrounding the bladder (*arrows*). The bladder wall also appears a little thickened.
These findings constitute the so called "bladder within bladder" sign (8). (*B*) Retrograde cystogram demonstrates the bladder (*B*) and extravasated contrast material (*arrow*). This patient had a perforation through the
dome of the bladder. (*C*) *Hematoma around bladder.* Note the increased soft tissue space between the contrast-
filled bladder and surrounding bony pelvis. There is a fracture through the pubic bone *on the right.* (*D*) Typical
elongated, almost pear-shaped bladder resulting from extensive perivesical hematoma formation. Note multiple
fractures of the pelvis.

Rupture of a diaphragmatic leaflet secondary to blunt abdominal trauma is not exceptionally common in childhood but by the same token frequently is overlooked (1–3, 6, 7). Most often, such rupture occurs on the left, but since in many cases there is nothing more to see than a slightly elevated or obscured diaphragmatic leaflet (1, 3, 5), the findings are missed. Of course, if atelectasis or a pleural effusion exists on the ipsilateral side, more attention is focused on the diaphragmatic leaflet, and when loops of distended intestine or stomach are seen in the chest, the diagnosis is virtually assured (Fig. 3.138). In these latter cases, the findings are quite similar to those seen with congenital diaphragmatic hernia, and often a nasogastric tube can be seen to head into the chest (6).

On the right side, since the liver protects the right diaphragmatic leaflet, even with tears of the diaphragm, one usually sees only elevation of the right diaphragmatic leaflet. Associated rib fractures can be seen on either side, and contrast studies may be necessary to determine that intestines or stomach are present in the chest. Much more rarely, abdominal contents can herniate into the pericardial sac (4). Delayed herniation weeks or months after initial injury also can occur, but initially simple awareness of the possibility of diaphragmatic injury is the most important factor (4).

Vascular injury often is catastrophic, and there is no time for roentgenograms to be obtained. In those less severe cases where such studies are obtained, the find-

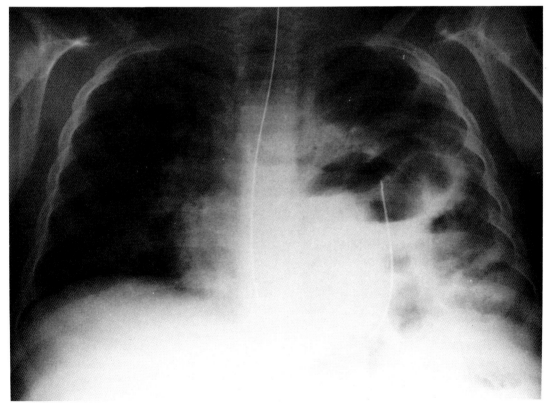

Figure 3.138. *Traumatic diaphragmatic hernia.* Note numerous collections of intestine in the left chest and note the position of the nasogastric tube as it heads into the stomach, herniated into the chest.

ings often are nonspecific and consist of nothing more than one or two loops of isolated, dilated intestine. Angiography, of course, is the procedure of choice in such cases.

Abdominal injury in the battered child syndrome usually is given less attention than it deserves. However, very often these children are dead on arrival to the emergency room and, interestingly enough, may show little in the way of skeletal injury (Fig. 3.139). One of the most commonly injured organs is the pancreas, and, indeed, acute pancreatitis and subsequent pseudocyst formation are very common in the battered child syndrome (1, 7, 9, 10). Duodenal trauma, usually with duodenal hematoma formation (4, 6–8) also is a common injury in the battered child syndrome and, interestingly enough, so is

small intestinal trauma. In addition, colon injuries are probably more common than generally appreciated. These can result from blunt trauma or insertion of various objects into the rectum with perforation (Fig. 3.140A). Traumatic mesenteric avulsion also has been reported in a case of presumed battered child (2), and, actually, when one encounters a child with any abdominal injury that is inadequately explained, one should suspect that the child has been battered.

Another interesting feature of the battered child syndrome, although not usually seen in the acute phase, is the post-traumatic development of lytic lesions in the long bones secondary to fat necrosis. These lesions, although not particularly common, can be perplexing unless one is aware of the phenomenon (2, 3, 5, 7).

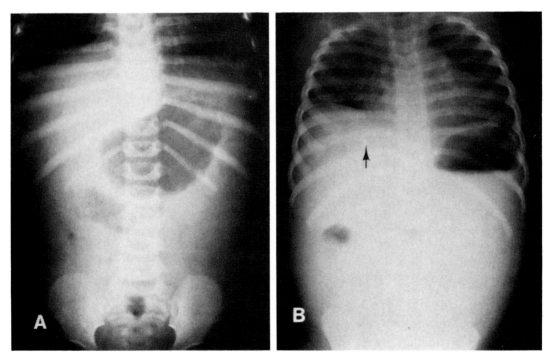

Figure 3.139. *Abdominal trauma; battered child syndrome.* (*A*) Supine film demonstrating generalized opacity of the abdomen and absence of visualization of the psoas shadows and liver edge. The findings suggest peritoneal fluid. (*B*) Upright view demonstrating similar findings and a slightly elevated right diaphragmatic leaflet. There was a small subpulmonic effusion on the right. Also note an almost invisible fresh rib fracture on the right (*arrow*). This was the only sign of skeletal injury in this battered child who had peritonitis secondary to perforation of the colon.

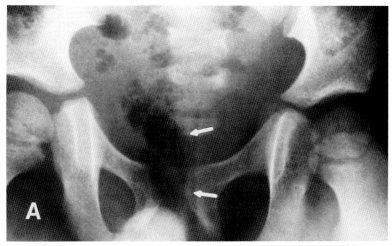

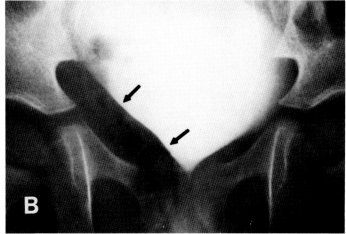

Figure 3.140. *Battered child syndrome; intestinal perforation.* (*A*) Note the bubbles of gas in the right groin area (*arrows*). This abscess resulted from a rectal perforation after insertion of an object into the rectum. (*B*) Cystogram demonstrates displacement of the bladder by the abscess (*arrows*).

REFERENCES

Spleen

1. Ascher, W., Parvin, S., Virgilio, R., and Haber, K.: Echographic evaluation of splenic injury after blunt trauma. Radiology 118: 411–415, 1976.
2. Brindle, M.J.: Radiological evaluation of splenic injury after blunt trauma. J. Can. Assoc. Radiol. 22: 3–9, 1971.
3. Cimmino, C.V.: Ruptured spleen: Some refinements in its roentgenologic diagnosis. Radiology 82: 57–62, 1964.
4. Kittredge, R.D., and Finby, N.: Infrapulmonary effusion in traumatic rupture of the spleen. A.J.R. 91: 891–895, 1964.
5. Korobkin, M., Moss, A.A., Callen, P.W., De-Martini, W.J., and Kaiser, J.A.: Computed tomog-

raphy of subcapsular splenic hematoma: Clinical and experimental studies. Radiology 129: 441–445, 1978.
6. Mall, J.C., and Kasier, J.A.: CT diagnosis of splenic laceration. A.J.R. 134: 265–269, 1980.
7. Schwartz, S.S., Boley, S.J., and McKinnon, W.M.P.: The roentgen findings in traumatic rupture of the spleen in children. A.J.R. 82: 505–509, 1959.

Liver, Gallbladder, and Bile Ducts

1. Abramson , S.J., Berdon, W.E., Kaufman, R.A., and Ruzal-Shapiro, C.: Case report. Hepatic parenchymal and subcapsular gas after hepatic laceration caused by blunt abdominal trauma. A.J.R. 153: 1031–1032, 1989.

2. Bourfque, M.D., Spigland, N., Bensoussan, A.L., Garel, L., and Blanchard, H.: Isolated complete transection of the common bile duct due to blunt trauma in a child. J. Pediatr. Surg. 24: 1068–1070, 1989.

3. Caro, A.M., and Losa, J.M.O.: Complete avulsion of the common bile duct as a result of blunt abdominal trauma: Case report of a child. J. Pediatr. Surg. 5: 60–62, 1970.

4. Evans, J.P.: Traumatic rupture of the gallbladder in a three-year-old boy. J. Pediatr. Surg. 11: 1033–1034, 1976.

5. Jander, H.P., Laws, H.L., Kogutt, M.S., and Mihas, A.A.: Emergency embolization in blunt hepatic trauma. A.J.R. 129: 249–252, 1977.

6. Rubin, B.E., and Katzen, B.T.: Selective hepatic artery embolization to control massive hemorrhage after trauma. A.J.R. 129: 253–256, 1977.

7. Shorthouse A.J., Singh, M.P., Treasure, T., and Franklin, F.H.: Isolated complete transection of the common bile duct by blunt abdominal trauma. Br. J. Surg. 65: 543, 1978.

8. Stalker, H.P., Kaufman, R.A., and Towbin, R.: Patterns of liver injury in childhood: CT analysis. A.J.R. 147: 1100–1205, 1986.

9. Susan, E.M., Klotz, D., Jr., and Kottmeier, P.K.: Liver trauma in children. J. Pediatr. Surg. 10: 411–417, 1975.

10. Vock, P., Kehrer, B., and Tschaeppeler, H.: Blunt liver trauma in children: The role of computed tomography in diagnosis and treatment. J. Pediatr. Surg. 21: 413–418, 1986.

11. Wolfel, D.A., and Brogdon, B.G.: Intrahepatic air—a sign of trauma. Radiology 91: 952–953, 1968.

Pancreas

1. Berger, J., Sauvage, P., Levy, M., Graf, H., Olive, B., Reinhardt, W., Sauvage, M.R., and Buck, P.: Pancreatic trauma in childhood. Ann. Chir. Inf. 13: 379–390, 1972.

2. Dahman, B., and Stephens, C.A.: Pseudocysts of the pancreas after blunt abdominal trauma in children. J. Pediatr. Surg. 16: 17–21, 1981.

3. Ekengren, K., and Soderlund, S.: Radiological findings in traumatic lesions of pancreas in childhood. Ann. Radiol. 9: 379–385, 1966.

4. Harkanyi, Z., Vegh, M., Hittner, I., and Popik, E.: Grayscale echography of traumatic pancreatic cysts in children. Pediatr. Radiol. 11: 81–82, 1981.

5. Leistyna, J.A., and Macaulay, J.C.: Traumatic pancreatitis in childhood: Report of case and review of literature. Am. J. Dis. Child. 107: 644–648, 1964.

6. Pellerin, D., Bertin, P., and Harouchi, A.: Pancreatic trauma in childhood. Ann. Chir. Inf. 13: 391–394, 1972.

7. Sivit, C.J., Eichelberger, M.R., Taylor, G.A., Bulas, D.I., Gotschall, C.S., and Kushner, D.C.: Blunt pancreatic trauma in children: CT diagnosis. A.J.R. 158: 1097–1100, 1992.

8. Stone, H.H.: Pancreatic and duodenal trauma in children. J. Pediatr. Surg. 7: 670–675, 1972.

9. Young, L.W., and Adams, J.T.: Roentgenographic findings in localized trauma to pancreas in children. A.J.R. 101: 639–648, 1967.

Duodenum

1. Andersson, A., and Bergdahl, L.: Hematoma of the duodenum in children: Review of the literature and report of two cases. Am. Surg. 39: 402–405, 1973.

2. Felson, B., and Levin, E.: Intramural hematoma of the duodenum. Radiology 63: 823–831, 1954.

3. Hayashi, K., Futgagawa, S., Kozaki, S., Hirao, K., and Hombo, Z.: Ultrasound and CT diagnosis of intramural duodenal hematoma. Pediatr. Radiol. 18: 167–168, 1988.

4. Raby, N., and Meire, H.: Duodenal haematoma mimicking traumatic pancreatic pseudocyst. Br. J. Radiol. 59: 279–280, 1986.

5. Slonim, L.: Duodenal haematoma. Aust. Radiol. 15: 236–242, 1971.

6. Winthrop, A.L., Wesson, D.E., and Filler, R.M.: Traumatic duodenal hematoma in the pediatric patient. J. Pediatr. Surg. 21: 757–760, 1986.

7. Woolley, N.M., Mahour, G.H., and Sloan, T.: Duodenal hematoma in infancy and childhood: Changing etiology treatment. Am. J. Surg. 136: 8–14, 1978.

8. Young, L.W.: Pancreatic and/or duodenal injury from blunt trauma in childhood: Radiopaque examinations and radiological review. Ann. Radiol. 18: 377–390, 1975.

Stomach, Esophagus, Small Intestines, and Colon

1. Bradpiece, H.A., and Kissin, M.W.: Massive traumatic hemomentocele. J. Pediatr. Surg. 19: 209, 1984.

2. Braun, P., and Dion, Y.: Intestinal stenosis following seat belt injury. J. Pediatr. Surg. 8: 549–550, 1973.

3. DeBeugny, P., Canarelli, L., and Bonevalle, M.: Intestinal perforations related to blunt abdominal trauma in children. Chir. Pediatr. 29: 7–10, 1988.

4. Doersch, K.B., and Dosjer, W.E.: The seat belt syndrome. The seat belt sign, intestinal and mesenteric injuries. Am. J. Surg. 116: 831, 1968.

5. Garrett, J.W., and Braunstein, P.W.: The seat belt syndrome. J. Trauma 1: 220, 1962.

6. Hardacre, J.M., II, West, K.W., Rescorla, F.R., Vane D.W., and Grosfeld, J.L.: Delayed onset of intestinal obstruction in children affter unrecognized seat belt injury. J. Pediatr. Surg. 25: 967–969, 1990.

7. Shalaby-Rana, E., Eichelberger, M., Kerzner, B.,

and Kapur, S.: Case report. Intestinal stricture due to lap-belt injury. A.J.R. 158: 63–64, 1992.

8. Shuck, J.M., and Lowe, R.J.: Intestinal disruption due to blunt abdominal trauma. Am. J. Surg. 136: 668–673, 1978.

9. Silver, S.F., Nadel, H.R., Flodmark, O.: Case report. Pneumorrhachis after jejunal entrapment caused by a fracture dislocation of the lumbar spine. A.J.R. 150: 1129–1130, 1988.

10. Sivit, C.J., Taylor, G.A., Newman, K.D., Bulas, D.I., Gotschall, C.S., Wright, C.J., and Eichelberger, M.R.: Safety-belt injuries in children with lap-belt ecchymosis: CT findings in 61 patients. A.J.R. 157: 111–114, 1991.

11. Ting, Y.M., and Reuter, S.R.: Hollow viscus injury in blunt abdominal trauma. A.J.R. 119: 408–413, 1973.

12. Westcott, J., and Smith, J.: Mesentery and colon injuries secondary to blunt trauma. Radiology 114: 597–600, 1975.

Urinary Tract

1. Barlow, B., and Gandhi, R.: Renal artery thrombosis following blunt trauma. J. Trauma 20: 614–617, 1980.

2. Baron, R.L., Stark D.D., McClennan, B.L., Shanes, J.G., Davis, G.L., and Koch, D.D.: Intrathoracic extension of retroperitoneal urine collections. A.J.R. 137: 37–41, 1981.

3. Beckley, D.E., and Walters, E.A.: Avulsion of pelviureteric junction: Rare consequences of nonpenetrating trauma. Brit. J. Radiol. 45: 423–426, 1972.

4. Boston, V.E., and Smyth, B.T.: Bilateral pelviureteric avulsion following closed trauma. Br. J. Urol. 47: 149–151, 1975.

5. Glassberg, K.I., Tolete-Velcek, F., Ashley, R., and Waterhouse, K.: Partial tears of prostatomembranous urethra in children. Urology 13: 500–504, 1979.

6. Hutchison, R.J., and Nogrady, M.B.: Late sequelae of renal trauma in the pediatric age group. J. Can. Assoc. Radiol. 24: 3–11, 1973.

7. Itoh, S., Yoshioka, H., Kaeriyama, M., Taguchi, T., Oka, R., Oka, T., and Okamura, Y.: Ultrasonographic diagnosis of uriniferous perirenal pseudocyst. Pediatr. Radiol. 12: 156–158, 1982.

8. Kauzlaric, D., and Barmeir, E.: Sonography of traumatic rupture of the bladder: "Bladder within a bladder" appearance of extra-peritoneal extravasation. J. Ultrasound Med. 5: 97–98, 1986.

9. Kokihova, E., Obenbergerova, D., and Apetaurova, B.: Total severance of renal pedicle caused by blunt trauma in children. Pediatr. Radiol. 1: 59–62, 1973.

10. Macpherson, R.I., and Decter, A.: Pediatric renal trauma. J. Can. Assoc. Radiol. 22: 10–21, 1971.

11. Mandour, W.A., Lai, M.K., Linke, C.A., and Frank, I.N.: Blunt renal trauma in the pediatric patient. J. Pediatr. Surg. 16: 669–676, 1981.

12. McInerney, D., Jones, A., and Roylance, J.: Urinoma. Clin. Radiol. 28: 345–351, 1977.

13. Palavatana, C., Graham, S.R., and Silverman, F.N.: Delayed sequels to renal injury in childhood. A.J.R. 91: 659–665, 1964.

14. Perskey, L.: Childhood urethral trauma. Urology 2: 603–606, 1978.

15. Ready, L.B., Wright, C., and Baltzan, R.B.: Bilateral traumatic renal artery thrombosis. Can. Med. Assoc. J. 109: 885–891, 1973.

16. Reid, I.S.: Renal trauma in children: A ten-year review. Aust. N.Z.J. Surg. 42: 260–266, 1973.

17. Sandler, C.M., and Toombs, B.D.: Computed tomographic evaluation of blunt renal injuries. Radiology 141: 461–466, 1981.

18. Schaner, E.G., Balow, J.E., and Doppman, J.L.: Computed tomography in the diagnosis of subcapsular and perirenal hematoma. A.J.R. 129: 83–88, 1977.

19. Stalker, H.P., Kaufman, R.A., and Stedje, K.: The significance of hematuria in children after blunt abdominal trauma. A.J.R. 154: 569–571, 1990.

20. Wan Y-L, Hsieh, H., Lee, T-Y., and Tsai, C-C.: Wall defect as a sign of urinary bladder rupture in sonography. J. Ultrasound Med. 7: 511–513, 1988.

21. Yale-Loehr, A.J., Kramer, S.S., Quinlan, D.M., LaFrance, N.D., Mitchell, S.E., and Gearfhart, J.P.: CT of severe renal trauma in children: Evaluation and course of healing with conservative therapy. A.J.R. 152: 109–113, 1989.

22. Young, L.W., Wood, B.P., and Linke, C.A.: Renal injury from blunt trauma in childhood: Radiological evaluation and review. Ann. Radiol. 18: 359–376, 1975.

Diaphragm

1. Ball, T., McCrory, R., Smith, J.O., and Clements, J.L., Jr.: Traumatic diaphragmatic hernia: Errors in diagnosis. A.J.R. 138: 633–637, 1982.

2. Carter, B.N., Giuseffi, J., and Felson, B.: Traumatic diaphragmatic hernia. A.J.R. 69: 56–72, 1951.

3. Fataar, S., and Schulman, A.: Diagnosis of diaphragmatic tears. Br. J. Radiol. 52: 375–381, 1979.

4. Gelman, R., Mirvis, S.E., and Gens, D.: Diaphragmatic rupture due to blunt trauma: Sensitivity of plain chest radiographs. A.J.R. 156: 51–57, 1991.

5. Minagi, H. Brody, W.R., and Laing, F.C.: The variable roentgen appearance of traumatic diaphragmatic hernia. J. Can. Assoc. Radiol. 28: 124–128, 1977.

6. Perlman, S.J., Rogers, L.F., Mintzer, R.A., and Mueller, C.F.: Abnormal course of nasogastric tube in traumatic rupture of left hemidiaphragm. A.J.R. 142: 85–87, 1984.

7. Sharma, L.K., Kennedy, R.F., and Heneghan, W.D.: Rupture of the diaphragm resulting from blunt trauma in children. Can. J. Surg. 20: 553–556, 1977.

Battered Child Syndrome

1. Bonviovi, J.J., and Logosso, R.D.: Pancreatic pseudocyst occurring in the battered child syndrome. J. Pediatr. Surg. 4: 220–226, 1969.
2. Fournemont, E.: Traumatic mesenteric avulsion: Case report of presumed battered child. Ann. Radiol. 20: 517–521, 1977.
3. Goluboff, N., Cram, R., Ramgotra, B., Singh, A., and Wilkinson, G.W.: Polyarthritis and bone lesions complicating traumatic pancreatitis in two children. Can. Med. Assoc. J. 118: 924–928, 1978.
4. Gornall, P., Ahmed, A.J., and Cohen, S.J.: Intra-abdominal injuries in the battered baby syndrome. Arch. Dis. Child. 47: 211–214, 1972.
5. Keating, J.P., Shackelford, G.D., Shackelford, P.G., and Ternbert, J.L.: Pancreatitis and osteolytic lesions. J. Pediatr. 81: 350–353, 1972.
6. Kleinman, P.K., Brill, P.W., and Winchester, P.: Resolving duodenal-jejunal hematoma in abused children. Radiol. 160: 747–750, 1986.
7. Kleinman, P.K., Raptopoulos, V.D., and Brill, P.W.: Occult nonskeletal trauma in the battered child syndrome. Radiology 141: 393–396, 1981.
8. Orel, S.G., Nussbaum, A.R., Sheth, S., Yale-Loehr, A., and Sanders, R.C.: Case Report: Duodenal hematoma in child abuse: Sonographic detection. A.J.R. 151: 147–149, 1988.
9. Pena, S.D.J., and Medovy, H.: Child abuse and traumatic pseudocyst of the pancreas. J. Pediatr. 83: 1026–1028, 1973.
10. Slovis, T.L., Berdon, W.E., Haller, J.O., Baker, D.H., and Rosen, L.: Pancreatitis and the battered child syndrome. Report of 2 cases with skeletal involvement. A.J.R. 125: 456–461, 1975.

INGESTED AND INSERTED FOREIGN BODIES AND MATERIALS

Corrosive Substance Ingestion. The most frequently ingested corrosive substance is lye (sodium hydroxide). Lye results in deep, full-thickness thermal burns, causing coagulation necrosis of the entire wall of the hypopharynx and/or esophagus (1, 2, 5, 7, 9, 12). With such extensive tissue necrosis, perforation is not uncommon, and, in this regard, the most devastating corrosives are the highly concentrated liquid corrosives, some of which also contain potassium hydroxide. These substances produce the severest of burns (2, 9, 12), and because of their high specific gravity and slickness, can pass to the stomach with great rapidity. This being the case, it is not uncommon to have the entire esophagus involved and, in addition, to have associated gastric burns. In those cases where granular or pellet corrosives are ingested, focal, upper third, esophageal burns are more common.

Hypopharyngeal burns usually are detected clinically, but on lateral views of the neck, obliteration of the hypopharynx due to thickening of the pharyngeal soft tissues can be seen. In some cases, lye may spill over onto the vocal cords and produce edema of these structures. On chest films, one may note a distended (paralyzed) air-filled esophagus (5, 12) or, if acute esophageal perforation occurs, mediastinal widening, with or without associated pneumomediastinum, pneumopericardium, or pneumatosis of the esophagus (Fig. 3.141). In other cases, tracheoesophageal fistulas (1) or communications to the pericardial sac can be seen (Fig. 3.141). In those patients with gastric burns, air-filled gastric bullae may be seen on plain films of the abdomen (10). This manifestation is associated with the more severe alkali burns to the stomach and probably results from gastric air leaking into the wall of the stomach through damaged mucosa.

Other corrosive fluids ingested include ammonium hydroxide and a variety of acids. These substances, however, unlike sodium and potassium hydroxide, usually do not produce a deep thermal burn to the esophagus; their damage is more superficial. In addition, because acids induce less esophageal and hypopharyngeal muscle spasm than does lye, the child is able to drink more, and because of this, gastric rather than esophageal burns are more common (6, 8, 14, 15). This is especially true of substances such as sulfuric acid which possess a greater degree of slickness and a higher specific gravity. Often the end

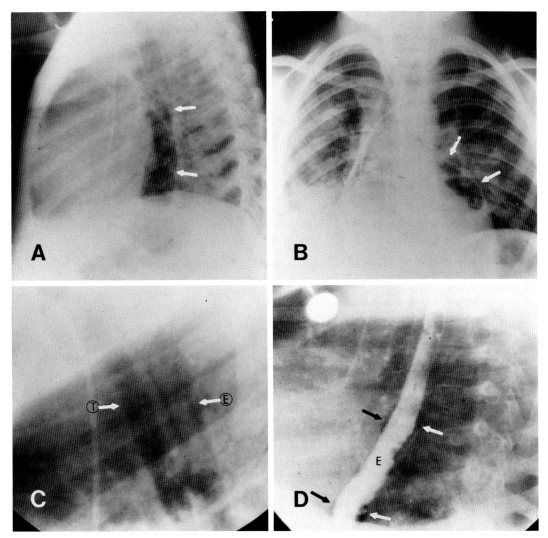

Figure 3.141. *Corrosive esophagitis.* (A) Note the paralyzed, distended, air-filled esophagus (*arrows*). (B) Same patient later with development of pneumopericardium (*arrows*). Also note that the mediastinum is widened, and that numerous infiltrates are present secondary to aspiration. (C) Preliminary barium swallow film demonstrates the trachea (*T*) and dilated, air-filled esophagus (*E*) (*arrows*). The central longitudinal density in the esophagus actually is the esophageal mucosa, and the air around it is due to pneumatosis of the esophagus. (D) Subsequent barium swallow demonstrates the esophageal lumen (*E*) and the presence of pneumatosis of the esophagus (*arrows*). Some contrast material is in the trachea secondary to aspiration.

result is pyloric scarring and stenosis (8, 15). Occasionally, with larger volumes of concentrated acids such as sulphuric acid, gastric wall damage can be more severe and the entire process can involve adjacent organs (4).

Other less common caustic agent burns to the esophagus are those sustained from the ingestion of Clinitest tablets (3) and, more recently, alkaline disk batteries (11, 13, 18). The latter, when impacted for prolonged periods of time, can lead to mucosal ulceration from sheer mechanical erosion, but it also has been determined that in some of these cases hydroxides within the battery are readily liberated into the esophagus and cause focal caustic burns. Interestingly enough, if these batteries pass into the stomach and distal gastrointestinal tract, little, if any, problem arises (13, 18). However, with lodgement in the esophagus, acquired tracheoesophageal fistula can result (16, 17).

The performance of a contrast study of the esophagus is of debatable value in the acute phase of a corrosive fluid ingestion problem. However, if perforation is suspected, a water-soluble contrast agent can be utilized to demonstrate the site of the leak. If no perforation is present, the contrast study of the esophagus shows little more than intense spasm and, in the more severe cases, evidence of mucosal ulceration. After a week or 10 days, a barium swallow can identify potential sites of stricture, for these sites will appear narrow, stiff, and aperistaltic.

REFERENCES

1. Amoury, R.A., Hrabovsky, E.E., Leonidas, J.C., and Holder, T.M.: Tracheoesophageal fistula after lye ingestion. J. Pediatr. Surg. 10: 273–276, 1975.
2. Ashcraft, K.W., and Padula, R.T.: The effect of dilute corrosives on the esophagus. Pediatrics 53: 226–232, 1974.
3. Burrington, J.D.: Clinitest burns of the esophagus. Ann. Thorac. Surg. 20: 400–404, 1975.
4. Canty, T.G., Sr.: Extensive multi-organ necrosis secondary to sulfuric acid ingestion. J. Pediatr. Surg. 23: 848–849, 1988.
5. Franken, E.A., Jr.: Caustic damage of the gastrointestinal tract: Roentgen features. A.J.R. 118: 77–85, 1973.
6. Gillis, D.A., Higgins, G., Kennedy, R.: Gastric damage from ingested acid in children. J. Pediatr. Surg. 20: 494–496, 1985.
7. Haller, J.A., Jr., Andrews, H.G., White, J.J., Tamer, M.A., and Cleveland, W.W.: Pathophysiology and management of acute corrosive burns of the esophagus: Results of treatment in 285 children. J. Pediatr. Surg. 6: 578–584, 1971.
8. Hognestad, J., and Ruud-Hansen, Th.W.: Stenosis of the gastric antrum after sulphuric acid ingestion. Z. Kinderchir. 21: 52–55, 1977.
9. Leape, L.L., Ashcraft, K.W., Scarpelli, D.G., et al.: Hazard to health-liquid lye. N. Engl. J. Med. 284: 578–581, 1971.
10. Levitt, R., Stanley, R.J., and Wise, L.: Gastric bullae: An early roentgen finding in corrosive gastritis following alkali ingestion. Radiology 115: 597–598, 1975.
11. Litovitz, T., and Schmitz, B.F.: Ingestion of cylindrical and button batteries. Pediatrics 89: 747–757, 1992.
12. Martel, W.: Radiologic features of esophagogastritis secondary to extremely caustic agents. Radiology 103: 31–36, 1972.
13. Maves, M.D., Lloyd, T.V., Carithers, J.S.: Radiographic identification of ingested disc batteries. Pediatr. Radiol. 16: 154–156, 1986.
14. Muhletaler, C.A., Gerlock, A.J., Jr., deSoto, L., and Halter, S.A.: Acid corrosive esophagitis: Radiographic findings. A.J.R. 134: 1137–1140, 1980.
15. Pinna, C.D.: Pyloric stenosis from acid burn in a six-year-old girl. Riv. Chir. Pediatr. 9: 384–395, 1967.
16. Sigalet, D., and Lees, G.: Tracheoesophageal injury secondary to disc battery ingestion. J. Pediatr. Surg. 23: 996–998, 1988.
17. Vaishnav, A., and Spitz, L.: Alkaline battery-induced tracheo-oesophageal fistula. Br. J. Surg. 76: 1045, 1989.
18. Votteler, T.P., Nash, J.C., and Rutledge, J.C.: The hazard of ingested alkaline disk batteries in children. J.A.M.A. 249: 2504–2506, 1983.

Ingested Foreign Bodies. Hypopharyngeal foreign bodies have been discussed in Chapter 2, and the discussion of ingested foreign bodies in this section is confined to esophageal, gastric, and intestinal foreign bodies. If such a foreign body is radiolucent, it will not be detected roentgenographically unless secondary signs of inflammation or perforation are present. Among other foreign bodies, this has become a problem with aluminum pop-top tabs from soft drink cans (5, 9, 16, 19, 20). However, it also is a problem with aluminum coins (11) and a wide variety of plastic objects (Fig. 3.142). Opaque foreign bodies, on the other hand, are readily detected roentgenographically (Fig. 3.143), and because of this a roentgenographic survey of the neck, chest, and abdomen is in order, indeed, mandatory (12, 31). This is especially true of infants and young children, for unlike older children, they cannot tell the physician exactly where they think the foreign body has lodged.

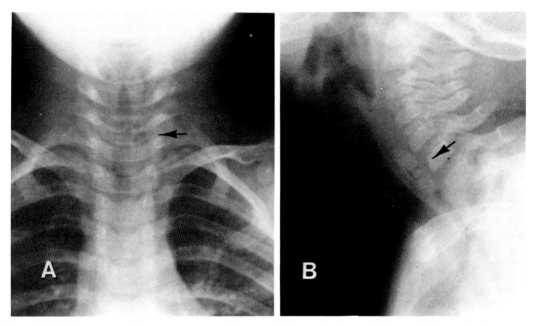

Figure 3.142. *Semiopaque button in upper esophagus.* (**A**) Note the four radiolucent holes in the button (*arrows*), lodged in the upper esophagus. (**B**) Lateral view demonstrates the button (*arrow*) and a mild degree of anterior displacement and compression of the trachea.

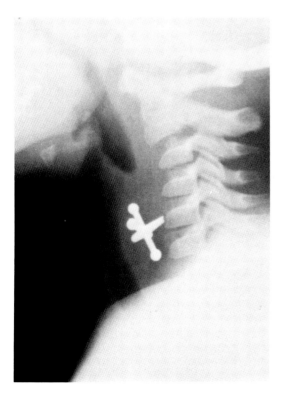

Figure 3.143. *Opaque foreign body (jack) in the upper esophagus.* Note the readily visible opaque jack in the upper esophagus of this infant.

Most round or oval foreign bodies pass down the esophagus into the stomach and through the intestine to cause little if any problem (29). On the other hand, larger or sharp foreign bodies (27) and those of irregular shape may well become impacted somewhere along the course of the GI tract. In the esophagus, foreign bodies commonly lodge at the level of the: (a) cricopharyngeal muscle, (b) aortic knob, or (c) gastroesophageal junction (Fig. 3.144). The least common site is at the gastroesophageal junction. If these foreign bodies are radiopaque they are not difficult to detect, but if they are radiolucent they will go undetected until a barium swallow is obtained. In this regard, many of these children have underlying esophageal strictures secondary to old tracheoesophageal fistula repairs, hiatus hernia problems, or lye burns (Fig. 3.145).

Animal bones impacted in the hypopharynx or esophagus are not as common in children as in adults. However, they still are encountered, and, in this regard, it should be noted that fishbones, although potentially visible (2) (Table 3.1), usually are difficult to visualize with certainty (6). Chicken and turkey bones, on the other hand, often contain enough calcium to allow them to be visible roentgenographically (Fig. 3.146). In those cases where a foreign body such as a fishbone is suspected but not visible, one may administer a cotton ball pledget soaked with barium to the patient. In many of these cases, the pledget becomes impaled on the bone, and thus aids in its localization. However, this maneuver does not work as often as one would first believe.

The misinterpretation of normally calcified laryngeal cartilages for a foreign body such as a chicken or fishbone is not a great problem in childhood. Apart from the hyoid bone, which ossifies early, about the only calcified cartilage presenting such a problem is the calcified cartilage triticei (Fig. 3.147). In teenagers and adults, of

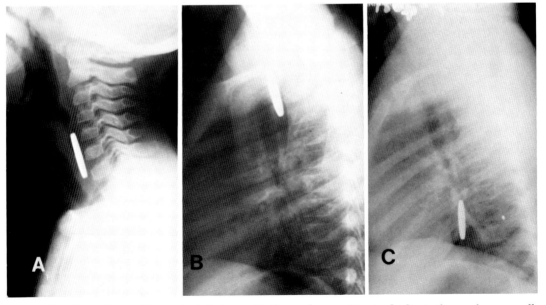

Figure 3.144. *Typical sites of foreign body lodgement in the esophagus.* Foreign bodies in the esophagus usually lodge at one of the following sites: (**A**) just above the level of the cricopharyngeal muscle; (**B**) just above the level of the aortic knob; (**C**) just above the gastroesophageal junction.

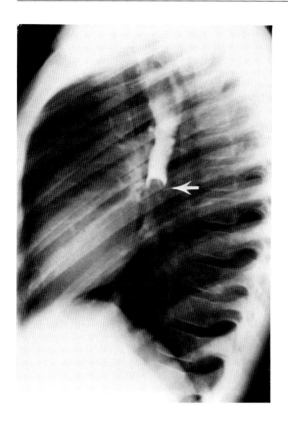

Figure 3.145. *Radiolucent foreign body in the esophagus.* Note the typical curvilinear filling defect (*arrow*) produced by a nonopaque foreign body in this barium-filled esophagus. This patient had underlying esophageal stenosis secondary to an old tracheo-esophageal fistula repair. The obstructing foreign body was a kernel of corn.

Table 3.1
Radiopacity of Bones of Various Fish Species[a]

Fish	No. Bones X-rayed	Definitely Diagnostic	Visible but Poorly Defined	Invisible
Bass	2	2		
Bluefish	4	3		1
Butterfish	3			3
Codfish	5	5		
Flounder	3	3		
Fluke	2	2		
Fresh salmon	4	4		
Gray sole	2	2		
Haddock	2	2		
Halibut	4	4		
Mackerel	4	1		3
Pompano	5		2	3
Porgie	3	3		
Red snapper	2	2		
Sea bass	2	2		
Smelt	1	1		
Smoked salmon	2	2		
Striped bass	2	2		
Trout	3		2	1
White perch	2	2		
Yellow pike	3	3		

[a]Reproduced from Bachman, A. L.: Radiology of fish foreign bodies in the hypopharynx and cervical esophagus. Mt. Sinai J. Med. 48: 212–220, 1981.

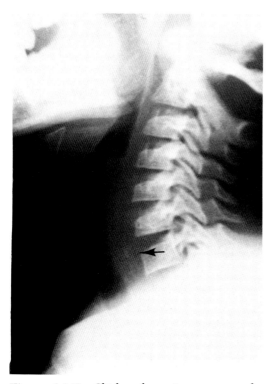

Figure 1.146. *Chicken bone is upper esophagus.* Note faint calcification in a chicken bone (*arrow*) lodged in the upper esophagus of this patient.

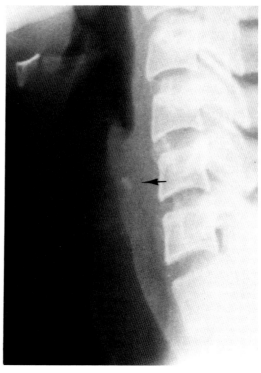

Figure 3.147. *Calcification in the cartilage triticei (arrow)* often is mistaken for an opaque foreign body.

course, laryngeal calcifications are much more common and the problem of differentiating them from an opaque foreign body is much greater.

In the past, removal of coins and other foreign bodies from the esophagus generally had been accomplished endoscopically. More recently, however, Foley catheter removal has become popular (7, 8, 25, 26, 32). When the Foley catheter is utilized, the deflated bulb of the catheter is inflated under fluoroscopic control, and opaque aqueous contrast material is utilized to distend the bulb so that it is visible roentgenographically. After inflation of the bulb, the catheter is withdrawn and the foreign body is retrieved. One must be careful that the patient does not reswallow or inhale the foreign body, and, of course, this procedure should be restricted to for-

eign bodies of recent impaction and to those that are not pointed or impaled in the esophageal wall. In addition, periesophageal edema (see Fig. 3.152) is a contraindication to catheter removal (37), and of course the entire procedure is not without hazard (22). Esophageal perforation always is a potential problem (2, 22). In this regard, an alternate approach has been suggested (1, 4), consisting of pushing the foreign body down into the esophagus rather than pulling it back (Fig. 3.148). Finally, it should be noted that metallic foreign bodies also can be retrieved with a magnet (14, 28, 36, 38, 39).

Those foreign bodies that pass into the stomach can pose a problem in terms of follow-up roentgenograms. However, if the foreign body is small or of such a shape that almost surely it should pass uneventfully,

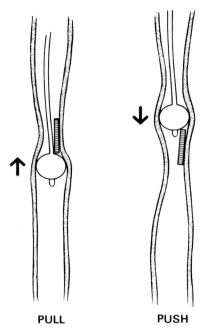

PULL **PUSH**

Figure 3.148. *Foley catheter foreign body removal.* Two methods are available. Pulling the foreign body is more popular, but we have found that pushing the foreign body can be quite productive. (From A.A. Alexander, C.E. Hayden, and L.E. Swischuk: Catheter removal of esophageal foreign bodies: Push or pull? A.J.R. 151: 835, 1988.)

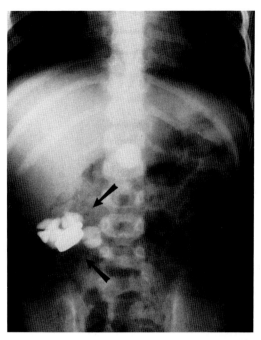

Figure 3.149. *Foreign bodies trapped in duodenal web.* Note numerous opaque foreign bodies on the right (*arrows*). These changed little in position from view to view, and ultimately were demonstrated to be trapped behind a duodenal web. There also is a foreign body in the gastric antrum.

follow-up roentgenograms are not required. On the other hand, should such a foreign body not pass with normal stooling, one might obtain a follow-up roentgenogram on the slight possibility that one might be dealing with an underlying, previously unsuspected, obstructing lesion such as gastric or duodenal web or diverticulum (18, 21) (Fig. 3.149). Obviously, this is a more remote consideration, but still one to considered under the proper circumstances.

The problem is quite different with the pointed, jagged, or long foreign body (27), for impaction of this type of foreign body is more common. Follow-up roentgenograms are most important in these cases, and if the foreign body fails to make progress or, even more significantly, if it does not change its position at all, one should suspect impaction and consider surgical intervention (Fig. 3.150). Another time when a foreign body may cease to make progress is when it lodges in the appendix. In some of these cases, no symptoms arise (17), but in others acute appendicitis eventually may develop.

Finally, it should be noted that ***upper esophageal foreign bodies can present with stridor or pneumonia*** and little in the way of dysphagia (3, 10, 13, 16, 23, 24, 30, 33–35). Many of these patients are young infants, and they seem to adapt to the esophageal obstruction with deceptive ease. They do this primarily by changing their diet to a more acceptable liquid one. ***Such a change often is so subtle that it eludes the parent and physician, and overall the presenting symptoms will cause one to focus on the respiratory tract (i.e., stridor,*** *wheezing, cough, etc.).* It is only with the knowledge that this can occur, and adequate examination of the lateral neck, chest, and esophagus that many of these foreign bodies are finally discovered (Fig. 3.151). In some cases ulceration or actual perforation of the esophagus eventually results (15, 33). However, initially only periesophageal edema occurs, and it is in-teresting to see how quickly such edema can develop. It is this edema that pro-duces compression of the adjacent trachea and often is still present after the foreign body has been removed (Fig. 3.152). Such edema, when present, con-stitutes a contraindication to removal of the foreign body with a Foley cath-eter (37).

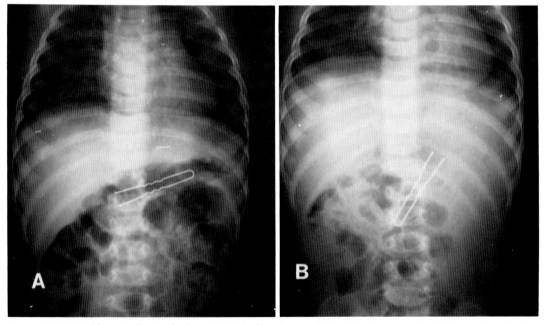

Figure 3.150. *Problematic foreign body.* (**A**) Early film showing hairpin in the stomach. (**B**) Later film showing complete change in position of the pin which thereafter remained lodged at this site. At laparotomy this turned out to be at the duodenal-jejunal junction.

Figure 3.151. *Upper esophageal foreign body presenting with stridor.* (**A**) Note the overdistended hypopharynx and upper trachea in this young infant presenting with stridor. Also note that the trachea below the level of the clavicles is narrowed (*arrows*). (**B**) With the neck fully extended, a semiopaque foreign body is demonstrated in the upper esophagus (*arrow*). The site of this foreign body corresponds to the site of tracheal narrowing noted in (**A**). (**C**) Barium swallow demonstrates the foreign body (*solid arrow*) in the esophagus and the deep anterior ulcer which it produced (*open arrow*). It is easy to see why this portion of the trachea appeared narrowed on the other studies. (Reprinted with permission from P.C. Smith, L.E. Swischuk, and C.J. Fagan: An elusive and often unsuspected cause of stridor or pneumonia [the esophageal foreign body]. A.J.R. 122: 80–89, 1974.)

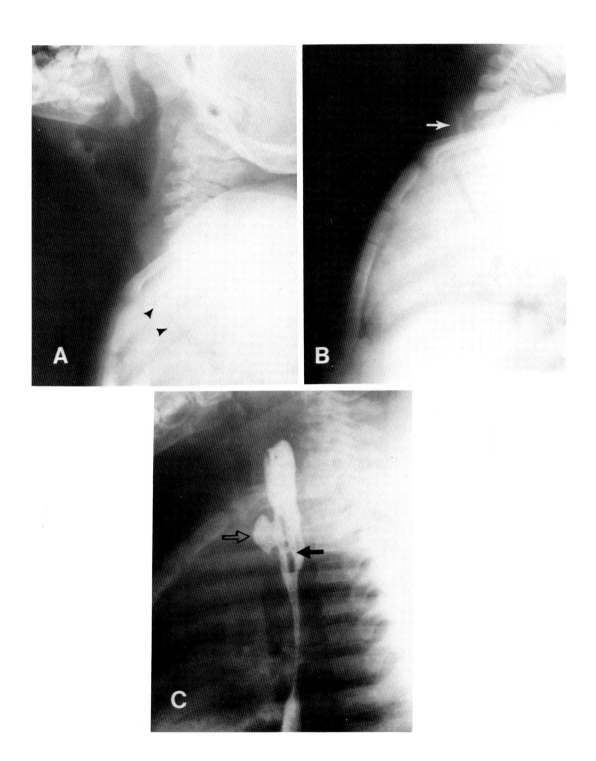

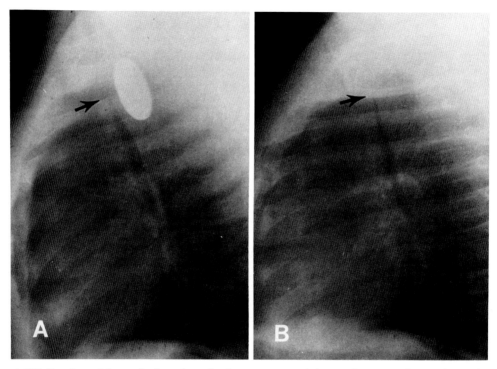

Figure 3.152. *Esophageal foreign body with tracheal compression.* (A) Note the coin in the esophagus (*arrow*). Also note that the trachea just adjacent to it is narrowed. This is due to periesophageal edema. (B) After removal of the coin, the trachea still is narrowed (*arrow*).

REFERENCES

1. Alexander, A.A., Hayden, C.K., and Swischuk, L.E.: Catheter removal of esophageal foreign bodies: Push or pull? A.J.R. 151: 835, 1988.
2. Bachman, A.L.: Radiology of fish foreign bodies in the hypopharynx and cervical esophagus. Mt. Sinai J. Med. 48: 212–220, 1981.
3. Beer, S., Avidan, G., Viure, E., and Starinsky, R.: A foreign body in the oesophagus as a cause of respiratory distress. Pediatr. Radiol. 12: 41–42, 1982.
4. Bonadio, W.A., Zona, J.Z., Glicklich, M., and Cohen, R.: Esophageal bougienage technique for coin ingestion in children. J. Pediatr. Surg. 23: 917–918, 1988.
5. Burrington, J.D.: Aluminum pop-tops: A hazard to child health. J.A.M.A. 235: 2614–2617, 1976.
6. Campbell, D.R., Brown, S.J., and Manchester, J.A.: An evaluation of the radio-opacity of various ingested foreign bodies in the pharynx and esophagus. J. Can. Assoc. Radiol. 19: 183–186, 1968.
7. Campbell, J.B., Quattromani, F.L., and Foley, L.C.: Foley catheter removal of blunt esophageal foreign bodies. Experience with 100 consecutive children. Pediatr. Radiol. 13: 116–119, 1983.
8. Carlson, D.H.: Removal of coins in the esophagus using a Foley catheter. Pediatrics 50: 475–476, 1972.
9. Eggbli, K.D., Potter, B.M., Garcia, V., Altman, R.P., and Breckbill, D.L.: Delayed diagnosis of esophageal perforation by aluminum foreign bodies. Pediatr. Radiol. 16: 511–513, 1986.
10. Glas, W.M., and Goodman, M.: Unsuspected foreign bodies in the young child's esophagus presenting with respiratory symptoms. Laryngoscope 76: 605, 1966.
11. Heller, R.M., Reichelderfer, T.E., Dorst, J.P., and Oh, K.S.: The problem with replacement of copper pennies by aluminum pennies. Pediatrics 54: 684–688, 1974.
12. Hodge, D., III, Techlenburg, F., and Fleisher, G.: Coin ingestion: Does every child need a radiograph? Ann. Emerg. Med. 14: 443–446, 1985.
13. Humphry, A., and Holland, W.G.: Unsuspected esophageal foreign bodies. J. Can. Assoc. Radiol. 32: 17–20, 1981.
14. Ito, Y., Ihara, N., and Sohma, S.: Magnetic re-

moval of alkaline batteries from the stomach. J. Pediatr. Surg. 20: 3: 250–251, 1985.

15. Janik, J.S., Bailey, W.C., and Burrington, J.D.: Occult coin perforation of the esophagus. J. Pediatr. Surg. 21: 794–797, 1986.

16. Jeffers, R.G., Weir, M.R., Wehunt, W.D., and Carter, S.C.: Pull-tab the foreign body sleeper. J. Pediatr. 92: 1023–1024, 1978.

17. Kassner, E.G., Mutchler, R.W., Jr., Klotz, D.H., Jr., and Rose, J.S.: Uncomplicated foreign bodies of the appendix in children: Radiologic observations. J. Pediatr. Surg. 9: 207–211, 1974.

18. Kassner, E.G., Rose, J.S., Kottmeier, P.K., Schneider, M., and Gallow, G.M.: Retention of a small foreign object in the stomach and duodenum: A sign of partial obstruction caused by duodenal anomalies. Radiology 114: 683–686, 1975.

19. Keating, J.P., Weldon, C.S., Connors, J.P., and McAlister, W.H.: The "pop-top" tab. J. Pediatr. 86: 111–112, 1975.

20. Levick, R.K., Spitz, L., and Robinson, A.: The "invisible" can top. Br. J. Radiol. 50: 596, 1977.

21. Mandell, G.A., Rosenberg, H.K., and Schnaufer, L.: Prolonged retention of foreign bodies in the stomach. Pediatrics 60: 460–462, 1977.

22. Myer, C.M., III: Potential hazards of esophageal foreign body extraction. Pediatr. Radiol. 21: 97–98, 1991.

23. Naftzger, J.B., and Gittens, T.R.: Foreign bodies in esophagus with respiratory symptoms complicating diagnosis. Laryngoscope 36: 370–376, 1926.

24. Newman, D.E.: The radiolucent esophageal foreign body: An often forgotten cause of respiratory symptoms. J. Pediatr. 92: 60–63, 1978.

25. Nixon, G.W.: Foley catheter method of esophageal foreign body removal: Extension of applications. A.J.R. 132: 441–442, 1979.

26. Ong, T.H.: Removal of blunt oesophageal foreign bodies in children using a Foley catheter. Aust. Paediatr. J. 18: 60–62, 1982.

27. Paul, R.I., and Jaffe, D.M.: Sharp object ingestions in children: Illustrative cases and literature review. Pediatr. Emerg. Care 4: 245–248, 1988.

28. Paulson, E.K., and Jaffe, R.B.: Metallic foreign bodies in the stomach: Fluoroscopic removal with a magnetic orogastric tube. Radiology 174: 191–194, 1990.

29. Pellerin, D., Fortier-Baeulieu, M., and Gueguen, J.: The fate of swallowed foreign bodies: Experience of 1250 instances of sub-diaphragmatic foreign bodies in children. In Progress in Pediatric Radiology, H.J. Kaufman (ed.), pp. 286–302. Year Book, Chicago, 1969.

30. Schidlow, D.V., Palmer, J., Balsara, R.K., Trutz, M.G., and Williams, J.L.: Chronic stridor and anterior cervical "mass" secondary to an esopha-

geal foreign body. Am. J. Dis. Child. 135: 869–870, 1981.

31. Schunk, J.E., Corneli, H., and Bolte, R.: Pediatric coin ingestions. Am. J. Dis. Child. 143: 546–548, 1989.

32. Shackelford, G.D., McAlister, W.H., and Robertson, C.L.: The use of a Foley catheter for removal of blunt esophageal foreign bodies from children. Radiology 105: 455–456, 1972.

33. Smith, P.C., Swischuk, L.E., and Fagan, C.J.: An elusive and often unsuspected cause of stridor or pneumonia (the esophageal foreign body). A.J.R. 122: 80–89, 1974.

34. Spitz, L., and Hirsig, J.: Prolonged foreign body impaction in the oesophagus. Arch. Dis. Child. 57: 551–553, 1982.

35. Tauscher, J.W.: Esophageal foreign body: An uncommon cause of stridor. Pediatrics 61: 657–658, 1978.

36. Towbin, R.B., Dunbar, J.S., and Rice, S.: Technical note. Magnet catheter for removal of magnetic foreign bodies. A.J.R. 154: 149–150, 1990.

37. Towbin, R., Lederman, H.M., Dunbar, J.S., Ball, W.S., and Strife, J.L.: Esophageal edema as a predictor of unsuccessful balloon extraction of esophageal foreign body. Pediatr. Radiol. 19: 359–360, 1989.

38. Volle, E., Hanel, D., Beyer, P., and Kaufmann, H.J.: Ingested foreign bodies: Removal by magnet. Radiology 160: 407–409, 1986.

39. Volle, E., Beyer, P., and Kaufmann, H.J.: Therapeutic approach to ingested button-type batteries: Magnetic removal of ingested button-type batteries. Pediatr. Radiol. 19: 114–118, 1989.

Miscellaneous Ingested Foreign Bodies and Substances. Pills or capsules are usually not identified unless they contain substances such as iron or calcium (1, 7, 8), and in such cases they may be seen, but not always clearly (4), on abdominal films (Fig. 3.153). This is important, for *iron intoxication* is not uncommon in children and can result in extensive gastrointestinal damage with bleeding, necrosis, and perforation (1, 5–8). *Pica in childhood* most often is accounted for by the eating of dirt or clay (1, 3). In these children, flecks of opaque material can be seen scattered throughout the GI tract, while in other cases actual pebbles may be noted (Fig. 3.154). Of course, fragments of *lead paint* also can be seen on roentgenograms and

Figure 3.153. *Iron tablet inges-*
tion. Note numerous, opaque tablets
scattered in the abdomen of this toxic infant with iron tablet ingestion.

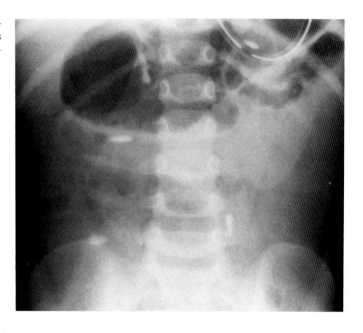

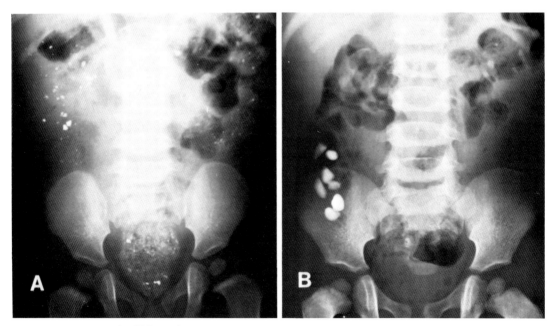

Figure 3.154. *Dirt and pebbles in the GI tract.* (**A**) Note scattered opacities throughout the GI tract in this patient. A good many of them are mixed with fecal material in the colon. Similar findings can be seen with lead
poisoning, but most often the findings represent those of dirt eating. (**B**) Note pebbles in the cecum of this patient.

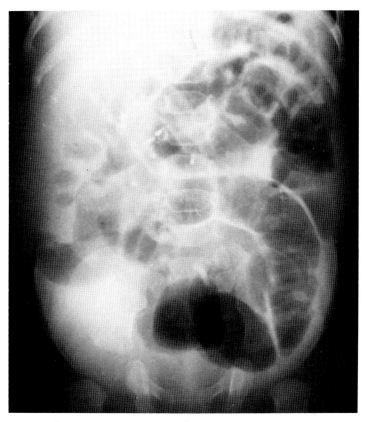

Figure 3.155. *Opacities in the GI tract in a patient with gastroenteritis.* Note numerous opacities in the distended intestines of this infant with gastroenteritis. Such opacities are common in these patients and represent bismuth in certain antacid preparations.

occasionally such infants will present in the emergency room with acute lead intoxication. Acute lead intoxication also has been seen with a North American Indian medicine known as Azarcon, utilized for a variety of illnesses (2).

Another opaque substance sometimes encountered in the emergency room setting is a bismuth-containing antacid. Such medications frequently are administered for gastroenteritis and commonly show up as irregular opacities in the intestines of these children (Fig. 3.155). Other foreign materials include dental fillings, teeth, mercury, plaster, erasers, modeling clay, and bubble gum (1, 5).

Finally, an interesting recent study has shown that a significant number of patients who ingest foreign bodies have increased lead levels in the blood (9). This emphasizes the concept that some infants and children simply are chronic ingestors of foreign materials, and that among these materials may be lead.

REFERENCES

1. Alexander, W.J., Kadish, J.A., and Dunbar, J.S.: Ingested foreign bodies in children. In *Progress in Pediatric Radiology*, H.J. Kaufmann (ed.), pp. 256–285. Year Book, Chicago, 1969.
2. Bose, A., Vashistha, K., and O'Loughlin, B.J.: Azarcon por Empancho: Another cause of lead toxicity. Pediatrics 72: 106–108, 1983.
3. Clayton, R.S., and Goodman, P.H.: Roentgenographic diagnosis of geophagia (dirt eating). A.J.R. 73: 203, 1955.
4. Everson, G.W., Oudjhane, J., Young, L.W., and Krenzelok, E.P.: Effectiveness of abdominal radiographs in visualizing chewable iron supple-

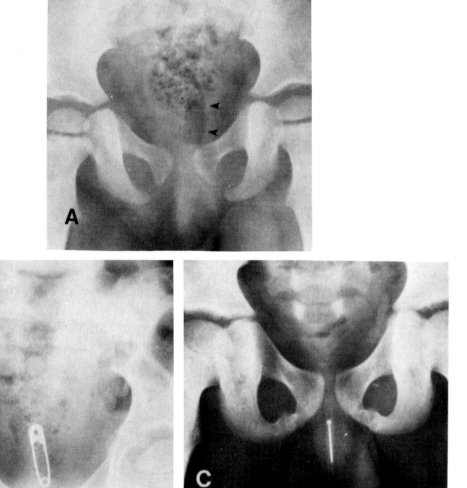

Figure 3.156. *Genitourinary foreign bodies.* (*A*) Note the radiolucent (plastic pen cap) foreign body (*arrows*) in the vagina of this girl. (*B*) Closed safety pin in the bladder of another girl. (*C*) Straight pin in the urethra of a young boy.

ments following overdose. Am. J. Emerg. Med. 7: 459–463, 1989.

5. Geller, E., and Smergel, E.M.: Bubble gum simulating abdominal calcifications. Pediatr. Radiol. 22: 298–299, 1992.

6. Gleason, W.A., Jr., de Mello, D.E., de Castro, F.J., and Connors, J.J.: Acute hepatic failure in severe iron poisoning. J. Pediatr. 95: 138–140, 1979.

7. Knott, L.H., and Miller, R.C.: Acute iron intoxication with intestinal infarction. J. Pediatr. Surg. 13: 720–721, 1978.

8. Smith, W.L., Franken, E.A., Jr., Grosfeld, J.L., and Ballantine, T.V.N.: Radiological quiz. Radiology 122: 192, 1977.

9. Staple, T.W., and McAlister, W.H.: Roentgenographic visualization of iron preparation in the gastrointestinal tract. Radiology 83: 1051, 1964.

10. Wiley, J.R., II, Henretig, F.M., and Selbst, S.M.: Blood lead levels in children with foreign bodies. Pediatrics 89: 593–596, 1992.

Genitourinary Foreign Bodies. Genitourinary foreign bodies (1, 2) inserted by the patient are more common than is generally appreciated. In girls, these foreign bodies often are inserted into the vagina, and occasionally they are demonstrable on plain films (Fig. 3.156). Urinary bladder foreign bodies also can be encountered in girls, but in boys one more often encounters such foreign bodies in the urethra (Fig. 3.156C). Patients with these foreign bodies can present with hematuria and/or urinary tract infection.

REFERENCES

1. Paradise, J.E., and Willis, E.D.: Probability of vaginal foreign body in girls with genital complaints. Am. J. Dis. Child. 139: 472–478, 1985.

2. Swischuk, L.E.: Acute, non-traumatic, genitourinary pediatric problems. Radiol. Clin. North Am. 16: 147–157, 1978.

MISCELLANEOUS ABDOMINAL PROBLEMS

Bezoars. Bezoars most frequently occur in the stomach, (1–3, 7, 10, 13) but in some cases also may be seen in the small bowel. Most likely, these latter instances represent cases wherein portions of the gastric bezoar break off and pass into the small intestine. Once a bezoar enters the small bowel, obstruction with or without intussusception (4, 9) may occur (Fig. 3.157).

The most common bezoar in childhood is a trichobezoar resulting from ingestion of hair, usually from the patient's own head. While usually considered to be the result of psychiatric difficulties, iron deficiency, much as with clay eating, has also been shown to be a potential contributing factor (8). Next most common is a phytobezoar, but currently in very young infants, lactobezoars are more common (2, 5, 6, 11, 12, 14). In these instances, a dense milk coagulation results when powdered milk is mixed with inadequate amounts of water. It is especially likely to occur in premature infants. Bezoars secondary to persimmon seed ingestion are not as common in childhood as in adulthood. In this type of bezoar, the protein material of the persimmon, after being acted upon by gastric acid, is converted to a shellac-like substance.

Plain film findings of a gastric bezoar consist of amorphous, granular, or at times whirlpool-like configurations of solid and gaseous material in the stomach (Fig. 3.157A). In other instances, the bezoar is so compact that a layer of air is seen to surround it (Fig. 3.157B). Barium studies confirm the presence of a bezoar and the presence of a gastric ulcer if such a complication is present. On plain films, bezoars must be differentiated from food in the stomach.

On ultrasound, the echogenic arc of air between the bezoar and gastric wall is characteristic (7, 10). In addition, an actual mass can be seen if fluid is administered to these patients (Fig. 3.158). CT also can demonstrate these masses very vividly (10).

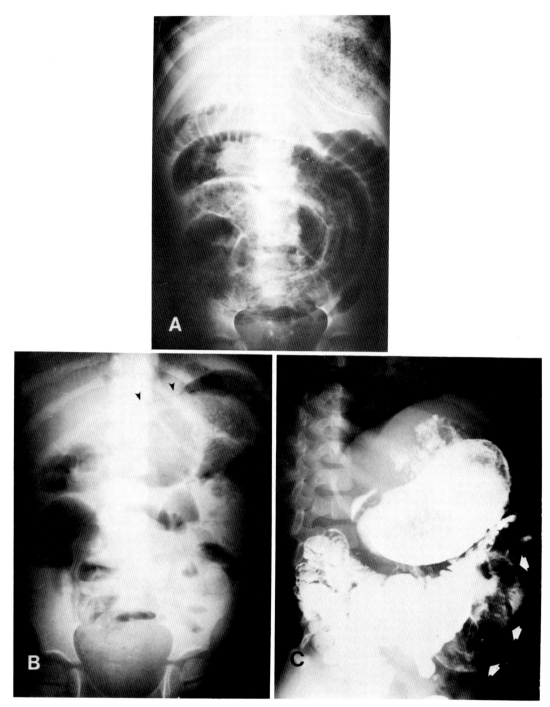

Figure 3.157. *Bezoars.* (*A*) Note the granular appearance of a bezoar in the stomach (*left upper quadrant*). Also note the presence of a classic small bowel obstruction and numerous granular, linear, and curvilinear densities within the small bowel. This patient had a large bezoar, part of which had become detached to produce a small bowel obstruction. (*B*) Another bezoar somewhat less well defined. However, note the thin rim of air trapped between it and the gastric wall (*arrows*). (*C*) Subsequent GI series demonstrates the large bezoar in the stomach, but in addition, note that a portion of it has become detached and is present in the distal small bowel (*arrows*). It was causing a moderate degree of obstruction.

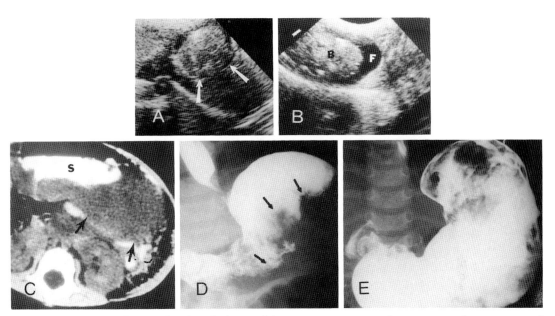

Figure 3.158. *Bezoar: ultrasound and CT findings.* (*A*) Transverse sonogram demonstrates echogenic material in the stomach (*arrows*). (*B*) With a little fluid (*F*) added to the stomach, the echogenic bezoar (*B*) is clearly visualized. (*C*) In this patient, an abdominal mass (*arrows*) displacing the stomach (*S*) was believed to be present. (*D*) Subsequent GI series demonstrates large, nodular filling defects in the stomach (*arrows*). (*E*) With the patient now in prone condition, barium coats the entire large nodular bezoar.

REFERENCES

1. DeBackey, M., and Ochsner, A.: Bezoars and concretions. Surgery 5: 132–160, 1939.
2. Grosfeld, J.L., Schreiner, R.L., Franken, E.A., Lemons, J.A., Ballantine, T.V.N., Weber, T.R., and Gresham, E.L.: The changing pattern of gastrointestinal bezoars in infants and children. Surgery 88: 425–432, 1980.
3. Eshel, G., Broide, E., and Azizi, E.: Phytobezoar following raisin ingestion in children. Pediatr. Emerg. Care 4: 192–193, 1988.
4. Harris, V.J., and Hanley, G.: Unusual features and complications of bezoars in children. A.J.R. 123: 742–745, 1975.
5. Levkoff, A.H., Gadsden, R.H., Hennigar, G.R., and Webb, C.M.: Lactobezoar and gastric perforation in a neonate. J. Pediatr. 77: 875–877, 1970.
6. Majd, M., and LoPresti, J.M.: Lactobezoar. A.J.R. 116:575–576, 1972.
7. McCracken, S., Jongeward, R., Silver, T.M. and Jafri, Z.H.: Gastric trichobezoar: Sonographic findings. Radiology 161: 123–124, 1986.
8. McGehee, F.T., Jr., and Buchanan, G.R.: Trichophagia and trichobezoar: Etiologic role of iron deficiency. J. Pediatr. 97: 946–948, 1980.
9. Mehta, M.H., and Patel, R.V.: Intussusception and perforations caused by multiple trichobezoars. J. Pediatr. Surg. 27: 1234–1235, 1992.
10. Newman, B., and Girdany, B.R.: Gastric trichobezoars: Sonographic and computed tomographic appearance. Pediatr. Radiol. 20: 526–527, 1990.
11. Singer, J.I.: Lactobezoar causing an abdominal triad of colicky pain, emesis and mass. Pediatr. Emerg. Care 4: 194–196, 1988.
12. Wexler, H.A., and Poole, C.A.: Lactobezoar, a complication of overconcentrated mild formula. J. Pediatr. Surg. 11: 261–262, 1976.
13. Wholey, M.H., Zikria, E.A., and Mansoor, M.: Instrument for the removal of a gastric bezoar. Acta Radiol. 15: 333–336, 1974.
14. Wolf, R.S., and Bruce, J.: Gastrotomy for lactobezoar in a newborn infant. J. Pediatr. 54: 811–812, 1959.

Abdominal Ascariasis. Ascariasis may be encountered as an incidental finding, but in other cases intestinal obstruction or even intestinal perforation can occur (1, 7, 9, 10). In addition, during the early phase

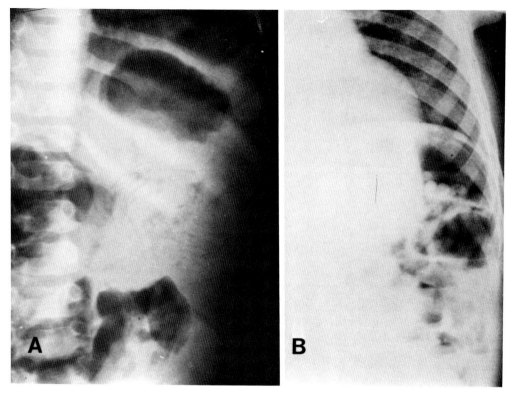

Figure 3.159. *Abdominal ascariasis.* (*A*) Note the whirlpool-like effect of worms in the intestines on the left side of the abdomen. (*B*) Another patient demonstrating worms visualized in air-filled loops of intestine.

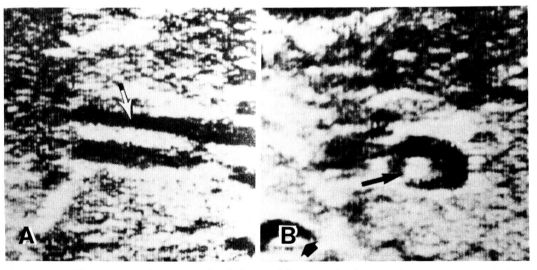

Figure 3.160. *Biliary ascaris: ultrasonographic findings.* (*A*) Longitudinal section demonstrating a dilated common bile duct with a worm in the center (*arrow*). (*B*) Cross-section demonstrating the bull's-eye sign with the echogenic worms in the center (*arrows*) of the dilated bile duct. (From G.G. Cerri, G.J. Leite, J.B. Simoes, D.J.C. DaRocha, F.P. Albuquerque, M.C.C. Machado, and A. Magalhaes: Ultrasonographic evaluation of ascaris in the biliary tract. Radiology 146: 753–754, 1983.)

of the infection, larvae can pass through the lymphatic system or portal system to the right side of the heart and be filtered out in the lungs, causing nonspecific infiltrates. Respiratory distress may be the presenting symptom in these patients (7).

On abdominal roentgenograms (2, 4, 6, 7), the adult *Ascaris* worm can be seen as a linear or circular filling defect in a loop of dilated bowel, but more commonly infestation is massive and a whirlpool, bezoar-like mass of linear, opaque, and radiolucent shadows is seen (Fig. 3.159). If barium is administered, the worms will ingest the barium and can be identified by the linear collections of barium in their GI tracts. *Ascaris* infection of the biliary system and pancreatic ducts also can occur, but is relatively rare. The findings in these cases are readily demonstrable with ultrasound (3, 5, 8). The worm in the dilated bile ducts is echogenic and produces a bull's-eye configuration (Fig. 3.160).

REFERENCES

1. Bar-Maor, J.A., deCarvalho, J.L.A.F., and Chappell, J.: Gastrografin treatment of intestinal obstruction due to *Ascaris lumbricoides*. J. Pediatr. Surg. 19: 174–176, 1984.
2. Bean, W.J.: Recognition of ascariasis by routine chest or abdomen roentgenograms. A.J.R. 94: 379–384, 1965.
3. Cerri, G.G., Leite, G.J., Simoes, J.B., DaRocha, D.J.C., Albuquerque, F.P., Machado, M.C.C., and Magalhaes, A.: Ultrasonographic evaluation of ascaris in the biliary tract. Radiology 146: 753–754, 1983.
4. Cremin, B.J., and Fisher, R.M.: Biliary ascariasis in children. A.J.R. 126: 352–357, 1976.
5. Cremin, B.J.: Ultrasonographic diagnosis of biliary ascariasis: "A bull's eye in the triple O." Br. J. Radiol. 55: 683–684, 1982.
6. Isaacs, I.: Roentgenographic demonstration of intestinal ascariasis in children without using barium. A.J.R. 76: 558–561, 1956.
7. Litt, R.E., Altman, D.H., and Greenberg, L.A.: Radiologic evaluation of the common parasitic diseases of childhood. South. Med. J. 62: 773–778, 1969.
8. Price, J., and Leung, J.W.C.: Ultrasound diagnosis of Ascaris lumbricoides in the pancreatic duct: The "four-lines" sign. Br. J. Radiol. 61: 411–413, 1988.
9. Rode, H., Cullis, S., and Millar, A.: Abdominal complications of Ascaris lumbricoides in children. Pediatr. Surg. Int. 5: 397–401, 1990.
10. Surendran, N., and Paulose, M.O.: Intestinal complications of round worms in children. J. Pediatr. Surg. 23: 931–935, 1988.

Abdominal Masses, Tumors, and Pseudotumors. Abdominal masses in the emergency setting are not a particularly common problem. However, occasionally, with hemorrhage into a tumor, trauma to a hydronephrotic kidney, etc., acute abdominal pain may be the presenting problem, and in such cases, ultrasonography is the most rewarding screening procedure (2–4). Although certain information can be obtained from plain films, ultrasonography usually provides ready information regarding whether the lesion is solid or cystic and its precise location (Fig. 3.161). CT scanning also can be utilized, but ultrasound usually is the first imaging modality employed.

In the emergency patient, one of the most commonly encountered problems is that of a normal structure presenting as a pseudotumor on abdominal roentgenograms. These so-called "pseudotumors" are quite common, and among the most common are the distended urinary bladder and the fluid-filled fundus or antrum of the stomach. The fluid-filled fundus appears as a soft tissue "tumor" in the left upper quadrant, while the fluid-filled antrum produces a similar configuration just to the right of the upper lumbar spine (1). In children, another type of pseudotumor occasionally is produced by a peculiar configuration of the stomach on upright view (Fig. 3.162). Pseudotumors anywhere in the abdomen can be seen as a result of fortuitous visualization of fluid-filled loops of normal intestine. Finally, it should be mentioned that one of the most common pseudotumors in infancy is that produced by an umbilical hernia (Fig. 3.163).

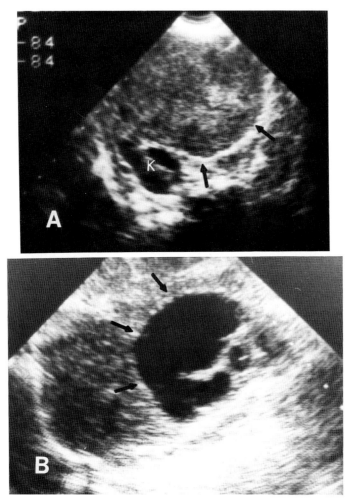

Figure 3.161. *Abdominal masses: ultrasound.* (**A**) Solid Wilm's tumor (*arrows*) in patient with abdominal pain and hematuria; compressed kidney (*K*). (**B**) Classic ureteropelvic junction obstruction (*arrows*) in patient with abdominal trauma and hematuria.

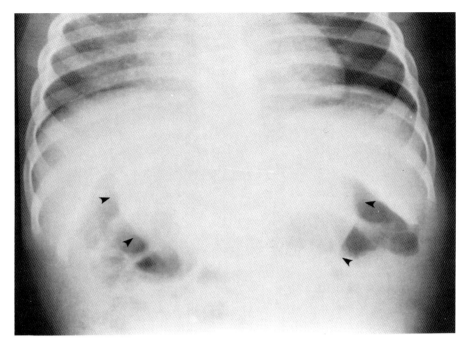

Figure 3.162. *Gastric pseudotumor.* Note the fluid-filled stomach presenting as a peculiar midabdominal pseudotumor (*arrows*). The *arrows on the right* outline the fluid-filled antrum, while those on the *left* outline the fluid-filled body. This configuration almost always is seen on upright views.

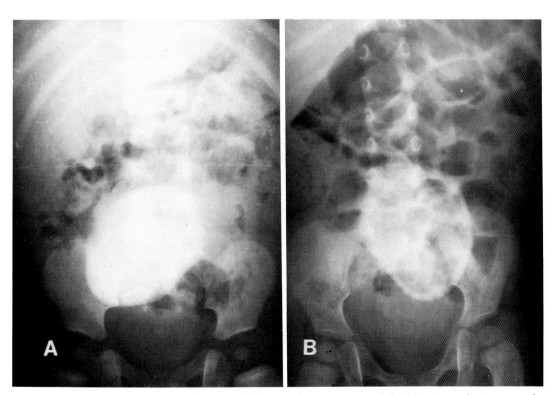

Figure 3.163. *Umbilical hernia: pseudotumor.* (**A**) Note a large opaque umbilical hernia producing a pseudotumor in the midabdomen. (**B**) Similar appearance in another patient, but this time the umbilical hernia contains air-filled loops of intestine.

REFERENCES

1. Balthazar, E.: Right upper quadrant pseudotumor, a fluid-filled viscus. Radiology 112: 11–12, 1974.
2. Goldberg, B.B., Capitanio, M.A., and Kirkpatrick, J.A.: Ultrasonic evaluation of masses in pediatric patients. A.J.R. 116: 677–684, 1972.
3. Goldberg, B.B., Pollack, H.M., Capitanio, M.A., and Kirkpatrick, J.A.: Ultrasonography: An aid in the diagnosis of masses in pediatric patients. Pediatrics 56: 421–428, 1975.
4. Stuber, J.L., Leonidas, J.C., and Holder, T.M.: Abdominal ultrasonography in pediatrics. Am. J. Dis. Child. 129: 1096–1101, 1975.

Rectus Sheath and Psoas Muscle Hematomas. Hematomas of the abdominal wall in the rectus muscle can present with acute abdominal pain and may be mistaken for conditions such as appendicitis or cholecystitis. In other cases, they may be mistaken for an abdominal mass. Because the abdomen often is so tense in these patients that physical examination is difficult to accomplish, ultrasonography has become the best modality with which to demonstrate these hematomas (1, 2). Psoas muscle hematomas are less common but can be seen with trauma and in hemophiliacs. They are demonstrable with ultrasound and CT (Fig. 3.164). Hematomas

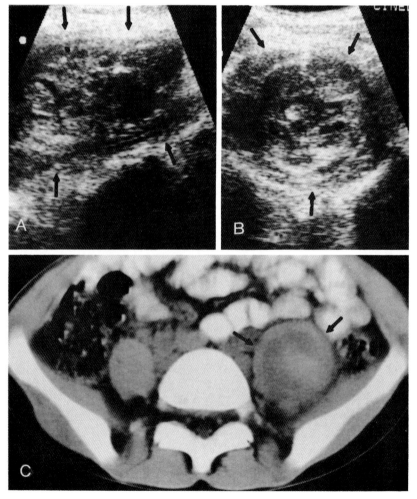

Figure 3.164. *Psoas hematoma.* (*A*) Longitudinal ultrasonogram demonstrates a large, heterogeneous mass (*arrows*) in the left psoas muscle. (*B*) Cross-sectional view of the same mass. (*C*) CT study demonstrates the enlarged left psoas muscle (*arrows*) and the hypodense hematoma within it. This patient was a hemophiliac.

are echogenic on ultrasound in their early stages, but as they mature and liquify, they become more anechoic.

REFERENCES

1. Benson, M.: Rectus sheath haematomas simulating pelvic pathology: The ultrasound appearances. Clin. Radiol. 33: 651–655, 1982.
2. Kaftori, J.K., Rosenberger, A., Pollack, S., and Fish, J.H.: Rectus sheath hematoma: Ultrasonographic diagnosis. A.J.R. 128: 283–285, 1977.

Abdominal Calcifications. Overall, abdominal calcifications are not particularly common in children, but one must realize the significance of those that are seen from time to time. In this regard, one of the most common *incidental calcification* found in the abdomen of a child is that *in the adrenal gland* (5). Such calcifications usually result from a previous, but often undocumented, neonatal adrenal hemorrhage, and when seen in the older child are of no clinical significance. Characteristically, the calcification lies above the kidney and is of triangular or near-triangular shape (Fig. 3.165A). Another innocuous calcification in the abdomen is the so-called "mulberry" or "popcorn" type calcification of old, inflamed mesenteric or retroperitoneal lymph nodes (Fig. 3.165B). Old healed tuberculosis or histoplasmosis often causes round, punctate,

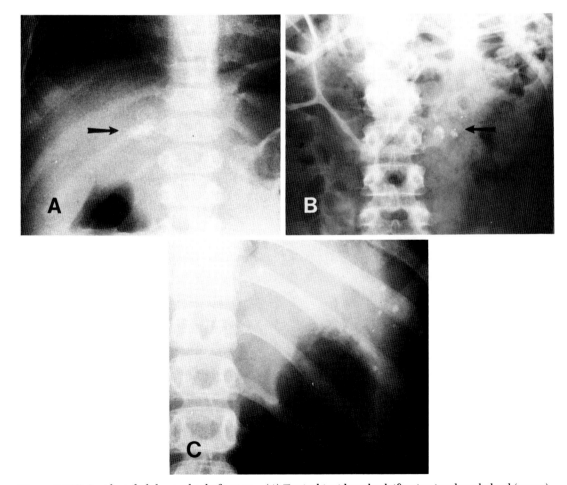

Figure 3.165. *Incidental abdominal calcification.* (A) Typical incidental calcification in adrenal gland (*arrow*). (B) Typical mulberry calcification in retroperitoneal lymph nodes (*arrow*). (C) Typical punctate calcification in the spleen. These calcifications often are secondary to healed histoplasmosis or tuberculosis.

frequently multiple calcifications in the liver or spleen (Fig. 3.165C).

Urinary tract calcifications are not as common in children as in adults, but they do occur (1–4, 7, 10, 11). Although in the past such calcifications usually were considered secondary to some type of metabolic disease, it is becoming increasingly apparent that most are due to other causes, including infection and idiopathic causes (10). Bladder calculi are seen in patients with neurogenic disease and in other chronically immobilized patients. However, in the emergency patient, the urinary tract calcification of most concern is the calcified renal calculus producing *renal colic* (see p. 276).

Diffuse calcifications such as those seen with renal tubular acidosis, oxalosis, and chronic glomerulonephritis and those resulting from renal cortical and medullary necrosis are seldom encountered other than as incidental findings or in patients presenting with renal failure.

Pancreatic calcifications usually are midabdominal and irregular, but on the whole are uncommon in childhood. They can be seen in cystic fibrosis, pancreatitis, and in association with protein malnutrition (6, 9). They usually are stippled and frequently outline the entire pancreas. Calcification of an *appendiceal fecalith* is of clear-cut significance and is dealt with under the section on appendicitis. Calcification of a *stone in a Meckel's diverticulum* is uncommon, but can mimic an appendiceal fecalith. *Other* abdominal calcifications may occur in teratomas, hemangiomatous tumors of the liver or other organs, hamartomas of the liver, and tumors of the adrenal glands such as neuroblastomas or adrenal cortical carcinoma. Massive calcification of a large adrenal gland is seen in Wolman's disease (8), and curvilinear or amorphous abdominal calcifications are seen with meconium peritonitis. Calcified phleboliths in the pelvis are not common in the pediatric population.

REFERENCES

1. Bennett, A.H., and Colodny, A.H.: Urinary tract calculi in children. J. Urol. 109: 318–320, 1973.
2. Daeschner, C.W., Singleton, E.B., and Curtis, J.C.: Urinary tract calculi and nephrocalcinosis in infants and children. J. Pediatr. 57: 721–732, 1960.
3. Ghazali, S., Barratt, T.M., and Williams, D.I.: Childhood urolithiasis in Britain. Arch. Dis. Child. 48: 291–295, 1973.
4. Hyams, B.B.: The signs of a passed ureteral stone. J. Can. Assoc. Radiol. 28: 270–273, 1977.
5. Jarvis, J.L., and Seaman, W.B.: Idiopathic adrenal calcification in infants and children. A.J.R. 82: 510–520, 1959.
6. Joffe, N.: Pancreatic calcification in childhood associated with protein malnutrition. Br. J. Radiol. 36: 758–761, 1963.
7. Paulson, D.S., Lenn, J.S., Hughes, J., Roberts, L.C., and Coppridge, A.J.: Pediatric urolithiasis. J. Urol. 108: 811–814, 1972.
8. Queloz, J.M., Capitanio, M.A., and Kirkpatrick, J.A.: Wolman's disease: Roentgen observations in 3 siblings. Radiology 104: 357–359, 1972.
9. Rajasuriya, K., Thenabadu, P.N., and Leanage, R.U.: Pancreatic calcification following prolonged malnutrition. Am. J. Dis. Child. 119: 149–151, 1970.
10. Walther, P.C., Lamm, D., and Kaplan, G.W.: Pediatric urolithiases: A ten-year review. Pediatrics 65: 1068–1072, 1980.
11. Wenzl, J.E., Burke, E.C., Strickler, G.B., and Utz, D.C.: Nephrolithiasis and nephrocalcinosis in children. Pediatrics 41: 57–61, 1968.

GI Bleeding. GI bleeding is not as common in childhood as in adulthood, but by no means is it rare (8). Unfortunately, however, as many as 30% of cases remain undiagnosed (6). Arteriography in acute bleeders is often helpful and should be performed on an emergency basis when required. However, bleeding must be brisk, probably at a rate of 1 ml/minute for the study to be fruitful.

Upper GI bleeding, of a massive nature, is usually due to portal hypertension (1), but also can be seen with esophagitis, peptic ulcer disease, and hemangiomas of the hypopharynx or GI tract. Bleeding from the rectum is very frequently secondary to juvenile polyps of the colon, either single or multiple (2, 9). In other instances, bleeding may result from colonic tumors

(7) and conditions such as ulcerative colitis and the hemolytic uremic syndrome. Indeed, colonic bleeding may be the presenting problem in the hemolytic uremic syndrome.

Bleeding in the form of red currant jelly stools is a classic feature of intussusception, but in some of these cases bright red bleeding or, indeed, no bleeding may be seen. Meckel's diverticula are notorious for presenting with painless lower GI bleeding as are so-called "benign" colonic or small intestinal ulcers of unknown etiology (3–6). Bright red rectal bleeding also occasionally is seen in peptic ulcer disease, especially in young infants where GI transit times may be rapid.

REFERENCES

1. Buonocore, E., Collmann, I.R., Kerley, H.E., and Lester, T.L.: Massive upper gastrointestinal hemorrhage in children. A.J.R. 115: 289–296, 1972.
2. Franken, E.A., Bixler, D., Fitzgerald, J.F., Gamet, D.J., and Russ, M.A.: Juvenile polyposis of the colon. Ann. Radiol. 18: 499–504, 1975.
3. Grosfeld, J.L., Schiller, M., Weinberger, M., and Clatworthy, H.W., Jr.: Primary nonspecific ileal ulcers in children. Am. J. Dis. Child. 120: 447–450, 1970.
4. Harrison, H.E., Spear, G.S., and Dorst, J.P.: Chronic idiopathic ulcerative ileitis in infancy. J. Pediatr. 78: 538–546, 1971.
5. Howard, E.R., and Whimster, W.F.: Benign rectal ulceration of unknown origin: An unusual cause of rectal bleeding. Arch. Dis. Child. 51: 156–157, 1976.
6. Shah, M.J.: Primary nonspecific ulcer in ileum presenting with massive rectal hemorrhage. Br. Med. J. 3: 474, 1968.
7. Skovgaard, S., and Sorensen, F.H.: Bleeding hemangioma of the colon diagnosed by coloscopy. J. Pediatr. Surg. 11: 83–84, 1976.
8. Spencer, R.: Gastrointestinal hemorrhage in infancy and childhood: 476 cases. Surgery 55: 718, 1961.
9. Toccalino, H., Guastavino, E., dePinni, F., and O'Donnell, J.C., and Williams, M.: Juvenile polyps of rectum and colon. Acta Paediatr. Scand. 62: 337–340, 1973.

Acute Urinary Retention. Acute urinary retention problems are uncommon in infancy and childhood. Occasionally, however, one can encounter a patient with a lower urinary tract obstruction and acute distension of the bladder presenting as an abdominal mass. Acute urinary retention also can be seen in severely injured children and those who might be comatosed.

REFERENCE

1. Swischuk, L.E.: Acute, non-traumatic, genitourinary pediatric problems. Radiol. Clin. North Am. 16: 147–157, 1978.

Hematuria. Hematuria can result from renal trauma, calculi, parenchymal disease, infection, or neoplasms. It also may be idiopathic and, as such, is not uncommon. Neoplasms leading to hematuria are seldom encountered in childhood as most Wilms's tumors do not present with hematuria. Hematuria is more often associated with urinary tract infection when cystitis is the problem. In such cases, ultrasound often can demonstrate thickened bladder mucosa. Renal parenchymal disease leading to hematuria, usually glomerulonephritis, may manifest in increased echogenicity and enlargement of the kidneys on ultrasound. With renal trauma, CT with contrast enhancement is much more productive than ultrasonography, and with renal colic, plain films and intravenous pyelography usually are utilized to supplement initial ultrasonographic examination. Nonetheless, overall, ultrasonography is a good screening examination for hematuria in the pediatric age group (1).

REFERENCE

1. Jequier, S., Cramer, B., and Pititjeanroget, T.: Ultrasonographic screening of childhood hematuria. J. Can. Assoc. Radiol. 38: 170–176, 1987.

Hydrometrocolpos. Although not a common cause of acute abdominal pain in girls, the condition does occur every so often. Classically, it is seen either in the neonatal period or in adolescence. Two types exist, simple imperforate hymen or actual vaginal atresia. The former is more likely to be the problem in the adolescent, but is not the exclusive cause. With the onset of menses, blood accumulates in the obstructed uterus and a painful abdominal mass develops. It can be seen on plain films, but is more specifically diagnosed with ultrasonography, where a sonolucent, elongated mass usually is seen behind the bladder (Fig. 3.166). Occasionally the mass is more solid as uterine and vaginal secretions predominate.

Acute Scrotal Problems. Acute scrotal problems include epididymo-orchitis, orchitis, testicular abscess, and testicular torsion. Testicular torsion occurs abruptly and may at first mimic testicular inflam-

mation. In the past, these problems were best assessed with technetium-99 pertechnetate nuclide imaging (4, 6, 7, 11), but currently ultrasonography with color flow Doppler is preferred (1, 3, 8, 10, 12–15). With epididymo-orchitis, increased perfusion and scintigraphic activity in the involved testicle are seen (Fig. 3.167A), while with testicular torsion in the early stages, decreased flow to the involved testes is noted (Fig. 3.167B). After a few days, in the so-called "missed" torsion, the involved testicle shows a cold center and increased activity around the rim of the tes-

Figure 3.166. *Hydrometrocolpos.* (A) Note typical central pelvic mass displacing the ureters and bladder. (B) Sagittal sonogram demonstrating fluid and debris in an enlarged vagina (V) and uterus (U). Note the position of the cervical os (*os*).

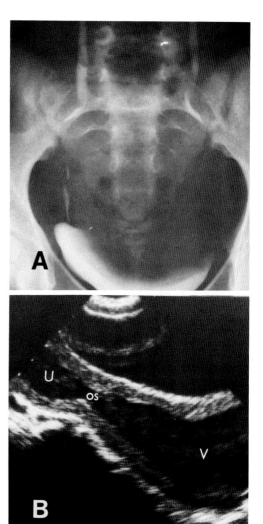

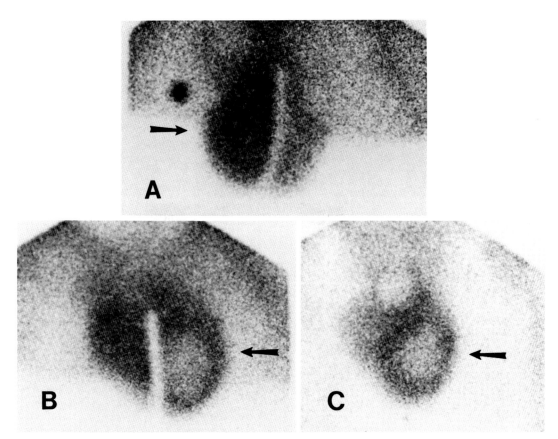

Figure 3.167. *Acute testicular problems: scintigraphy.* (*A*) *Epididymo-orchitis.* Note increased isotope activity in the enlarged right testicle (*arrows*). (*B*) *Early testicular torsion.* Note decreased isotope uptake in the left testicle (*arrow*). A scrotal rim is present, but it is not hyperemic. (*C*) *Missed torsion.* Characteristically with missed torsion, a similar cold testicular center is seen, but the scrotal wall around it becomes hyperemic (*arrow*).

ticle (Fig. 3.167C). Testicular abscesses are rather rare, but also produce cold spots on the isotope scan. Similar cold spots can be seen after trauma.

On ultrasonography, in the early stages of testicular torsion, decreased echogenicity of the enlarged testicle is seen (3). However, others have noted increased echogenicity (5). The epididymus, a highly echogenic structure, may be noted to be displaced from its normal position and, with color flow Doppler, absent blood flow to the torsed testicle is seen (1, 10, 12, 15) (Fig. 3.168A and B). With missed torsion, increased flow to the epididymis and tissues surrounding the testicle is seen, much as occurs with the nuclear scintigram (Fig.

3.168D). This is due to reactive hyperemia with blood flow coming from the external spermatic artery circulation. The testicle itself, however, remains bloodless. With spontaneous detorsion, blood flow will return to the testicle. In addition, with incomplete torsion, blood flow to the testicle still will be seen (12). Ultrasound also has been utilized to monitor manual, nonsurgical detorsion of the testicle (2). In these cases, once the testicle has been detorsed, blood flow returns to it. With epididymo-orchitis, blood flow is increased, both in the epididymus and the testicle (1, 8, 14, 15) (Fig. 3.168F and G). With epididymitis alone intratesticular blood flow may be sparse or not present at all (Fig. 3.168E),

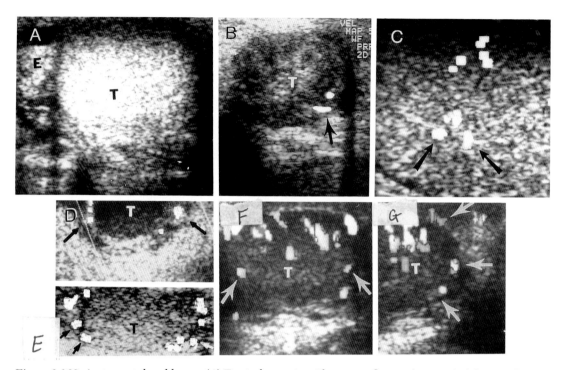

Figure 3.168. *Acute scrotal problems.* (**A**) Testicular torsion. There is no flow to the testicle (T). Note the epididymus (E). (**B**) Testicular torsion with minimal peripheral flow (*arrow*). Testicle (T). The testicle is somewhat hyperechoic. (**C**) Normal intratesticular blood flow (*arrows*). (**D**) Missed torsion. Note the hypoechoic testicle (T) and blood flow in the hyperemic rim (*arrows*). (**E**) Epididymitis. Note the enlarged testicle (T) and surrounding blood flow (*arrows*). (**F**) Epididymo-orchitis. Note exuberant blood flow (*arrows*) to the testicle (T). (**G**) Cross-sectional view demonstrates both peripheral and intratesticular increased blood flow (*arrows*). Testicle (T).

and the findings then may mimic those of missed torsion (Fig. 3.168*D*). With torsion of appendix testes (6), the findings most often mimic those of epididymo-orchitis. In the end, however, any testicle showing absent blood flow becomes a surgical problem. This is certainly true if, in addition, no peritesticular blood flow is seen. If peritesticular flow is seen, a dilemma results and close clinical correlation is required to determine whether one is dealing with: (1) missed torsion, (2) epididymitis without orchitis, or (3) very occasionally, torsion of the appendix testes. In the end, most of these testicles will undergo surgical exploration for it is best to be safe than sorry.

With trauma, ultrasound usually demonstrates disorganization of the normally uniform echogenicity of the testicle. In addition, there is loss of the testicular margins, demonstration of an associated hematocele (sonolucent area), and thickening of the scrotal wall (9).

REFERENCES

1. Atkinson, G.O., Jr., Patrick, L. E., Ball, T.I., Jr., Stephenson, C.A., Broecker, B.H., and Woodard, J.R.: The normal and abnormal scrotum in children: Evaluation with color Doppler sonography. A.J.R. 158: 613–617, 1992.
2. Betts, J.M., Norris, M., Cromie, W.J., and Duckert, J.W.: Testicular detorsion using Doppler ultrasound monitoring. J. Pediatric Surg. 18: 607–610, 1983.
3. Bird, K., Rosenfield, A.T., and Taylor, K.J.: Ultrasonography in testicular torsion. Radiology 147: 527–534, 1983.
4. Boedecker, R.A., Sty, J.R., and Jona, J.Z.: Testicular scanning as diagnostic aid in evaluating scrotal pain. J. Pediatr. 94: 760–762, 1979.
5. Chinn, D.H., and Miller, E.I.: Generalized testicular hyperechogenicity in acute testicular torsion. J. Ultrasound Med. 4: 495–496, 1985.

6. Cohen, H.L., Shapiro, M.A., Haller, J.O., and Glassberg, K.: Torsion of the testicular appendage. J. Ultrasound Med. 11: 81–83, 1992.

7. Hitch, D.C., Gilday, D.L., Shandling, B., and Savage, J.P.: New approach to diagnosis of testicular torsion. J. Pediatr. Surg. 11: 537–541, 1976.

8. Horstman, W.G., Middleton, W.D., and Melson, G.L.: Scrotal inflammatory disease: Color Doppler US findings. Radiology 179: 55–59, 1991.

9. Jeffrey, R.B., Laing, F.C., Hricak, H., and McAninch, J.W.: Sonography of testicular trauma. A.J.R. 141: 993–995, 1983.

10. Jensen, M.C., Lee, K.P., Halls, J.M., and Ralls, P.W.: Color Doppler sonography in testicular torsion. J. Clin. Ultrasound 18: 446–448, 1990.

11. Mendel, J.B., Taylor, G.A., Treves, S., Cheng, T.H., Retik, A., and Bauer, S.: Testicular torsion in children: Scintigraphic assessment. Pediatr. Radiol. 15: 110–115, 1985.

12. Meza, M.P., Amundson, G.M., Aquilina, J.W., and Reitelman, C.: Color flow imaging in children with clinically suspected testicular torsion. Pediatr. Radiol. 22: 370–373, 1992.

13. Middleton, W.D., and Melson, G.L.: Testicular ischemia: Color Doppler sonographic findings in five patients. A.J.R. 152: 1237–1239, 1989.

14. Middleton, W.D., Siegel, B.A., Melson, G.L., Yates, C.K., and Andriole, G.L.: Acute scrotal disorders: Prospective comparison of color Doppler US and testicular scintigraphy. Radiology 177: 177–181, 1990.

15. Mueller, D.L., Amundson, G.M., Rubin, S.Z., and Wesenberg, R.L.: Acute scrotal abnormalities in children: Diagnosis by combined sonography and scintigraphy. A.J.R. 150:643–646, 1988.

Pregnancy. Of course, it is well known that GI upsets are common in pregnancy, but often one does not think of pregnancy in the pediatric age group. Nevertheless, one should be aware of this possibility, for the first indication that a pregnancy is present may come from the abdominal roentgenogram wherein a pelvic mass or even a formed fetus will be demonstrated. Confirmation now is readily accomplished with ultrasonography (Figs. 3.169 and 3.170) and pregnancy tests.

NORMAL FINDINGS CAUSING PROBLEMS

Gastric and Colon Contents Mimicking Abscesses and Bezoars. This point seems straightforward, and yet in some cases, if

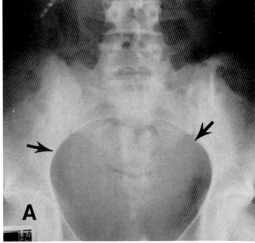

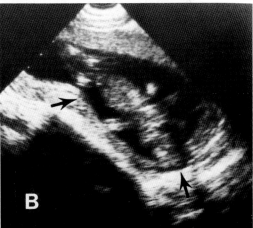

Figure 3.169. *Late pregnancy.* (*A*) Note fullness, or a mass in the pelvis (*arrows*). (*B*) Ultrasonogram demonstrating well-developed fetus (*arrows*).

gastric or colonic contents are visualized in just the right place, it is most difficult to differentiate them from the findings of an abdominal abscess or gastric bezoar (Fig. 3.171). Contents in the right side of the colon are especially problematic in patients with appendicitis and suspected perforation. Indeed, in some cases it is most difficult to determine whether one is dealing with an appendiceal abscess or fortuitous visualization of feces in the colon. In young infants, milk curds can conglomerate in the stomach to produce a bezoar or even mass-like configuration (Fig. 3.172).

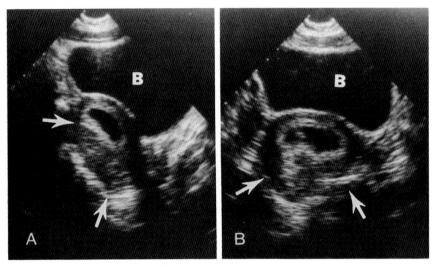

Figure 3.170. *Early pregnancy; ultrasound findings.* (*A*) On this sagittal view note the enlarged uterus (*arrows*) with an early decidual sac (sonolucent center) behind the bladder (*B*). (*B*) Transverse sonogram demonstrates the same findings within the enlarged uterus (*arrows*). Urinary bladder (*B*).

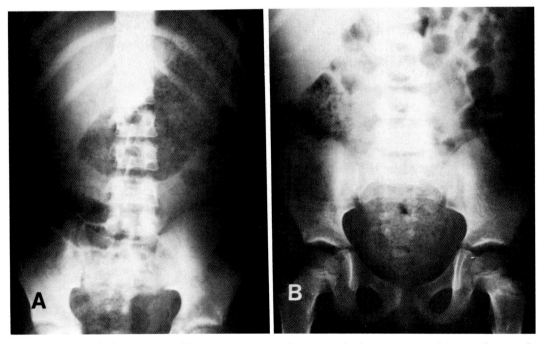

Figure 3.171. *Pseudoabscess or pseudobezoar appearance of gastric and colonic contents.* (*A*) Note the granular appearance of food and air mixed within the stomach of this patient. The pattern is similar to that seen with abdominal abscesses or gastric bezoars. (*B*) Another patient with fecal material mixed with air in the rectum and hepatic flexure. Either of these collections alone could be misinterpreted as an abscess.

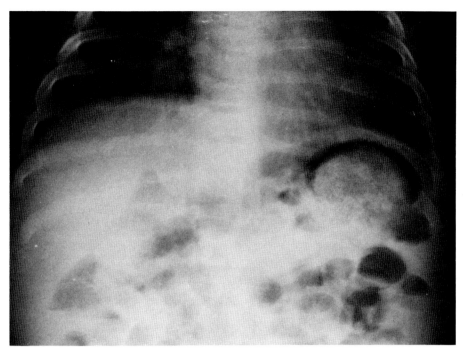

Figure 3.172. *Milk curds in stomach of infant.* Note the mass-like collection of milk curds in the fundus of the stomach of this young infant. The findings mimic those of a gastric bezoar, but they are normal and common.

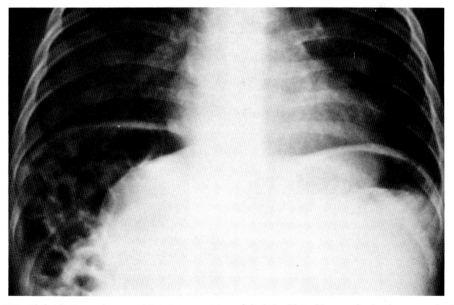

Figure 3.173. *Chilaiditi's syndrome.* Note interposition of slightly dilated loops of colon between the liver and the right diaphragmatic leaflet. The findings should not be misinterpreted as free air under the diaphragmatic leaflet, especially on chest films where the top of the abdomen only is included on the study.

Figure 3.174. *Normal duodenal air mimicking free air under the liver.* Note the linear collection of air in the duodenum (*arrows*). Such configurations usually are best visualized on upright views and can mimic the appearance of free air under the liver.

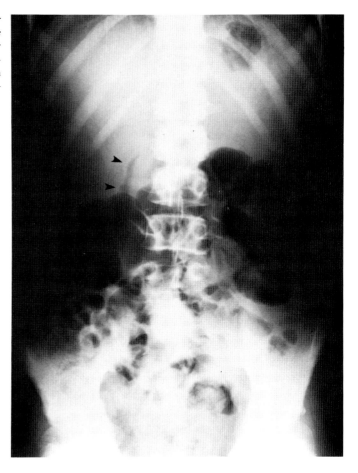

Abdominal Pseudotumors. These are discussed with abdominal masses on p. 347.

Chilaiditi's Syndrome (Hepatodiaphragmatic Interposition). This condition usually is considered a normal variation and consists of interposition of the colon between the liver and the diaphragm (1–3). Most often, it is seen on the right, but it can be seen bilaterally. The findings should not be misinterpreted as free peritoneal air (Fig. 3.173).

REFERENCES

1. Behlke, F.M.: Hepatodiaphragmatic interposition in children. A.J.R. 91: 669, 1964.

2. Jackson, A.D.M., and Hudson, C.J.: Interposition of colon between liver and diaphragm (Chilaiditi's syndrome) in children. Arch. Dis. Child. 32: 151, 1957.
3. Vessal, K., and Borhanmanesh, F.: Hepatodiaphragmatic interposition of the intestine (Chilaiditi's syndrome). Clin. Radiol. 27: 113–116, 1976.

Duodenal Air Mimicking Air under the Liver. In some cases, air trapped in the partially collapsed duodenal bulb is virtually indistinguishable from free air trapped under the liver. Only familiarity with this normal configuration will avoid physician misinterpretation (Fig. 3.174).

CHAPTER 4

The Extremities

This chapter addresses itself primarily to the detection of *the more subtle and frequently missed fractures and inflammatory lesions of the extremities.* There is no attempt to cover all fractures, especially those that require roentgenographic examination merely to confirm their presence or visualize the precise position of the fractured fragments. Although many of these injuries represent significant management problems, they offer no real problems with roentgenographic diagnosis. Furthermore, they are dealt with in whole or part in a number of excellent publications on the subject (2–4).

In addition to these aspects, *there also will be a greater than usual emphasis on evaluation of the soft tissues and periarticular fat pads.* These structures generally are underutilized and underestimated in importance. They are, however, invaluable in yielding data regarding the specific location and nature of a lesion, and their special usefulness in infants and young children will be stressed. This is especially important in this age group, as clinical history and physical examination often are less than optimal. Clinical history, however, is important in determining the nature and possible location of an injury (1), and physical examination is most predictive of a fracture when point tenderness, deformity, and extensive edema are present (5).

REFERENCES

1. Berbaum, K.S., El-Khoury, G.Y., Franken, E.A., Jr., Kathol, M., Montgomery, W.J., and Hesson, W.: Impact of clinical history on fracture detection with radiography. Radiology 168: 507–511, 1988.
2. Blount, W.P.: *Fractures in Children*, Ed. 2. Williams & Wilkins, Baltimore, 1980.
3. Pollen, A.G.: *Fractures and Dislocations in Children.* Williams & Wilkins, Baltimore, 1973.
4. Rang, M.: *Children's Fractures*, Ed. 2. J.B. Lippincott, Philadelphia, 1982.
5. Rivara, F.P., Parish, R.A., and Mueller, B.A.: Extremity injuries in children: Predictive value of clinical findings. Pediatrics 78: 803–807, 1986.

GENERAL CONSIDERATIONS

What Views Should Be Obtained? At least two views, usually at right angles to each other, are necessary. Most often these views consist of a *frontal* and *lateral* projection of the involved extremity, and in this regard it cannot be stated too forcefully that *true frontal and lateral projections are required. One cannot settle for a "sort of" frontal or lateral view,* for if one does, one will come to regret it. If these views fail to yield useful information *oblique* or other *special* views should be obtained.

In addition, it is of the utmost benefit to obtain *comparative views* of the other (normal) side, especially in cases where abnormal findings are subtle. These views are extremely useful, for, generally speaking, symmetry from side to side in the normal patient is very consistent and, because of this, any asymmetry, no matter how subtle, should be treated with the greatest suspicion.

Over the years, there has been movement toward discouraging the routine use of comparative views (1–3). The publications addressing this point all deliver the message that such views, on a generalized basis, are not required. While there is some merit to this attitude, most experienced radiologists, especially those not sustained on a steady diet of pediatric films, still probably prefer to obtain comparative views. *Indeed, at our institution, even though a pediatric facility, we obtain comparative views rather liberally, for we do not feel we can detect subtle bony injury or evaluate the soft tissues satisfactorily without them.* In terms of the publications that express opposition to obtaining comparative views, it might be noted that *in a summary report, the Committee on Radiology of the American Academy of Pediatrics provided so many loopholes in the premise that comparative views are not required, that the loopholes virtually destroyed the original premise.* For example, with direct quotation from their report (3), we have the following statements:

"Injury to the hip joint is a notable exception to the selective approach; at least one view should routinely include the normal hip, with the gonads shielded. Hip injuries in children are most frequently associated with joint effusion, which can be detected only with comparing similar measurements of the opposite joint space.

Other specific areas of appendicular skeleton may require more comparative views. The elbow, with a relatively large number of ossification centers appearing at widely varying times, may prove confusing even to the experienced radiologist; comparison view of this joint may be requested frequently. Detection of joint effusion in the knee and ankle may necessitate a comparison view, in at least one projection. Comparison views may also be helpful in evaluating the tissue planes and subcutaneous fat in suspected inflammatory conditions of the soft tissues or bones."

Finally, a conclusion from another of these communications (1) suggests that no one uniform policy can be expected for all individuals dealing with pediatric trauma. To quote from that communication:

"A number of theoretical and practical considerations will continue to determine the use of comparison views. Personal conviction based on experience and training is the major theoretical consideration. Practical considerations include the availability of radiologic consultation, the expertise of the physician who initially interprets the study and clinical demands. An individual's policy toward the use of comparison images is a balance of these considerations."

The latter paragraph probably is the most important in this ongoing controversy. *Do what you have to do, but be sure in your mind that you will not miss any fractures when you obtain views of the injured side only. In this regard one might ask, "How sure are you that you are not missing a bending fracture, a subtle Salter-Harris type I injury, or a minimal buckle fracture?"*

REFERENCES

1. Committee on Radiology: Comparison radiographs of extremities in childhood: Recommended usage. Pediatrics 65: 646–647, 1980.
2. McCauley, R.G.K., Schwartz, A.M., Leonidas, J.C., Darling, D.B., Bankoff, M.S., and Swan, C.S., II: Comparison views in extremity injury in children: An efficacy study. Radiology 131: 95–97, 1979.
3. Merten, D.F.: Comparison radiographs in extremity injuries of childhood: Current application in radiological practice. Radiology 126: 209–210, 1978.

Utilizing the Soft Tissues. Evaluating soft tissue changes in trauma and infection of the extremities in childhood, and even adulthood (1), is invaluable. The findings one should look for include: (a) localized or generalized swelling of the soft tissues, (b) obliteration of the muscle-fat interfaces, and (c) displacement or obliteration of the periarticular fat pads. These latter structures are displaced when fluid accumulates within the joint and obliterated when edema surrounds the joint. Evaluating the soft tissues in this manner can serve to localize the site of injury or infection, and such an evaluation should be undertaken before the bones themselves are examined (Fig. 4.1). Of course, the changes will differ a little from joint to joint and bone to bone, but basically abnormality can be as-

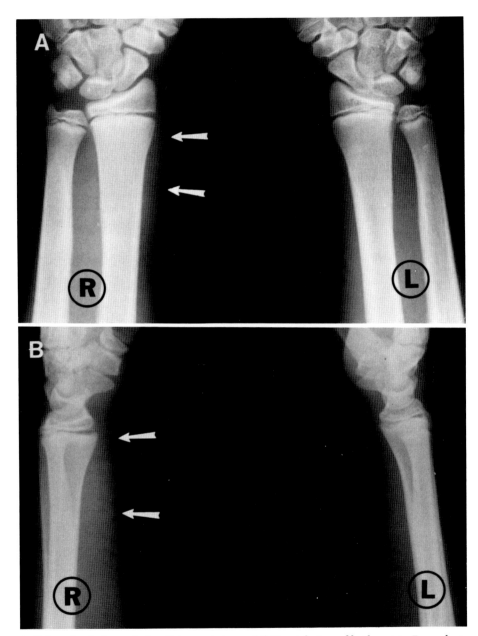

Figure 4.1. *Value of soft tissues in localizing an injury.* (**A**) Frontal view of both wrists. Bony abnormality is subtle and consists primarily of a little widening of the distal right radial epiphyseal line. This should signify the presence of a Salter-Harris type I epiphyseal-metaphyseal injury, but the finding is subtle and could be missed. However, when it is noted that soft tissue swelling also is present *(arrows)* the finding takes on more significance. (**B**) Soft tissue swelling also is noted on the lateral view *(arrows)*. Note that not only are the soft tissues thicker, but that edema and swelling have obliterated the normal fat-muscle interfaces. Compare with the normal appearance of the left wrist. Note the slightly wider epiphyseal line and mininally displaced (posteriorly) distal, right radial epiphysis.

sessed under one of the three categories just proposed. A more detailed discussion of the soft tissue changes for each joint of the body is presented at subsequent points throughout this chapter.

REFERENCE

1. Curtis, D. J., Downey, E.F., Jr., Brower, A.C., Cruess, D.F., Herrington, W.T., and Ghaed, N.: Importance of soft tissue evaluation in hand and wrist trauma: Statistical evaluation. A.J.R. 142: 781–788, 1984.

Significance of Intra-articular Fluid. As a general rule, in children, fluid in the joint in the absence of trauma should be presumed pus until proven otherwise. In the elbow and ankle, fluid in the joint is manifested by outward displacement of the anterior and posterior fat pads, while in the shoulder and hip, fluid accumulation causes lateral displacement of the humerus or femur and concomitant joint space widening. Knee fluid produces bulging of the suprapatellar bursa, just behind the quadriceps tendon, while in the wrist, joint fluid is manifested simply by the presence of swelling around the wrist.

In the presence of trauma, fluid in the joint should cause one to look more diligently at the bones for evidence of a fracture in this area. However, not always will one see such a fracture, and indeed in our study on the subject (1), the incidence of missed fracture was surprisingly low (Table 4.1). It is important to emphasize,

however, that *these figures were compiled on the basis of liberal use of comparison views and close scrutiny of the bones for subtle fractures,* frequently missed by the inexperienced observer.

REFERENCE

1. Swischuk, L.E., Hayden, C.K., and Kupfer, M.C.: Significance of intra-articular fluid without visible fracture in children. A.J.R. 142: 1261–1262, 1984.

What Type of Bony Injuries Are Seen in Children? The types of fractures most peculiar to childhood are: (a) cortical, buckle, or torus fractures; (b) greenstick fractures; (c) bent or bowed bones without a visible fracture line (i.e., acute plastic, bending fractures); and (d) epiphyseal-metaphyseal fractures (Fig. 4.2). Of course, typical midshaft, transverse, spiral, oblique, and comminuted fractures also occur in children, but none are especially peculiar to childhood and most are not difficult to detect. One might make some exception when these fractures are of the so-called "hairline" variety, but other than this these fractures are readily demonstrable roentgenographically and not difficult to diagnose. Hairline fractures occur most commonly in the tibia and small bones of the hands and feet. In the tibia, both transverse (upper metaphysis) and spiral, shaft (toddler's fracture) occur (Fig. 4.3).

Buckle or torus fractures are simple compression fractures which manifest

Table 4.1
Occult Fracture—Percent Probability[a]

Fracture	Total No. of Cases	Total Cases with No X-ray Follow-up	Total Cases with X-ray Follow-up	No. of Cases with Fracture Detected	Percent Fracture Probability
Shoulder	0	0	0	0	0
Elbow	46	20	26	4	15.8
Wrist	5	2	3	2	67
Hip	0	0	0	0	0
Knee	16	9	7	0	0
Ankle	61	34	27	3	11
Total	128	65	63	8	12.6

[a]Reproduced from: Swischuk, L.E., Hayden, C.K., and Kupfer, M.C.: Significance of intraarticular fluid without visible fracture in children, A.J.R. 142: 1261–1262, 1984.

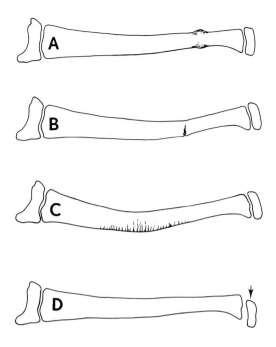

Figure 4.2. *Fractures peculiar to children.* (*A*) Typical torus or buckle fracture with buckling of the cortex. (*B*) Greenstick fracture with the fracture visible through one aspect of the cortex only. The fracture is incomplete and a certain degree of bending coexists. (*C*) Bending or plastic bowing fracture of long bone. No fracture line is visible roentgenographically but numerous microfractures exist along the outer aspect of the bent bone. (*D*) Epiphyseal-metaphyseal injury with or without displacement of the epiphysis *(arrow)*.

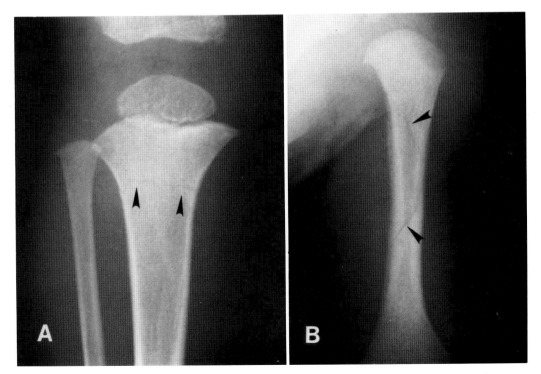

Figure 4.3. *Hairline fractures.* (*A*) Note the hairline fracture *(arrows)* traversing the upper right tibia. It is not easy to see. (*B*) Spiral hairline fracture *(arrows)* in a battered infant. The presence of periosteal new bone indicates early healing. Hairline fractures often become more readily visible at this stage.

themselves by buckling, kinking, or notching of the cortex. They occur most frequently in the metaphyseal regions of long bones, for this is where the cortex is weakest. However, they also can be seen in the clavicles, pubic bones, and even the scapulae. Some of these buckle or torus fractures are quite subtle, but if one follows the rule that the distal ends of the long bones should possess smooth, continuous curves, then one will not accept even the slightest bump, dent, buckle, or cortical irregularity as normal (Fig. 4.4). Nonetheless, some of these fractures do elude initial detection, and when follow-up films are obtained, signs of healing in the form of sclerosis along the fracture line and periosteal new bone deposition can be seen (Fig. 4.5).

Greenstick fractures are bending fractures with a fracture line extending through one cortex of the bone only (Fig. 4.6). The term "greenstick" comes from the comparison of this type of fracture to the manner in which a "green," supple tree branch breaks when it is bent. True *bending or bowing (plastic) fractures, without a visible fracture line* (1–4, 10, 18) can be considered the precursor of the classic greenstick fractures (*i.e., the greenest of greenstick fractures*). These fractures frequently are missed unless comparative views of the normal extremity are obtained, and although a fracture line is not visible roentgenographically, numerous microfractures exist along the outer surface of the bent bone. In these cases, the fracture force is not dissipated at any one site, and thus a single fracture line is not visualized. With enough bending, a single fracture line develops, but until then, only bending is seen (Fig. 4.6). Most often these fractures occur in the forearm (1–4, 17), but they also can be seen in the lower extremity (3, 16), clavicle, and indeed almost any long bone in the body of the infant or young child. These fractures are discussed in more detail in later sections, but it might be noted at this point that seldom, if ever, do they show classic

signs of healing. In other words, whereas with a greenstick fracture one will see sclerosis and periosteal new bone formation, with the usual bending fracture, nothing but the deformity persists (Fig. 4.7).

Epiphyseal-metaphyseal fractures are very common in childhood and, of course, occur exclusively in the child. Because the junction between the epiphysis and metaphysis is a weak area, if a shearing force is applied to the end of a long bone, it is quite natural that epiphyseal-metaphyseal slippage or separation results. A variety of injuries can be sustained at this junction, and to facilitate their understanding and categorization, the Salter-Harris classification (15) of five types usually still is employed (Fig. 4.8). More complicated classifications have been suggested, but the Salter-Harris classification is more than adequate and probably will not be replaced.

As far as the radiologist is concerned, the greatest challenge comes from the Salter-Harris type I and II injuries (14). The reason for this is that if in these cases, the epiphysis is not displaced, bony changes are subtle, and one must rely more on soft tissue changes and widening of the epiphyseal line. Salter-Harris type I and II fractures heal in characteristic fashion, and thus, should they not be detected in their acute phase, repeat roentgenograms 10 days to 2 weeks later show sclerosis and irregularity of the epiphyseal-metaphyseal junction and periosteal new bone deposition along the metaphysis (Fig. 4.9). Salter-Harris type III and IV fractures usually are relatively easy to detect, for often some degree of epiphyseal displacement exists and, in any case, the fracture lines are more readily visible. Type III fractures occur most commonly in the distal tibia, followed by the small bones of the hands and feet.

The type V Salter-Harris injury, that is, the one in which epiphyseal plate compression only occurs (11), is the least common of all. Indeed, a question has been raised as to whether the type V fracture occurs at all (12). It is, however, considered

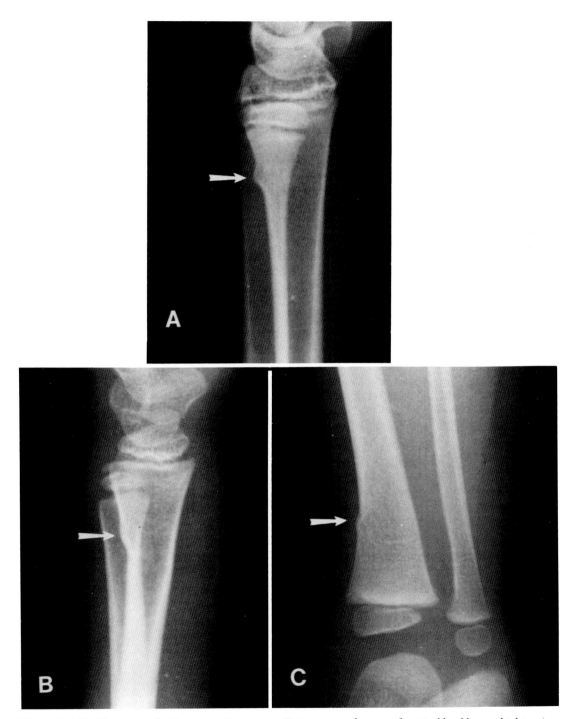

Figure 4.4. *Buckle or torus fractures—various types.* Note varying degrees of cortical buckling or kinking *(arrows)* in these typical torus fractures of the wrist (*A* and *B*) and ankle (*C*).

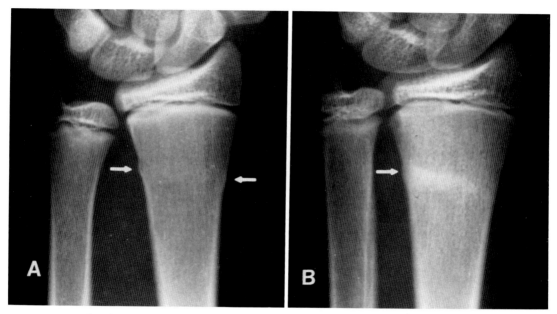

Figure 4.5. *Healing buckle or torus fracture.* (*A*) Note typical, but subtle, bulging of the cortex *(arrows)*. Also note that the trabecular pattern along the fracture line has been disturbed. (*B*) Two weeks later note sclerosis along the fracture line *(arrow)*.

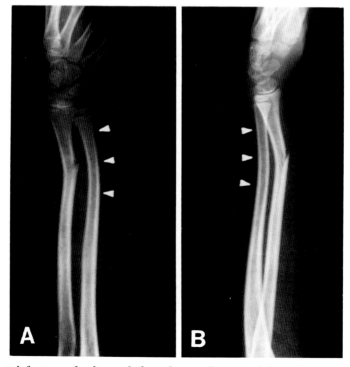

Figure 4.6. *Greenstick fracture of radius and plastic bowing fracture of ulna.* Anteroposterior (*A*) and lateral (*B*) views. Note the greenstick fracture of the distal radius. In addition, however, note bending of the ulna *(arrows)*. This latter finding represents an acute plastic bending fracture of the ulna. Some concomitant bending of the fractured radius also is present.

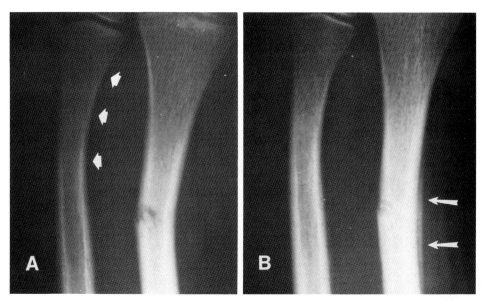

Figure 4.7. *Greenstick and plastic bending fracture; healing phase.* (*A*) Note the greenstick fracture of the distal radius. In addition, note bending of the ulna *(arrows)*. (*B*) Follow-up films demonstrate classic healing of the radial fracture *(arrows)*, but in the ulna, nothing but residual bending is seen.

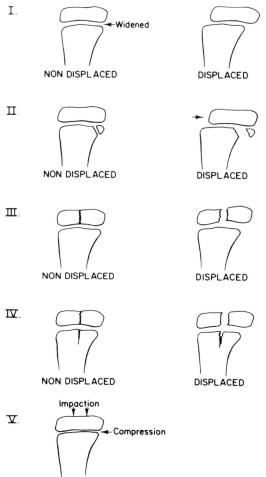

Figure 4.8. *Salter-Harris classification of epiphyseal-metaphyseal fractures.* *Type I:* the epiphyseal line (physis) is widened secondary to some degree of epiphyseal separation. The epiphysis may or may not be displaced. *Type II:* there is a small or large metaphyseal fracture fragment in association with widening of the epiphyseal line. The epiphysis and fracture fragment may or may not be visibly displaced. *Type III:* in this type, the fracture occurs through the epiphysis and the fracture may or may not be displaced. When displacement occurs, usually only part of the fractured epiphysis is displaced. *Type IV:* fractures exist through the epiphysis and the metaphysis; displacement of the fragments may or may not be present. *Type V:* an impaction fracture with compressive injury of the epiphyseal plate only is present. No roentgenographic findings other than swelling around the involved epiphyseal-metaphyseal junction usually are present.

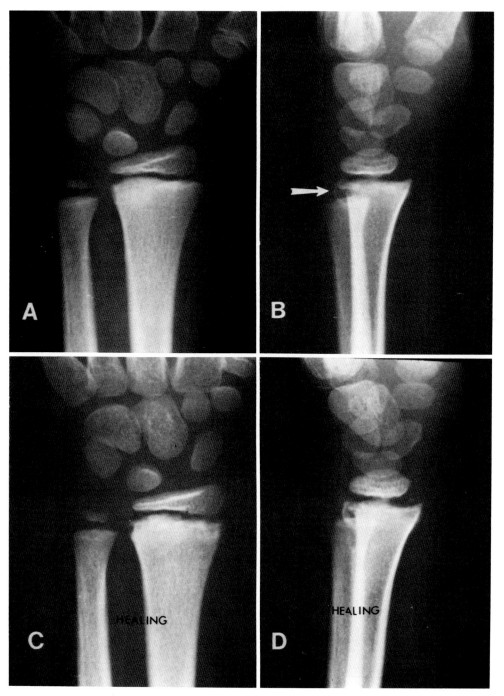

Figure 4.9. *Healing epiphyseal-metaphyseal injury.* (**A**) Frontal view demonstrating little if any abnormality of the epiphyseal-metaphyseal junction. (**B**) Lateral view demonstrates posterior displacement of the radial epiphysis and a corner fracture of the posterior metaphysis *(arrow)*. These findings are consistent with a Salter-Harris type II injury. (**C**) Two weeks later note how sclerotic and irregular the radial metaphyseal margin has become. This is characteristic of the healing phase of these fractures. (**D**) Lateral view showing similar findings.

one of the more serious injuries a child can sustain, for epiphyseal plate damage and subsequent impaired epiphyseal growth are common (7, 11, 13, 15). Growth abnormalities also are a significant complication of the type IV fracture, but are a lesser problem with the other Salter-Harris epiphyseal-metaphyseal injuries. Roentgenographically, in the type V fracture the films usually are void of bony abnormality.

Although the fractures just outlined constitute the major portion of childhood fractures, one also can see *stress fractures* with considerable frequency (8, 16, 19) and, to a lesser extent, *pathologic fractures.* Stress fractures usually, but not always, occur in perfectly normal individuals, and the most common site for such a fracture to occur in a child is the upper tibia. However, they can occur in almost any bone of the lower extremity. Stress fractures of the second metatarsal usually are referred to as "march fractures."

It is unusual to detect stress fractures in their initial stages, for unless a fracture line is seen through the involved cortex, one will not even suspect that such an injury is present. Consequently, these fractures frequently go undetected for days or weeks, and finally come to the attention of the physician in their healing phase, replete with sclerosis along the fracture line and periosteal new bone deposition over the fracture site (Fig. 4.10A). Indeed, so striking are these changes that very often they are misinterpreted for more serious lesions such as a bone tumor (Fig. 4.10B).

Nuclear scintigraphy also is very useful in the detection of stress fractures (5, 13, 18). Although the findings are nonspecific, they do localize the site of injury. Stress fractures also now can readily be detected with MR imaging (6, 9). However, in most cases plain films and nuclear scintigraphy suffice.

The classic *pathologic fracture* in childhood is the one occurring through a unicameral bone cyst. Unicameral bone cysts are common in children, and most often are located in the metaphyses of long bones, especially the upper humerus. Indeed, in the spring when field and track, and baseball practice begin, many a child has come to the emergency room with a pathologic fracture through such a cyst (Fig. 4.10C). Not as common, but nonetheless quite important, is the pathologic fracture through a malignant bone lesion (Fig. 4.10D). Most often the underlying lesion is one of the so-called "round cell" tumors, i.e., Ewing's sarcoma, lymphoma, leukemia, or metastatic neuroblastoma. Pathologic fractures through weakened or dysplastic bones such as those seen with osteopetrosis, osteogenesis imperfecta, hyperparathyroidism, rickets, hypophosphatasia, etc., also occur but are not within the scope of this book.

REFERENCES

1. Borden, S., IV: Traumatic bowing of the forearm in children. J. Bone Joint Surg. 56A: 611–616, 1974.
2. Borden, S., IV: Roentgen recognition of acute plastic bowing of the forearm in children. A.J.R. 125: 524–530, 1975.
3. Cail, W.S., Keats, T.E., and Sussman, M.D.: Plastic bowing fracture of the femur in a child. A.J.R. 130: 780–782, 1978.
4. Crowe, J.E., and Swischuk, L.E.: Acute bowing fractures of the forearm in children: A frequently missed injury. A.J.R. 128: 981–984, 1977.
5. Geslien, G.E., Thrall, J.H., Espinosa, J.L., and Older, R.A.: Early detection of stress fracture using 99m Tc-polyphosphate. Radiology 121: 683–687, 1976.
6. Horev, G., Korenreich, L., Ziv, N., and Grunebaum, M.: The enigma of stress fractures in the pediatric age: Clarification or confusion through the new imaging modalities. Pediatric Radiol. 20: 469–471, 1990.
7. Keret, D., Mendez, A.A., Harcke, H.T., and MacEwen, G.D.: Type V physeal injury: A case report. J. Pediatr. Orthop. 10: 545–548, 1990.
8. Kroening, P.M., and Shelton, M.L.: Stress fractures. A.J.R. 89: 1281–1286, 1963.
9. Lee, J.K., and Yao, L.: Stress fractures: MR imaging. Radiology 169: 2217–2220, 1988.
10. Mabry, J.D. and Fitch, R.D.: Plastic deformation in pediatric fractures: Mechanism and treatment. J. Pediatr. Orthop. 9: 310–314, 1989.
11. Mendez, A.A., Bartal, E., Grillot, M.B., and Lin,

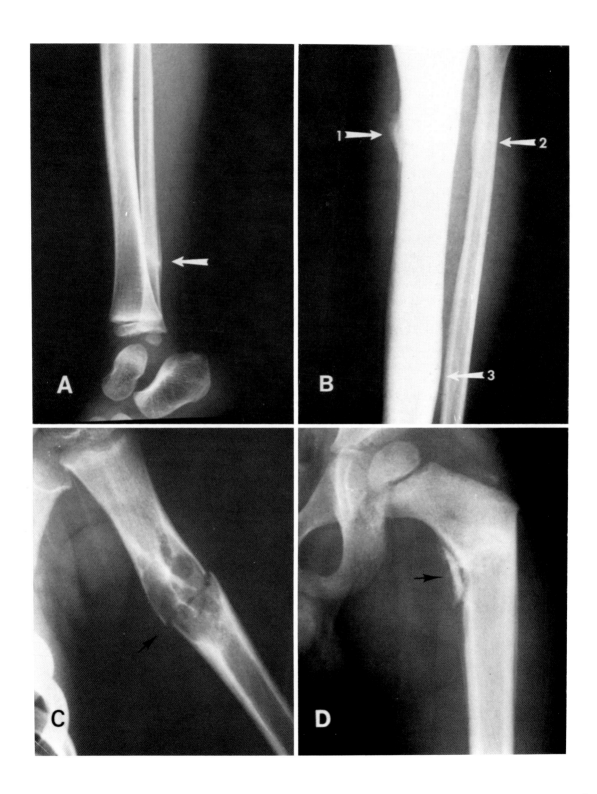

J.J.: Compression (Salter-Harris type V) physeal fracture: An experimental model in the rat. J. Pediatr. Orthop. 12: 29–37, 1992.

12. Peterson, H.A., and Burkhart, S.S.: Compression injury of the epiphyseal growth plate: Fact or fiction? J. Pediatr. Orthop. 1: 377–384, 1981.

13. Prather, J.L., Nusynowitz, M.L., Snowdy, H.A., Hughes, A.D., McCartney, W.H., and Bagg, R.J.: Scintigraphic findings in stress fractures. J. Bone Joint Surg. 59: 869–874, 1977.

14. Rogers, L.F.: The radiography of epiphyseal injuries. Radiology 96: 289–299, 1970.

15. Salter, R.B., and Harris, W.R.: Injuries involving the epiphyseal plate. J. Bone Joint Surg. 45A: 587–622, 1963.

16. Savoca, C.J.: Stress fractures: A classification of the earliest radiographic signs. Radiology 100: 519–524, 1971.

17. Strenstrom, R., Gripenberg, L., and Bergius, A.R.: Traumatic bowing of forearm and lower leg in children. Acta Radiol. 19: 243–249, 1978.

18. Wilcox, J.R., Jr., Moniot, A.L., and Green, J.P.: Bone scanning in the evaluation of exercise-related stress injuries. Radiology 123: 699–702, 1977.

19. Wilson, E.S., Jr., and Katz, F.N.: Stress fractures. An analysis of 250 consecutive cases. Radiology 92: 481–486, 1969.

Occult Fractures and Obscure Extremity Pain.

Often one is presented with a patient who has obscure skeletal pain and who may in fact may have an occult fracture. Nuclear scintigraphy has proven to be the best screening modality for this problem (1, 3, 7, 8, 10–12). Bone scintigraphy can demonstrate the presence of a bony injury or even infection before plain film radiographic findings become apparent. It is especially useful in detecting early osteomyelitis, occult fractures, and stress fractures (Fig. 4.11A–D). Recently MR imaging also has proven useful in detecting occult fractures (2, 5, 6). However, it is not in widespread use on an emergent

basis. Occult fractures also can be detected with CT (4) and even with ultrasound (9), where the cortical break can be imaged.

Finally, it should be remembered that patients with underlying malignancies such as leukemia (6), lymphoma, and metastatic neuroblastoma can present with obscure bone pain. With leukemia trophic lines may be the only finding (Fig. 4.11E). However, bone destruction also can be seen (Fig. 4.11F) as it is with metastatic neuroblastoma (Fig. 4.11G).

REFERENCES

1. Aronson, J., Garvin, K., Seibert, J., Glasier, C., and Tursky, E.A.: Efficiency of the bone scan for occult limping toddlers. J. Pediatr. Orthop. 12: 38–44, 1992.

2. Berger, P.E., Ofstein, R.A., Jackson, D.W., Morrison, D.S., Silvino, N., and Amador, R.: MRI demonstration of radiographically occult fractures: What have we been missing? RadioGraphics 9: 407–436, 1989.

3. Graif, M., Stahl-Kent V., Ben-Ami, T., Strauss, S., Amit, Y., and Itzchak, Y.: Sonographic detection of occult bone fractures. Pediatr. Radiol. 18: 383–385, 1988.

4. Hindman, B.W., Kulik, W.J., Lee, G., and Avolio, R.E.: Occult fractures of the carpals and metacarpals demonstration by CT. A.J.R. 153: 529–532, 1989.

5. Jaramillo, D., Hoffer, F.A., Shapiro, F., and Rand, F.: MR imaging of fractures of the growth plate. A.J.R. 155: 1261–1265, 1990.

6. Jonsson, O.G., Sartain, P., Ducore, J.M., and Buchanan, G.R.: Bone pain as an initial symptom of childhood acute lymphoblastic leukemia: Association with nearly normal hematologic indexes. J. Pediatr. 117: 233–237, 1990.

7. Marty, R., Denney, J.D., McKamey, M.R., and Rowley, M.J.: Bone trauma and related benign disease: Assessment by bone scanning. Semin. Nucl. Med. 6: 197–220, 1976.

8. Park, H.M., Rothschild, P.A., Kernek, C.B.: Scintigraphic evaluation of extremity pain in chil-

---

Figure 4.10. *Other fractures in childhood.* (**A**) Stress fracture of fibula. Note the area of increased sclerosis and periosteal new bone deposition in the lower fibula *(arrow)*. (**B**) Another patient demonstrating multiple stress fractures. First note the large "lump" of periosteal new bone adjacent to the tibial fracture (*1*). Then note a similar, but much less pronounced, finding in the fibula just across from the tibia (*2*), and, finally, note the old healed stress fracture of the lower tibia (*3*). (**C**) Pathologic fracture through unicameral bone cyst of the humerus *(arrow)*. (**D**) Pathologic fracture in Ewing's sarcoma with avulsion of the lesser trochanter *(arrow)*. Note that there is destruction of the medullary portion of the bone, and that reactive periosteal new bone is present circumferentially. This patient experienced acute hip pain while running.

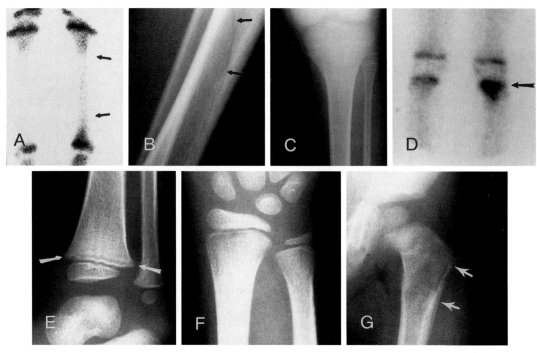

Figure 4.11. *Obscure skeletal pain.* (A) *Occult fracture.* Nuclear scintigraphy demonstrates an area of increased activity throughout the left tibia *(arrows).* (B) X-ray demonstrates a spiral (toddler's) fracture of the tibia *(arrows).* (C) *Occult osteomyelitis.* This patient had acute pain but virtually no swelling in the upper leg on the left. The roentgenographic changes are completely normal and there was little in the way of soft tissue swelling. (D) Subsequent bone scan, however, shows marked focal increase in uptake of the isotope in the upper left tibia *(arrow).* (E) Patient with leukemia presenting with vague bone pain demonstrates a classic, trophic line in the distal tibia *(arrows).* These trophic lines are nonspecific but highly suggestive of leukemia when bone pain is present. (F) Another patient with leukemia demonstrating diffuse bony destruction in the distal radius and ulna. The findings could be mistaken for simple demineralization. (G) Metastatic neuroblastoma presenting as hip pain. Note the moth-eaten permeated destruction in the upper femur with some early periosteal new bone *(arrows).*

dren: Its efficacy and pitfalls. A.J.R. 145: 1079–1084, 1985.

9. Patten, R.M., Mack, L.A., Wang, K.Y., and Lingel, J.: Nondisplaced fractures of the greater tuberosity of the humerus: Sonographic detection. Radiology 182: 201–204, 1992.

10. Rosenthal, L., Hill, R.O., and Chuang, S.: Observation on the use of 99m Tc-phosphate imaging in peripheral bone trauma. Radiology 119: 637–641, 1976.

11. ter Meulen, D.C., and Majd, M.: Bone scintigraphy in the evaluation of children with obscure skeletal pain. Pediatrics 79: 587–592, 1987.

12. Wilcox, J.R., Jr., Moniot, A.L., and Green, J.P.: Bone scanning in the evaluation of exercise-related injuries. Radiology 123: 699–702, 1977.

Osteomyelitis. Roentgenographic bony changes in osteomyelitis take 10 days to 2 weeks to develop; therefore in the early stages one can only infer the diagnosis from soft tissue changes. In this regard, osteomyelitis manifests in deep soft tissue edema, while superficial cellulitis demonstrates findings reflective of superficial edema (Fig. 4.12) and deep edema should suggest the presence of osteomyelitis until proven otherwise. Soft tissue abscesses also can produce deep edema, but osteomyelitis is more common and is manifest in enlargement of the deep muscle bulk (Fig. 4.12). In addition, at sites such as the distal femur and elbow, displacement of the fat pads overlying the involved metaphyses also can be seen (5, 11).

After 10–14 days, bony destruction is

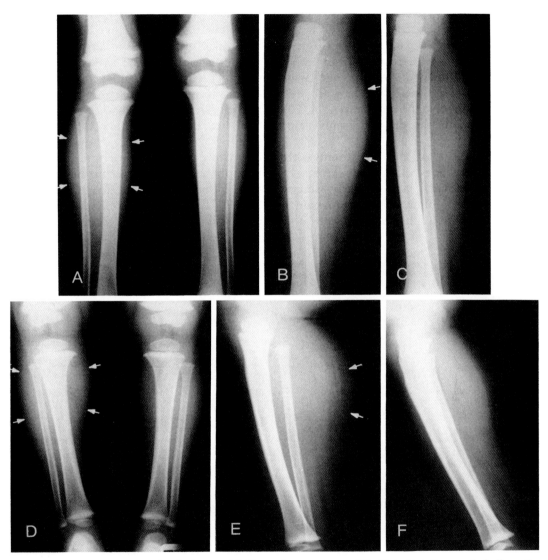

Figure 4.12. *Deep versus superficial edema.* (*A*) *Deep edema: osteomyelitis.* Note that the muscle bulk on the right is enlarged *(arrows)* and yet the subcutaneous soft tissues show little in the way of edema. The edge of the muscle is sharp. All of this should point towards a deep inflammatory process (i.e., osteomyelitis or deep abscess). (*B*) Lateral view demonstrating the same phenomenon with marked enlargement of the deep muscle bulk of the calf *(arrows)*. The edge of the muscle is sharp. (*C*) Normal side for comparison. Note that the muscle bulk is smaller and less dense. (*D*) *Superficial edema: cellulitis.* In this patient, note enlargement of the right calf *(arrows)*. (*E*) Lateral view shows extensive superficial edema *(arrows)* with thickening and reticulation of the subcutaneous fat. The interface between the muscle and subcutaneous fat is indistinct. (*F*) Normal side for comparison. Compare the muscle bulk with that in (*D*). Note that there is no real difference attesting to the fact that enlargement of the calf on the right is due primarily to superficial edema (i.e., cellulitis).

seen and can manifest as an acute destructive process or a low-grade smoldering problem. More aggressive permeative and "moth-eaten" changes are seen with the former while with the latter more reactive bony healing or sclerosis is seen (Fig. 4.13). In addition, while osteomyelitis usually is a metaphyseal problem, it frequently can involve the epiphysis (2, 4, 16) and occasionally the diaphysis only (Fig. 4.13E).

Clinically, in advanced osteomyelitis the extremity is swollen and extremely tender. However, in the early stages edema may be minimal even though pain is marked, and in such cases an elevated erythrocyte sedimentation rate is a valid positive indicator of underlying infection (17).

If one suspects the presence of osteomyelitis clinically and plain film changes do not support the diagnosis, then one should turn to nuclear scintigraphy. Nuclear scintigraphy is the single most effective method with which to detect early underlying bone infection. Although the findings are nonspecific, when one utilizes the three-phase technetium-99m pyrophosphate study consisting of the blood flow, blood pool, and static imaging phases (9, 17, 19), occult osteomyelitis usually is detected and differentiated from cellulitis

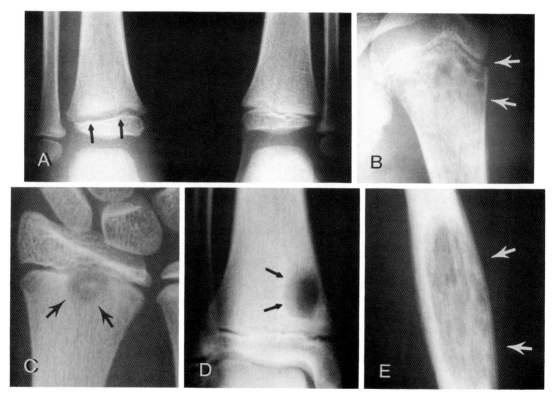

Figure 4.13. *Osteomyelitis; various roentgenographic changes.* (**A**) In this patient, only increased lucency and width of the epiphyseal line on the right, due to adjacent metaphyseal destruction, is seen *(arrows)*. Compare with the normal side. (**B**) Another patient demonstrating more aggressive changes in the upper humeral metaphysis consisting of irregular, permeative bone destruction *(arrows)*. (**C**) Low-grade osteomyelitis of the distal radius *(arrows)* with a small central sequestrum. The process has crossed the epiphyseal line and is extending into the epiphysis. (**D**) Low-grade, clean-appearing lytic lesion *(arrows)* with some adjacent sclerosis characteristic of a low-grade Brodie's abscess. (**E**) Unusual middiaphyseal low-grade osteomyelitis *(arrows)*. The findings could be mistaken for a Ewing's tumor.

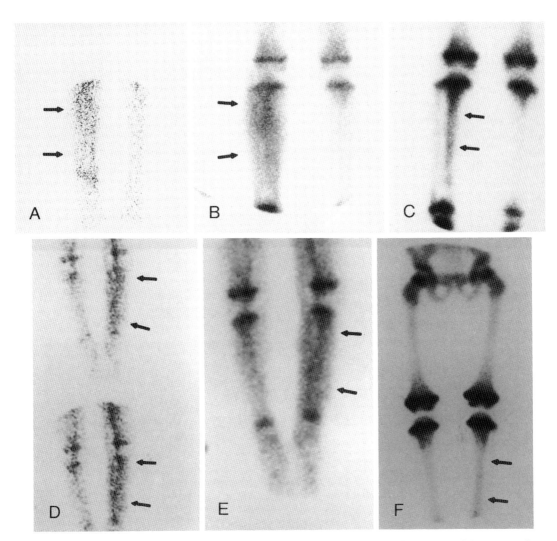

Figure 4.14. *Osteomyelitis verus cellulitis; nuclear scintigraphy technetium-99m bone scan.* **(A)** *Osteomyelitis.* Flow phase demonstrates increased flow to the right lower leg *(arrow)*. **(B)** Blood pool phase demonstrates pooling of isotope in the right lower extremity *(arrow)*. **(C)** Static scan demonstrates diffusely increased uptake over the entire right tibia *(arrows)*. **(D)** *Cellulitis.* Flow phase demonstrates increased flow to the left lower leg *(arrows)*. **(E)** Blood pool phase demonstrates pooling of isotope into the right lower extremity *(arrows)*. **(F)** Static scan, however, fails to demonstrate significant accumulation of isotope in the tibial shaft *(arrows)*. There is a faint ghost of the shaft suggested. This speaks against osteomyelitis and in favor of cellulitis, for while there always is a minor degree of reactive periosteal activity with adjacent soft tissue inflammation, for the bone scan to be positive for osteomyelitis, it must show markedly increased uptake of the isotope as seen in **(C)**.

(Fig. 4.14A–C). It should be remembered, however, that the pyrophosphate bone scan measures reactive (healing) bone activity and not the development of a purulent exudate per se. It is for this reason that in some cases imaging with gallium- or indium-labeled white blood cells (6, 15) may be required to determine whether an infection is actually present. However, in the pediatric age group osteomyelitis is a relatively clean and a first-time focal event, and thus the technetium-99m pyrophosphate study usually suffices. On the other hand, it should be remembered that in many cases, the technetium bone scan, in the very early stages of the infection, may appear falsely normal (3, 7, 10, 18).

The reason for the bone scan being normal in these early stages is that there is so much congestion of the bone marrow by the developing infection that blood flow, and hence the delivery of the isotope to the bone, is impaired. Usually within 24–48 hours results of the bone scan turn positive. Therefore if one can make the presumptive diagnosis of osteomyelitis on the basis of clinical and plain film roentgenographic (deep edema) findings, then one should assume that such infection is present and begin therapy. The bone scan, primarily for confirmation, can then be delayed for a day or two.

Because of the problem of the falsely negative bone scan, CT and MRI also have been utilized in the detection of early osteomyelitis (6, 8, 12, 13). In addition, ultrasonography has been utilized for this purpose (1). With ultrasound the findings depend on demonstration of hypoechoic purulent exudate between the periosteum and the cortex of the bone (Fig. 4.15). Of all imaging modalities, however, it is the least useful. On CT, bone marrow changes are subtle with the normally radiolucent bone marrow showing increased density or signal. Bone destruction, however, is very precisely delineated (Fig. 4.15C). With MRI the normal high signal of fat on the T_1-weighted images is lost, and on the proton density or T_2-weighted im-

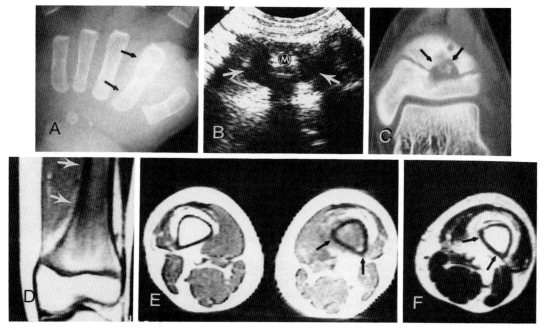

Fig. 4.15. *Osteomyelitis: Demonstration with various imaging modalities.* (*A*) Note mixed destruction and reactive sclerosis of the second metatarsal *(arrows)* in this infant with osteomyelitis. There is considerable soft tissue swelling. (*B*) Sonogram demonstrates a ring of hypoechoic pus *(arrows)* around the metacarpal (*M*). (*C*) CT study in another patient demonstrates a discrete focus of destruction in the distal tibia *(arrows)* with a suggestion of a small bony sequestrum. (*D*) MR, T_1-weighted image in another patient demonstrates decreased signal in the bone marrow of the distal left femur *(arrows)*. The plain film changes in this patient were near normal. Only a small focus of suspicious bony destruction was seen on the lateral view. (*E*) Axial images, T_1-weighted, demonstrate decreased signal of the marrow of the involved femur *(arrows)*. There is surrounding soft tissue edema. (*F*) Proton density image demonstrates increased signal in the involved marrow *(arrows)* indicating the presence of pus. In addition, surrounding edema now shows increased signal.

ages, increased signal is seen (Fig. 4.15*D–F*).

Nuclear scintigraphy also can be utilized to differentiate osteomyelitis from cellulitis (9). While in both conditions the blood flow and blood pool findings may be identical, with cellulitis there is no significant accumulation of the isotope agent in the bone itself. Only a ghost of the bone may be seen (Fig. 4.14*D–F*).

Most cases of osteomyelitis in childhood are hematogenous in origin, but some result from puncture wounds with secondary involvement of the underlying bone. A very small number result from osteomyelitis superimposed on a previous fracture (14). In any event, the bony changes are the same but it should be noted that osteomyelitis in flat bones (i.e., pelvic bones, clavicle, ribs, scapula) is much more difficult to detect with plain films, and it is in these instances that nuclear scintigraphy has a major role (12). In addition, CT (12) and MRI (8) can be utilized, but nuclear scintigraphy is less expensive.

REFERENCES

1. Abiri, M.M., Kirpekar, M., and Ablow, R.C.: Osteomyelitis: Detection with US. Work in progress. Radiology 169: 795–797, 1988.
2. Andrew, T.A., and Porter, K.: Primary subacute epiphyseal osteomyelitis: A report of three cases. J. Pediatr. Orthop. 5: 155–157, 1985.
3. Berkwitz, I.D., and Wenzel, W.: "Normal" technetium bone scans in patients with acute osteomyelitis. Am. J. Dis. Child. 134: 828–830, 1980.
4. Bogoch, E., Thompson, G., and Salter, R.B.: Foci of chronic circumscribed osteomyelitis (Brodie's abscess) that traverse the epiphyseal plate. J. Pediatr. Orthop. 4: 162–169, 1984.
5. Capitanio, M.A., and Kirkpatrick, J.A.: Early roentgen observation in acute osteomyelitis. A.J.R. 108: 488–496, 1970.
6. Dangman, B.C., Hoffer, F.A., Rand, F.F., and O'Rourke, E.J.: Osteomyelitis in children: Gadolinium enhanced MR imaging. Radiology 182: 743–747, 1992.
7. Fleisher, G.R., Paradise, J.E., Plotkin, S.A., and Borden, S., IV: Falsely normal radionuclide scans for osteomyelitis. Am. J. Dis. Child. 134: 499–502, 1980.
8. Fletcher, B.D., Scoles, P.V., and Nelson, A.D.: Osteomyelitis in children: Detection by mag-

netic resonance. Pediatr. Radiol. 150: 57–60, 1984.
9. Gilday, D.L., and Paul, D.J.: The differentiation of osteomyelitis and cellulitis in children using a combined blood pool and bone scan. J. Nucl. Med. 15: 494, 1974.
10. Handmaker, H.: Acute hematogenous osteomyelitis: Has the bone scan betrayed us? Radiology 135: 787–789, 1980.
11. Hayden, C.K., Jr., and Swischuk, L.E.: Para-articular soft tissue changes in infections and trauma of the lower extremity in children. A.J.R. 134: 307–311, 1980.
12. Hernandez, R.J., Conway, J.J., Poznanski, A.K., Tachdjian, M.O., Dias, L.S., and Kelikian, A.S.: The role of computed tomography and radionuclide scintigraphy in the localization of osteomyelitis in flat bones. J. Pediatr. Orthop. 5: 151–154, 1985.
13. Kuhn, J.P., and Berger, P.E.: Computed tomographic diagnosis of osteomyelitis. Radiology 130: 503–506, 1979.
14. Morrissy, R.T., and Haynes, D.W.: Acute hematogenous osteomyelitis: A model with trauma as an etiology. J. Pediatr. Orthop. 9: 447–456, 1989.
15. Raptopoulos, V., Dohery, P.W., Goss, T.P., King, M.A., Johnson, K., and Gantz, N.M.: Acute osteomyelitis: Advantage of white cell scans in early detection. A.J.R. 139: 1077–1082, 1982.
16. Rosenbaum, D.M., and Blumhagen, J.D.: Acute epiphyseal osteomyelitis in children. Radiology 156: 89–92, 1985.
17. Scott, R.J., Christofersen, M.R., Robertson, W.W. Jr., Davidson, R.S., Rankin, L., and Drummond, D.S.: Acute osteomyelitis in children: A review of 116 cases. J. Pediatr. Orthop. 10: 649–652, 1990.
18. Sullivan, D.C., Rosenfield, N.S., Ogden, J., and Gottschalk, A.: Problems in the scintigraphic detection of osteomyelitis in children. Radiology 135: 731–736, 1980.
19. Treves, S., Khettry, J., Broker, F.H., Wilkinson, R.H., and Watts, H.: Osteomyelitis: Early scintigraphic detection in children. Pediatrics 57: 173–186, 1976.

Osteomyelitis versus Bone Infarction in Sickle Cell Disease. The problem of differentiating bone infection from bone infarction in patients with sickle cell disease is difficult (1). Clinically and roentgenographically the findings may be similar in the early stages, but extremity swelling is usually more marked in osteomyelitis. Nuclear scintigraphy is of value in some of

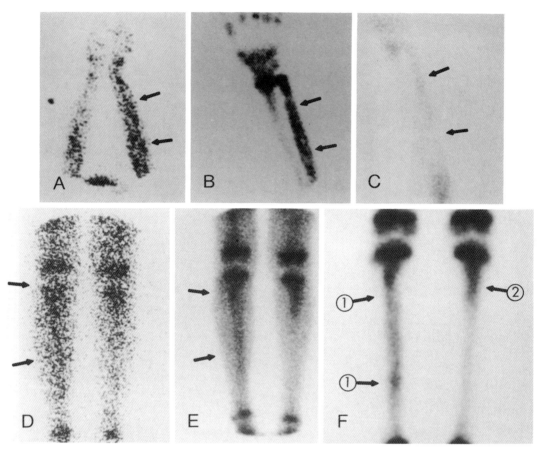

Figure 4.16. *Nuclear scintigraphy—Bone infarct.* (*A*) Blood flow phase demonstrates increased flow to the right upper extremity *(arrows)*. (*B*) Static scans demonstrate markedly increased uptake of isotope throughout the entire ulna *(arrows)* on the right. (*C*) Subsequent gallium bone scan shows vague and very subtle increase in activity in the left ulna. If this patient had osteomyelitis, the signal in the left ulna would be significantly increased. (*D*) Another patient with increased flow to a painful right lower extremity *(arrows)*. (*E*) Blood pool phase demonstrates the same findings *(arrows)*. However, note that the upper left tibial metaphysis also shows increased uptake of isotope. (*F*) Subsequent static scan demonstrates diffuse, but spotty, uptake of isotope throughout the right tibia (*1*). However, the uptake is irregular. In addition, there is increased uptake in the upper left tibia (*2*). A gallium scan would have been most helpful in this patient; otherwise it is difficult to interpret the findings, for some are due to old healing infarctions. This patient had no signs or symptoms referable to the left leg. Presumably the findings in the upper left tibia were due to an old healing infarct. In view of this, how can one be certain that the increased areas of activity in the right tibia are due to osteomyelitis? The answer is: one cannot and that is why these cases are so puzzling and why additional scans are necessary.

these cases (2, 3), for with a fresh infarct the bone scan will show decreased uptake in the area of infarction. Later, the area will become positive, for the bone scan will record reactive, healing bone activity. In this regard, however, the findings are no different than in osteomyelitis. Therefore, one should then proceed to a bone marrow imaging agent such as gallium citrate or in-

dium-labeled white blood cells. These studies can yield further data as to whether an infarction or an infection is present. With infarction the gallium- or indium-labeled white blood cell studies will be negative (Fig. 4.16A–C).

If a patient has sustained multiple episodes of bone infarction the findings on nuclear scintigraphy can be very confusing.

Indeed, they can be more confusing than helpful (Fig. 4.16D–F). Therefore, very often on must make one's final determination on the basis of clinical, laboratory, and other imaging findings. In this regard, if pronounced and extensive swelling of the extremity is present, simple infarction is unlikely. However, if only focal pain with minimal swelling is present, the problem can be due to either infection or infarction. Furthermore, it is quite likely that infarction precedes infection in many if not most of these cases and this only adds to the confusion. Even when CT (4) and MR are employed, they may not be helpful, for with both infection and infarction, bone marrow and bone insult occur. If one process affected the bone only and the other the marrow only, then the problem would, for the most part, be resolved. In the end, there is no simple answer to the problem.

REFERENCES

1. Mallouh, A., and Talab, Y.: Bone and joint infection in patients with sickle cell disease. J. Pediatr. Orthop. 5: 158–162, 1985.
2. Majd, M., and Frenkel, R.S.: Radionuclide imaging in skeletal inflammatory and ischemic disease in children. A.J.R. 126: 832–841, 1976.
3. Rao, S., Solomon, N., Miller, S., and Dunn, E.: Scintigraphic differentiation of bone infarction from osteomyelitis in children with sickle cell disease. J. Pediatr. 107: 685–688, 1985.
4. Stark, J.E., Glasier, C.M., Blasier, R.D., Aronson, J., and Seibert, J.J.: Osteomyelitis in children with sickle cell disease: Early diagnosis with contrast-enhanced CT. Radiology 179: 731–733, 1991.

Septic Arthritis. The roentgenographic assessment of septic arthritis centers around the detection of fluid in the involved joint and periarticular soft tissue edema. For the most part, this is accomplished by noting: (a) increased width of the joint space, (b) displacement of fat pads where applicable, and (c) comparing the suspicious findings on the abnormal side to those on the normal side. Assessment of all of the bony and soft tissue structures is especially important in the very young infant in whom little in the way of

systemic response to infection often is present. In other words, fever is not high, leukocytosis is not striking, toxicity is not marked, and the only finding may be an inability to move the involved extremity (pseudoparesis). However, with properly positioned roentgenograms and an evaluation of the joint space and soft tissues, one usually will detect the problem. In this regard, *in the absence of trauma, a good rule to follow is: fluid in the joint should be considered pus until proven otherwise.*

In the past, nuclear scintigraphy has been advocated for the differentiation of septic arthritis from other inflammatory processes around the joint, but generally speaking it is not overly productive in this role. In the end, one must rely on clinical findings and plain films in most cases, and then, if suspicion is high, arthrocentesis is required. Ultrasonography, however, has now become useful, especially in the hip joint where plain films often are unrewarding. More detailed discussions of the findings of septic arthritis for each joint are undertaken at later points.

UPPER EXTREMITY PROBLEMS

SHOULDER

Normal Soft Tissues of the Shoulder. There are no specific fat pads to evaluate around the shoulder, but over the clavicle the companion shadow can be of some use. This shadow represents the edge of the skin and subcutaneous tissues as they pass over the clavicle, and the edge can become obliterated by the edema associated with clavicular fractures (see Fig. 4.18C). Other than this, evaluation of the soft tissues of the shoulder is nonspecific.

Detecting Fluid in the Shoulder Joint. Fluid in the shoulder joints (i.e., pus or blood) causes the humerus to be displaced laterally and the joint space to be widened (Fig. 4.17). Associated swelling, edema, and bulging of the soft tissues around the shoulder may or may not be present, and are more prone to occur in young infants.

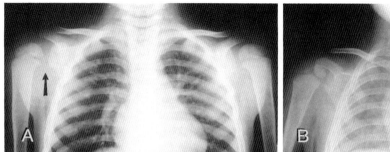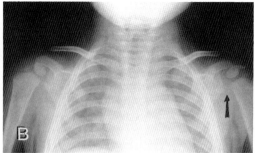

Figure 4.17. *Detecting fluid in the shoulder joint.* (**A**) Note widening of the joint space on the right *(arrow)*. The upper humerus and humeral head are displaced laterally from the glenoid fossa. This signifies the presence of intra-articular fluid. This child had *Haemophilus influenzae* septic arthritis. (**B**) Another patient with joint widening on the left *(arrow)* due to a Salter-Harris epiphyseal-metaphyseal fracture. Note that the epiphyseal line between the humeral head and metaphysis is wider than the one on the normal right side (i.e., Salter-Harris type I fracture).

As far as positioning the shoulder for examination in these cases, one can accept almost any reasonable anteroposterior position, as long as both the involved and noninvolved extremities are examined in the same position. In other words, one wants to avoid the situation where one extremity is examined in internal rotation while the other is examined in external rotation. On a practical basis, it often is best to examine the involved extremity in whichever position the patient holds that extremity and then to match that position in the normal extremity.

Clavicular Injuries. Overall, the clavicle is the most commonly injured bone of the shoulder in infants and young children. Injury usually results from: (a) falling on an outstretched extremity, (b) falling directly on the shoulder, or (c) a direct blow to the clavicle. By far the most common location for a clavicular fracture is the midshaft, and while many are easy to identify (Fig. 4.18*A*), others are more elusive. One reason for this is that many *clavicular fractures are greenstick or plastic bowing fractures or other fractures with a poorly visible fracture line.* In all of these cases, one should learn to look first for abnormal angulation or curvature of the injured clavicle. This is best accomplished by comparing one clavicle with the other, and any dis-

crepancy should be treated with suspicion. In addition, one also should assess the soft tissues for: (a) a general increase in density due to edema and bleeding, (b) obliteration of the companion shadow of the clavicle, and (c) obliteration of the supraclavicular fat-muscle interfaces (Fig. 4.18*B* and *C*).

Complete fractures through the midshaft of the clavicle, with displacement of the fracture fragments also are common, but are not a problem as far as roentgenographic detection is concerned. However, even in these cases, very often the position of the fracture is such that it is hidden by the first or second ribs. It is only with oblique or lordotic views that one can actually see the fracture (Fig. 4.19).

The most important pitfall in the evaluation of suspected clavicular fractures lies in the misinterpretation of a clavicle distorted by poor positioning or patient rotation, for a fractured clavicle (Fig. 4.20).

Acromioclavicular separations are not particularly common in infancy, but do occur in the older child and adolescent. In such cases, one should first look for soft tissue prominence over the acromioclavicular joint and then for separation of the joint itself. In this regard, although the acromioclavicular joint will be widened, one often also will note widening between the clavicle and the coracoid process of the scapula (Fig. 4.21). Indeed, separation at this site due to ligamentous sprain often is easier to detect than is acromioclavicular separation. Furthermore, in some of these cases it has been noted that an associated cora-

coid process fracture can occur (6). In the infant and young child, rather than acromioclavicular separation, an isolated fracture through the lateral end of the clavicle usually is sustained. However, even in some of these cases, a certain degree of

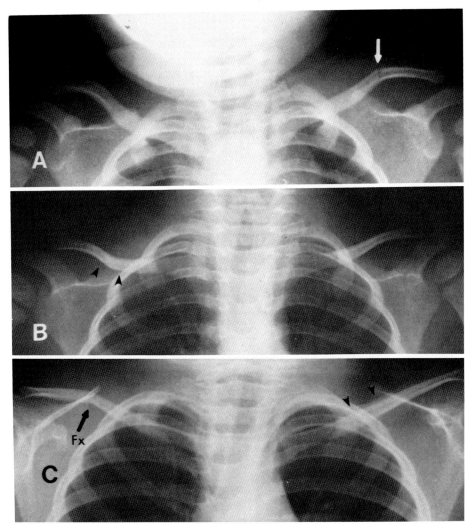

Figure 4.18. *Clavicular fractures.* (**A**) Typical fracture of clavicle. Note the easily identified fracture (arrow) of the bent left clavicle. (**B**) Subtle bending fracture. The only signs of a clavicular injury in this patient are those of unusual downward bending of the right clavicle (arrows) and a generalized increase in soft tissue density (edema) of the soft tissues around it. (**C**) Subtle bending fracture with soft tissue changes. In this patient, there is unusual bending of the right clavicle, but the fracture line *(Fx)* is difficult to see because it is obscured by the overlying scapular tip. However, note that there is a generalized increase in soft tissue density of the soft tissues in the right supraclavicular region, and that the companion shadow on the right is absent. Compare these findings with the normal findings on the left, including the presence of a normal companion shadow *(arrows)*. The companion shadow represents the interface between the air and the skin and subcutaneous tissues overlying the clavicle. With edema and swelling, these soft tissues thicken and the companion shadow is lost.

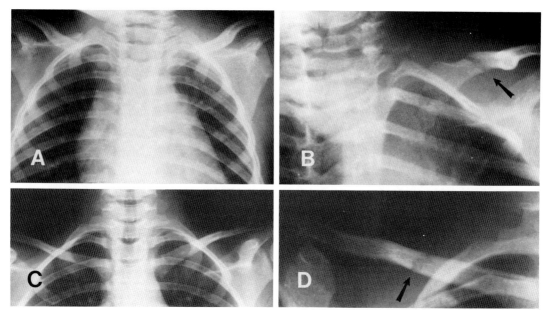

Figure 4.19. *Occult clavicular fractures.* (*A*) The clavicles are quite symmetric, but note soft tissue swelling over the left clavicle. Also note that it might be more bent than the right. (*B*) Oblique view demonstrates a clear-cut fracture through the medial portion of the left clavicle *(arrow)*. (*C*) Curvature of the clavicles is asymmetric. This is important. This patient had injury to the right shoulder, but one cannot see the fracture behind the second rib. (*D*) Another view, more oblique, demonstrates the fracture *(arrow)*.

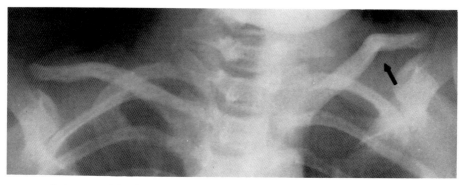

Figure 4.20. *Pseudofracture of the clavicle due to rotation.* This patient is rotated to the left, and this causes the left clavicle to telescope and appear bent *(arrow)*.

acromioclavicular separation and coraco-clavicular ligament sprain exists (Fig. 4.22).

Medial clavicular injuries usually consist of *anterior or posterior dislocations,* for fracturing in this area is relatively uncommon (4). With anterior displacement, a clinically visible and palpable bulge is present over the involved sternoclavicular

joint. With posterior displacement, such a bulge is not present, but a more serious problem arises in that tracheal compression occurs (Fig. 4.23). On frontal view, dislocation of the medial end of the clavicle, either anterior or posterior, can be suspected when it is noted that the medial end of the involved clavicle is lower than the medial end of the normal clavicle (Fig.

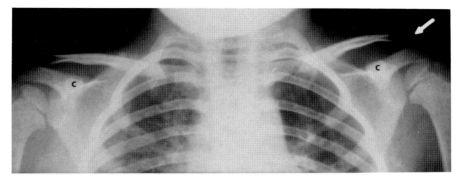

Figure 4.21. *Acromioclavicular separation.*   First note that the left clavicle is higher than the right, and then note that the acromioclavicular joint on the left is widened *(arrow)*. However, in addition, note that the space between the clavicle and the coracoid process *(c)* also is increased (coracoclavicular ligament sprain).

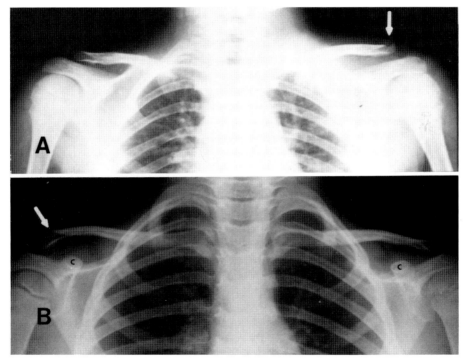

Figure 4.22. *Lateral clavicular fracture with varying degrees of acromioclavicular and coracoclavicular separation.*   (*A*) Note the fracture of the lateral end of the left clavicle *(arrow)*. The space between the fracture fragment and acromial process of the scapula is barely widened. Minimal if any associated acromioclavicular separation exists. (*B*) Note the fracture of the lateral end of the right clavicle *(arrow)*. However, also note that the space between the clavicle and coracoid process *(c)* is widened secondary to associated coracoclavicular ligament sprain. Although not visible on this illustration, a mild degree of acromioclavicular separation also was present in this patient.

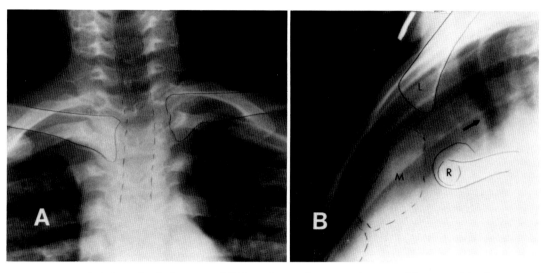

Figure 4.23. *Medial clavicular dislocation.* (A) Frontal view demonstrating typical downward displacement of the medial end of the right clavicle. This can occur with either posterior or anterior dislocations. (B) Oblique view demonstrating the posteriorly displaced right clavicle (R), and normally aligned left clavicle (L). Note associated anterior indentation of the trachea *(arrow)*. Manubrium, (M). (Reprinted with permission from F.A. Lee and J.L. Gwinn: Retrosternal dislocation of the clavicle. Radiology 110: 631–634, 1974.)

4.23). Occasionally the clavicle is displaced upward (Fig. 4.24), but in any case CT should be the next study to be performed. It very clearly can delineate the position of the clavicle and detect any associated avulsion fractures (Fig. 4.24).

Injuries of the Upper Humerus. In childhood, one of the more common injuries of the upper humerus is the Salter-Harris type I or II epiphyseal-metaphyseal injury (Figs. 4.25–4.27). Salter-Harris type III epiphyseal injuries are less common (Fig. 4.27C) and types IV and V are quite uncommon in the shoulder. In those type I and II injuries where the epiphysis is completely separated, the diagnosis never is in doubt (5), but in the more subtle cases, one should look for widening of the epiphyseal line and/or the presence of a metaphyseal corner fracture. In chronic form, this same injury is the one seen in young boys (epiphyseal) playing baseball and partaking in overexuberant stressful pitching. It is termed *"little leaguer's shoulder"* (1, 2, 3, 8).

Other fractures occurring through the upper humerus include the easily identi-

fied surgical neck fracture, transverse or oblique upper humeral shaft fractures, and the more subtle buckle or torus fractures (Fig. 4.28). In addition, *it should be noted that pathologic fractures through unicameral bone cysts quite commonly occur in the upper humerus (see Fig. 4.10C).*

A major pitfall in the evaluation of the upper humeral fractures is to misinterpret the normal epiphyseal line for a fracture. This can occur when the epiphyseal line is open and wide or when it is closing and narrow (Fig. 4.29). Of course, when comparative views of the normal extremity are obtained, almost always the line appears exactly the same, and the problem is solved. However, this simple solution notwithstanding, it is still very common to miscall this normal finding for a fracture.

Dislocations of the shoulder are not common in the young infant and child, for it is only after the epiphysis closes that it becomes a problem. The dislocations, of course, can be either anterior (i.e., subglenoid or subcoracoid) or posterior. The posterior dislocations are more difficult to detect, for overlapping of the humeral

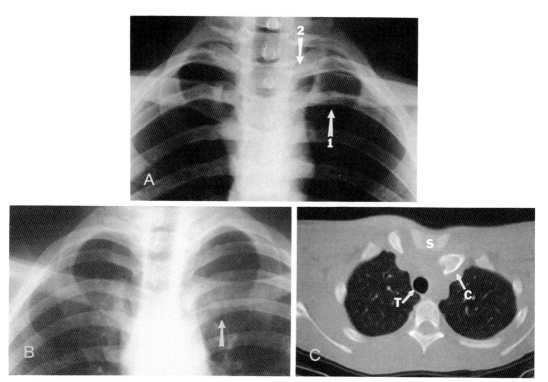

Figure 4.24. *Superior medial dislocation of clavicle.* (*A*) Note the elevated medial end of the left clavicle (*1*). The sternoclavicular joint is disrupted and widened (*2*). (*B*) Another patient with an elevated medial end of the left clavicle (*C*). (*C*) Axial CT study demonstrates the posteriorly displaced left medial clavicle *(arrow)*. Sternum (*S*); trachea (*T*). Note that the trachea is not compressed. Also note the normal position of the medial end of the right clavicle.

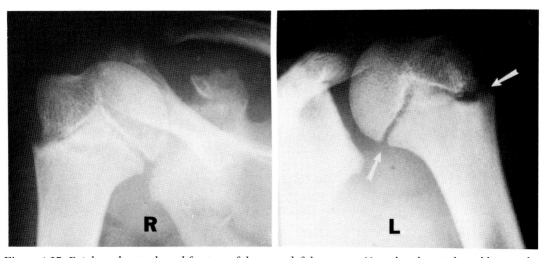

Figure 4.25. *Epiphyseal-metaphyseal fracture of the upper left humerus.* Note that the epiphyseal line on the left is wider and more radiolucent *(arrows)* than the one on the right. Such widening of the epiphyseal line denotes the presence of a Salter-Harris type injury, either I or II. The findings above are those of a Salter-Harris type I injury. In addition, note that on the normal side the humeral head along its lateral aspect appears offset or displaced on the metaphysis. This is normal and should not be misinterpreted as a displaced epiphyseal fracture.

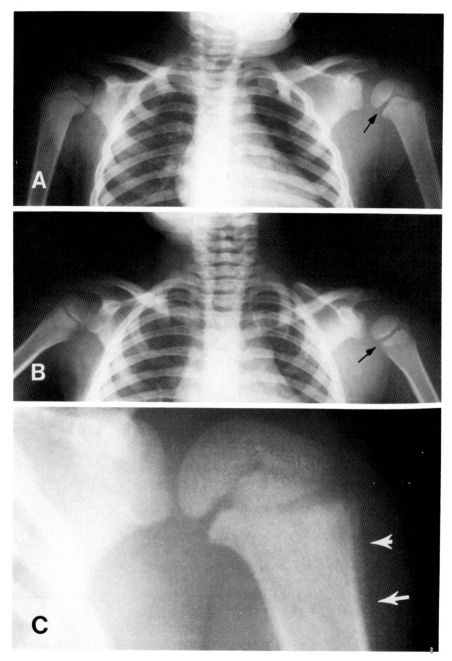

Figure 4.26. *Epiphyseal-metaphyseal fracture—shoulder.* (*A*) Note widening of the epiphyseal line of the upper left humerus *(arrow)*. Also note that the joint space is widened, suggesting fluid (blood) in the joint. (*B*) Another view demonstrating similar findings. Note especially that the epiphyseal line remains widened *(arrow)*. (*C*) Follow-up film 2 weeks later demonstrates healing of the fracture with periosteal new bone along the upper humeral shaft *(arrows)*.

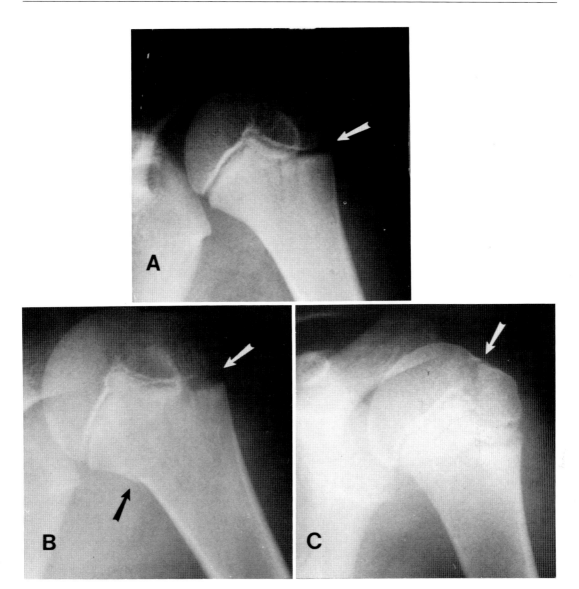

Figure 4.27. *Other epiphyseal-metaphyseal fractures of the upper humerus.* (**A**) Salter-Harris type II injury with a widened epiphyseal line laterally *(arrow)* and two poorly defined vertical fracture lines extending into the upper humeral shaft. (**B**) Salter-Harris type II injury with a widened epiphyseal line laterally *(white arrow)* and a cortical break medially *(black arrow).* The metaphyseal fracture fragment is rather large in this patient. (**C**) Salter-Harris type III injury. Note the fracture *(arrow)* through the nondisplaced epiphysis.

head and the glenoid fossa can be subtle. Anterior dislocations usually present a rather characteristic appearance, with the humeral head being displaced downward and resting under the coracoid process or glenoid fossa (Fig. 4.30). In any case, and especially with posterior dislocations, transaxillary views of the shoulder should

be obtained for clearer definition (Fig. 4.30). Of course, CT studies now can also be obtained, and are especially useful for locating the humeral head and any associated glenoid avulsions.

Scapular Fractures. These can occur through the body of the scapula or the acromial or coracoid processes of the scap-

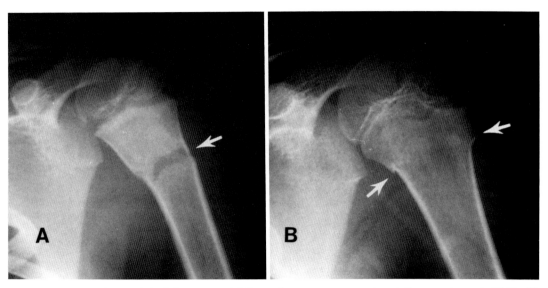

Figure 4.28. *Upper humeral shaft fractures.* (*A*) Typical transverse surgical neck fracture *(arrow)*. (*B*) Buckle compression-type fracture of the upper humerus *(arrows)*. This type of fracture is quite common in infants and young children, for the cortex in this area is still relatively weak.

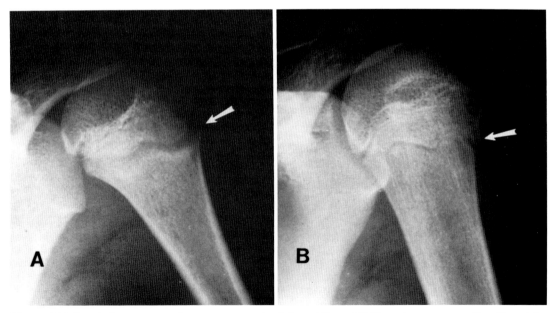

Figure 4.29. *Pseudofracture upper humerus—normal epiphyseal line.* (*A*) Normal appearance of a wide epiphyseal line *(arrow)* often misinterpreted as a fracture. (*B*) Older child with narrower epiphyseal line mimicking a fracture *(arrow)*.

ula. Fractures through the body of the scapula usually result from direct blows and can be linear, curvilinear (Fig. 4.31), or stellate. Fractures through the acromial and coracoid processes of the scapula can result from direct blows or falls on the outstretched extremity and may be difficult to detect (Fig. 4.31). Comparative views are of the utmost importance here, especially with the more peculiar fractures (Fig.

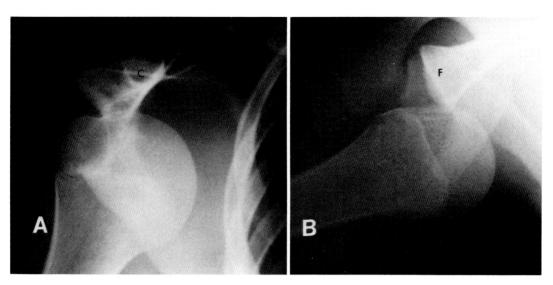

Figure 4.30. *Anterior dislocation of the shoulder.* (*A*) Note abnormal position of the upper humerus. It is located below the coracoid process (*C*). This is a subcoracoid dislocation. (*B*) Transaxillary view showing dislocated humerus anterior to the glenoid fossa (*F*). With subglenoid dislocations, the humeral head lies under the glenoid fossa, while with posterior dislocations it lies posterior to the scapula.

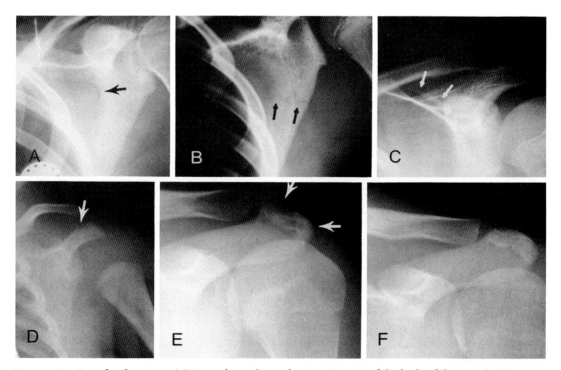

Figure 4.31. *Scapular fracture.* (*A*) Typical curvilinear fracture *(arrow)* of the body of the scapula. (*B*) Transverse, linear fracture *(arrow)* of the scapula. (*C*) Avulsion fracture *(arrows)* of the upper scapular edge in an older child. (*D*) Acromial fracture *(arrow)* in a battered infant. (*E*) Bending fracture of acromion. Note peculiar shape of acromial process *(arrows)*. This was a bending fracture of the acromion resulting from a direct fall on the tip of the shoulder. (*F*) Normal side for comparison.

4.31*E* and *F*), and of course CT studies are invaluable in analyzing fractures of the scapula, especially those of the glenoid fossa (Fig. 4.32).

Septic Arthritis, Osteomyelitis, and Cellulitis of the Shoulder. With septic arthritis, the most important roentgenographic features are joint space widening and lateral displacement of the upper humerus (Fig. 4.33*A* and *B*). These findings denote the presence of pus in the shoulder joint (7), and in the very young infant, the adjacent soft tissues may appear edematous and cause the whole shoulder to bulge. In the older child, however, the only finding usually is joint space widening, and in many cases nothing is seen. Ul-

trasound may be useful for demonstrating occult pus in these cases, for much as it is in the hip, increase in the width of the joint space may be more difficult to detect in older children.

When osteomyelitis or cellulitis of the shoulder is present, there usually is little in the way of joint space widening, except in the young infant, where septic arthritis and osteomyelitis frequently occur together. In such cases, of course, features of both conditions will be present (Fig. 4.33*C* and *D*). With osteomyelitis alone, however, early stage findings usually consist of nothing more than soft tissue edema and obliteration of the normal fat-muscle tissue planes. This causes the soft tissues to ap-

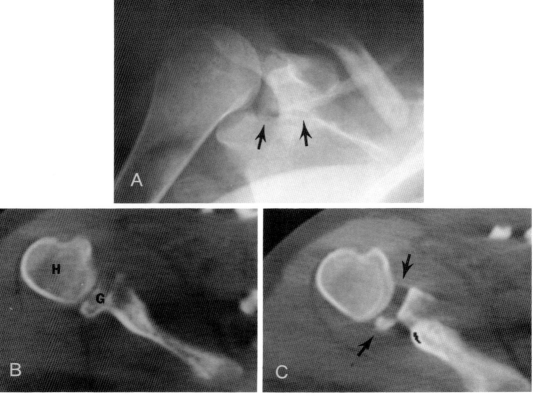

Figure 4.32. *Shoulder dislocation with scapular fracture—CT findings.* (**A**) Note the superiorly dislocated humerus and the associated fracture through the acetabulum *(arrows)*. The humeral head is still articulating with the superior fragment. (**B**) Upper CT cut demonstrates the humeral head (*H*) articulating with the superior portion of the glenoid fossa (*G*). (**C**) Lower cut demonstrates widening of the joint space *(upper arrow)* and a small avulsed bony fragment *(lower arrow)*.

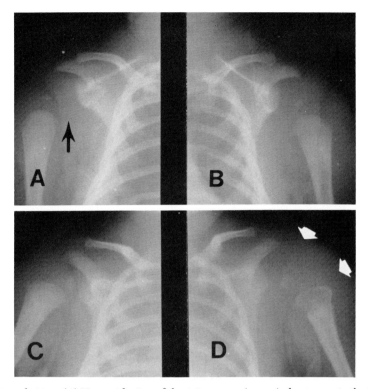

Figure 4.33. *Septic arthritis.* (**A**) Note widening of the joint space *(arrow)*, due to pus in the joint. (**B**) Normal left side for comparison. (**C**) Septic arthritis and osteomyelitis. Normal right shoulder. (**D**) On the *left,* note bulging of the soft tissues of the left shoulder *(arrows)* and widening of the joint space due to pus in the joint. Destruction of the upper humerus also is present. If this patient had osteomyelitis alone, little if any joint space widening would occur. Contrarily, if septic arthritis were the only problem, no bone destruction of the metaphysis would be seen and soft tissue swelling would be less pronounced.

pear more homogeneously opaque than normal (Fig. 4.34*A* and *B*) and, later on, bony destruction can be seen (Fig. 4.34*C*). Cellulitis around the shoulder is not a particularly common problem in children.

Miscellaneous Shoulder Problems. Occasionally, one can encounter a patient who does not move his or her upper extremity because of: (a) scapular or clavicular involvement by Caffey's disease (infantile cortical hyperostosis), (b) osteomyelitis of the scapula or clavicle, (c) metastatic disease, (d) histiocytosis X of the bones of the shoulder (Fig. 4.35*A*), or a rotator cuff injury. The latter currently is best evaluated with **MR** but is not a common problem in childhood. With **MRI**, tears of the supraspinatus muscle and tendon, produce focal high signal because of the edema and bleeding in the supraspinatus tendon (Fig. 4.35*B*).

Normal Findings Causing Problems. Misinterpretation of the upper humeral epiphyseal line for a fracture has been dealt with earlier and is demonstrated in Figure 4.29. Other normal structures frequently misinterpreted for abnormalities include a bony exostosis along the inferior aspect of the clavicle just at the site of the costoclavicular ligament (Fig. 4.36*A*) and a normal accessory ossification center at the medial end of the clavicle (Fig. 4.36*B*). Still other normal structures causing problems include the various ossification centers of the scapula (Fig. 4.37) and, in this regard, the secondary center for the coracoid process can be very large and surely suggestive of a fracture in some individuals

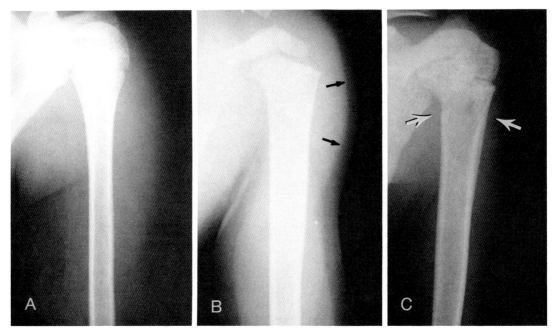

Figure 4.34. *Osteomyelitis.* (*A*) Early changes in older child. Note that the humerus is intact, but that there is extensive deep and superficial edema of the adjacent soft tissues. No muscle-fat planes are identified, and the soft tissues are of increased, homogeneous density. (*B*) Normal shoulder for comparison demonstrating the normal interface between the muscle and the subcutaneous fat *(arrows)*. Note that the other fat-muscle interfaces also are clearly visible. (*C*) Later notice destruction of the upper humeral metaphysis and some early periosteal new bone deposition *(arrows)*.

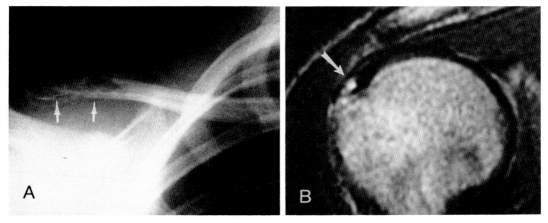

Figure 4.35. (*A*) *Histiocytosis X of clavicle.* Note the expanding, lytic, somewhat bubbly appearing lesion of the distal right clavicle *(arrows)*. (*B*) *Rotator cuff injury.* Coronal MR image demonstrates a focus of high signal in the supraspinatus tendon *(arrow)*.

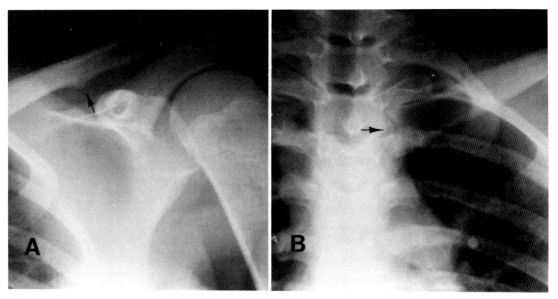

Figure 4.36. *Normal variations of the clavicle.* (*A*) Note the bony exostosis *(arrow)* at the site of the insertion of the costoclavicular ligament. (*B*) Normal medial accessory ossification center *(arrow)*. The wire loop just below and medial to it is a wire suture in the sternum from a prior thoracotomy.

(Fig. 4.37*C* and *D*). In addition the ring apophysis of the glenoid fossa, if caught tangentially, can erroneously suggest a glenoid rim avulsion fracture (Fig. 4.38).

Vascular grooves in the scapula also can create problems and be misinterpreted for fractures (Fig. 4.39). Finally, one might mention the normal deltoid notch, a finding frequently misinterpreted for a destructive lesion, and the vacuum joint phenomenon around the shoulder, as examples of other findings causing uncertainties in interpretation (Fig. 4.40).

REFERENCES

1. Adams, J.E.: Little league shoulder: Osteochondrosis of proximal humeral epiphysis in boy baseball pitchers. Calif. Med. 105: 22–25, 1966.
2. Bowerman, J.W., and McDonnell, E.J.: Radiology of athletic injuries: Baseball. Radiology 116: 611–615, 1975.
3. Dotter, W.E.: Little leaguer's shoulder—a fracture of the proximal epiphyseal cartilage of the humerus due to baseball pitching. Guthrie Clin. Bull. 23: 68, 1953.
4. Lee, F.A., and Gwinn, J.L.: Retrosternal dislocation of the clavicle. Radiology 110: 631–634, 1974.
5. Nicastro, J.F., and Adair, D.M.: Fracture-dislocation of the shoulder in a 32-month-old child. J. Pediatr. Orthop. 2: 427–429, 1982.
6. Protass, J.J., Stampfli, F.V., and Osmer, J.C.: Coracoid process fracture diagnosis in acromioclavicular separation. Radiology 116: 61–64, 1975.
7. Schmidt, D., Mubarak, S., and Gelberman, R.: Septic shoulders in children. J. Pediatr. Orthop. 1: 67–72, 1981.
8. Torg, J.S., Pollack, H., and Sweterlitsch, P.: The effect of competitive pitching on the shoulders and elbows of preadolescent baseball players. Pediatrics 49: 267–272, 1972.

HUMERAL SHAFT

Midshaft fractures of the humerus commonly occur in infancy and childhood. The most common is the spiral or oblique fracture, but transverse fractures also are seen. Usually these fractures are so obvious that there is no problem in their roentgenographic detection, but occasionally they are hairline and undisplaced and more difficult to detect. Cortical buckling or torus fractures do not usually occur in the midshaft of the humerus, for the cortex is thick in this area, and the only normal finding

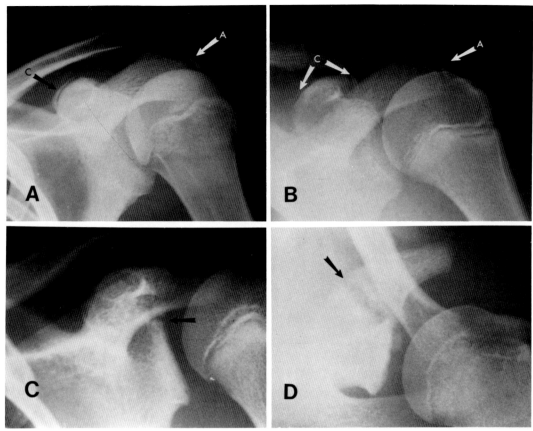

Figure 4.37. *Normal findings—scapular ossification centers.* (*A* and *B*) Usual accessory centers. Note the variable appearance of the accessory ossification centers of the acromion (*A*) and coracoid (*C*) process. (*C*) Large coracoid secondary center. Note the junction between the large coracoid secondary center and the scapula (*arrow*) simulating a fracture. (*D*) Special oblique view demonstrating that the fracture fragment actually is a large coracoid secondary center, and that the junction between it and the scapula produces a pseudofracture line (*arrow*). These large secondary centers should not be misinterpreted for fractures. This patient had a similar center in the other scapula.

Figure 4.38. *Glenoid rim; secondary ossification center.* Note the fracture fragment-like secondary center (*arrows*) of the glenoid fossa.

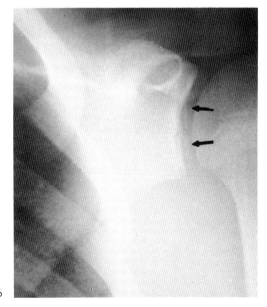

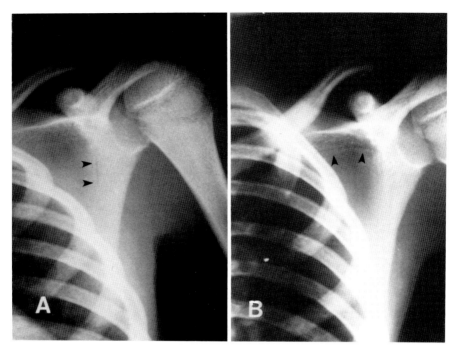

Figure 4.39. *Normal vascular grooves of scapula.*   (*A* and *B*) Demonstration of vascular grooves of the scapula *(arrows)*, frequently misinterpreted as fractures.

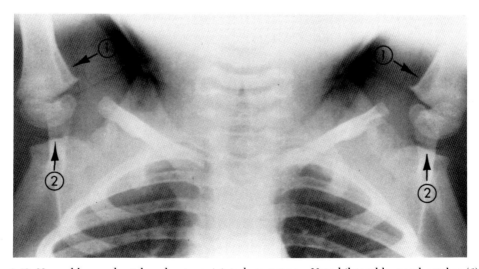

Figure 4.40. *Normal humeral notch and vacuum joint phenomenon.*   Note bilateral humeral notches (*1*) often misinterpreted as destructive lesions of the proximal humerus. These notches represent a normal depression of the bone in the region of insertion of the deltoid muscle. The notch is characteristically visualized when the extremity is upwardly extended. Also note the normal vacuum joint phenomenon in both shoulders (*2*). This phenomenon occurs when the upper extremities are stretched and is normal. Although the term "vacuum joint" is used to describe this finding, there is debate as to whether the radiolucent area actually represents a vacuum, or a space filled with nitrogen or water vapor.

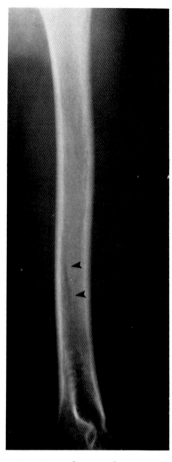

Figure 4.41. *Normal vascular groove of humerus.* Note the vascular groove *(arrows)* in the distal humerus. These vascular grooves can be confused with linear or spiral fractures. However, when one notes that the radiolucent line is rather wide and that there is slight sclerosis along either edge, one should make the diagnosis of normal vascular groove.

that can be misinterpreted for a fracture is a normal vascular groove (Fig. 4.41).

ELBOW

Normal Soft Tissues and Fat Pads. In the elbow, the most important fat pads to assess are the anterior and posterior fat pads (2, 3, 13, 18, 19). The anterior fat pad is located in the coronoid fossa, while the posterior fat pad is located in the olecranon fossa. These fat pads must be evaluated on true lateral, flexed views of the elbow, for

with any degree of rotation, their usefulness diminishes or is totally invalidated. Normally, on the true lateral flexed view of the elbow, the anterior fat pad is visible, but the posterior fat pad is not (Fig. 4.42A). The reason for the lack of visualization of the posterior fat pad is that it lies deep in the olecranon fossa. It becomes visible only when fluid in the joint displaces it posteriorly. On extension, however, it may be visible normally, but never on a flexed view. These fat pad configurations are very consistent, and consequently, any deviation from the configurations illustrated in Figure 4.42 should be considered abnormal.

The supinator fat pad (24) is another normal fat pad around the elbow. It also is seen on true lateral views and overlies the anterior aspect of the supinator muscle (Fig. 4.42B). Overall, however, this fat pad is less useful than the other elbow fat pads, for it is less consistently visualized, especially in infants and young children. Nonetheless, it can be obliterated, and/or displaced with fractures of the proximal radius. It also can be obliterated with generalized edema around the elbow.

Evaluation of the soft tissues around the elbow, other than the fat pads, is nonspecific. Basically, it consists of noting whether the fat-muscle interfaces are distinct or indistinct. If they are indistinct, edema is present.

Detecting Fluid in the Elbow Joint—Displaced Fat Pads. Fluid in the elbow joint usually produces upward and outward displacement of the anterior and posterior fat pads (Fig. 4.43A). These fat pads overlie the capsule of the elbow joint, and their displacement is very accurate in reflecting the presence of intra-articular fluid. Indeed, evaluation of the fat pads is the only way to roentgenographically determine whether fluid is present in the elbow joint, for the ligaments and muscles around the elbow are too strong to allow distraction of the articulating bones. Consequently, significant joint space widening

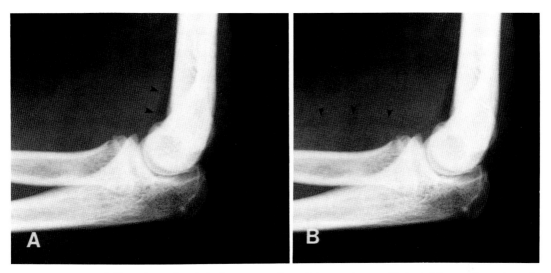

Figure 4.42. *Normal elbow fat pads.* (A) The anterior fat pad *(arrows)* normally is visible as a thin, triangular radiolucency anterior to the humerus. The posterior fat pad, on true lateral flexed views of the elbow, is not visible under normal circumstances. (B) The supinator fat pad *(arrows)* is thin and more often visible in older children.

seldom, if ever, is seen. Ultrasonography also can be used to detect fluid in the elbow joint (15) but seldom is needed as the findings on lateral elbow films are very sensitive. It should be noted, however, that if edema also surrounds the elbow, the displaced fat pads will be obliterated, or just faintly visible (Fig. 4.43).

Injuries of the Distal Humerus. Injuries of the distal end of the humerus most commonly include: (a) supracondylar fractures, (b) lateral condylar fractures, and (c) medial epicondylar fractures. The most common of these, however, is the *supracondylar fracture* and generally this fracture results from a fall on the outstretched upper extremity. The classic, clearly visible, supracondylar fracture with angulation and posterior displacement of the distal fragment is not difficult to recognize (Fig. 4.44). However, very often even though a fracture is visible on lateral view it is not seen on frontal view (Fig. 4.45). In addition, when the fracture is hairline or merely a plastic, bending fracture, little angulation occurs. In such cases, one must rely more on fat pad abnormalities and an abnormal anterior humeral line. The anterior humeral line is a line drawn along the anterior aspect of the distal humerus and should be applied on true lateral views. Under normal circumstances, it intersects the ossified capitellum somewhere through its middle third (26). If it intersects the capitellum through the anterior third, or if it misses it entirely, a supracondylar fracture should be present (Fig. 4.46). The anterior humeral line is a little more difficult to apply in the young infant where the capitellum is incompletely ossified, but even in these cases, if the findings are compared to those on the normal side, posterior displacement will be detected. In addition, in almost every instance, the fat pads are elevated and/or obliterated in these patients, and if they are, one should assume that an elbow injury has occurred. Not always will it be a supracondylar fracture, but since this fracture is so common, in the absence of other visible fractures, one should assume that it is present. In many of these cases, on follow-up healing phase films, one's original suspicions will be confirmed (Fig. 4.47). There will, of

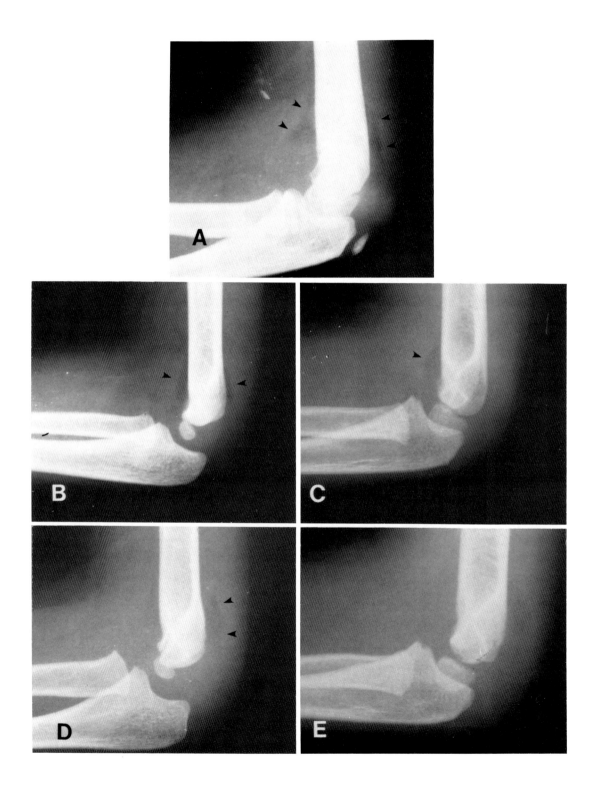

course, be cases where no such evidence of healing is present, and in such cases one assumes that a traumatic joint effusion only was present. However, it is better to have a few of these cases than to miss those with occult supracondylar fractures.

Although most fractures through the supracondylar region are of the type demonstrated in Figures 4.44 through 4.47, in the young infant where the cortex is relatively thin and weak, one can encounter buckle fractures in this region (Fig. 4.48). Of course, as with any buckle type fracture, one view may be better than the other for fracture visualization and, indeed, one often requires oblique views for full demonstration of these fractures. Finally, it should be noted that in some cases a supracondylar fracture with faulty alignment results in a cubitus varus (gunstock) deformity of the elbow (14), which may need surgical correction.

In terms of *condylar* and *epicondylar* injuries of the distal humerus, it is the medial epicondyle and lateral condyle that most commonly are injured (6, 23). Medial condylar and lateral epicondylar fractures are rare (20). *Lateral condylar fractures tend to occur in young infants and children while medial epicondylar fractures more often occur in older children.*

Unfortunately, many of these fractures are rather subtle and, once again, examination of the soft tissues becomes most important. In this regard, an abnormality of the fat pads of the elbow usually is present

but, more importantly, there will be telltale unilateral swelling and edema of the soft tissues. With medial epicondylar fractures, of course, such swelling occurs medially, while with lateral condylar fractures, it occurs laterally. The presence of such unilateral soft tissue change is especially important in the assessment of those medial epicondylar injuries where minimal or no displacement of the epicondyle occurs (Fig. 4.49), or in children under 5–7 years of age where the epicondyle is not yet ossified.

A wide range of medial epicondylar injuries occur, and injuries seen range from those with simple separation of the epicondyle to those with complete dislocation and/or intra-articular entrapment of the epicondyle (Fig. 4.50). Medial epicondylar injuries result from avulsion secondary to the pull of the flexor pronator tendon. Thus, the more severe the wrenching injury, the more severe the displacement. In some cases minimal or no displacement is seen (Fig. 4.51A), while in others not only will displacement be present, but the medial epicondyle also will be rotated (Fig. 4.51B). When entrapment of the medial epicondyle occurs, the medial epicondyle is not visible in its normal position (Fig. 4.52). In addition to these injuries of the medial epicondyle, it should be noted that avulsion of this secondary center frequently accompanies dislocations of the elbow. In these cases, the fact that the medial epicondyle is displaced can elude de-

---

Figure 4.43. *Abnormal fat pad configurations.* Elevation and displacement denotes the presence of fluid in the joint; obliteration denote periarticular edema and swelling. Both can occur together. (**A**) Elevation and displacement only. Note that both the anterior and posterior fat pads are visible and displaced upward and outward (*arrows*). This patient had an occult supracondylar fracture of the humerus. (**B**) Less pronounced displacement of the fat pads (*arrows*). The fact that the posterior fat pad is even visible is abnormal in itself, for when it is visible, it is displaced. (**C**) Anterior fat pad displacement only. The anterior fat pad is displaced and elevated (*arrow*), while the posterior fat pad is not displaced and not visible. This patient had a minimal fracture of the lateral condyle. (**D**) Displacement and obliteration. The posterior fat pad is markedly displaced (*arrows*) and a little hazy (obliterated) because of edema around the elbow. The anterior fat pad also is displaced, but because of edema, also is obliterated. Only a subtle suggestion of its presence, in its abnormally elevated position, is noted. (**E**) Displacement and marked obliteration. Both fat pads are displaced and elevated, but both are barely visible because of extensive edema around the elbow. Both this patient and the patient in (**D**) had subtle distal humerus fractures.

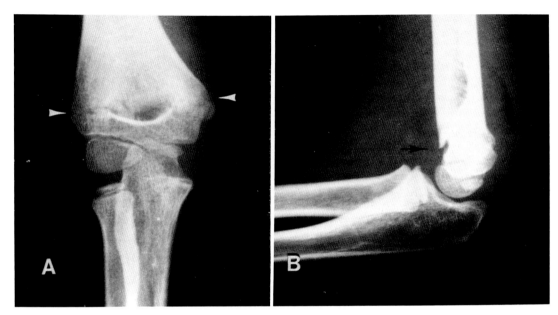

Figure 4.44. *Typical supracondylar fractures.*   (*A*) Frontal view: note the transverse fracture line *(arrows)*. (*B*) Lateral view: note the anterior fracture *(arrow)* and posterior tilting of the distal fracture fragment. In addition, note that the anterior fat pad is elevated and obliterated, and that the posterior fat pad is markedly elevated.

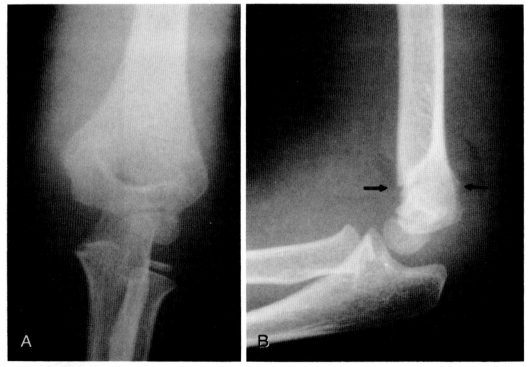

Figure 4.45. *Supracondylar fracture not visible on anteroposterior view.*   (*A*) On the anteroposterior view there is considerable soft tissue swelling, but the fracture through the supracondylar region is not visible. (*B*) Lateral view demonstrates the typical fracture *(arrows)*, with obliteration and elevation of the anterior fat pad and elevation of the posterior fat pad.

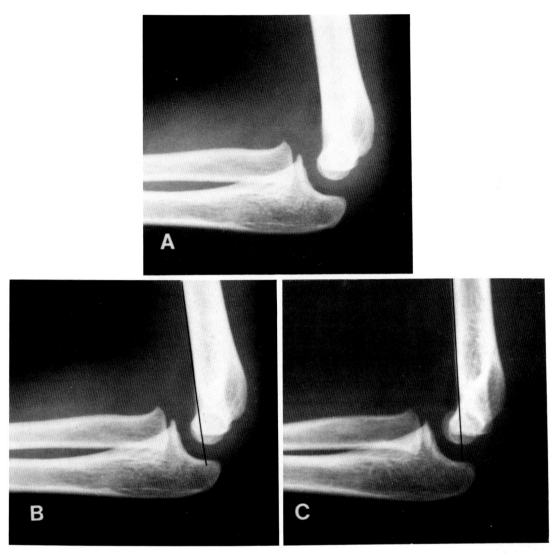

Figure 4.46. *Subtle supracondylar fractures—value of soft tissues and anterior humeral line.*   (*A*) Young child with elbow injury. Note soft tissue swelling around the elbow and a partially obliterated and elevated anterior fat pad. (*B*) Same elbow. The anterior humeral line intersects the capitellum through its anterior third. An occult, greenstick, or bending fracture should be suspected. (*C*) Normal elbow for comparison. Note the position of the normal anterior fat pad and the normal position of the anterior humeral line. It intersects the capitellum through its middle third.

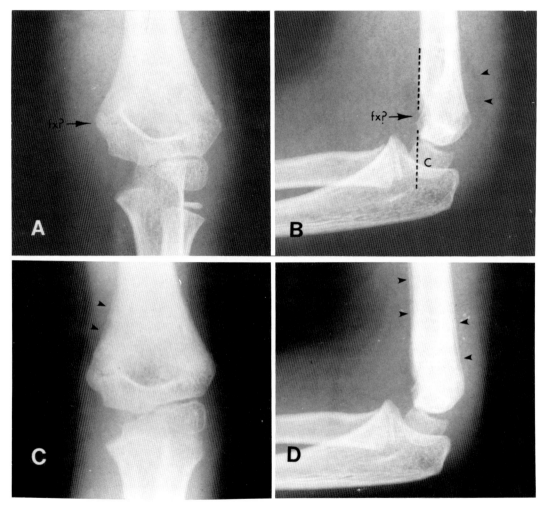

Figure 4.47. *Subtle supracondylar fracture with healing.*   (*A*) Frontal view demonstrating little or no abnormality. A subtle fracture line *(fx)* is suggested medially. (*B*) Lateral view demonstrating abnormal fat pads and an anterior humeral line that intersects the capitellum (*c*) through its anterior third. This should suggest posterior displacement of the capitellum and an underlying supracondylar fracture. A fracture line *(arrow)* also is suggested, but it is not definitely visible. (*C*) Two weeks later, note periosteal new bone deposition along both sides of the distal humerus *(arrows)*. The fracture line is more clearly visible. (*D*) Lateral view demonstrating periosteal new bone deposition along the shaft of the humerus *(arrows)*. Also note that the fat pads have returned to normal, but that the capitellum still is posteriorly displaced.

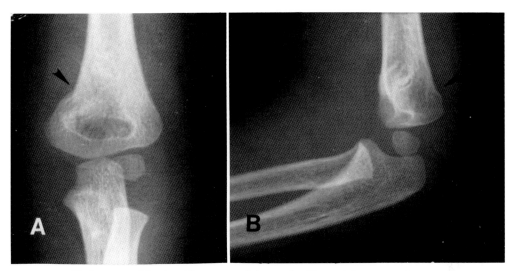

Figure 4.48. *Buckle fracture of the distal humerus.* (*A*) Note buckling of the cortex along the medial aspect of the distal humerus *(arrowhead)*. (*B*) Lateral view demonstrating buckling of the cortex posteriorly *(arrowhead)*, and posterior displacement of the capitellum. Also note the faintly visible but definitely displaced posterior fat pad. The anterior fat pad is, for the most part, obliterated.

tection until postreduction films are obtained (Fig. 4.53).

With lateral condylar injuries, it is most important to determine whether they are displaced or undisplaced. When displacement occurs, it occurs upward and outward, and does so when the fracture extends through the articular cartilage of the distal humerus. In these cases, the stabilizing, hinge-like function of the nondisplaced fracture fragment is lost and the injury becomes unstable (Fig. 4.54). Such fractures require internal fixation, and thus it is most important to identify them accurately. Examples of displaced and nondisplaced lateral condylar fractures are presented in Fig. 4.55. Another variation of the lateral condylar fracture occurs in young infants in whom only a small sliver of the metaphysis is avulsed. In these cases, which actually are very common, close inspection of roentgenograms and assessment of the fat pads and adjacent soft tissues is most worthwhile (Fig. 4.56), but in other cases oblique views become more important (Fig. 4.57).

Lateral epicondylar and medial condylar fractures (20), as noted earlier, are much less common than the fractures just discussed, but in those cases where they occur, similar subtle bony and unilateral soft tissue changes should serve to alert one to their presence. *Total fractures through the condylar regions of the humerus* can present clinically with apparent dislocation of the elbow (9, 17, 25). Roentgenographically, however, the misconception is readily corrected, for the findings are completely different from those of true dislocation of the elbow (Fig. 4.58).

The *little leaguer's elbow* usually is devoid of significant soft tissue or bony abnormalities on the roentgenograms (4, 5, 27). It is a traumatic lesion resulting from too much pitching at too young an age, and if long-term bony changes occur, they consist of fragmentation and enlargement of the medial epicondyle. In other cases, if such stress on the elbow continues, the following can occur: overgrowth and fragmentation of various other epiphyses and secondary centers around the elbow (11),

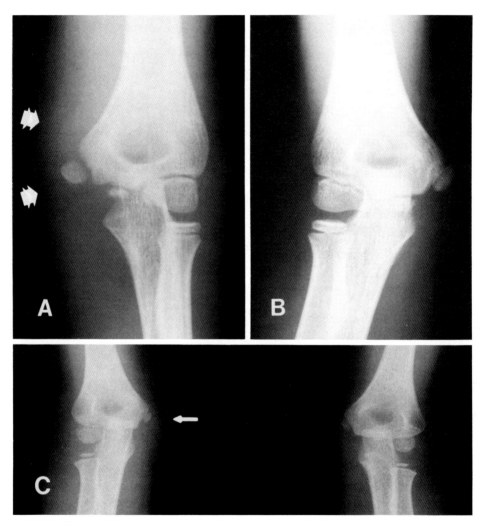

Figure 4.49. *Medial epicondyle injury—value of soft tissue changes.* (*A*) Note prominence of the soft tissues over the medial epicondyle *(arrows)* and that the medial epicondyle appears displaced. (*B*) Comparative view of the other side demonstrates normal position of medial epicondyle and lack of soft tissue swelling. (*C*) More subtle case. Note swelling over the right medial epicondyle *(arrow)*. However, the epicondyle itself does not appear particularly displaced. On the normal side, note that there is no soft tissue swelling over the medial epicondyle.

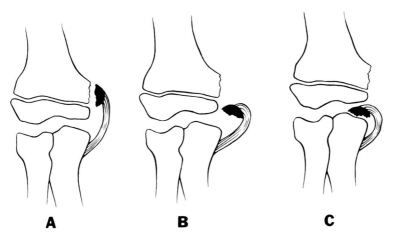

Figure 4.50. *Range of medial epicondylar injuries; diagrammatic representation.* (**A**) Simple separation. (**B**) Separation with rotation. (**C**) Separation with entrapment in joint space.

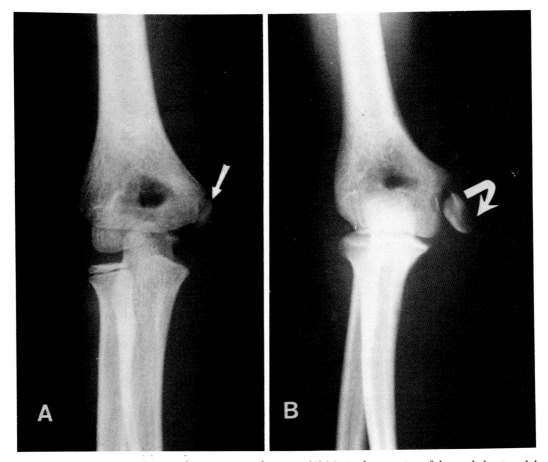

Figure 4.51. *Medial epicondylar avulsions; varying degrees.* (**A**) Minimal separation of the medial epicondyle with slight downward displacement *(arrow)*. Note that the soft tissues over the area are a little thickened. (**B**) Markedly displaced and completely rotated medial epicondyle *(arrow)*.

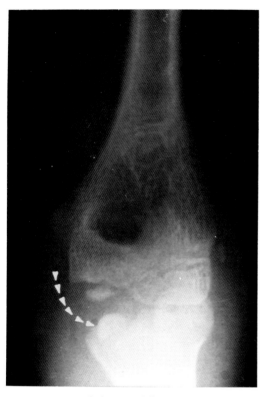

Figure 4.52. *Medial epicondylar entrapment.* Note the abnormal position of the entrapped medial epicondyle. It has been displaced from its normal position, and now lies in the intra-articular space *(arrows)*. (Courtesy of Lee Rogers, M.D., and Harvey White, M.D.)

chronic anterior angulation of the radial head (10, 11), and nonunion of the olecranon epiphysis (21).

Injuries of the Radial Head. Gross, fragmented, or displaced fractures of the radial head are not difficult to detect, but the more *subtle corner fracture* frequently is missed (Fig. 4.59). Of course, in most cases, abnormalities of the soft tissues and fat pads around the elbow can alert one to the presence of this fracture, but still, the fracture commonly remains elusive. Equally important as not missing the fracture, however, is misinterpreting a normal notch in the radial head of many young infants for an actual fracture (Fig. 4.60). The notch defect in question usually is seen in infants and young children in whom the ra-

dial head epiphysis is not ossified. In the older child, it usually is not a problem.

Most radial head fractures are impaction fractures with the capitellum hammering the radial head. Again, many of these are subtle and, in such cases, it is of the utmost importance to obtain comparative views of the normal extremity and then to look for any subtle evidence of cortical buckling, radial head tilting, or cortical fracturing (Fig. 4.61). Even then, the most subtle of these fractures will elude one's initial detection, and only when follow-up films are obtained will it come to one's attention that such a fracture existed in the first place (Fig. 4.62).

Dislocation of the radius (radial head) obviously occurs when the entire elbow is dislocated, but dislocation of the radius alone usually occurs in association with a fracture of the ulna (i.e., Monteggia fracture). The ulnar fracture can occur through the proximal end of the ulna (Fig. 4.63) or the midshaft of the ulna (see Fig. 4.76). In assessing the radius for dislocation, one should determine whether the radial head and capitellum line up in a straight line. If they do not, the radius is dislocated (Fig. 4.63). This rule is valid on both lateral and anteroposterior views.

Dislocation of the radial head from the annular ligament, or the so-called "pulled," "curbstone," or "nursemaid's" elbow, is not true dislocation (12, 23). Rather, there is subluxation of the radial head from the annular ligament, incomplete tearing of the ligament, and subsequent entrapment of a portion of the ligament in the joint space (Fig. 4.64). This is a very common elbow injury in infancy and early childhood and results from a brisk pull on the elbow such as occurs when lifting the child by one arm. The condition produces exquisite pain and a most unhappy child. The clinical picture is absolutely characteristic: a previously well child suddenly refuses to move the involved extremity. Clinical examination is

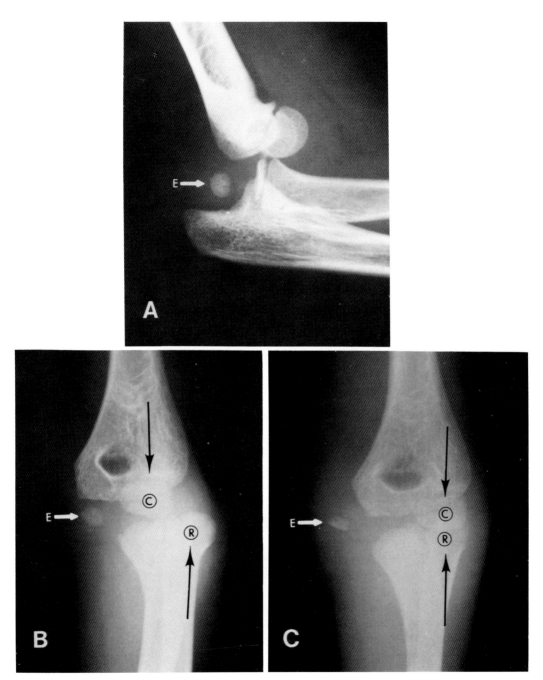

Figure 4.53. *Medial epicondyle separation secondary to elbow dislocation.* (*A*) Lateral view; total dislocation of the elbow. Note position of the medial epicondyle (*E*). (*B*) Frontal view demonstrating complete dislocation of the elbow. Note that the capitellum (*C*) does not line up with the proximal radial head (*R*). However, also note the position of the displaced medial epicondyle (*E*). Just beneath it is a small avulsed sliver-like metaphyseal bony fragment. (*C*) Postreduction film demonstrates extensive edema of the elbow and persistent separation of the medial epicondyle (*E*). Now note that the capitellum (*C*) is in a straight line relationship with the head of the radius (*R*).

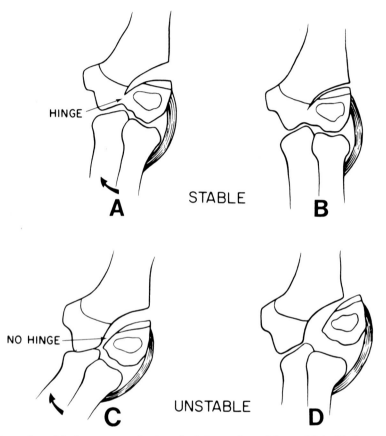

Figure 4.54. *Lateral condyle fractures; mechanics of stability and instability.* (*A*) Stable fracture. Twisting forces *(arrow)* cause separation of the lateral condyle from the humeral metaphysis. The articular cartilage, however, is incompletely broken and a stabilizing hinge remains. (*B*) When the fracture-causing forces are removed, the fracture fragment returns to a nearly normal position. It is stable. (*C*) Unstable fracture. Same twisting forces *(curved large arrow)* causing complete fracture through the articular cartilage with no residual hinge. (*D*) With removal of the forces, the totally separated lateral condyle rotates upward and outward. Because there is no hinge remaining, the fracture is unstable. (Redrawn from M. Rang: *Children's Fractures,* J.B. Lippincott Co., Philadelphia, 1974.)

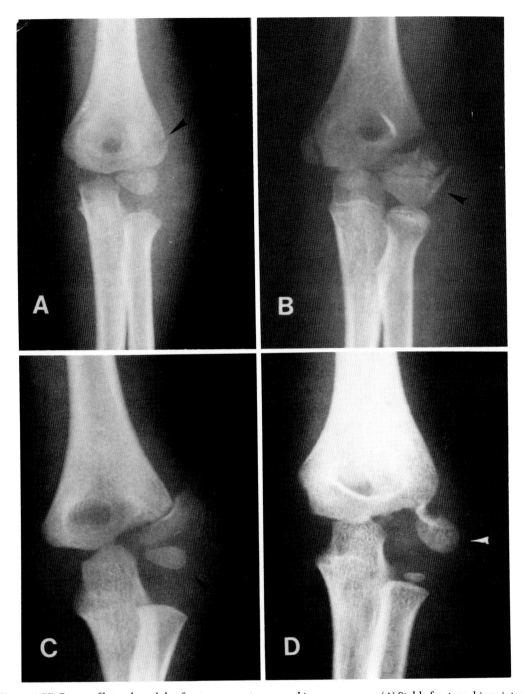

Figure 4.55. *Range of lateral condylar fractures; roentgenographic appearance.* (*A*) Stable fracture, hinge intact. Note the undisplaced lateral condylar fracture *(arrow)*. Also note the presence of adjacent unilateral edema of the soft tissues. (*B*) Stable fracture hinge intact. In this case, however, there is more downward displacement of the fractured fragment *(arrow)*. (*C*) Unstable fracture, hinge not intact. Note pronounced lateral and upward displacement of the fractured lateral condyle *(arrows)*. (*D*) Unstable fracture, hinge not intact. Note complete rotation and marked upward displacement of the lateral condyle *(arrow)*.

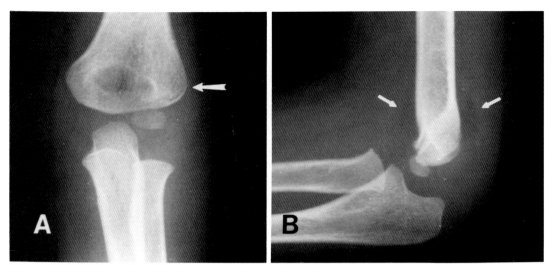

Figure 4.56. *Subtle lateral condylar fracture.*   (**A**) Frontal view demonstrating a subtle fracture line through the lateral condyle *(arrow)*. A sliver-like piece of bone has been avulsed. (**B**) Lateral view demonstrating abnormal displacement of both the anterior and posterior fat pads *(arrows)*. This is a stable, and very common fracture.

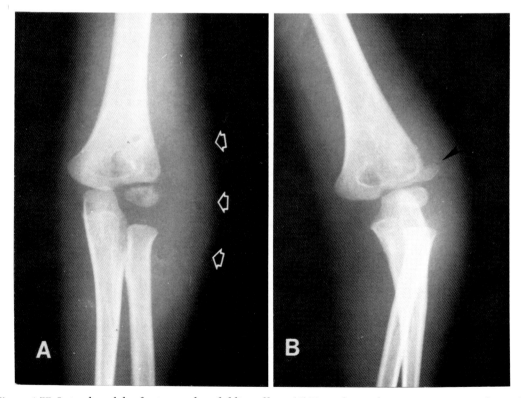

Figure 4.57. *Lateral condylar fracture; value of oblique film.*   (**A**) Frontal view demonstrating no significant abnormality in the bones. However, note prominent unilateral swelling of the soft tissues over the lateral aspect of the elbow *(arrows)*. This should signify the presence of an injury to the lateral condyle. (**B**) Oblique view demonstrates the displaced fracture fragment with greater clarity *(arrow)*.

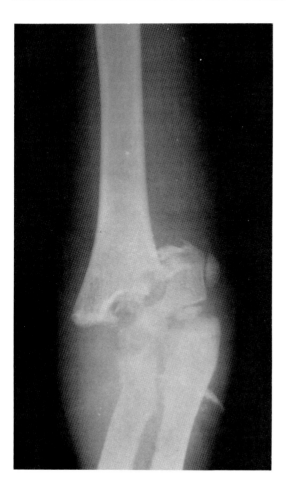

Figure 4.58. *Complete fracture distal elbow; clinical pseudodislocation.* Note the completely displaced fracture of the distal humerus. Clinically, this type of injury can cause the elbow to appear dislocated, but in actual fact, no dislocation is present. Note that the displaced distal humeral fracture fragment is in normal alignment with both the radius and ulna. Compare with true dislocation of the elbow in Figure 4.53.

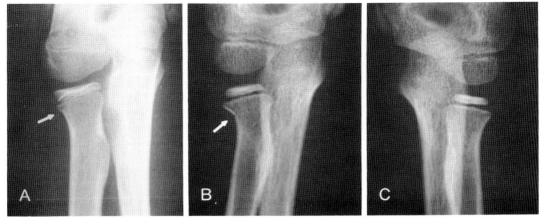

Figure 4.59. *Radial head corner: impaction fracture.* (**A**) Note the minimally impacted corner fracture of the radial head *(arrow)*. (**B**) Another patient with a more pronounced impaction *(arrow)*. (**C**) Normal side for comparison.

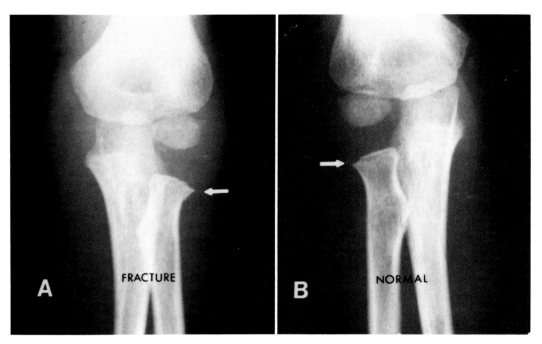

Figure 4.60. *Radial head corner fracture versus normal notch.*   (**A**) Note typical, slightly impacted corner fracture of the proximal radial head *(arrow)*. (**B**) Normal side for comparison. Note normal notch in radial head *(arrow)*, frequently misinterpreted for a fracture. Also note that the soft tissues in (**A**) (fracture side) are fatter and more opaque due to edema and swelling.

not productive, for any way you move the arm or, indeed, even touch the arm, the child seems to hurt. The arm is held in slight flexion and pronation, and supination is impossible without great pain. Occasionally the problem can be bilateral (16).

The roentgenographic findings in "pulled" elbow usually are negative, both in terms of bony and soft tissue abnormality. Usually, however, the views obtained are suboptimal for it is very difficult to position these patients for adequate roentgenograms. On the other hand, many times while trying to position the arm properly, such manipulation leads to reduction. Indeed, almost as if by magic, there is an immediate full return to normal movement of the extremity, and a previously crying, tormented child is all smiles. In other cases, mild discomfort may persist for 30 minutes to 1–2 hours. Actually, if one is cognizant of this injury, it can be reduced before

roentgenograms ever are obtained, for with the thumb over the radial head, supination and slight flexion of the elbow will result in a palpable click and reduction of the radial head (23). After reduction, one can encounter, in some cases, evidence of edema and fat pad displacement suggesting minimal fluid accumulation in the joint.

Fractures of the Proximal Ulna and Olecranon. Fractures of the proximal ulna can occur with elbow dislocations, direct blows to the olecranon, or falls on the outstretched extremity. The latter are most common. Gross fractures of the olecranon are not difficult to detect, but more subtle fractures may elude one's initial inspection. Fortunately, most of these fractures are associated with some abnormality of the elbow fat pads (Fig. 4.65). However, one should remember that since it is the trochlea jamming the trochlear notch in most cases, a splitting, impacting force causes peculiar linear and transverse frac-

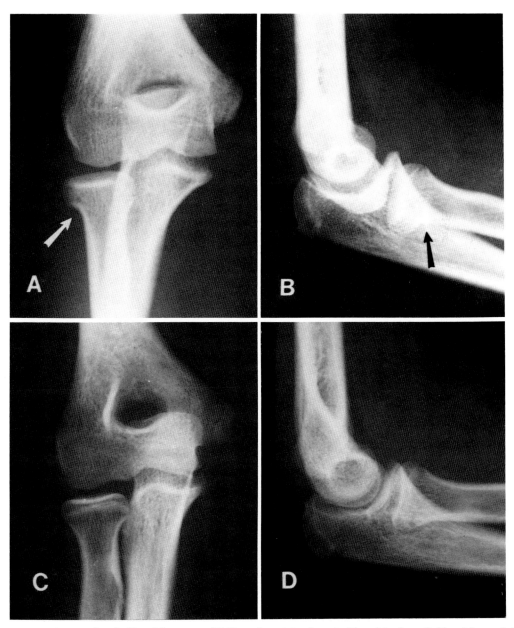

Figure 4.61. *Impacted radial head fracture.* (**A**) Note the minimal cortical break in the radial head *(arrow)*. (**B**) Lateral view demonstrating displaced fat pads and subtle suggestion of the same fracture in the radial head *(arrow)*. The findings on both views might be overlooked unless compared with the same area on the normal side. (**C**) Normal frontal view for comparison. Compare the configuration of the normal radial head with the tilted and slightly impacted head in (**A**). (**D**) Normal lateral view for comparison. Compare again this normal radial head with the slightly impacted and tilted head in (**B**).

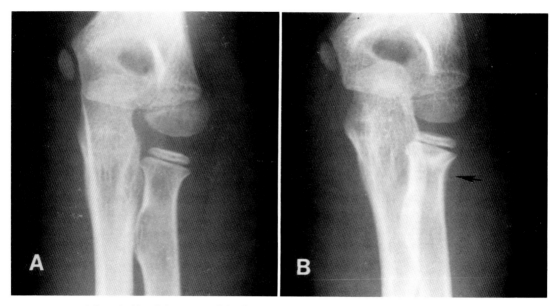

Figure 4.62. *Subtle radial head fracture with healing.*   (A) The radial head appears normal, but the elbow in this patient was painful. (B) Two weeks later, note periosteal new bone deposition *(arrow)* and sclerosis of the metaphysis indicating the presence of a healing, impacted radial head fracture.

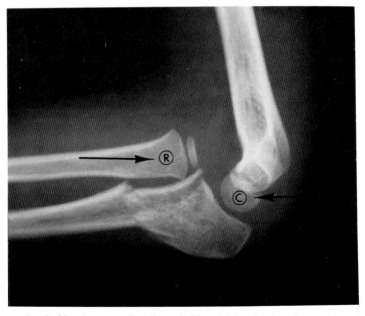

Figure 4.63. *Dislocated radial head.*   Note that the radial head (R) is displaced upward. It does not line up in a straight line relationship with the capitellum (C). Also note the angulated fracture of the proximal ulna. The ulna is not dislocated.

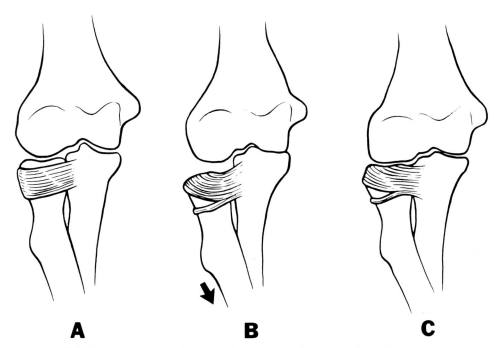

A   **B**   **C**

Figure 4.64. *Pulled elbow mechanics.* (**A**) Note the position of the normal annular ligament. It is wrapped around the radial head. (**B**) With pulling on the elbow, the annular ligament is torn, and some of the fibers roll over the radial head. (**C**) When pulling stops, the fibers which rolled over the radial head remain in that position and the elbow becomes painful. (Redrawn and modified from M. Rang: *Children's Fractures,* J. B. Lippincott Co., Philadelphia, 1974.)

tures to occur (Fig. 4.66). Osteochondral avulsion fractures (1) also are not uncommon and result from additional twisting forces (Fig. 4.65*B*). Transverse hairline fractures also can be seen (Fig. 4.65*A*).

Dislocation of the Elbow. Total dislocation of the elbow is not particularly common and usually is associated with a fracture of one or more of the bones of the elbow. Occasionally no fractures exist, but more often one will see transverse or spiral fractures of one of the bones of the elbow or avulsion fractures of the condyles and epicondyles (see Fig. 4.53). The clinical deformity in these patients is striking, but a similar deformity can occur with completely displaced fractures through the distal humerus. In these cases, there is no dislocation of the elbow, but the markedly displaced fracture causes the clinical findings to suggest true dislocation. Roentgen-ographically, however, the two conditions usually are readily differentiated (see Fig. 4.58 and compare with Fig. 4.53).

Osteochondritis of the Elbow. Although not a common problem, osteochondritis of the elbow can involve the capitellum, trochlear epiphysis (7, 28), or radial head. Involvement of the capitellum perhaps is most common and produces a bony defect with subtle adjacent sclerosis (Fig. 4.67). MRI is useful in determining the exact position of the fragment, if required.

Septic Arthritis, Osteomyelitis, and Cellulitis of the Elbow. Septic arthritis of the elbow is not as common as is septic arthritis of the shoulder and hip. However, when it occurs, it produces marked swelling around the elbow and displacement or obliteration of the elbow fat pads (Fig. 4.68*A* and *B*). Usually, however, there is little in the way of joint space widening.

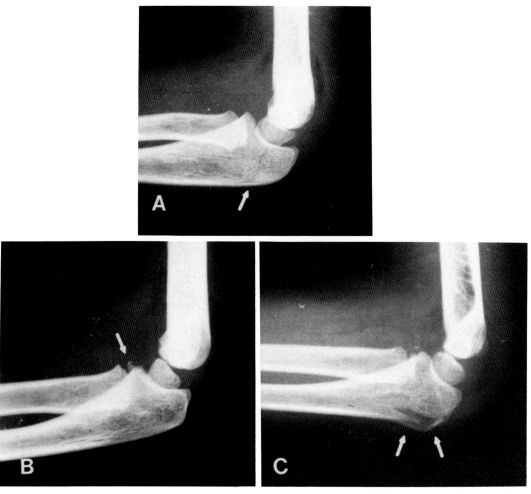

Figure 4.65. *Proximal ulnar fractures.*   (*A*) Note linear fracture *(arrow)* through the olecranon. There is no bony displacement, but both fat pads are displaced outward. (*B*) Avulsion fracture of the coronoid process of the ulna *(arrow)*. Once again note that both elbow fat pads are displaced. (*C*) Cortical buckling, impaction fracture of the proximal ulna *(arrows)*. The fat pads are elevated, indicating the presence of interarticular bleeding.

Osteomyelitis of the bones around the elbow usually produces extensive deep soft tissue swelling and obliteration of the normal soft tissues and fat pads (Fig. 4.68C and D). In the early stages, there is little in the way of bony destruction, but after 10–14 days or so bone destruction and periosteal new bone deposition appear.

With cellulitis of the elbow, if edema is circumferential, the findings are difficult to differentiate from those of early osteomyelitis. However, if edema is superficial and localized to one side of the elbow, the di-

agnosis of localized cellulitis can be made with greater confidence (Fig. 4.69). In many such cases, one actually is dealing with an acute epitrochlear lymphadenitis (8), which frequently is due to cat-scratch disease.

Normal Variations Causing Problems. The most common normal variations misinterpreted for a fracture are the various secondary ossification centers around the elbow (Fig. 4.70). Of these, the sliver-like lateral epicondyle and the frequently, irregularly ossified medial condyle are the

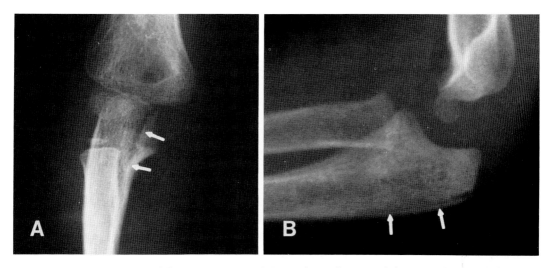

Figure 4.66. *Linear fractures of olecranon process.* (**A**) Note linear fracture of olecranon *(arrows).* (**B**) Another patient with a peculiar linear fracture of the olecranon *(arrows).*

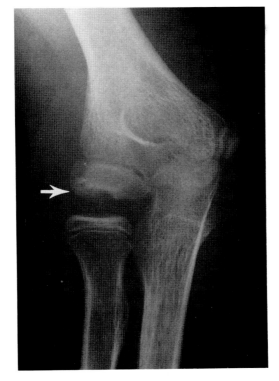

Figure 4.67. *Osteochondritis of capitellum.* Note lytic defect with sclerotic border in the capitellum *(arrow).*

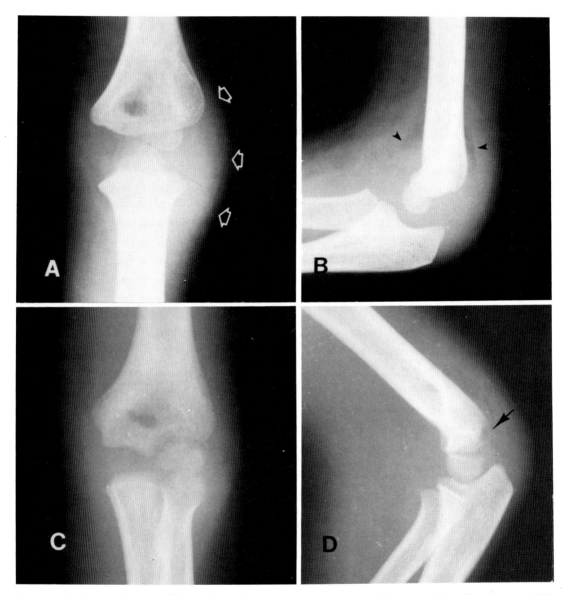

Figure 4.68. *Septic arthritis.* (*A*) Frontal view demonstrating extensive swelling around the elbow *(arrows)*. (*B*) Lateral view demonstrating elevation of both the anterior and posterior fat pads *(arrows)*. This indicates the presence of fluid (pus) in the elbow joint. (*C*) Frontal view of osteomyelitis of the distal humerus. Note extensive circumferential deep swelling around the elbow. The soft tissues are homogeneously opaque and no normal muscle-fat interfaces are seen. (*D*) Lateral view demonstrating extensive deep edema around the elbow and an area of destruction in the distal humerus *(arrow)*. Note that the anterior fat pad has been totally obliterated by edema, and that the indistinct posterior fat pad is displaced.

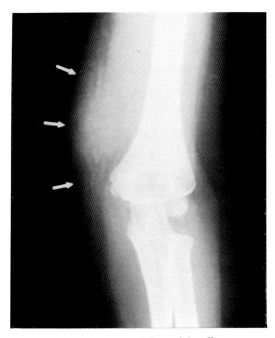

Figure 4.69. *Localized cellulitis of the elbow.* Note the localized area of superficial edema *(arrows)* and reticulation of the subcutaneous fat. These findings are secondary to adenopathy (i.e., epitrochlear adenitis) and soft tissue inflammation in this area. They are quite different from the pattern of generalized soft tissue swelling seen in the patient with osteomyelitis in Figure 4.68*C* and *D*.

two most problematic bones. However, they are followed in short order by the accessory center of the olecranon (Fig. 4.70*B*). Another normal finding misinterpreted as abnormality is the circular radiolucency in the distal humerus, representing an area of normal thinning of the floor of the olecranon fossa (Fig. 4.70*A*). In young infants, this radiolucency can erroneously suggest osteomyelitis. Finally, it should be reiterated that the normal radial head notch demonstrated in Figure 4.60 should not be misinterpreted as a radial head corner fracture.

REFERENCES

1. Blamoutier, A., Klaue, K., Damsin, J.P., and Carlioz, H.: Osteochondral fractures of the glenoid fossa of the ulna in children: Review of four cases. J. Pediatr. Orthop. 11: 638–640, 1991.
2. Bledsoe, R.C., and Izenstark, J.L.: Displacement of fat pads in disease and injury of the elbow. Radiology 73: 717–724, 1959.
3. Bohrer, S.P.: The fat pad sign following elbow trauma. Its usefulness and reliability in suspecting "invisible" fractures. Clin. Radiol. 21: 90–94, 1970.
4. Bowerman, J.W., and McDonnell, E.J.: Radiology of athletic injuries: Baseball. Radiology 116: 611–615, 1975.

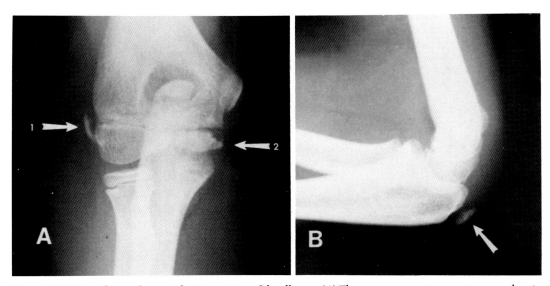

Figure 4.70. *Normal secondary ossification centers of the elbow.* (*A*) The accessory centers most commonly misinterpreted as fractures are the lateral epicondyle (*1*) and the irregularly ossified medial condyle (*2*). The central radiolucency in the humerus is due to normal thinning of the base of the olecranon fossa. (*B*) The accessory ossification center of the olecranon *(arrow)* also often is misinterpreted as a fracture.

5. Brogden, B.G., and Crow, N.E.: Little leaguer's elbow. A.J.R. 83: 671–675, 1960.

6. Chessare, J.W., Rogers, L.F., White, H., and Tachdjian, M.O.: Injuries of the medial epicondylar ossification center to the humerus. A.J.R. 129: 49–55, 1977.

7. Clarke, N.M.P., Blakemore, M.E., and Thompson, A.G.: Osteochondritis of the trochlear epiphysis. J. Pediatr. Orthop. 3: 601–604, 1983.

8. Currarino, G.: Acute epitrochlear lymphadenitis. Pediatr. Radiol. 6: 160–163, 1977.

9. DeLee, J.C., Wilkins, K.E., Rogers, L.F., et al.: Fracture-separation of the distal humeral epiphysis. J. Bone Joint Surg. 62A: 46–51, 1980.

10. Ellman, H.: Anterior angulation deformity of the radial head: an unusual lesion occurring in juvenile baseball players. J. Bone Joint Surg. 11: 281, 1976.

11. Gore, R.M., Rogers, L.F., Bowerman, J., Suker, J., and Compere, C.L.: Osseous manifestations of elbow stress associated with sports activities. A.J.R. 134: 971–977, 1980.

12. Illingworth, C.M.: Pulled elbow: Study of 100 patients. Br. Med. J. 2: 672–674, 1975.

13. Kohn, A.M.: Soft tissue alteration in elbow trauma. A.J.R. 82: 867–875, 1959.

14. Labelle, H., Bunnell, W.P., Duhaime, M., and Poitras, B.: Cubtius varus deformity following supracondylar fracture of the humerus in children. J. Pediatr. Orthop. 2: 539–546, 1982.

15. Markowitz, R.I., Davidson, R.S., Harty, M.P., Bellah, R.D., Hubbard, A.M., and Rosenberg, H.K.: Pictorial essay. Sonography of the elbow in infants and children. A.J.R. 159: 829–833, 1992.

16. Michaels, M.G.: A case of bilateral nursemaid's elbow. Pediatr. Emerg. Care 5: 226–227, 1989.

17. Mizuno, K., Hirohata, K., and Kashiwagi, D.: Fracture-separation of the distal humeral epiphysis in young children. J. Bone Joint Surg. 61A: 570–573, 1979.

18. Murphy, W.A., and Siegel, M.J.: Elbow fat pads with new signs and extended differential diagnosis. Radiology 124: 659–665, 1977.

19. Norell, H.G.: Roentgenologic visualization of the extracapsular fat: Its importance in the diagnosis of traumatic injuries to the elbow. Acta Radiol. 42: 205–210, 1954.

20. Papavasiliou, V., Nenopoulos, S., and Venturis, T.: Fractures of the medial condyle of the humerus in childhood. J. Pediatr. Orthop. 7: 421–423, 1987.

21. Pavlov, H., Torg, J.S., Jacobs, B., and Vigorita, V.: Non-union of olecranon epiphysis: Two cases in adolescent baseball pitchers. A.J.R. 136: 819–829, 1981.

22. Quan, L., and Marcuse, E.K.: The epidemiology and treatment of radial head subluxation. Am. J. Dis. Child. 139: 1194–1197, 1985.

23. Rang, M.: *Children's Fractures*, pp. 93–123. J.B. Lippincott, Philadelphia, 1974.

24. Rogers, S.L., and MacEwan, D.W.: Changes due to trauma in the fat plane overlying the supinator muscle: A radiologic sign. Radiology 92: 954–958, 1969.

25. Rogers, L.F., and Rockwood, C.A.: Separation of the entire distal humerus epiphysis. Radiology 106: 393–399, 1973.

26. Rogers, L.F., Malave, Jr. S., White, H., and Tachdjian, M.O.: Plastic bowing, torus and greenstick supracondylar fractures of the humerus: Radiographic clues to obscure fractures of the elbow in children. Radiology 128: 145–150, 1978.

27. Torg, J.S., Pollack, H., and Sweterlitsch, P.: The effect of competitive pitching on the shoulders and elbows of preadolescent baseball players. Pediatrics 49: 267–272, 1972.

28. Vanthournout, I., Rudelli, A., Valenti, Ph., and Montagne, J. Ph.: Osteochondritis dissecans of the trochlea of the humerus. Pediatr. Radiol. 21: 600–601, 1991.

FOREARM

Injuries of the Forearm. Fractures through the midshaft of the radius and ulna are common, and either both bones or one bone only can be fractured. In this regard, *when a midshaft fracture is encountered in one bone, it is worthwhile to look for a fracture in the other bone*—not only in its midshaft, but at either end (Fig. 4.71). The types of fractures that can occur through the midshaft of the bones of the forearm include clearly visible transverse, spiral, and oblique fractures and the more subtle hairline, greenstick, and plastic bending or bowing fractures. Buckle or torus fractures are uncommon in the midshaft of these bones, for as compared to the metaphyseal regions, the cortex of the midshaft is rather sturdy and not prone to buckling. Many overt midshaft fractures result from direct blows, but many also result from falls on the outstretched extremity.

Acute *plastic or bowing* fractures of the forearm are commonly missed in spite of the fact that pain and deformity are present clinically (1, 2, 5, 7). In these patients,

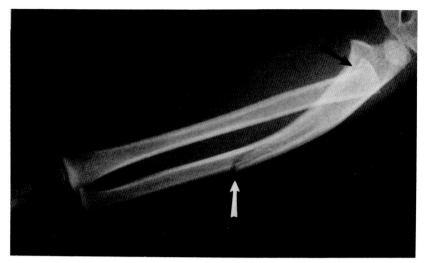

Figure 4.71. *Ulnar fracture with occult radial head fracture.* Note the clearly visible fracture through the mid-shaft of the ulna *(white arrow)*. It is a greenstick fracture with considerable bending of the ulna. In addition, note that there has been a metaphyseal fracture of the proximal radius *(black arrow)*. The radial head is not dislocated in this patient, but the fracture could be overlooked because of the potentially distracting ulnar fracture.

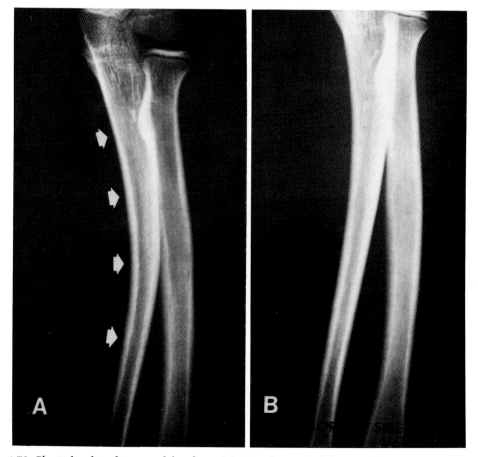

Figure 4.72. *Plastic bending fracture of the ulna.* (**A**) Note the marked degree of bending of the entire ulna *(arrows)*. No fracture line is visible, but unless a comparative view of the normal side is examined, the bony deformity could be missed. (**B**) Normal side for comparison. Note the configuration of the normal ulna and compare it with the bent ulna in (**A**).

there often is loss of supination-pronation function, but when roentgenograms are obtained, a classic fracture with a visible fracture line is not detected. Rather, one notes only a variable degree of bowing of one or another, or both, of the bones of the forearm (Figs. 4.72 and 4.73). In this regard, one should note that the entire bone or just one part of it can be bent. These fractures can be considered the *"greenest of greenstick"* fractures, and although numerous microfractures exist along the outer surface of the bones (2–4), none are large enough to be visualized as a single fracture roentgenographically (1, 3, 4). Because of this, the entire injury may go undetected unless comparative views of the other arm are obtained and, when they

are, the curvature of the involved bone should be compared inch for inch with the normal contralateral bone (Fig. 4.74). This is most important, for if only one extremity is examined, normal bowing can be misinterpreted as a plastic bending fracture (Fig. 4.75).

Overall, acute plastic bowing or bending fractures of the forearm are more common than generally believed and, at the same time, are quite variable. In some cases, both bones are involved in the bending process, while in others only one is involved. In still other cases, one bone may be bent and the other frankly fractured (5). Another interesting feature of these fractures is that, unlike other fractures of the forearm, when they heal they usually pro-

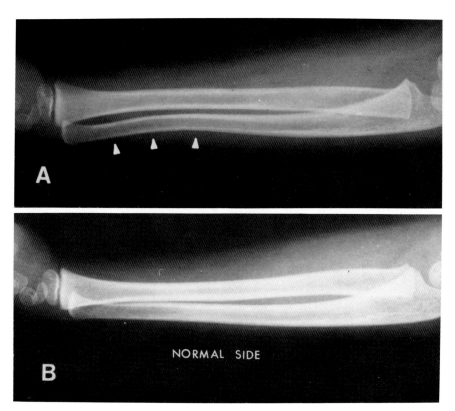

Figure 4.73. *Acute plastic bending fracture of the distal ulna and radius.* (**A**) Note bending of the distal ulna *(arrows)* and, to a lesser extent, of the distal radius. (**B**) Normal side for comparison. Although the views are not exactly the same in terms of positioning, one still can see that the normal ulna and radius are not bent.

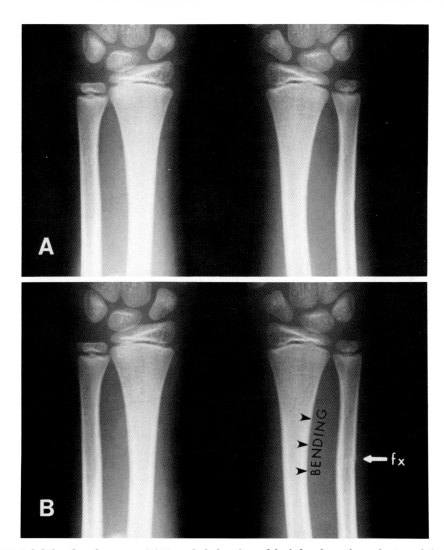

Figure 4.74. *Subtle bending fracture.*   (*A*) Note slight bending of the left radius. There also is a subtle greenstick fracture of the distal ulna. (*B*) Fractures are labeled. Bending fracture of radius *(black arrow)*. Fracture of ulna *(fx)*.

duce little in the way of periosteal bone reaction. However, if bone scans are obtained they will be positive, but usually they are not required. Clinically there is no attempt to reduce these fractures and thus residual bowing with supination-pronation motion impairment can persist well after healing is complete.

The other noteworthy fracture of the bones of the forearm is the *Monteggia* frac-

ture. This fracture consists of a fracture of the ulna and a dislocation of the radial head (Fig. 4.76). Both anterior and posterior Monteggia fractures occur, and in either case, it is the associated dislocation of the radial head that is the missed portion of this injury (6). *In this regard, it cannot be restated often enough that one always should line up the radial head and capitellum to determine whether they are in a*

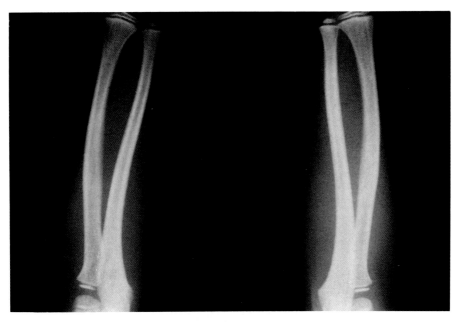

Figure 4.75. *Normal bowing of bones of the forearm.* Note the normal degree of bowing of the bones of the forearm on both sides. This is the reason why comparative views should always be obtained when a bending fracture is suspected. Only with comparative views will one be certain that such a fracture exists. If only one of these extremities were examined, the degree of bending could be misconstrued as being abnormal.

straight line relationship. If they are not, dislocation of the radial head is present.

Normal Variations Causing Problems. The only normal finding in the midshaft of the radius and ulna which can be misinterpreted as a fracture is a vascular groove in either bone. These vascular grooves are diaphyseal and appear no different from those in other long bones.

REFERENCES

1. Borden, S.: Traumatic bowing of the forearm in children. J. Bone Joint Surg. 56A: 611–616, 1974.
2. Borden, S.: Roentgen recognition of acute plastic bowing of the forearm in children. A.J.R. 125: 524–530, 1975.
3. Chamay, A.: Mechanical and morphological aspects of experimental overload and fatigue in bone. J. Biomech. 3: 263–270, 1970.
4. Chamay, A., and Tschantz, P.: Mechanical influences in bone remodeling, experimental research on Wolff's law. J. Biomech. 5: 173–180, 1972.
5. Crowe, J.E., and Swischuk, L.E.: Acute bowing fractures of the forearm in children: A frequently missed injury. A.J.R. 128: 981–984, 1977.
6. Giustra, P.E., Killoran, P.J., Furman, R.S., and Root, J.A.: Missed Monteggia fracture. Radiology 110: 45–47, 1974.
7. Stenstrom, R., Gripenberg, L., and Bergius, A.-R.: Traumatic bowing of forearm and lower leg in children. Acta Radiol. 19: 243–249, 1978.

Wringer Injuries. For the most part, washing machine wringer arm injuries are uncommon in this day and age, but some still do occur (1). However, bone injury is very uncommon, and although an occasional epiphyseal dislocation may be encountered, these injuries are mainly soft tissue injuries.

REFERENCE

1. Stone, H.H., Cantwell, D.V., and Fullenwider, J.T.: Wringer arm injuries. J. Pediatr. Surg. 11: 375–379, 1976.

WRIST

Normal Fat Pads. There are two fat pads around the wrist which can be uti-

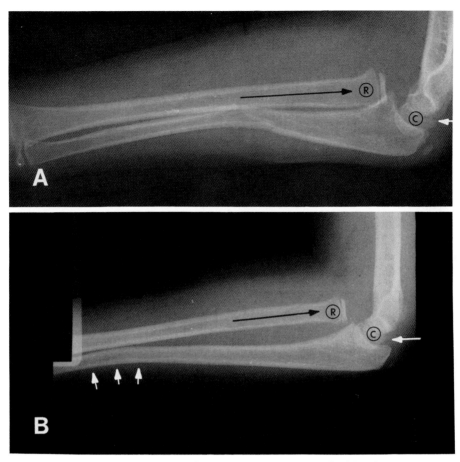

Figure 4.76. *Monteggia fracture.* (*A*) Note the fracture through the midshaft of the ulna. There is considerable associated bending of the ulna. Also note that the radial head (*R*) is dislocated and does not line up in a straight line with the capitellum (*C*). (*B*) Another patient with a dislocated radial head (*R*). This time, however, the only other fracture is a subtle bending fracture of the ulna *(arrows)*. Capitellum (*C*).

lized in the assessment of wrist injuries. The first is the pronator quadratus fat pad, and the second is the navicular fat pad (8, 14). The pronator quadratus fat pad is seen on lateral views of the wrist and lies along the pronator quadratus muscle (Fig. 4.77). The navicular fat stripe lies just medial to the navicular bone and is seen on postero-anterior views of the wrist (Fig. 4.78). In young infants, this latter fat stripe is not visualized with as much consistency as it is in older children. This is not so unfortunate, however, for obliteration of the navicular fat pad is utilized primarily for the detection of navicular fractures, and these frac-

tures are not particularly common in infancy. Distal, radial, and ulnar fractures, on the other hand, are quite common, and it is in this regard that displacement and obliteration of the pronator quadratus fat pad become most useful.

Determining the Presence of Fluid in the Wrist Joint. Determining the presence of fluid in the wrist joint simply amounts to noting whether the soft tissues around the wrist are swollen. Apart from this, there is little else to look for, for the joint space seldom becomes widened, and except for the navicular fat pad, no other useful fat pads are present. With wrist joint

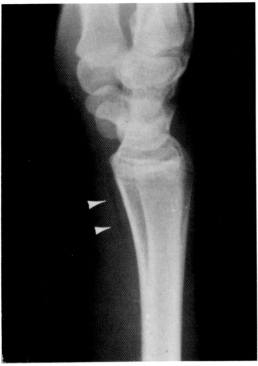

Figure 4.77. *Normal pronator quadratus fat pad.* Note the normal appearance and location of the pronator quadratus fat pad *(arrows).*

fluid, most of the swelling occurs distal to the radial and ulnar epiphyseal lines (Fig. 4.79A). When edematous swelling is due to a distal radioulnar fracture, such swelling is primarily located proximal to the epiphyseal lines (Fig. 4.79B).

Injuries of the Distal Radius and Ulna. Although a variety of *transverse* and *oblique fractures* commonly occur through the distal third of the radius and ulna, with or without angulation or displacement, these fractures usually are not difficult to detect (Fig. 4.80). On the other hand, if they are hairline or subtle *greenstick fractures*, they may elude early diagnosis unless one studies the soft tissues first (Fig. 4.81). The same can be said for subtle bending fractures (see Fig. 4.74).

Cortical buckle or torus fractures and epiphyseal-metaphyseal injuries also are common in this area, and most often are sustained from falls on the outstretched ex-

tremity. The cortical buckles and kinks are of an almost endless variety of configurations, and usually are more clearly visible on one view than another (Fig. 4.82). This is especially true of posterior buckle fractures of the distal radius where the fracture and associated posterior tilting of the articular surface frequently are seen on the lateral view only (Fig. 4.83). With regard to Salter-Harris epiphyseal-metaphyseal injuries, the type I and II injuries are most common. Types III and IV and even the type V injury are relatively uncommon. Most often the Salter-Harris type I or II fracture involves the epiphyseal-metaphyseal junction of the radius, but occasionally the ulna also is similarly involved. In detecting these injuries, one should look for one or more of the following changes: (a) soft tissue edema, (b) obliteration or displacement of the pronator quadratus fat pad, (c) widening of the involved epiphyseal line, (d) an associated metaphyseal corner fracture, and (e) displacement of the epiphysis (Figs. 4.84–4.86). Widening of the epiphyseal line, however, is most important.

When the ulna is involved in these in-

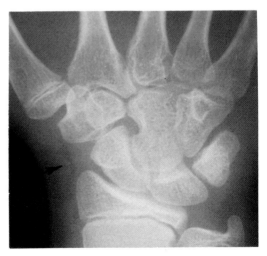

Figure 4.78. *Normal navicular fat pad.* The navicular fat pad *(arrow)* is best visualized in older children. It can be obliterated or displaced with navicular bone injuries.

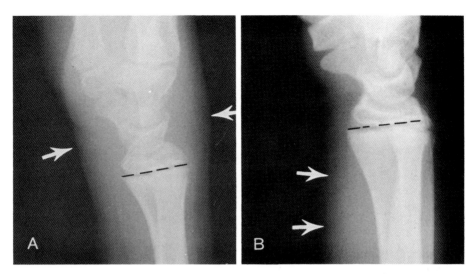

Figure 4.79. *Joint fluid in the wrist.* *(A) Navicular fracture.* In this patient with joint fluid secondary to a navicular fracture, note that most of the swelling *(arrows)* is located above the epiphyseal line of the distal radius *(dotted line)*. *(B) Distal radial fracture.* Wrist swelling is again present, but most of the swelling *(arrows)* is located below the epiphyseal line of the distal radius *(dotted arrow)*. This speaks against the presence of any significant wrist joint fluid.

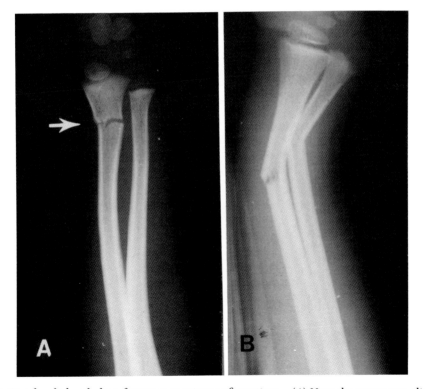

Figure 4.80. *Distal radial and ulnar fractures; varying configurations.* *(A)* Note the transverse, slightly angulated fracture through the distal radius *(arrow)*. *(B)* Markedly angulated fractures through both bones of the forearm.

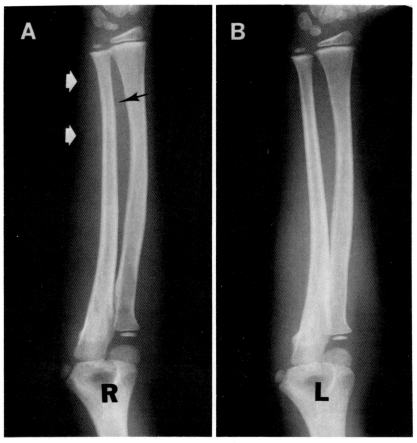

Figure 4.81. *Subtle ulnar fracture; value of soft tissues.* (A) First, note thickening and prominence of the soft tissues along the distal ulna *(white arrows)*. A greenstick fracture through the distal ulna basically is invisible *(black arrow)*, and slight generalized bending of the ulna is subtle. (B) Normal side for comparison. Note the normal appearance of the soft tissues. Also note that the normal ulna is straighter than the fractured ulna, further attesting to the presence of the ulnar fractures on the right.

juries, very often rather than an epiphyseal-metaphyseal injury, there is a *fracture of the ulnar styloid process* (12). Indeed, if the radial epiphyseal-metaphyseal fracture is subtle, there is a distinct tendency for the often more readily visible styloid fracture to distract one's attention. One should avoid this trap, for virtually always, when an ulnar styloid process fracture is present, a radial fracture also is present (12). If there is enough force to fracture the ulnar styloid process, the radius also fractures, for the ligaments surrounding the two bones are too strong to allow for isolated ulnar styloid injuries. Therefore,

the ulnar styloid fracture, no matter how subtle, should be regarded as a major clue for the presence of an associated radial fracture. These latter fractures may be overt, but it is most important to appreciate that many also are subtle buckle or epiphyseal-metaphyseal injuries (Fig. 4.87).

Old, ununited styloid avulsion fractures may erroneously suggest the presence of a secondary ossification center (Fig. 4.88A), but such a center does not exist. The distal ulnar epiphysis may be bifed, but this occurs through its midpoint and not through the styloid process (Fig. 4.88B). Isolated

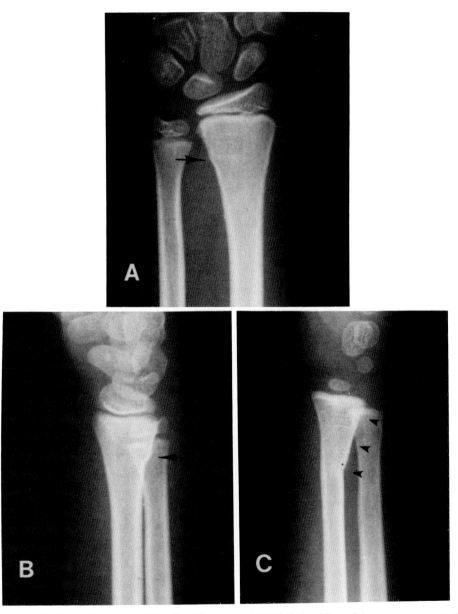

Figure 4.82. *Buckle (torus) fractures of the distal forearm.* (**A**) Subtle buckling of the cortex is seen in the distal radius *(arrows)*. (**B**) Lateral view more clearly demonstrates the buckling *(arrow)*. Note that the soft tissues are swollen and that the pronator quadratus fat pad has been obliterated. (**C**) Another infant with a buckle fracture of the distal radius *(arrows)*.

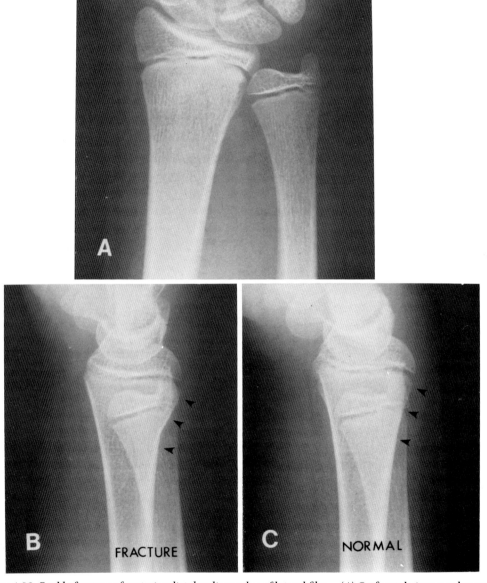

Figure 4.83. *Buckle fracture of posterior distal radius; value of lateral film.* (**A**) On frontal view, no abnormality is seen. (**B**) On lateral view, however, note the subtle buckle fracture of the distal radius *(arrows)*. There is slight posterior tilting of the articular surface of the distal radius. (**C**) Normal side for comparison. Compare the normal smooth curve of the posterior aspect of the distal radius *(arrows)*. This is the most commonly missed fracture of the distal radius.

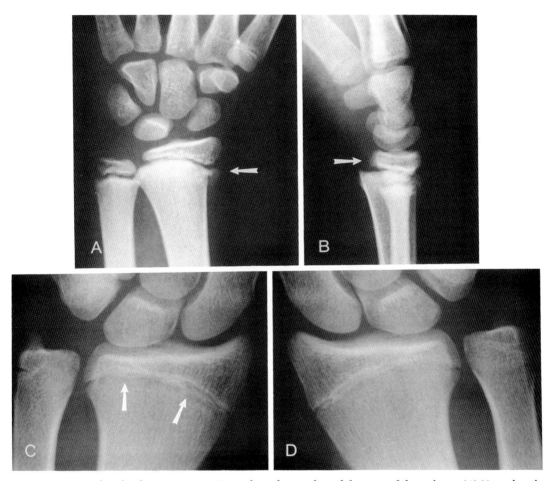

Figure 4.84. *Displaced Salter-Harris type II epiphyseal-metaphyseal fracture of the radius.* (**A**) Note that the distal radial epiphysis is displaced laterally, and that there is a small metaphyseal corner fracture *(arrow)*. (**B**) Lateral view demonstrates the marked degree of posterior displacement of the distal radial epiphysis *(arrow)*. There is slight impaction of the posterior corner of the distal radial metaphysis. (**C**) *Subtle Salter-Harris type I fracture of radius (arrows)* in older child with epiphysis almost closed. (**D**) Normal side for comparison.

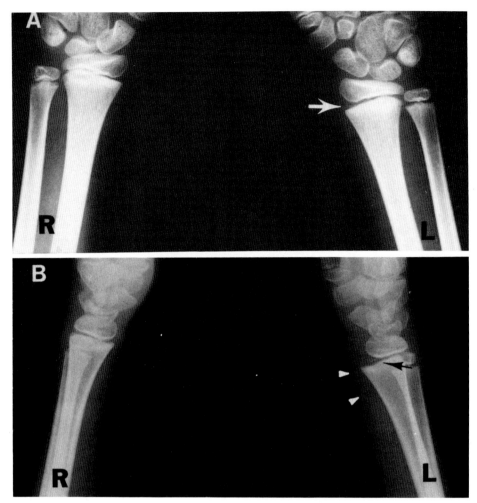

Figure 4.85. *Epiphyseal-metaphyseal fracture of the wrist with small avulsed fragment (Salter-Harris type II injury).* (*A*) On frontal view, note that the left distal radial epiphysis is slightly displaced, and that the epiphyseal line is a little wider than the normal epiphyseal line on the right. Also note the thin sliver-like avulsed metaphyseal fragment *(arrow)*. (*B*) Lateral view demonstrating swelling of the soft tissues around the left wrist, anterior displacement of the pronator quadratus fat pad *(white arrows)*, posterior displacement of the distal radial epiphysis, and the sliver-like avulsed metaphyseal fragment *(black arrow)*.

ulnar styloid fractures can be seen when direct blows to the styloid process are sustained (12).

Finally it should be noted that chronic stress-induced epiphyseal-metaphyseal fractures of the distal radius and ulna can be seen in gymnasts (1, 3, 10). These fractures appear no different than classic Salter-Harris epiphyseal-metaphyseal injuries. The Galeazzi fracture, which often is associated with radioulnar disassocia-tion, is rare in childhood (6). The radioulnar disassociation is best evaluated on lateral views and thereafter is usually is finally delineated with CT scanning (11).

Injuries of the Carpal Bones. Fractures and/or dislocations of the carpal bones in infants and young children are quite uncommon. In the older child, one may encounter *fractures of the navicular,* but even this injury is relatively uncommon. Nonetheless, it can occur, and when it does the clinical findings are similar to those seen in adults (i.e., acute tenderness in the anatomic snuff box). Roentgenographically, this fracture can be suspected when there is: (a) localized soft tissue swelling and/or obliteration of the navicular fat pad (4, 8), (b) shortening or telescoping of the navicular bone, (c) rotation and resultant increase in density of one of the fracture fragments, or (d) a visible fracture line (Fig. 4.89). In some cases, oblique (navicular) views may be necessary for clearer visualization of the suspected fracture, and in those cases where the fracture is in doubt, nuclear scintigraphy can be of value (9). Aseptic necrosis as a complica-

tion of these fractures also can occur in children but is rare (2, 12). Overall, navicular fractures are quite variable and often subtle (Fig. 4.90).

The only other bones in the wrist to fracture with any frequency in childhood are the pisiform and triquetrum (7). These fractures usually result from direct blows to the bones, and with the pisiform it is quite important to realize that it tends to ossify irregularly, and as such should not be mistaken for a fracture (see Fig. 4.94).

The occasional case of *lunate or perilunate dislocation* of the wrist in the older child presents with malalignment of the proximal row of carpal bones and associ-

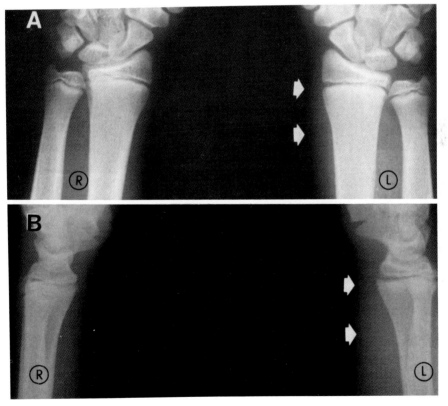

Figure 4.86. *Salter-Harris type I epiphyseal-metaphyseal fracture of the wrist; value of soft tissues.* (**A**) On frontal view, one might suspect that the epiphyseal line through the distal left radius is a little wider than the one on the right, but if one first notes that soft tissue swelling in the area also is present *(arrows)*, then the finding becomes even more suspicious. (**B**) Confirmation is present on the lateral view where one can see marked swelling of the soft tissues anterior to the wrist *(arrows)* and complete obliteration of the pronator quadratus fat pad. In addition, the distal radial epiphysis probably is slightly posteriorly displaced.

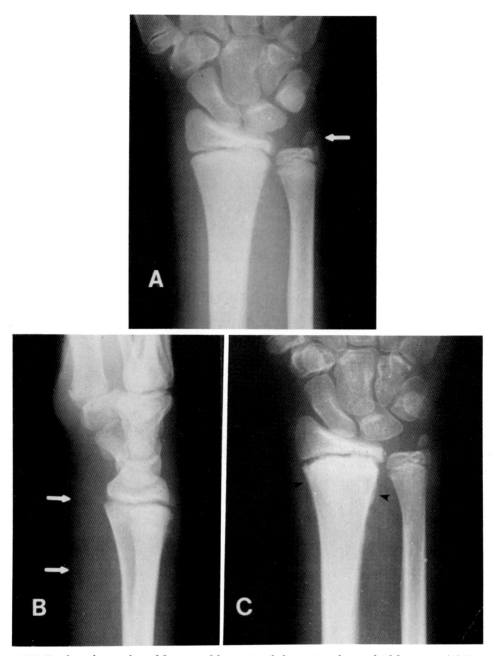

Figure 4.87. *Epiphyseal-metaphyseal fracture of the wrist with distracting ulnar styloid fracture.*   (**A**) Note swelling around the wrist and a fractured ulnar styloid process *(arrow)*. At first one might think this is the only injury present. However, on lateral view, (**B**), one can see that there is considerable swelling anterior to the wrist *(arrows)*, and that the pronator quadratus fat pad is totally obliterated. Under these circumstances, one should suspect an underlying epiphyseal-metaphyseal injury of the radius, for an isolated ulnar styloid process fracture would not result in this much swelling. In **C**, 2 weeks later, note evidence of healing of the occult epiphyseal-metaphyseal fracture of the distal radius. Some periosteal new bone is seen along the distal radial shaft *(arrows)*, and sclerosis along the epiphyseal-metaphyseal junction is clearly evident. The ununited ulnar styloid process fracture is noted again.

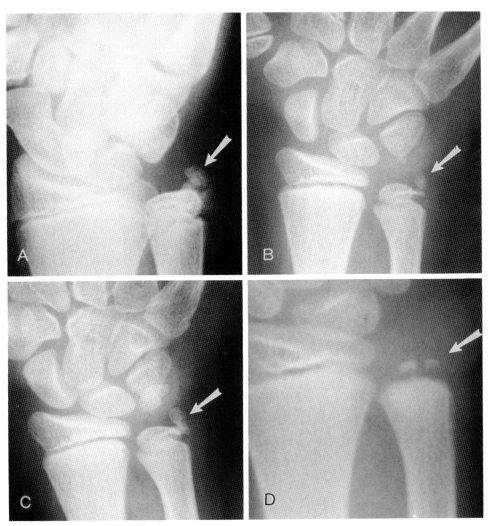

Figure 4.88. *(A) Ununited styloid fracture.* Note the smooth, ununited styloid tip fracture *(arrow)* and note that the ulnar epiphysis is normal in configuration. *(B) Separate ulnar styloid ossification center.* Note the accessory ossification center *(arrow)*. The underlying epiphysis is dysplastic and flat. *(C)* As the child grows older the accessory epiphysis is beginning to unite *(arrow)*. The ulnar epiphysis itself remains thin and dysplastic. *(D)* Bifed normal ulnar epiphysis *(arrow)*. (Parts *A–C* from S.D. Stansberry, L.E. Swischuk, J.L. Swischuk, and W.T. Midgett: Significance of ulnar styloid fractures in childhood. Pediatr. Emerg. Care 6: 99–103, 1990.)

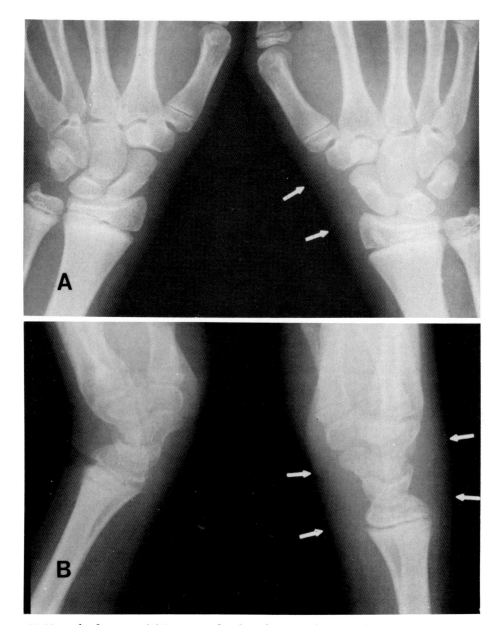

Figure 4.89. *Navicular fracture.* (*A*) First, note that the soft tissues adjacent to the navicular bone are thickened and edematous *(arrows)*. In addition, note that the navicular bone on the left is shorter (impacted) than the normal one on the right. A subtle fracture line through its upper third also is suggested. (*B*) Lateral view demonstrating extensive swelling around the wrist. Swelling extends both anteriorly and posteriorly *(arrows)*. Note that the site of the swelling is located primarily around the carpal bones. With distal radial injuries, it usually is located more proximally and there is more displacement of the pronator quadratus fat pad (i.e., see Figure 4.79*B*).

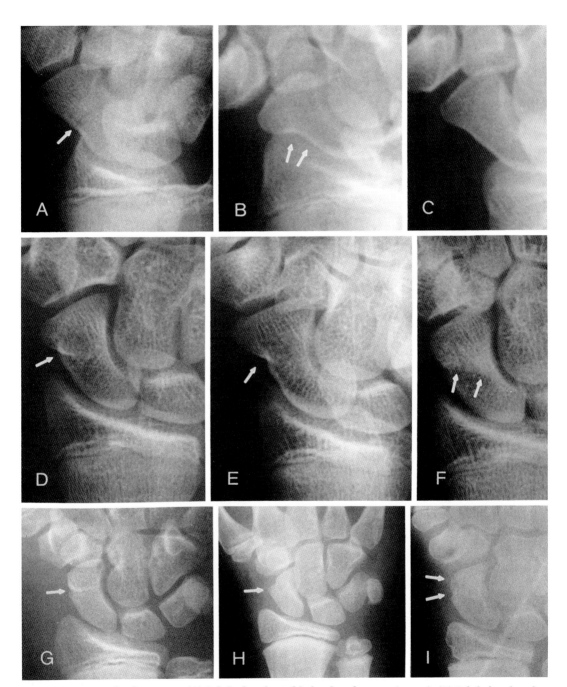

Figure 4.90. *Navicular fractures.* (**A**) Subtle, barely visible hairline fracture *(arrow)*. (**B**) Subtle bending fracture *(arrows)*. (**C**) Normal side for comparison. (**D**) Another patient with a buckle fracture *(arrow)*. (**E**) Oblique view in this patient demonstrates the same fracture *(arrow)*. (**F**) Later, with healing, note the area of sclerosis *(arrow)*. (**G**) Transverse fracture *(arrow)* with slight tilting of the upper fragment in another patient. (**H**) Markedly angulated fracture with a small avulsed fragment *(arrow)*. (**I**) Another fracture with multiple fragments.

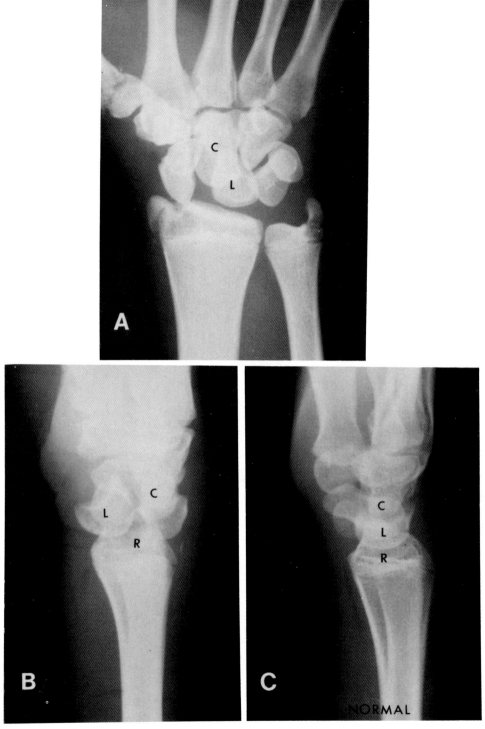

Figure 4.91. *Dislocation of the lunate.* (*A*) Note that the joint spaces to either side of the lunate bone (*L*) are unequal. This should alert one to the dislocation. In addition, note that the lunate bone overlies the capitate (*C*) and that the wrist is foreshortened. Also note fractures of the ulnar styloid process, distal radial epiphysis, proximal thumb, and navicular bone (foreshortening and rotation). (*B*) Lateral view demonstrating abnormal anterior location of the lunate bone (*L*). The capitate (*C*) and distal radial epiphysis (*R*) lie behind the lunate bone. (*C*) Normal view for comparison showing the normal vertical, sequential arrangement of the capitate (*C*), lunate (*L*), and distal radial epiphysis (*R*).

ated discrepancy in the width of the peri-lunate joint spaces. In other words, the joint spaces will be narrower or completely obliterated on one side, and wider on the other (Fig. 4.91A). Obliteration of the joint space is due to overlap of the dislocated carpal bones, and widening, of course, is due to distraction of the involved bones. On lateral view, the normal vertical, sequential arrangement of the capitate, lunate, and distal radial epiphysis is lost in these cases (Fig. 4.91B). This latter point is most important, for any deviation from this arrangement of the carpal bones should indicate an underlying dislocation. Of course, with a lunate dislocation, the lunate will lie anterior to the capitate and distal radial epiphysis, while with a perilunate dislocation both the lunate and distal radius and its epiphysis move forward and lie anterior to the other bones of the wrist.

Other dislocations in the wrist are quite uncommon. These include isolated rotatory subluxation of the navicular (5) (Fig. 4.92) and dislocation of the carpal-meta-carpal joints. However, *when assessing the wrist for a suspected underlying dislocation of any of the bones, one should follow two rules.* First, one should identify each of the carpal bones with clarity, and, second, one should note whether the individual joint spaces are uniform and delineated by parallel lines. In other words, one should try to determine whether any bony overlap or joint widening is present. If any of the individual bones are not clearly visualized and if any of the joint spaces appear suspiciously narrow or wide, one should turn to oblique and lateral views for further delineation and verification.

Sprained Wrist. There is a good rule to follow with wrist injuries, and it goes as follows: *"a sprained wrist is a fractured wrist until proven otherwise."* This rule taught to me by Bill Miller, M.D., an Oklahoma City orthopaedic surgeon, has proven most trustworthy. This is not to say that simple sprains of the wrist do not occur, but rather that many so-called "sprains" actually turn out to be Salter-Harris epiphyseal-metaphyseal or cortical

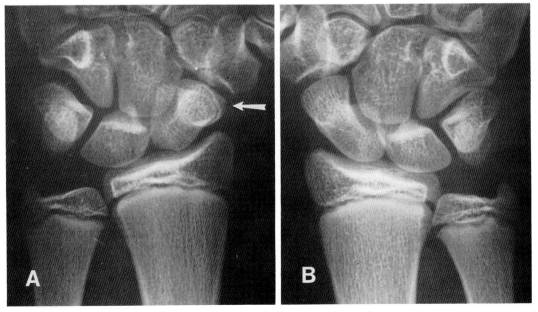

Figure 4.92. *Rotatory subluxation of navicular.* (**A**) Note slight increase in the navicular-lunate joint space and also telescoping (due to rotation) of the navicular bone resulting in the circle sign *(arrow)*. (**B**) Normal side for comparison.

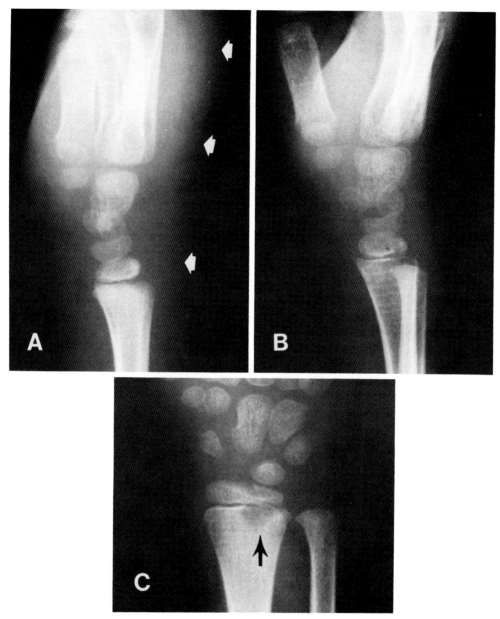

Figure 4.93. *Osteomyelitis; distal radius.*   (A) Note extensive swelling of the hand, wrist, and distal forearm *(arrows).* (B) Normal side for comparison. (C) Frontal view demonstrating metaphyseal defect due to osteomyelitis *(arrow).*

buckle injuries. Even in those cases where the radiographic findings are confined to soft tissue swelling and obliteration of the quadratus pronator fat pad, clinical tenderness along the epiphyseal line or distal radius will belie the presence of an epiphyseal-metaphyseal injury. It is quite a different problem from the one encountered in the ankle, where a sprained ankle more often than not turns out to be just a sprained ankle.

Septic Arthritis, Osteomyelitis, and Cellulitis of the Wrist.   Generally speaking, all of these conditions lead to pronounced swelling in and around the wrist joint. The various normal soft tissue structures are obliterated and, in early cases, soft tissue swelling is most pronounced around the area of primary involvement. In less advanced cases, less bone destruction is seen (Fig. 4.93), and nuclear scintigraphy often is required.

Normal Findings Causing Problems. For the most part, the carpal bones ossify as single smooth foci, but occasionally irregular ossification of one or another of the carpal bones can be misinterpreted for a fracture. This occurs with the pisiform bone more that any other (Fig. 4.94A). Another problem in the wrist, although far less common, is that of misinterpreting a bipartite navicular bone as a fractured navicular bone (Fig. 4.94B). In the distal radius and ulna, an incompletely obliterated but normally closing epiphyseal line (14) can be misinterpreted for a fracture (Fig.4.94C), and occasionally normal bony spicules extending into the epiphyseal line

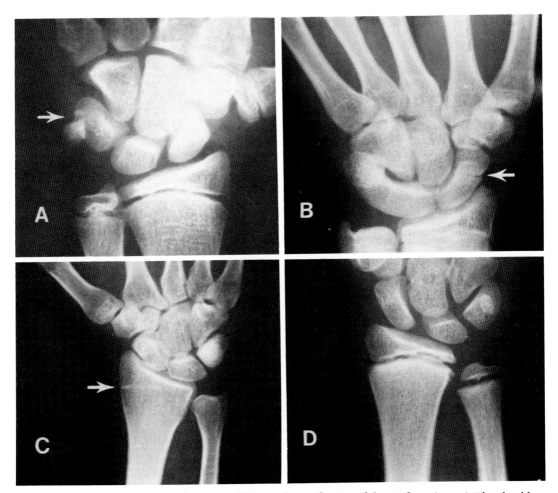

Figure 4.94. *Normal variations in the wrist.* (*A*) Irregular ossification of the pisiform *(arrow)*. This should not be misinterpreted for a fracture of the pisiform. (*B*) Bipartite navicular. Note the bipartite navicular *(arrow)*. Also note that the lunate and triquetral bones are fused. The bipartite navicular should not be misinterpreted for a fracture. (*C*) *Incompletely obliterated radial epiphysis.* Note the incompletely obliterated epiphysis of the distal radius *(arrow)*, often misinterpreted for a fracture. (*D*) Epiphyseal-metaphyseal spicules. Note normal spicules extending from the ulnar epiphysis and normal metaphyseal spicules and irregularity along the inner aspect of the distal radial metaphysis.

can suggest an epiphyseal-metaphyseal injury (Fig. 4.94*D*).

REFERENCES

1. Carter, S.R., Aldridge, M.J., Fitzgerald, R., and Davies, A.M.: Stress changes of the wrist in adolescent gymnasts. Br. J. Radiol. 61: 109–1112, 1988.
2. Christodoulou, A.G., and Colton, C.L.: Scaphoid fractures in children. J. Pediatr. Orthop. 6: 37–39, 1986.
3. Fliegel, C.P.: Stress-related widening of the radial growth plate in adolescents. Ann. Radiol. 29: 374–376, 1986.
4. Haverling, M., and Sylven, M.: Soft tissue abnormalities at fracture of the scaphoid. Acta Radiol. 19: 497–501, 1978.
5. Hudson, T.M., Caragol, W.J., and Kaye, J.J.: Isolated rotatory subluxation of the carpal navicular. A.J.R. 126: 601–611, 1976.
6. Landfried, M.J., Stenclik, M., and Susi, J.G.: Variant of Galeazzi fracture-dislocation in children. J. Pediatr. Orthop. 11: 332–335, 1991.
7. MacEwan, D.W.: Changes due to trauma in the fat plane overlying the pronator quadratus muscle: A radiologic sign. Radiology 82: 879–886, 1964.
8. Rolfe, E.B., Garvie, N.W., Khan, M.A., and Ackery, D.M.: Isotope bone imaging in suspected scaphoid trauma. Br. J. Radiol. 54: 762–767, 1981.
9. Roy, S., Caine, D., and Singer, K.M.: Stress changes of the distal radial epiphysis in young gymnasts: A report of twenty-one cases and a review of the literature. Am. J. Sports Med. 13: 301–308, 1985.
10. Scheffler, R., Armstrong, D., and Hutton, L.: Computed tomographic diagnosis of distal radioulnar joint disruption. J. Can. Assoc. Radiol. 35: 212–213, 1984.
11. Southcott, R., and Rosman, M.A.: Nonunion of carpal scaphoid fractures in children. J. Bone Joint Surg. 59B: 20–23, 1977.
12. Stansberry, S.D., Swischuk, L.E., Swischuk, J.L., and Midgett, T.A.: Significance of ulnar styloid fractures in childhood. Pediatr. Emerg. Care 6: 99–103, 1990.
13. Teates, C.D.: Distal radial growth plate remnant simulating fracture. A.J.R. 110: 578–581, 1970.
14. Terry, D.W., Jr., and Ramin, J.E.: The navicular fat stripe: A useful roentgen feature for evaluating wrist trauma. A.J.R. 124: 25–28, 1975.

HAND

Evaluation of the Fat Pads and Soft Tissues. There are no specific fat pads to evaluate in the hand and evaluation of the

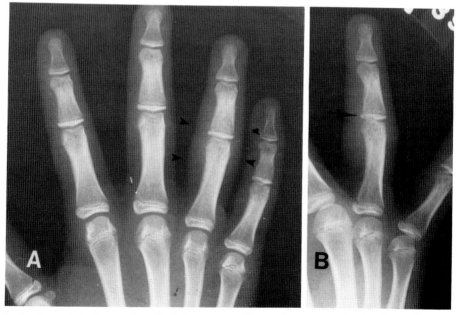

Figure 4.95. *Phalangeal fracture; value of soft tissues.* (**A**) Note soft tissue swelling localizing the site of injury to the proximal interphalangeal joint of the ring finger *(arrows)*. (**B**) Oblique view demonstrates the swelling again, but in addition also demonstrates the presence of a small chip fracture of the epiphysis *(arrow)*. This is a Salter-Harris type III injury with bleeding into the joint and associated periarticular soft tissue swelling.

soft tissues consists primarily of noting whether localized soft tissue edema and swelling are present. However, this latter finding, as non-specific as it is, is very helpful in localizing the site of injury in the fingers (Fig. 4.95).

Detecting Fluid in the Small Joints of the Hand. Detection of fluid in the small joints of the hand depends primarily on noting the presence of swelling around the joint. In some cases, the joint space may be widened (7), but this finding often is subtle (Fig. 4.96). There are no specific fat pads to evaluate and, thus, in most cases, one is left only with generalized swelling around a knuckle (Fig. 4.95).

Injuries of the Metacarpals and Phalanges. Crush injuries to the terminal phalanges are hardly worth obtaining roentgenograms for, because unless the fracture is a compound fracture, little needs to be done for these injuries. The typically comminuted terminal phalangeal tuft is not difficult to detect roentgenographically, and even if it is missed, no dire sequelae develop. Other injuries to the fingers and thumb result from hyperextension, twisting, or direct blows to the digits. The *types of fractures sustained include buckle (torus) fractures, epiphyseal-metaphyseal injuries, fracture dislocations, and linear, transverse, or spiral fractures.* They come in an almost endless assortment of configurations, and some are illustrated in Figure 4.97. In addition, although rare, plastic bending fractures can occur (Fig. 4.98).

An important point regarding cortical buckle (torus) fractures occurring at the proximal end of the phalanges or distal ends of the metacarpals is that if one sees one such fracture, then one should look at the neighboring digits for other similar fractures. In addition, usually all of these fractures are more clearly defined on oblique views (Fig. 4.99). Direct blows to the dorsum of the hand resulting in transverse fractures through the metacarpal bones often elude initial observation. The reason for this is that many times the frac-

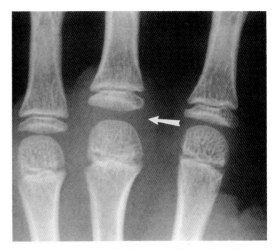

Figure 4.96. *Joint fluid.* Note the widened joint space *(arrow)* at the metacarpal joint. This was due to traumatic hemarthrosis.

ture line is barely visible, and little or no displacement of the fracture fragments occurs. In such cases, it is of great benefit to examine the soft tissues first, and then, when edema and swelling are noted, to focus one's attention on the underlying bones (Fig. 4.100).

Dislocations of the fingers and thumb (Fig. 4.101) are not particularly common in childhood, for rather than a dislocation, an epiphyseal-metaphyseal separation occurs (see Fig. 4.97B). However, clinically these separations often appear to be true dislocations. The classic fracture dislocation of the base of the first metacarpal (Bennett's fracture) occurs only after the epiphysis of the thumb has fused. Until this time, the equivalent of this fracture is a Salter-Harris type I or II injury (Fig. 4.97E). This, however, is not to say that the thumb never dislocates in childhood, for indeed it does, but usually it occurs at the metacarpal-phalangeal joint. Frequently, this dislocation is associated with an epiphyseal-metaphyseal fracture (Fig. 4.101), and in the older child where the epiphysis has fused or is near fusion, the same injury can result in the so-called "gamekeeper's thumb." In this injury, the avulsion fracture indicates the presence of a severe collateral ligament injury leading

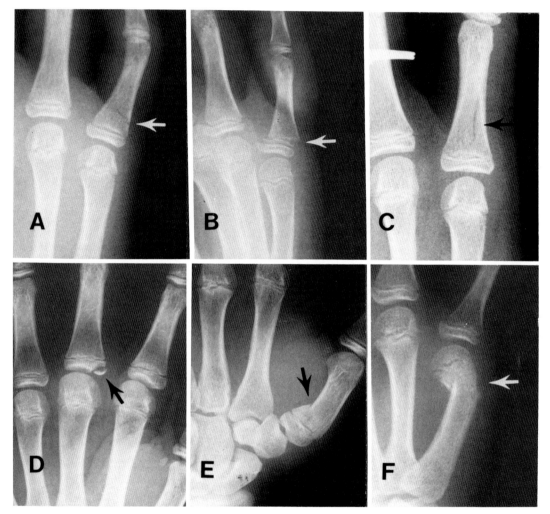

Figure 4.97. *Phalangeal and metacarpal fractures; various types.* (**A**) Typical transverse fracture *(arrow)*. (**B**) Epiphyseal-metaphyseal fracture with displacement *(arrow)*. Clinically, this type of fracture can be mistaken for a true dislocation. (**C**) Longitudinal fracture through phalanx *(arrow)*. (**D**) Epiphyseal chip fracture *(arrow)*. (**E**) Epiphyseal-metaphyseal fracture (Salter-Harris type II injury) of the base of the first metacarpal *(arrow)*. (**F**) Typical angulated fracture *(arrow)* through the head of the fifth metacarpal. This fracture usually is sustained by punching someone or something and often is termed the "boxer's" fracture.

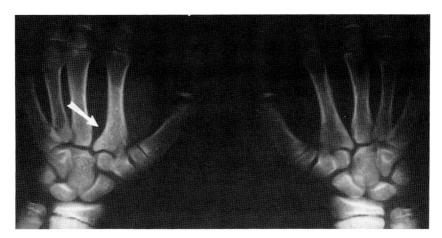

Figure 4.98. *Plastic bending fracture; metacarpal.*   Note swelling over the left hand and a wavy, bent appearance of the first metacarpal *(arrow).* Compare with its normal, straight appearance on the other side.

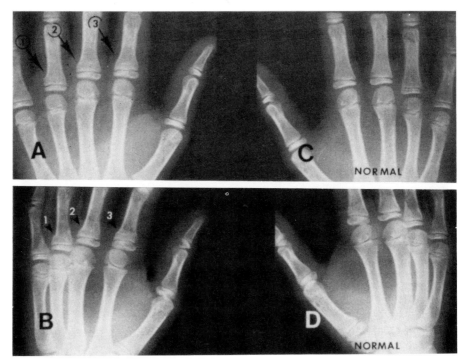

Figure 4.99. *Buckle (torus) fractures of the base of the phalanges.*   (*A*) Frontal view demonstrating a buckle fracture through the base of the proximal phalanx of the fourth digit (*1*). A more subtle but similar fracture is present through the base of the proximal phalanx of the third digit (*2*). An even more subtle fracture is present through the base of the proximal phalanx of the second digit (*3*). This latter fracture is most subtle and might not be appreciated on this view alone. (*B*) Oblique view more clearly demonstrates all three fractures. (*C* and *D*) Normal frontal and oblique views for comparison. Specifically, compare the contour of the cortices of the involved bones.

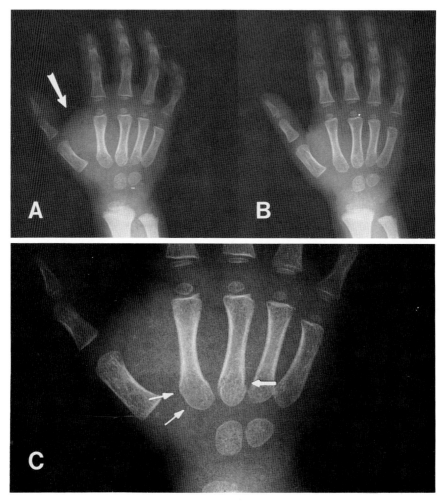

Figure 4.100. *Subtle metacarpal cortical fractures; value of soft tissues.* (**A**) First, note soft tissue swelling (increased thickness and density of the soft tissues between thumb and index finger) *(arrow)*. (**B**) Normal side for comparison. Look back at the right hand in (**A**) and note that there is a subtle bending-buckle fracture through the base of the second metatarsal and a transverse fracture through the base of the third metatarsal. (**C**) Closeup view demonstrating the buckle-bending fracture of the second metacarpal and the transverse fracture through the base of the third metacarpal *(arrows)*.

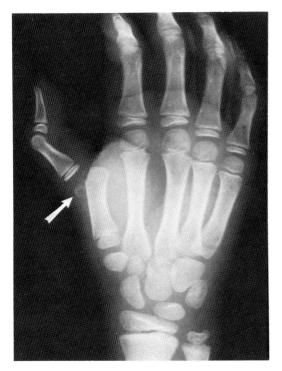

Figure 4.101. *Fracture dislocation of the thumb.* Note the dislocated metacarpal phalangeal joint of the first digit, and the avulsed bony fragment *(arrow).*

Septic Arthritis, Osteomyelitis, and Cellulitis of the Hand. Cellulitis of the fingers is very common and produces generalized soft tissue swelling without joint or bone abnormalities. Osteomyelitis of the small bones of the hands also produces soft tissue swelling, virtually indistinguishable from that seen with cellulitis. Of course, if bone destruction is present, the diagnosis becomes relatively easy. With septic arthritis, pronounced swelling around the involved joint will be noted, and if enough pus has accumulated in the joint space, one may see some widening of the joint space.

A note regarding the *hand-foot syndrome in sickle cell disease* is probably in

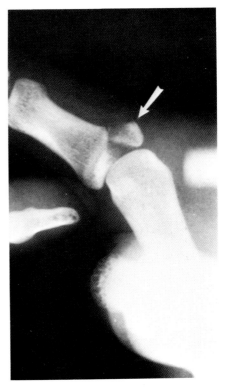

Figure 4.102. *Gamekeeper's thumb.* Note the avulsed epiphyseal-metaphyseal fragment *(arrow).* In this condition, there is an associated injury of the medial joint capsule and ligament, and the injury is unstable. The patient is unable to grasp anything with the thumb.

to instability and an inability to grasp objects with the thumb. In chronic cases, the injury can be quite disabling, and thus surgical intervention usually is required. Roentgenographically, the presence of this injury can be detected when the avulsed fragment is noted (Fig. 4.102).

In assessing the thumb for the presence of a dislocation, it is important to note that when the thumb is examined in oblique position, it can erroneously appear dislocated. This *pseudodislocated appearance of the thumb* is a common finding, for almost always the thumb is in oblique position when the remainder of the hand is being examined in true frontal projection. Under such circumstances, the first metacarpal joint appears dislocated, but with proper positioning one will soon see that the joint is normal (Fig. 4.103).

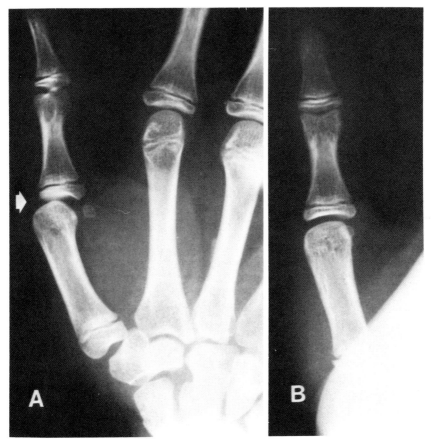

Figure 4.103. *Pseudodislocation of the thumb; pitfall.* (**A**) Note that the first metacarpal-phalangeal joint appears dislocated *(arrow)*. The small bony ossicle along the inner aspect of the joint is a normal sesamoid bone. (**B**) With proper anteroposterior positioning, one can see that the joint is not dislocated.

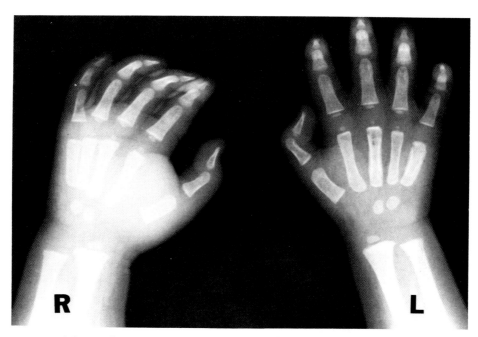

Figure 4.104. *Hand-foot syndrome.* Note extensive swelling of the entire right hand. These are acute soft tissue changes of the hand-foot syndrome. The bones are intact. On the left, however, note periosteal new bone deposition along the third and fifth metatarsals, providing evidence of previous infarcts. In addition, lytic lesions are noted through the distal ends of these bones. The findings are similar to those of osteomyelitis.

order at this point. In these cases, edema and swelling of the soft tissues of the hand can be extensive, and in some cases one may note the presence of healing changes from similar episodes in the past (Fig. 4.104). The bony changes are due to infarction and are indistinguishable from those of osteomyelitis where the organism often is *Salmonella* (1).

Frostbite. Frostbite injuries, on an acute basis, produce nothing more than soft tissue swelling. However, later on resorption of the involved bones and eventual autoamputation and deformity can be seen (2–6).

Normal Findings Causing Problems. The small bones of the hand have numerous epiphyses and pseudoepiphyses (apophyses) which commonly are misinterpreted as fractures (Fig. 4.105). Bipartite epiphyses also can be misinterpreted as epiphyseal fractures but are not particularly common in the hand. A number of

sesamoid bones also can be seen in the hand but seldom are they misinterpreted as fractures. Only if they are bipartite is there a tendency to make such a misinterpretation, and actually the problem is more common in the foot. The most common sesamoids of the hand are those located just over the heads of the first and second metacarpals (see Fig. 4.103).

REFERENCES

1. Bennett, O.M.: Salmonella osteomyelitis and the hand-foot syndrome in sickle cell disease. J. Pediatr. Orthop. 12: 534–538, 1992.
2. Brown, F.E., Spiegel, P.K., and Boyle, W.E., Jr.: Digital deformity: An effect of frostbite in children. Pediatrics 71: 955–959, 1983.
3. Mooney, W.R., and Reed, M.H.: Growth disturbances in the hands following thermal injuries in children. J. Can. Assoc. Radiol. 39: 91–94, 1988.
4. Reed, M.H.: Growth disturbances in the hands following thermal injuries in children: 2. Frostbite. Can. Assoc. Radiol. J. 39: 95–99, 1988.
5. Sweet, E.M., and Smith, M.G.H.: "Winter fingers!" Bone infarction in Scottish children as a

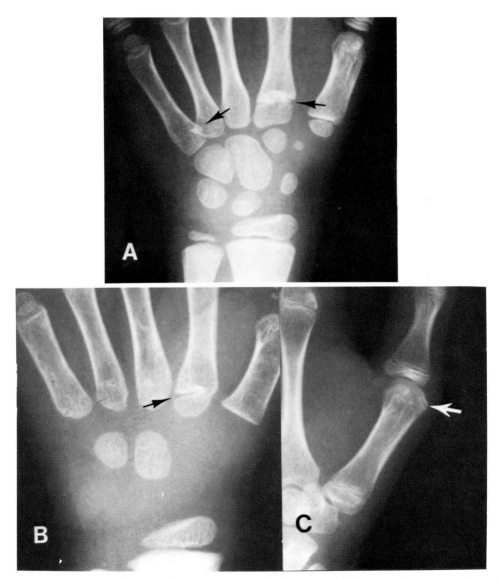

Figure 4.105. *Normal secondary ossification centers; pseudofractures.* (*A*) Note pseudofractures through the base of the fifth and second metatarsals *(arrows)*. (*B*) Another infant with an incompletely fused secondary center at the base of the second metacarpal *(arrow)*. (*C*) Incompletely fused accessory center producing fracture-like appearance through the distal end of the first metacarpal *(arrow)*.

manifestation of cold injury. Ann. Radiol. 22: 71–75, 1979.

6. Tishler, J.M.: The soft tissue and bone changes in frostbite injuries. Radiology 102: 511–513, 1972.

7. Weston, W.J.: Joint space widening with intracapsular fractures in joint of the fingers and toes of children. Australas. Radiol. 15: 367–371, 1971.

LOWER EXTREMITY PROBLEMS PELVIS AND SACRUM

Injuries of the Pelvis. Pelvic fractures frequently are multiple and can range from simple buckle or torus cortical fractures to extensive fracture-dislocations associated with internal organ or vascular injury (12, 15, 20, 22, 23, 25, 28). Most often these latter fractures are sustained in automobile accidents. Pelvic fractures resulting in separation of the symphysis pubis, fractures through the acetabulum, and so-called "diametric" fractures of the pelvis are considered unstable, while other fractures are not (23). With ring fractures, it is important to note whether the fracture forces were due to lateral compression, anteroposterior compression, or vertical shearing (32). With lateral compression diastasis of the symphysis pubis is rare, but, on the other hand, vertical fractures through the sacral ala are common as are vertical fractures through the iliac wing and horizontal fractures of the pubic bones. Sacroiliac diastasis is not as common as when anteroposterior compressive forces are at work. With the latter, however, separation of the symphysis pubis is more common. With vertical shearing forces, vertical fractures through the ischium and pubis are seen along with vertical disassociation of the sacroiliac joints (32).

Separation of the Symphysis Pubis. Gross separation of the symphysis pubis leading to pelvic instability often is associated with dislocation at the sacroiliac joints and is not difficult to detect. As just mentioned, the problem usually stems from anteroposterior compressive forces. With lesser degrees of diastasis, it may be more difficult to appreciate the problem ini-

tially, especially in young infants where underossification of the pubic bones leads to a normally wide space between them and a picture suggestive of separation (see Fig. 4.123). However, when looking for true separation, one should look for asymmetric alignment (offsetting) and associated fractures of the pubic bones (Fig. 4.106).

Diametric Fractures. In this type of injury, fractures exist both anteriorly and posteriorly (ring fracture), and they may be on the same, or opposite sides of the pelvis. The more severe diametric fractures tend to be unstable (27), and oblique views of the pelvis may be required for demonstration of all the individual fractures present. Posteriorly, these can occur through the iliac bone, sacrum, or sacroiliac joint, while anteriorly they occur through the pubic bone and/or anterior portion of the ischium (Fig. 4.107). These fractures usually result from lateral compressive forces (32).

Isolated Pelvic Fractures. Most often isolated fractures of the pelvis occur through the pubic bone or iliac wing (Fig. 4.108), but occasionally they can occur through the ischium or even the ischiopubic synchondrosis (Fig. 4.109). Isolated torus or buckle fractures of the cortex of the pubic bone also can be seen in childhood, and one can avoid missing them if one looks for subtle bends or kinks in the cortex and adjacent soft tissue edema (Fig. 4.110).

Acetabular Fractures. Acetabular rim fractures are not particularly common in childhood, but can be seen in association with posterior hip dislocations (Fig. 4.111). Fractures through the center of the acetabulum usually occur in older children and result from the femoral head being impacted into the acetabulum. Often they are difficult to detect on plain films (25). Indeed, the findings may consist of nothing more than widening of the joint space (hemarthrosis) and obliteration of the soft tissues along the obturator inter-

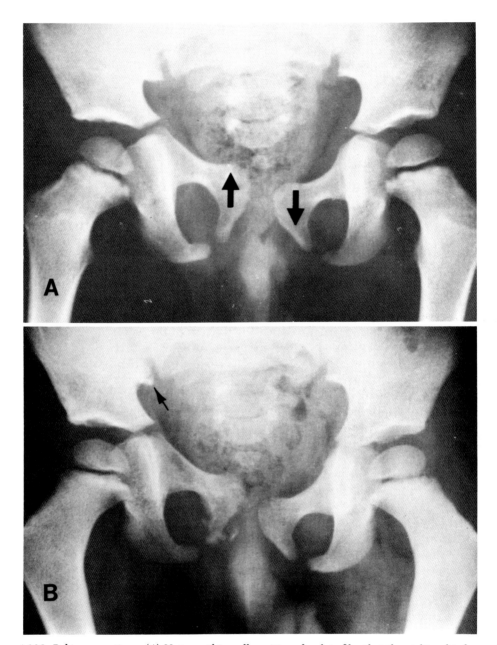

Figure 4.106. *Pubic separation.* (A) Note on this well-positioned pelvic film that the right pubic bone rides higher than the left *(arrows).* This boy was run over by a farm wagon and complained of right hip pain. (B) One month later, note persistent malalignment of pubic bones and signs of healing around the inferior right pubic ramus. Also note development of an osteophyte along the inferior aspect of the right sacroiliac joint *(arrow),* belying a previously suspected injury at this site. Most likely there was a mild degree of sacroiliac joint separation sustained at the time of initial injury.

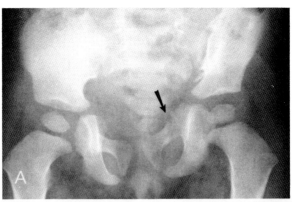

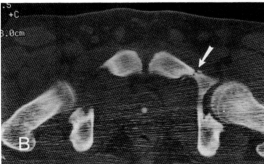 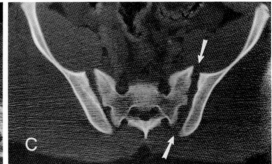

Figure 4.107. *Diametric pelvic fracture.* (A) Note the fracture of the left pubic bone *(arrow)*. Also note separation of the left sacroiliac joint and a small chip fracture along the inferior aspect of the joint. The left iliac wing is abnormally rotated and appears smaller than the right. (B) Another patient demonstrating a similar fracture on CT. Note the superior ramus fracture on the right. (C) A lower slice demonstrates diastasis of the right sacroiliac joint *(arrows)*.

nus fat pad (edema and bleeding). In the infant and young child, these fractures tend to occur through the triradiate cartilage (Fig. 4.112), but generally speaking they are not very common. Furthermore, care should be taken not to confuse the normal triradiate cartilage distorted by faulty positioning of the pelvis for one rendered abnormal by a fracture (Fig. 4.113). Most often, such faulty positioning is due to rotation but it also can result from a combination of rotation and utilization of the angled inlet view (30).

Many times, the first clue to the presence of an otherwise occult triradiate cartilage fracture is the presence of edema and soft tissue thickening along the inner aspect of the pelvis (Fig. 4.112). Then, when one notes this finding, one may also note that the triradiate cartilage is wider than normal, or that the bones on either side are displaced (Fig. 4.112).

CT, of course, is invaluable in the assessment of pelvic fractures. This is especially true of acetabular injuries (13) (Figs. 4.111 and 4.114). However, since CT images the pelvis in the axial plane, many fractures still are more clearly visualized with plain films (24). Therefore, one cannot rely on CT alone. It should be used in combination with plain films, so that all fractures are visualized adequately. Of course, with coronal or sagittal reconstruction one may obtain CT data in other than the axial plane, but, in any case, a combination of computerized tomography and plain films is invaluable in the assessment of pelvic injury.

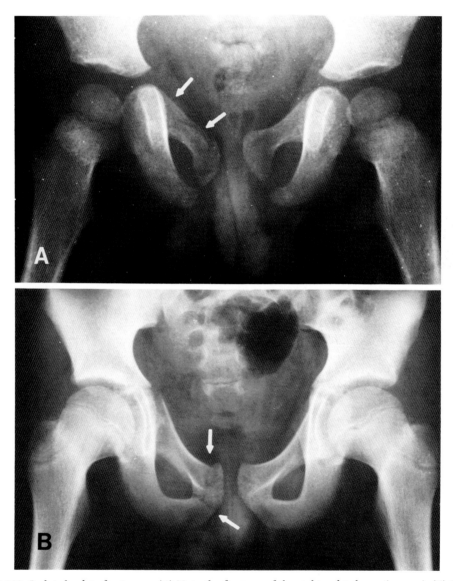

Figure 4.108. *Isolated pelvic fractures.*   (**A**) Note the fracture of the right pubic bone *(arrows)*. (**B**) Note the buckle fracture through the left pubic bone *(upper arrow)*. Also note soft tissue swelling causing obliteration of the obturator fat pad along the inner margin of the bony pelvis and a nondisplaced fracture through the ischio-pubic synchondrosis *(lower arrow)*.

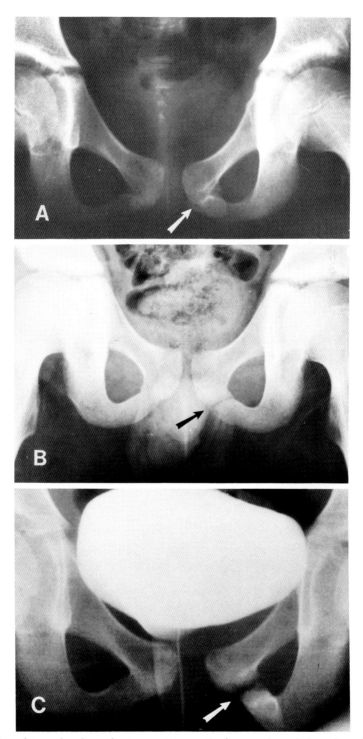

Figure 4.109. *Ischiopubic synchondrosis fractures.* (*A*) Note the fracture through the ischiopubic synchondrosis on the left *(arrow)*. It is most important to differentiate this fracture from the normal ischiopubic synchondrosis (see Fig. 4.123). (*B*) Another, more subtle fracture through the ischiopubic synchondrosis *(arrow)*. A similar fracture is seen in Figure 4.108*B*. (*C*) A displaced fracture through the ischiopubic synchondrosis *(arrow)*. Separation of the symphysis also is present.

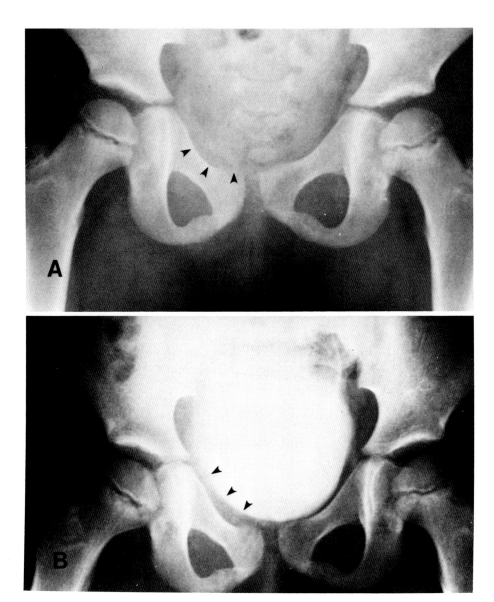

Figure 4.110. *Cortical-bending (plastic) fracture of superior pubic ramus.* (A) Note the abnormal curvature of the superior aspect of the right pubic ramus *(arrows)* as compared with the normal left pubic ramus. Also note the increase in soft tissue density over the right pubic ramus and obliteration of the fat pads and soft tissues in the area. (B) Followup cystogram demonstrates increased soft tissue thickness between the right pubic ramus and contrast-filled bladder *(arrows)*. This is due to bleeding and edema secondary to the cortical-bending fracture of the right pubic ramus.

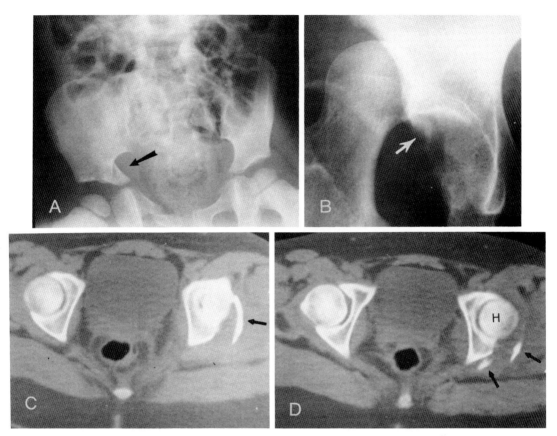

Figure 4.111. *Acetabular fracture.* (**A**) Note the fracture through the acetabular roof *(arrow)*. The fracture fragment is rotated and there is associated soft tissue thickening medially. The joint space also is widened due to blood in the joint. (**B**) Another patient with a hip dislocation and a barely visible acetabular fracture *(arrow)*. (**C**) CT scan, however, clearly demonstrates the avulsed acetabular fragment *(arrow)*. (**D**) A slightly lower cut demonstrates the femoral head (*H*) and the acetabular fracture *(arrows)*. Study obtained after reduction.

With extensive pelvic fractures, internal visceral and vascular injury is quite common. Indeed, as has been mentioned earlier, exsanguination and other catastrophic complications can result. Once again, CT is invaluable in the assessment of many of these injuries, and when the urinary tract is involved, positive contrast cystography, usually retrograde, is in order (Fig. 4.115). Arteriography can be utilized in certain cases if time permits.

Avulsion Fractures. Avulsion fractures of the pelvic bones commonly occur in children and most often they are seen along the outer aspect of the iliac wing, the anterior-inferior iliac spine (14), and inferior aspect of the ischium (Figs. 4.116 and 4.117). Less commonly, they occur over the upper portion of the superior pubic ramus (Fig. 4.116D), at the top of the iliac wing. In the femur, they occur over the greater and lesser trochanters (see Fig. 4.131). CT can be used to identify the more obscure of these fractures (11), but most often plain films suffice.

With most pelvic avulsion fractures, actual fracture fragments are seen, but in some cases not enough bone is avulsed for this to occur. This is especially common over the ischium, where often only bone

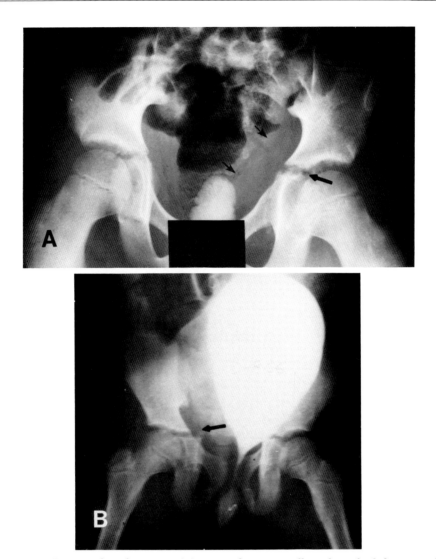

Figure 4.112. *Triradiate cartilage fractures.* (*A*) Note soft tissue swelling along the left inner pelvic margin *(multiple arrows)*. Also note that the triradiate cartilage is wider*(single arrow)* than the one on the right. (*B*) Note the dislocation through the triradiate cartilage on the right *(arrow)*. Also note that on this well-positioned anteroposterior view the joint space on the right is distorted and narrower than that on the left. Furthermore, the bladder has been displaced and elevated by a large intrapelvic hematoma. (Courtesy of Charles J. Fagan, M.D.)

resorption, causing a cortical defect, is seen in the early stages (Fig. 4.117A). Later, as this fracture heals, considerable intermixed bony resorption and osteoblastic reparative change occurs, and bizarre roentgenographic configurations result (Figs. 4.117 and 4.118). These healing avulsion fractures also can occur at other sites (Fig. 4.118), and it has always been

cautioned, and rightly so, that these bizarre configurations not be misinterpreted for those of a more serious lesion such as a bone tumor or osteomyelitis (3–7, 11, 28, 29, 31). *The key, here, is to keep in mind just where these very predictable avulsions occur.*

Before leaving the topic of pelvic avulsion fractures, it should be noted that the normal apophyses, along the inferior aspect of the ischium and superior aspect of the iliac wing, can mimic nondisplaced avulsion fractures (see Fig. 4.124). Of course, this does not mean that the apophyses themselves are never avulsed, for this would be untrue, but it does mean that one will see many more normal apophyses than avulsed ones.

Stress fractures of the pelvic bones are quite uncommon in children, and are more likely to occur in adolescents and adults (15). The key findings include an area of sclerosis and associated periosteal new bone (Fig. 4.119). They are positive on isotope bone scans and the main differential diagnosis is osteoid osteoma, which unfortunately also is positive on regular technetium-99m pyrophosphate bone scans. On indium or gallium bone scans, however, osteoid osteoma usually is not positive.

Fractures of the Sacrum. Sacral fractures commonly are associated with pelvic injuries and, overall, may be difficult to detect. However, if one systematically compares the cortical margins of the sacral foramina on one side to those on the other, disruption of their margins (arcuate lines) (8, 18) will provide a clue to the presence of a fracture (Fig. 4.120A). In addition to sacral fractures, many of these patients demonstrated associated sacroiliac joint separations. Once again, CT is useful in confirming, or initially detecting these sacral injuries (Fig. 4.120B and C). *Other injuries associated with pelvic fractures* include fractures of the femur or injuries to the bladder (see Fig. 4.115), urethra, and pelvic blood vessels. Indeed, rapid demise secondary to exsanguination associated with vascular injury is not uncommon at all (6, 15, 20).

Osteomyelitis of the Pelvic Bones and Sacroiliac Joints. Osteomyelitis of the pelvic bones is more common than generally appreciated but very often its diagnosis is delayed (1, 2, 5, 17, 27). In the early

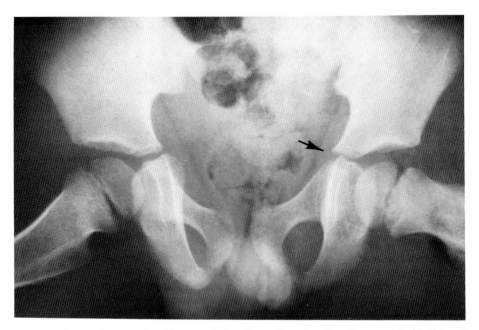

Figure 4.113. *Pseudotriradiate cartilage fracture-dislocation.*   Note that the pelvis is rotated in this patient (i.e., compare the size of the foramina outlined by the pubic and ischial bones on either side; they are unequal, indicating that rotation is present). Rotation causes apparent offsetting or pseudodislocation of the bones about the triradiate cartilage on the left *(arrow)*.

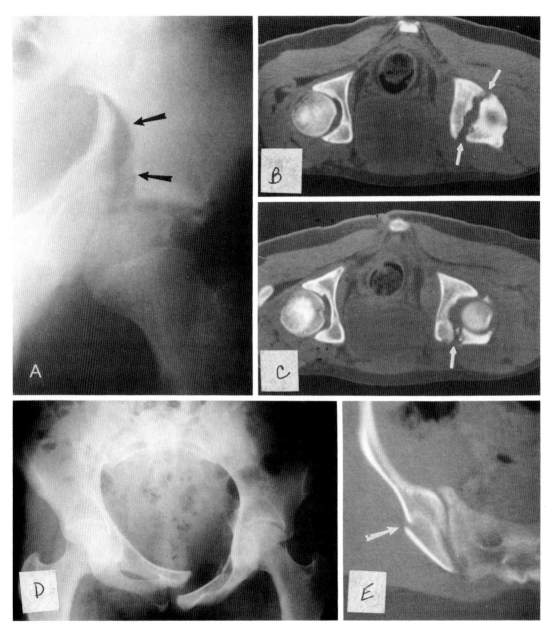

Figure 4.114. *Plain films and CT—complementary functions.* (*A*) Note the gross fracture through the acetabulum *(arrows)*. (*B*) High CT cut demonstrates the fracture through the iliac bone, above the acetabulum *(arrows)*. (*C*) Lower CT cut demonstrates the fracture *(arrow)* and, even more clearly, its relationship to the femoral head. Overall, the two studies provide a very accurate three-dimensional picture of the fracture. (*D*) Another patient with extensive displaced fractures of the pubic bones, overriding of the symphysis pubis, disruption of the right sacroiliac joint, and a vaguely apparent fracture through the right iliac wing. (*E*) CT study clearly demonstrates the iliac wing fracture *(arrow)*. Again, the two studies together provide a complete picture of the fractured pelvis.

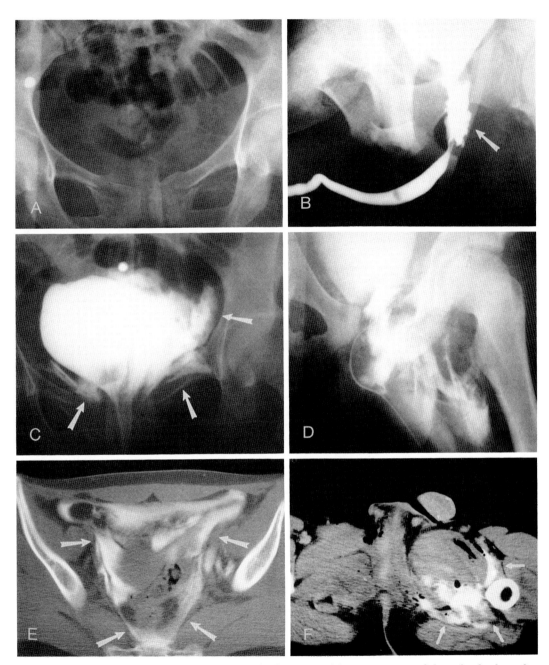

Figure 4.115. *Pelvic fractures with bladder and urethral trauma.* (**A**) Note numerous bilateral pubic bone fractures *(arrows)*. (**B**) Retrograde cystogram showing numerous sites of extravasation of contrast material *(arrows)*. (**C**) CT study through the upper pelvis demonstrates extensive contrast and urine extravasation throughout the peritoneal cavity *(arrows)*. (**D**) Another patient with a posterior urethral tear whose retrograde urethrogram demonstrates early extravasation of contrast material *(arrows)*. (**E**) CT scan demonstrates extensive extravasation of contrast material into the pelvic soft tissues. (**F**) A lower CT cut demonstrates contrast material extravasated into the left groin *(arrows)*. Air bubbles are seen scattered in the soft tissues.

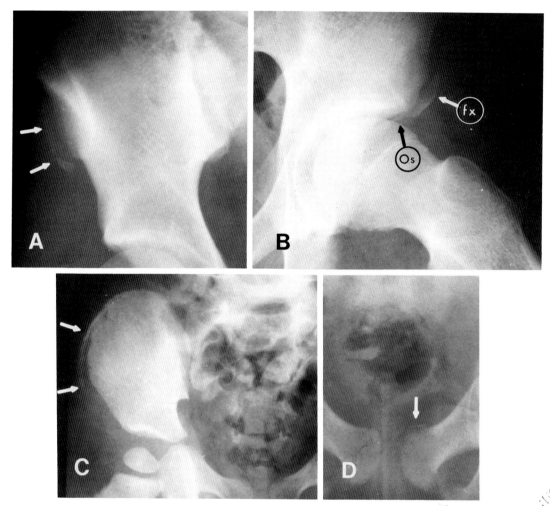

Figure 4.116. *Acute pelvic avulsion injuries.*   (*A*) Note typical iliac wing avulsion *(arrows)* of anterior superior. (*B*) Another iliac bone avulsion fracture *(fx)*, this time involving the anterior, inferior iliac spine. The normal os acetabulum *(Os)* should not be confused with these fractures (also see Fig. 4.125). The os acetabulum lies under the acetabular roof while fractures occur lateral to the acetabulum. (*C*) Long, linear avulsion of iliac wing *(arrows)*. (*D*) Small pubic bone avulsion *(arrow)*.

stages, one may see nothing more than nonspecific, but often extensive, soft tissue swelling around the area of bone involvement. Bone scans are invaluable in such cases and should be utilized whenever the possibility of osteomyelitis is even remotely suspected (Fig. 4.121). This is particularly important, since destruction of the bones of the pelvis may be very subtle in the early stages (Fig. 4.122).

Osteomyelitis of the sacroiliac joint (1, 18, 23) also can be very elusive and, once again, is more readily diagnosed in its early stages with bone scans (21) (Fig. 4.122C–D). Patients with sacroiliac joint infection can present with acute back pain, referred pain down the leg, a limp, or symptoms suggestive of an intra-abdominal problem. As with osteomyelitis of the flat bones of the pelvis, initial roentgenographic findings often are very subtle or nonexistent. Later, destruction along the sacroiliac joint becomes apparent, but in the meantime it is the isotope bone scan which de-

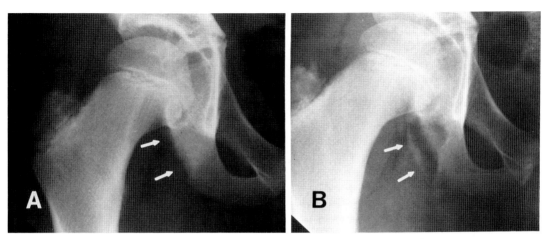

Figure 4.117. *Ischial avulsion with healing.* (*A*) Early phase shows nothing more than bone resorption *(arrows)*. (*B*) Later, with healing, the avulsed fracture fragment is visible *(arrows)*, as hypertrophic bone is beginning to form.

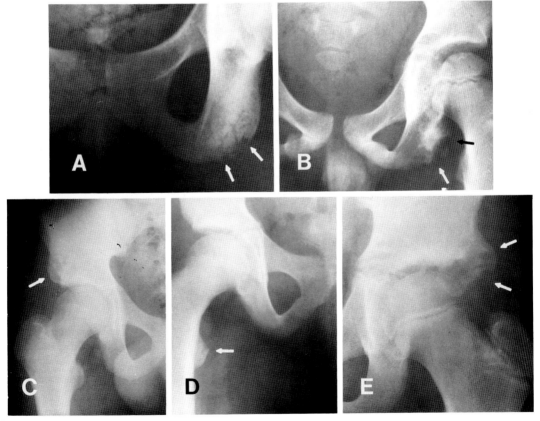

Figure 4.118. *Chronic avulsion injuries.* (*A*) Expanded ischium with irregular new bone formation *(arrows)*. (*B*) Tumor-like appearance of a healing ischial avulsion fracture *(arrows)*. (*C*) Chronic avulsion of the anterior, inferior iliac spine *(arrow)*. (*D*) Chronic avulsion of lesser trochanter *(arrow)*. (*E*) Marked hyperostosis due to chronic avulsion of the anterior, inferior iliac spine *(arrows)*.

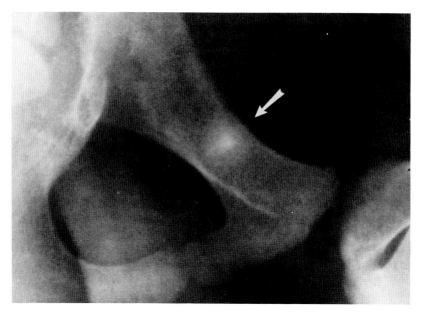

Figure 4.119. *Stress fracture—pubic bone.* (**A**) Note area of sclerosis in pubic bone *(arrow).* Later, periosteal new bone was seen and the bone scan was positive in this patient. (Courtesy of Jack Riley, M.D., Denver, Colorado.)

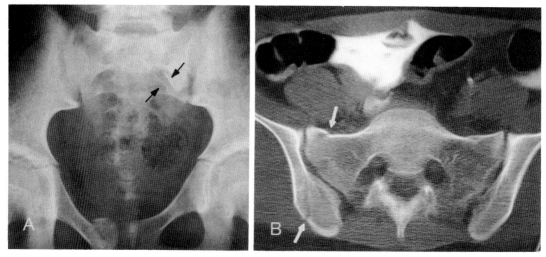

Figure 4.120. *Sacral fractures.* (**A**) Note the disrupted ala of the intervertebral foramina *on the left.* Two disrupted cortices are seen on edge *(arrows).* In addition, note the pubic bone fracture *on the right.* (**B**) CT study in another patient demonstrates a sacral fracture *on the right (upper arrow).* In addition, note the fracture through the iliac bone *(lower arrow).* Contrast material in the peritoneal cavity was secondary to a urinary bladder tear.

livers the most useful information. CT and MRI (18) also are useful in detecting early bone destruction around the sacroiliac joints and in fact are much more sensitive than plain films (Fig. 4.122*F* and *G*).

In addition to osteomyelitis of the pelvis and sacrum, one occasionally can encounter deep soft tissue abscesses, not associated with bone infection (19). These lesions usually are best demonstrated with

CT scanning, MRI, ultrasonography, or indium or gallium nuclear scintigraphy.

Normal Findings Causing Problems. There are a number of normal findings in the pelvis that frequently are misinterpreted for pathology. First of all, the normally wide space between the pubic bones in the infant and young child frequently is mistaken for a pubic bone separation (Fig. 4.123), and second, the exceedingly vari-

able and "pathology-suggesting" appearance of the ischiopubic synchondrosis is misinterpreted for a lesion (Fig. 4.123). The normal ischiopubic synchondrosis is positive on nuclear scintigraphy, but when osteomyelitis involves the synchondrosis, the activity over the area is more marked. This is important to appreciate, for osteomyelitis of the ischiopubic synchondrosis is not uncommon (9, 10) (see Fig. 4.122A).

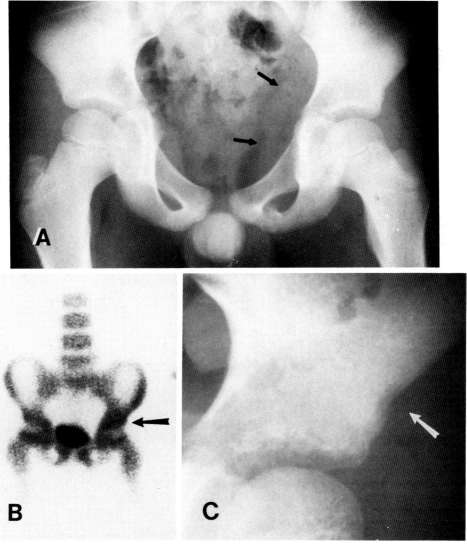

Figure 4.121. *Pelvic bone osteomyelitis with bone scan.* (**A**) Note soft tissue thickening along the inner left pelvic margin *(arrows)*. Bone changes are virtually nonexistent. (**B**) Anterior bone scan, however, demonstrates increased uptake in the left iliac bone *(arrow)*. (**C**) Film of the iliac wing obtained 2 weeks later shows bone destruction *(arrow)*.

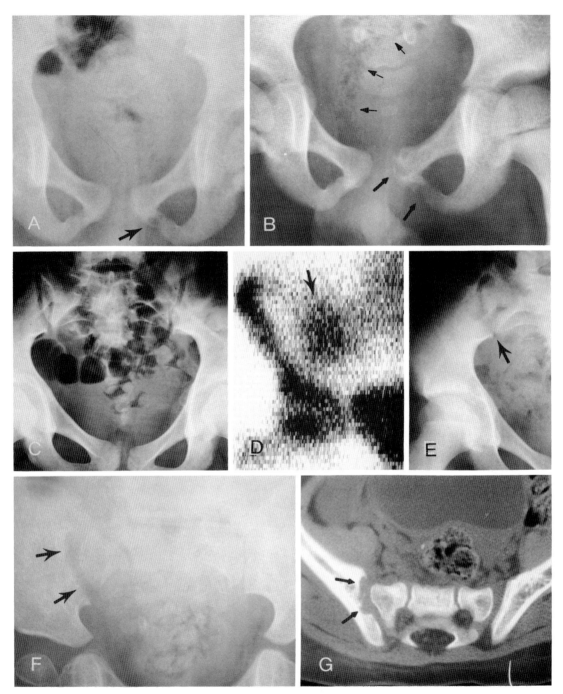

Figure 4.122. *Osteomyelitis: ischiopubic synchondrosis.* (**A**) Note faint radiolucency in the region of the left ischiopubic synchondroses *(arrow).* This finding could be normal but was the early lesion in this case. Also note that the obturator fat pad *on the left* is a little less distinct than the one *on the right.* This patient presented with acute left hip pain. (**B**) A few weeks later, note extensive destruction of the pubic bones *on the left (lower arrows),* consistent with extensive osteomyelitis. Also note the large, soft tissue mass (abscess) in the pelvis causing displacement of the gas and feces-filled rectum *to the right* (upper arrows). (**C**) *Osteomyelitis of sacroiliac joint.* This patient presented with back pain and a right limp. No abnormalities are noted, especially in the right sacroiliac joint. (**D**) Bone scan, however, demonstrates increased activity over the right sacroiliac joint *(arrow).* (**E**) Two weeks later, note complete destruction of the right sacroiliac joint *(arrows).* (**F**) Another patient with visible destruction of the right sacroiliac joint *(arrows).* (**G**) CT study demonstrates destruction of the iliac bone around the sacroiliac joint *(arrows).*

468

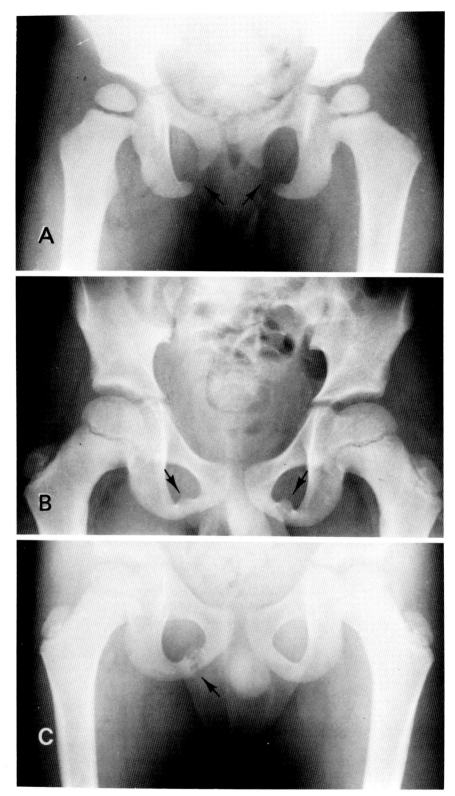

Figure 4.123. *Normal symphysis pubic and ischiopubic synchondroses.* (*A*) Note the normal width between the pubic bones in this young infant. Also note the normal width of the ischiopubic synchondroses *(arrows).* (*B*) Older patient showing normal appearance of the ischiopubic synchondroses *(arrows).* Also note that the space between the pubic bones still is wider than in adults. (*C*) Unilateral ischiopubic synchondrosis on the right *(arrow).*

Figure 4.124. *Normal iliac and ischial apophyses.* (***A***) Note the normal iliac wing apophysis *(arrows)*. (***B***) Normal ischial apophysis *(arrows)*.

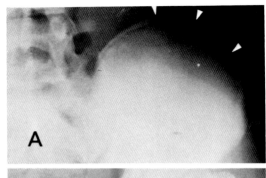

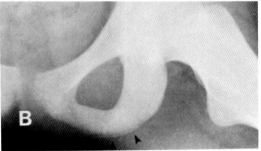

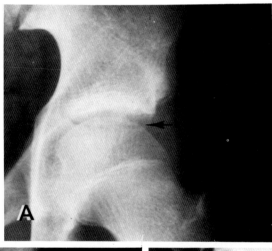

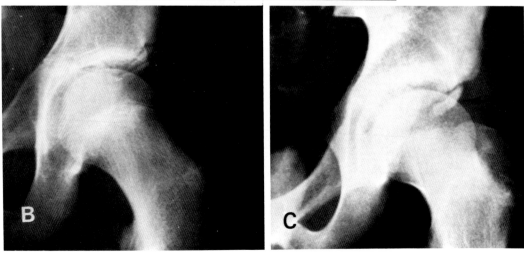

The apophyses along the superior aspect of the iliac bone and inferior aspect of the ischial bone are another source of erroneous interpretation (Fig. 4.124), and so are the numerous normal fragments of the lateral aspect of the normally ossifying acetabulum (Fig. 4.125). These normal bony fragments (os acetabulae) and apophyses can be misinterpreted for fractures, especially avulsion type fractures. Finally, the nearly obliterated triradiate cartilage remnant must not be misinterpreted for a central acetabular fracture (Fig. 4.125).

REFERENCES

1. Coy, J.T., Wolf, C.R., Brower, T.D., and Winter, W.G.: Pyogenic arthritis of the sacro-iliac joint. J. Bone Joint Surg. 58: 845–849, 1976.
2. Edwards, M.S., Baker, C.J., Granberry, W.M., and Barrett, F.F.: Pelvic osteomyelitis in children. Pediatrics 61: 62–67, 1978.
3. Eklof, O., Hugosson, C., and Lindham, S.: Normal variations and posttraumatic appearance of the tuberosity of ischium in adolescence. Ann. Radiol. 22: 77–84, 1979.
4. Ellis, R.E., and Green, A.G.: Ischial apophyseolysis. Radiology 87: 646–648, 1966.
5. Farley, T., Conway, J., and Shulman, S.T: Hematogenous pelvic osteomyelitis in children. Am. J. Dis. Child. 139: 946–949, 1985.
6. Finby, N., and Begg, C.: Traumatic avulsion of ischial epiphysis simulating neoplasm. N.Y. State J. Med. 67: 2488–2490, 1967.
7. Goergen, T.G., Resnick, D., and Riley, R.R.: Post-traumatic abnormalities of the pubic bone simulating malignancy. Radiology 126: 85–87, 1978.
8. Jackson, H., Kam, J., Harris, J.H., Jr., and Harle, T.S.: The sacral arcuate lines in upper sacral fractures. Radiology 145: 35–39, 1982.
9. Jarvis, J., McIntyre, W., Udjus, K., and Kloiber, R.: Osteomyelitis of the ischiopubic synchondrosis. J. Pediatr. Orthop. 5: 163–166, 1985.
10. Kloiber, R., Udjus, K., McIntyre, W., and Jarvis, J.: The scintigraphic and radiographic appearance of the ischiopubic synchondroses in normal

11. Kozlowski, K., Campbell, J.B., and Azouz, E.M.: Traumatized ischial apophysis: Report of six cases. Australas. Radiol. 33: 140–143, 1989.
12. Levine, J.I., and Crampton, R.S.: Major abdominal injuries associated with pelvic fractures. Surg. Gynecol. Obstet. 116: 223–226, 1963.
13. Mack, L.A., Harley, J.D., and Winquist, R.A.: CT of acetabular fractures: Analysis of fracture patterns. A.J.R. 138: 407–412, 1982.
14. Mader, T.J.: Avulsion of the rectus femoris tendon: An unusual type of pelvic fracture. Pediatr. Emerg. Care 6: 198–199, 1990.
15. Meurman, K.O.A.: Stress fracture of the pubic arch in military recruits. Br. J. Radiol. 53: 521–524, 1980.
16. Murphey, M.D., Wetzel, L.H., Bramble, J.M., Levine, E., Simpson, K.M., and Lindsley, H.B.: Sacroiliitis: MR imaging findings. Radiology 180: 239–244, 1991.
17. Nixon, G.W.: Hematogenous osteomyelitis of metaphyseal-equivalent locations. A.J.R. 130: 123–129, 1978.
18. Northrop, C.H., Eto, R.T., and Loop, J.W.: Vertical fracture of the sacral ala: Significance of non-continuity of the anterior superior sacral foraminal line. A.J.R. 124: 102–106, 1975.
19. Oliff, M., and Chuang, V.P.: Retroperitoneal iliac fossa pyogenic abscess. Radiology 126: 647–652, 1978.
20. Patterson, F.K., and Morton, K.S.: The cause of death in fractures of the pelvis. J. Trauma 13: 849–856, 1973.
21. Pope, T.L., Jr., Teague, W.G., Jr., Kossack, R., Bray, S.T., and Flannery, D.B.: Pseudomonas sacroiliac osteomyelitis: Diagnosis by gallium citrate [167]Ga scan. Am. J. Dis. Child. 136: 649–650, 1982.
22. Quinby, W.C., Jr.: Fractures of the pelvis and associated injuries in children. J. Pediatr. Surg. 1: 353–364, 1966.
23. Reed, M.H.: Pelvic fractures in children. J. Can. Assoc. Radiol. 27: 255–261, 1976.
24. Resnik, C.S., Stackhouse, D.J., Shanmuganathan, K., and Young, J.W.R.: Diagnosis of pelvic fractures in patients with acute pelvic trauma: Efficacy of plain radiographs. A.J.R. 158: 109–112, 1992.
25. Rogers, L.F., Novy, S.B., and Harris, N.F.: Oc-

Figure 4.125. *Normal triradiate cartilage remnant and acetabular ossicles (os acetabulae).* (**A**) Note the incompletely obliterated triradiate cartilage remnant (*1*) which might be misinterpreted for a central acetabular fracture. Also note the normal, small acetabular ossicle (os acetabulum) or accessory ossification center (*2*). (**B**) Multiple acetabular ossicles *(arrow).* (**C**) Large acetabular ossicle *(arrow),* which might be misinterpreted for an acetabular rim fracture. However note its classic location under the lateral acetabular margin. Fractures occur laterally, outside the acetabular roof (see Fig. 4.116B).

cult central fractures of the acetabulum. A.J.R. 124: 96–101, 1975.

26. Sauser, D.D., Billimoria, P.E., Rouse, G.A., and Mudge, K.: CT evaluation of hip trauma. A.J.R. 135: 269–274, 1980.

27. Schaad, U.B., McCracken, G.H., Jr., and Nelson, J.D.: Pyogenic arthritis of the sacroiliac joint in pediatric patients. Pediatrics 66: 375–379, 1980.

28. Schlonsky, J., and Olix, M.L.: Functional disability following avulsion fracture of the ischial epiphysis. J. Bone Joint Surg. 54A: 641–644, 1972.

29. Schneider, R., Kay, J.J., and Ghelman, B.: Abductor avulsive injuries near the symphysis pubis. Radiology 120: 567–569, 1976.

30. Shipley, R.T., Griscom, N.T., Kirkpatrick, J.A., and Gross, G.: Artifact of projection simulating a pelvic fracture. A.J.R. 141: 479–480, 1983.

31. Slayton, C.A.: Ischial epiphysiolysis. A.J.R. 76: 1161–1162, 1956.

32. Young, J.W.R., and Resnik, C.S.: Fracture of the pelvis: Current concepts of classification. A.J.R. 155: 1169–1175, 1990.

HIP

Normal Fat Pads and Joint Space. The two views generally obtained for evaluating the hip are the straight anteroposterior and anteroposterior frogleg views. The fat pads surrounding the hip and the joint space are best assessed on the straight anteroposterior view (Fig. 4.126). The fat pads around the hip include the obturator internus, iliopsoas, and gluteus (Fig. 4.126). These fat pads do not lie against the joint capsule directly, and thus are not displaced outwardly when fluid accumulates within the joint. The only exception occurs with the gluteus fat pad, which can be displaced outwardly with the femur, if it is displaced by joint fluid. With soft tissue edema, of course, the fat pads become obliterated.

Detecting Fluid in the Hip Joint. When fluid (blood, pus, serous fluid) accumulates in the hip joint, the femoral head is displaced laterally (Fig. 4.127). This is a natural and easily accomplished decompressive phenomenon, for outward displacement of the femur is the avenue of least resistance in the hip joint. When such decompression occurs, it causes the joint space to become widened medially, and

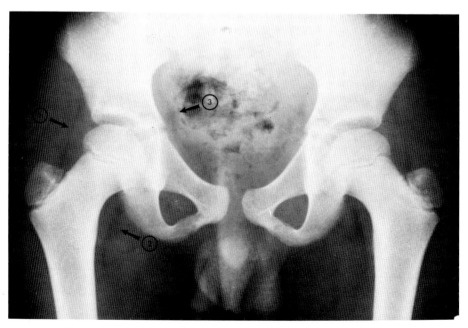

Figure 4.126. *Normal hip joint: soft tissues and fat pads.* Note that the joint space both superiorly and medially is of equal width on both sides. The visible fat pads include the gluteus (*1*), iliopsoas (2), and the obturator internus (3).

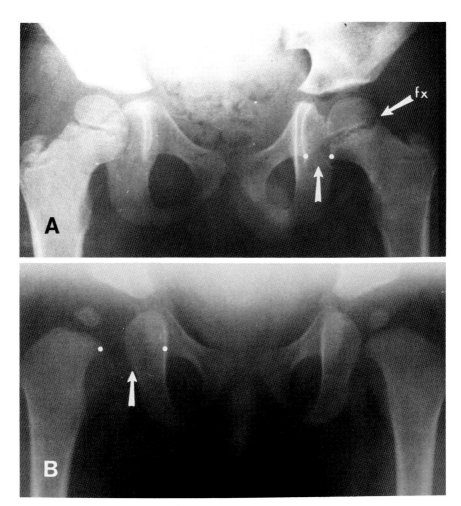

Figure 4.127. *Detecting fluid in the hip joint.* (*A*) Note that the left joint space is wider *(arrow)* than the right. Such lateral displacement of the femoral head with widening of the joint space is indicative of fluid in the joint. This patient sustained a mild Salter-Harris type I epiphyseal-metaphyseal injury (i.e., note subtle widening of the epiphyseal line *on the left (fx)*. The fluid, of course, was blood. (*B*) Young infant with septic arthritis on the right. Note marked widening of the joint space *(arrow)*. *Dots* mark the best place to make one's measurements.

this is the most important roentgeno-graphic finding in the detection of fluid in the hip joint. In addition, one may note displacement or bulging of the gluteus fat pad, but this latter finding is less consistent and dependable.

Proper positioning of the hips is mandatory for the evaluation of joint space widening, for any deviation from normal positioning can lead to erroneous interpretations. In this regard, optimal positioning of the hips is accomplished when the legs are internally rotated (i.e., the toes point

toward each other and the kneecaps point upward). If pelvic rotation occurs or if one leg is out of position, erroneous measurements surely will result.

With regard to joint space widening, it has been demonstrated that widening of the joint space secondary to the accumulation of joint fluid is less likely to occur in older children (47). This also has been our experience, and most likely this occurs because the ligaments are tighter in older children. In young children and infants, however, the femur is readily displaced laterally when joint fluid accumulation occurs, and thus, joint space widening in this age group is a reliable finding for the presence of fluid in the hip joint (47).

Currently, detecting fluid in the hip joint is best accomplished with ultrasonography (8, 39, 46, 49). By means of imaging in the sagittal plane through the hip joint, one easily can determine whether joint fluid is present. When joint fluid is present, the overlying iliopsoas muscle is displaced outwardly from the underlying femur (Fig. 4.128). To detect minimal displacement, it is always wise to compare the findings with the normal side. Blood and pus can produce echogenic debris from within the joint fluid.

Injuries of the Upper Femur. Fractures through the femoral neck and intertrochanteric region of the femur are distinctly less common in children than in adults (4, 16, 19, 22, 25). *Epiphyseal-metaphyseal injuries,* on the other hand, are more common and most often are Salter-Harris type I or II injuries. In assessing the upper femur for the presence of these fractures, one first should look for an increase in the width and radiolucency of the involved epiphyseal line, and then for widening of the medial joint space (Fig. 4.129A). The first finding indicates the presence of an epiphyseal-metaphyseal separation, while the second indicates the presence of associated bleeding into the joint. Of course, if dislocation of the femoral capital epiphysis also is present, the injury is not difficult to detect (Fig. 4.129B). With Salter-Harris type II injuries, an associated metaphyseal corner fracture also will be present.

Anterior or posterior *dislocation of the hip* is not particularly common in childhood (32, 33, 40). The reason for this is that since the epiphysis is still open, it represents the weakest point of the bone, and thus Salter-Harris type I or II injuries are more likely to result. Of course, in the older child, with epiphyseal closure a dislocation is more likely and, as in adults, posterior dislocations are much more common (Fig. 4.130). Acetabular rim fractures are a frequent associated injury and, indeed, a fragment of the acetabulum can become trapped in the joint space. Roent-

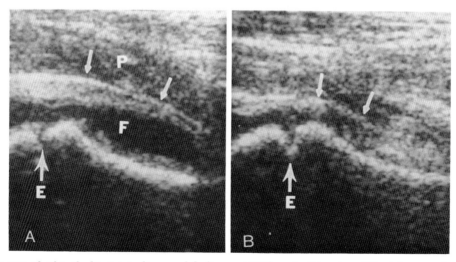

Figure 4.128. *Fluid in the hip joint; ultrasound findings.* (**A**) There is distension of the joint capsule *(arrows)* due to fluid (*F*) in the joint. The femoral neck and femoral head produce the echogenic curved line below. The break in the *curved line* represents the epiphyseal plate (*E*). Psoas muscle (*P*). (**B**) Normal side for comparison. Compare the width of the joint space. The joint capsule *(arrows)* is not bulging. Epiphyseal plate (*E*).

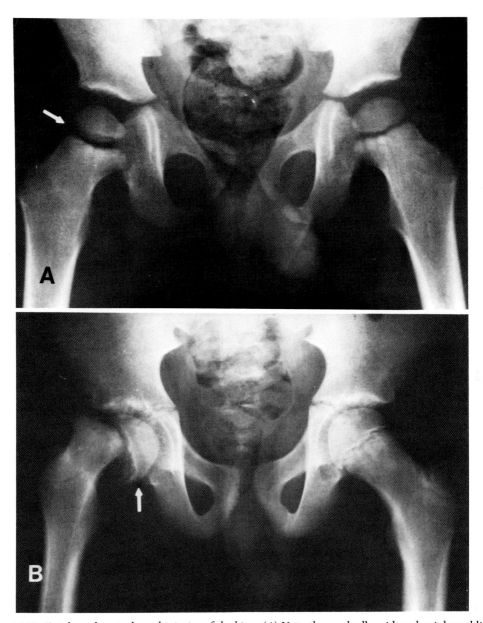

Figure 4.129. *Epiphyseal-metaphyseal injuries of the hip.* (**A**) Note the markedly widened epiphyseal line *on the right (arrow).* The joint space is minimally widened because of associated hemarthrosis. This is a Salter-Harris type I injury, undisplaced. Also see Figure 4.127A for a more subtle fracture. Note the clearly detached epiphysis *on the right (arrow).* (**B**) This is a displaced Salter-Harris type I epiphyseal-metaphyseal injury.

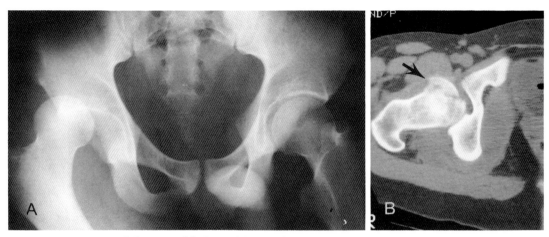

Figure 4.130. *Posterior dislocation of the hip.* (**A**) Note the typical position of a posteriorly dislocated femur in this teenager. The injury was sustained in an automobile accident. (**B**) Another patient who sustained a dislocated hip which was then relocated. A CT scan demonstrates an underlying femoral head fracture *(arrow)*.

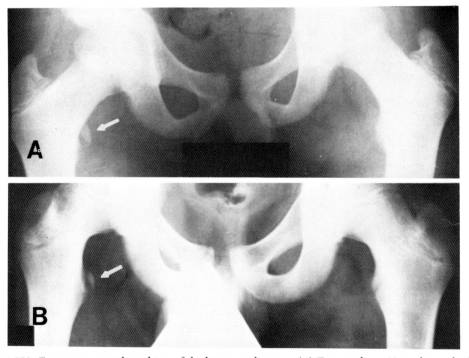

Figure 4.131. *True versus pseudoavulsion of the lesser trochanter.* (**A**) *True avulsion.* Note the avulsed lesser trochanter *on the right (arrow)*. Compare the position of both hips. Both are held in internal rotation. In this position, the lesser trochanter should not be visualized on edge; it should appear as it does *on the left.* (**B**) *Pseudoavulsion.* Note the avulsed appearance of the lesser trochanter *on the right (arrow)*. However, note that the position of the right hip is different from that on the left. The left is internal rotation while the right is an external rotation. External rotation causes the hip to assume a coxa valga configuration, and under such circumstances, the lesser trochanter is seen on edge and can appear avulsed.

genographically, this complication can be suspected when the joint space fails to return to its normal width after reduction. This can be a most important observation, for the fragment frequently is cartilaginous and not visible, and thus, only a high index of suspicion will lead to subsequent CT or MR scanning for definitive diagnosis.

Trochanteric Avulsion Fractures. Avulsion fractures of the trochanteric apophyses, especially of the lesser trochanter, are not particularly common (Fig. 4.131A). These latter avulsions, however, often are difficult to diagnose and/or differentiate from the normal lesser trochanter apophysis which is not avulsed. In this regard, an important point to remember is that if the lesser trochanter apophysis is visible and appears avulsed on the normal anteroposterior view of the hips (i.e., with the hips in internal rotation), then an avulsion probably is present. However, if the femur is externally rotated, or held in the frogleg position, the apophysis of the

lesser trochanter normally is visualized on edge and then erroneously "appears" avulsed (Fig. 4.131B).

Stress fractures are not particularly common in the femur but most often occur in the femoral neck (6). The characteristic findings on plain films consist of sclerosis along the fracture line or, more often, nonspecific sclerosis (Fig. 4.132).

Septic Arthritis, Toxic Synovitis, Osteomyelitis, and Cellulitis of the Hip. The differentiation of these conditions often is a difficult task (15, 32), for the clinical and roentgenographic findings can be very similar. In most cases plain films and ultrasonography lead to the correct diagnosis, but these two studies can be augmented by the three-phase bone scan (1). Plain films can provide information regarding the presence of joint fluid, and, of course, bony destruction with osteomyelitis, but it is ultrasound that is most effective in demonstrating the presence of joint fluid (8, 9, 39, 46, 49). With transient synovitis the

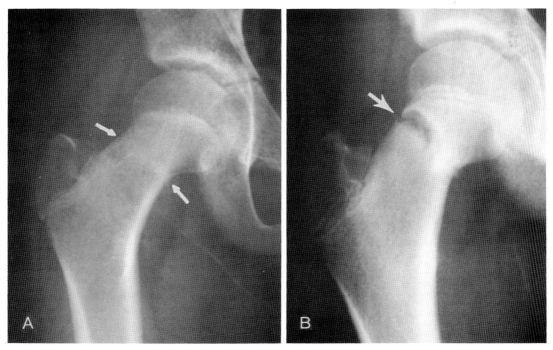

Figure 4.132. *Stress fracture.* (*A*) Note the subtle sclerotic line *(arrows)* through the right femoral neck in this patient with a stress fracture. (*B*) Another patient with a healing and refractured stress fracture *(arrow)*.

fluid usually is clear, but with bacterial infection debris in the fluid and, in some cases, thickening of the joint capsule can be seen. Ultrasonographically the findings depend on demonstrating an increase in the distance between the femoral neck and the overlying iliopsoas muscle (see Fig. 4.128).

With *toxic or transient synovitis*, systemic symptoms usually are less pronounced than with septic arthritis. Indeed these infants often smile as they limp and hobble along, but with septic arthritis, well-established pain rules. The precise etiology of toxic synovitis is unknown, but it probably is a viral joint infection that can afflict older infants and children. It seldom occurs below the age of 2 years. Roentgenographically, the findings are normal in most cases, but in a few, more pronounced cases, there will be widening of the joint space, bulging of the gluteus fat pad, and obliteration of the obturator fat pad (13, 18, 29, 32, 42) (Fig. 4.133). These latter findings are very similar, if not identical, to those of septic arthritis, and similarly, the ultrasonographic findings demonstrating the presence of fluid are the same.

Transient synovitis is usually a one-time affair. However, recurrences do occur (15) and then one should consider the possibility of a more indolent disease process. In this regard, Legg-Perthes disease is the

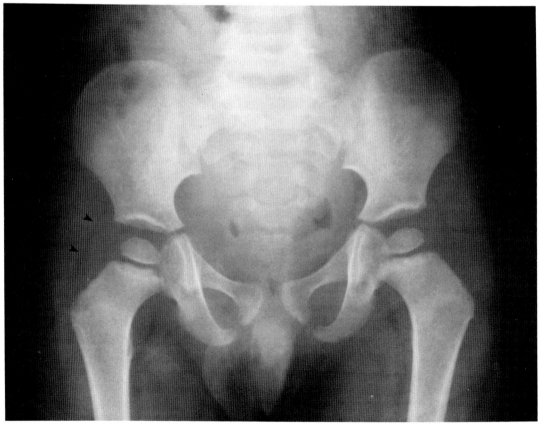

Figure 4.133. *Toxic synovitis—right hip.*   First, note that the joint space *on the right is a little wider than that on the left* (fluid). Then, note that the right gluteus fat pad shows slight bulging *(arrows)*. In addition, there is complete obliteration of the obturator internus fat pad (edema). Compare these findings with those on the normal left side. For detection of fluid in these joints, see Figure 4.128.

problem in some of these patients but the incidence is low, probably no more than 10%. Another possible cause for apparent recurrence of the condition may be the presence of a problem such as rheumatoid arthritis. However, this is quite rare and thus, most often, once one diagnoses transient synovitis, it is treated conservatively and never recurs.

In the classic case of *septic arthritis of the hip,* there is considerable pain secondary to capsular distension, marked diminution in the range of motion of the hip, and in some cases swelling and redness over the hip. The systemic reaction usually is pronounced and both fever and a marked leukocytosis are common (20, 28, 45). An exception to the latter statement occurs in the newborn and very young infant, in whom the lesion may be surprisingly silent. Indeed, in these patients the systemic reaction may be very mild, a leukocytosis may not be present, and the only problem may be a loss of motion of the hip. It is in these cases that the roentgenographic and ultrasonographic examination of the hip becomes of paramount importance.

Roentgenographically, the hallmark of septic arthritis of the hip is widening of the joint space due to lateral displacement of the femoral head and upper femur (Fig. 4.134). This occurs sooner and more often in infants and young children. In older children joint pus may be present, but due to tighter ligaments the joint is not widened (47). With larger collections of pus in the hip joint, the obturator fat pad often is obliterated, and in infants and younger children there also will be a generalized increase in the density of the soft tissues around the hip secondary to associated edema (Fig. 4.134). With ultrasonography distension of the joint space will be seen (Fig. 4.135).

Acute, fulminant, osteomyelitis of the upper femur is common in children and, in very young infants, often is accompanied by septic arthritis. This occurs because in the young infant the blood supply to the femoral metaphysis and epiphysis is contiguous and, thus, spread of infection from one side of the epiphyseal cartilage to the other is readily accomplished. This is not unique to the hip joint, of course, but definitely unique to the young infant. In such cases, roentgenographic changes of both conditions are present, but in the older child, where osteomyelitis alone exists, there usually are no signs of joint involvement. Absence of joint space widening, plus obliteration of the iliopsoas fat pad, serve to differentiate septic arthritis from osteomyelitis, even in those cases of osteomyelitis where a small sympathetic joint effusion occurs. In such cases, periarticular soft tissue changes so outweigh the slight degree of joint space widening that one is forced to conclude that septic arthritis could not be the primary problem. If it were, and were causing so much soft tissue change, joint space widening would be pronounced. Later on, of course, bony destruction of the metaphysis occurs, and the diagnosis of osteomyelitis is more readily established (Fig. 4.136). Low-grade osteomyelitis also can occur in the upper femur and, in some cases, it can appear as a frank Brodie's abscess, but in the area of the greater trochanter, it often has a less specific and more subtle appearance (Fig. 4.137). Indeed, because the infection often is so low grade, it may elude initial detection (10, 30, 45). It is in such cases, and in early cases, that nuclear scintigraphy is most valuable, and should be employed promptly.

Cellulitis of the soft tissues around the hip, in the absence of underlying bone infection also can occur. Most often such infection is due to inflammation of the inguinal lymph nodes, and the findings may be difficult to differentiate from those of osteomyelitis or septic arthritis. However, ultrasound now can be of assistance for it can clearly identify joint fluid with septic arthritis and enlarged lymph nodes with increased blood flow with inflammatory adenopathy (see Fig. 4.245).

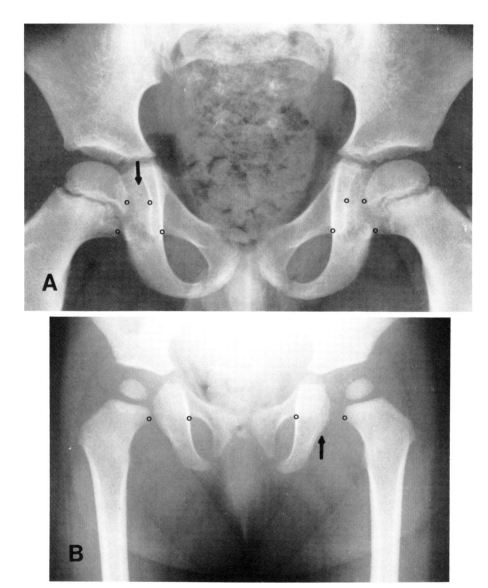

Figure 4.134. *Septic arthritis.*   (*A*) Note widening of the joint space *on the right (arrow).* In this older child, widening is more apparent through *the upper dots.* (*B*) Infant with more pronounced widening of the left joint *(arrow).* The distance *between the dots* is more easily assessed. Also note that there is increased density of the soft tissues along the inner aspect of the acetabulum, causing obliteration of the obturator internus fat pad. This is characteristic of more advanced cases of septic arthritis.

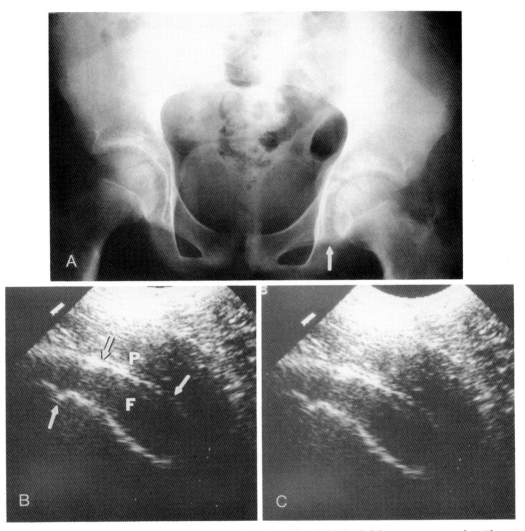

Figure 4.135. *Septic hip—value of ultrasound.* (*A*) In this older child the left hip was very tender. The joint space *(arrow)* may be slightly widened. (*B*) Ultrasound, however, clearly demonstrates a markedly bulging joint capsule *(arrows)* due to fluid (*F*) in the joint. The psoas muscle (*P*) lies above the capsule. The lower, curved echogenic line represents the femoral neck. The break in the line represents the epiphyseal line (*E*). Compare this with normal findings in Figure 4.128*B*. (*C*) Unlabeled scan for comparison.

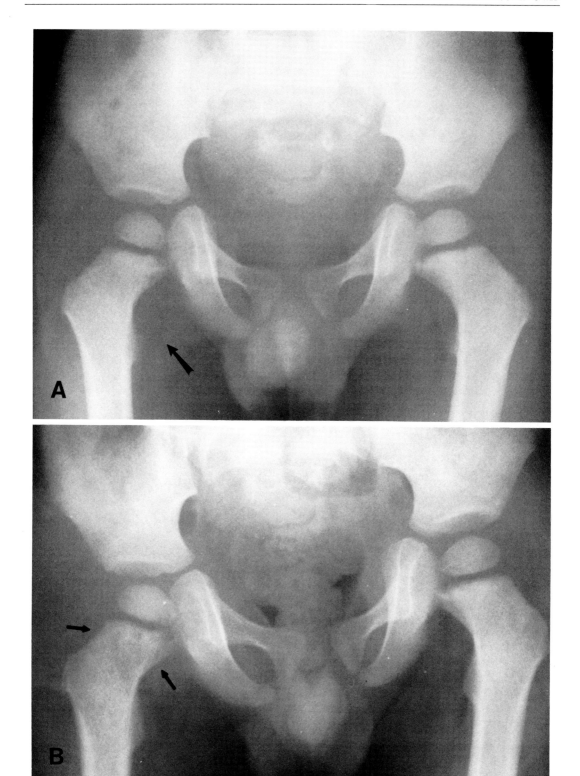

Miscellaneous Hip Problems. Occasionally, on an acute basis, one can be presented with a painful hip due to monoarticular rheumatoid arthritis, nonspecific synovitis, or early Legg-Perthes disease. Any of these conditions can present with findings resembling toxic synovitis or septic arthritis and, indeed, it is generally held that as many as 10% of patients with so-called "toxic synovitis" eventually are determined to have *Legg-Perthes* disease. This is not to say that the two are related, nor that one is necessarily a precursor of the other, but only to indicate that their initial presentations may be very similar (Fig. 4.138A). Early on, in Legg-Perthes disease, demineralization and smallness of the involved femoral head occur (43). These are the earliest bony findings of the disease (43), and while subchondral fractures also occur relatively early (4, 31) (Fig. 4.139), they are not nearly as common as are the other early findings (43). Intraepiphyseal gas also occasionally can be encountered (3) and, in all cases, the femoral head eventually shows increasing sclerosis and then fragmentation as the necrotic bone disintegrates and is absorbed (Fig. 4.138C). In many cases associated irregularities of the metaphyses occur (41). These changes are secondary and consist of reactive fibrous tissue extensions into the metaphysis with resultant irregular bone resorption. Generally they are considered a poor prognostic sign.

When the plain film findings are equivocal or when they are normal and one still suspects Legg-Perthes disease, one can turn to nuclear scintigraphy (2, 5, 7, 44) or MRI (26, 34). There are those who believe that MR imaging is more sensitive, but nuclear scintigraphy is less expensive. With nuclear scintigraphy, one looks for photon-deficient areas in the femoral head, usually laterally (Fig. 4.138D). With MRI, there is loss of the normal high signal of fatty marrow in the femoral head. Once again, the changes in the early stages tend to be more lateral than medial.

Aseptic necrosis also can occur with sickle cell disease and in patients on steroid therapy. Often the problem is bilateral in these patients while with idiopathic Legg-Perthes disease only about 10% of cases demonstrate bilateral involvement. Roentgenographically the changes are no different than in the idiopathic form but may be more acute in onset.

The so-called *"slipped capital femoral epiphysis"* of childhood is another lesion which may occasionally present on an acute basis. This occurs when a superimposed acute slip occurs (Fig. 4.140C and D). More often, however, these patients have a history of chronic hip pain or limp for a number of months (3, 17, 21, 35, 45). The symptoms often tend to be low grade, and in some cases very minimal, with virtually no pain (23). The classic early roentgenographic findings consist of: (a) smoothing of the curve of the epiphyseal line, (b) increased sclerosis on the epiphyseal side, and (c) widening and increased lucency of the epiphyseal line, and slight slipping of the epiphysis (Fig. 4.140A). Later these changes become more profound and are associated with more pronounced medial and posterior tilting of the epiphysis. The latter often is best seen on the frogleg view (Fig. 4.140B).

Figure 4.136. *Osteomyelitis, upper femur.* (A) First, note that the iliopsoas fat pad on the right is obliterated *(arrow)*. Compare with the normal fat pad on the left. The joint space is only minimally widened, and is due to a small sympathetic effusion. The fact that septic arthritis (i.e., joint space widening) is not the primary problem can be deduced from the roentgenographic findings. It would be most unusual for septic arthritis to cause enough edema to obliterate the iliopsoas fat pad and yet not cause any more widening of the joint space. (B) Follow-up films demonstrate irregular lytic lesions in the upper femur *(arrows)*, consistent with osteomyelitis (surgically confirmed).

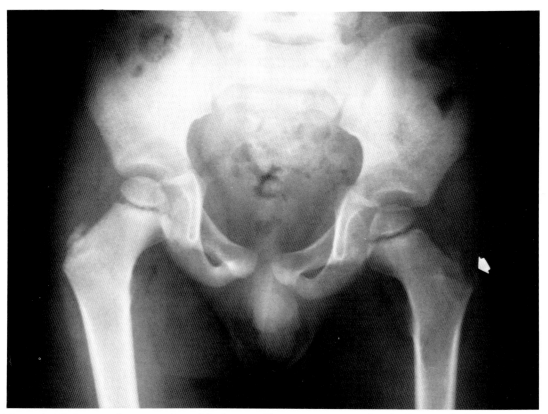

Figure 4.137. *Low-grade osteomyelitis of the femur.*   This patient presented with a limp on the left. Roentgenograms demonstrated a large lytic lesion just under the greater trochanter *(arrow)*. (Surgically proven low-grade osteomyelitis.)

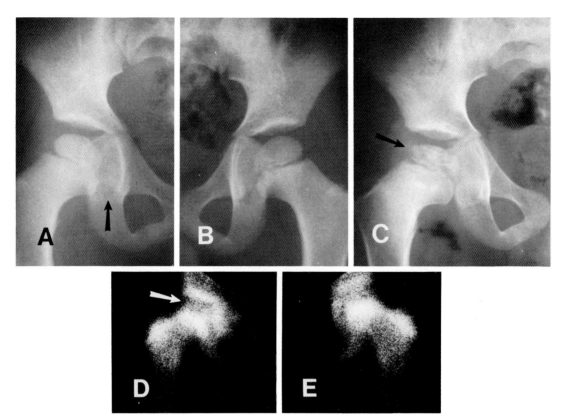

Figure 4.138. *Legg-Perthes disease mimicking acute arthritis.* (*A*) This patient presented with an acute limp and hip pain on the right. The roentgenographic findings suggest slight widening of the joint space *on the right (arrow)*, and a general increase in soft tissue density due to edema. The findings would be impossible to differentiate from toxic synovitis or early septic arthritis. (*B*) Normal side for comparison. (*C*) Months later, note typical changes of advanced Legg-Perthes disease, consisting of a small sclerotic femoral head and metaphyseal irregularity *(arrow)*. (*D*) Isotope study in another patient shows characteristic photon deficient area *(arrow)* in the epiphysis. (*E*) Normal side for comparison.

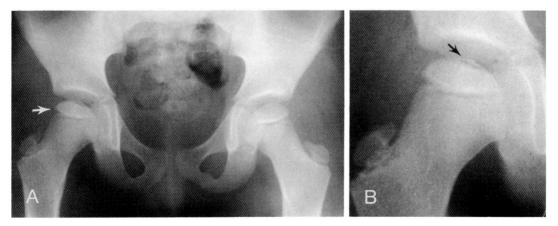

Figure 4.139. *Early findings in Legg-Perthes disease.* (*A*) Note the slightly smaller and slightly more sclerotic femoral head *(arrow)*. A subchondral fracture also is present. (*B*) Magnified view of the right hip demonstrates the subchondral fracture *(arrow)*. These are all early findings in Legg-Perthes disease, but smallness and sclerosis of the head are more common than the subchondral fracture.

485

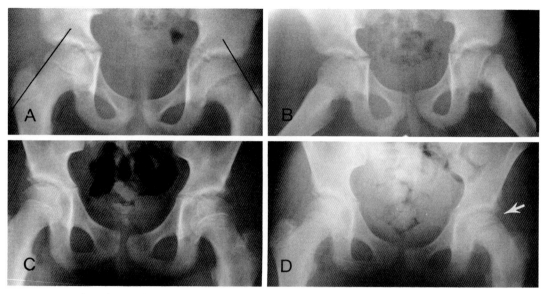

Figure 4.140. *Slipped capital femoral epiphysis.* (*A*) Note that *on the left* the epiphyseal line between the femoral capital epiphysis and femoral neck is wider than that *on the right.* In addition, note that the line applied along the outer aspect of the femoral neck fails to intersect the femoral capital epiphysis. On the normal right side, it intersects the epiphysis. (*B*) Frogleg view demonstrating posterior slippage of the left femoral head. In addition, note how much wider the epiphyseal line is when compared to the normal one on the right. (*C*) This patient had pain on the left. The findings are very subtle. There is some generalized demineralization of the bones secondary to disuse, and the epiphyseal line is just slightly more rounded and sclerotic than the one on the right. (*D*) Two weeks later, a frank slip on the left *(arrow)* has occurred. The findings in (*C*) represent the so-called "pre-slip" stage.

On frontal view, a line drawn along the outer aspect of the femoral neck can aid in determining whether the epiphysis has slipped medially, for in those cases where such slippage has occurred, the line does not intersect the femoral capital epiphysis (Fig. 4.140A). Posterior slippage of the femoral head usually accompanies medial slippage and, actually, often predominates. It is best detected, as noted earlier, on frogleg views of the hips (Fig. 4.140B).

The precise etiology of the slipped capital femoral epiphysis in childhood is unknown, but it probably represents a subclinical Salter-Harris type I epiphyseal-metaphyseal injury. In this regard, it has been suggested that in many of these patients the epiphyseal-metaphyseal junction is more vertical than normal (27, 36) and because of this, the epiphysis is more prone to such slippage. A lack of normal anteversion also has been noted to predispose to slippage (11, 12, 36) and, of course, so has obesity (11). It is also a little more common in males. In addition to these mechanical factors, the following predisposing hormonal factors have been identified: decreased growth hormone (37, 48), hypothyroidism (14, 48), and decreased testosterone levels (48).

Normal Variations Causing Problems. In and around the hip, irregularity of the acetabulum and femoral head are the most common normal variations to be misinterpreted for fractures or other abnormalities. Irregularity of femoral head ossification can be pronounced in children and, indeed, the normal femoral head can appear quite fragmented (Fig. 4.141). These findings often are misinterpreted as those of Legg-Perthes disease and have been referred to as Meyer's dysplasia (24).

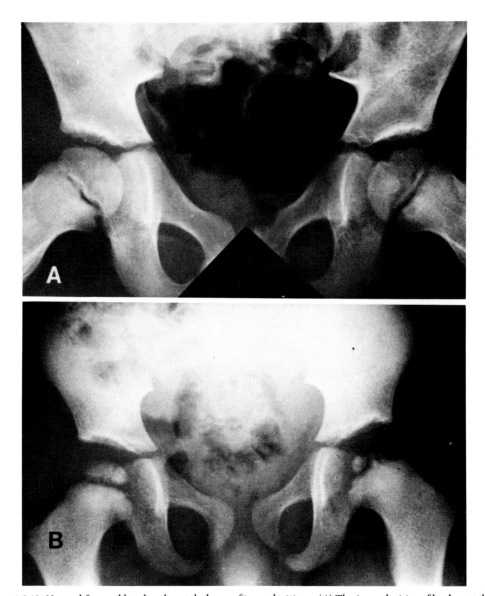

Figure 4.141. *Normal femoral head and acetabular roof irregularities.* (*A*) The irregularities of both acetabular roofs and of the femoral head on the left are normal. (*B*) Normal irregular and asymmetric ossification of the femoral heads.

The normal apophysis of the lesser trochanter being mistaken for an avulsion fracture has been dealt with earlier (see Fig. 4.131), but it also should be noted that the normal greater trochanter, because of its frequently very irregular appearance, also can be subject to misinterpretation for a chronic avulsion injury (Fig. 4.142B). Similarly, the cartilage remnant between the greater trochanter and femur, as visualized on frogleg views, can be mistaken for a fracture (Fig. 4.142). The vacuum joint phenomenon demonstrated in the shoulder (see Fig. 4.40B) also is common in the hip. It is especially prone to occur with stretching of the hips for the frogleg views.

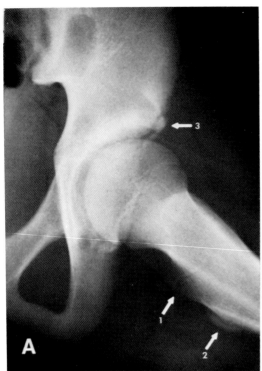

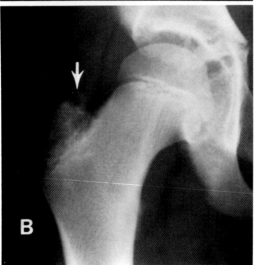

Figure 4.142. *Other normal upper femoral findings causing problems.* (*A*) Note: (*1*) the fracture-like cartilaginous remnant between the greater trochanter and femur; (*2*) normal lesser trochanter apophysis; and (*3*) normal acetabular ossicles. (*B*) Normal irregular greater trochanter *(arrow)*.

REFERENCES

1. Alexander, J.E., Seibert, J.J., Aronson, J., Williamson, L., Glasier, C.M., Rodgers, A.B., and Corbitt, S.L.: A protocol of plain radiographs, hip ultrasound and triple phase bone scans in the evaluation of painful pediatric hip. Clin. Pediatr. 27: 175–181, 1988.
2. Bensahel, H., Bok, B., Cavailloles, F., and Csukonyi, Z.: Bone scintigraphy in Perthes disease. J. Pediatr. Orthop. 3: 302–305, 1983.
3. Bloomberg, T.J., Nuttall, J., and Stoker, D.J.: Radiology in early slipped femoral capital epiphysis. Clin. Radiol. 29: 667, 1978.
4. Caffey, J.: The early roentgenographic changes in essential coxa plana. A.J.R. 103: 620–634, 1968.
5. Canale, S.T., and Bourland, W.L.: Fracture of the neck and intertrochanteric region of the femur in children. J. Bone Joint Surg. 59A: 431–443, 1977.
6. Coldwell, D., Gross, G.W., and Boal, D.K.: Stress fracture of the femoral neck in a child (stress fracture). Pediatr. Radiol. 14: 174–176, 1984.
7. Danigelis, J.A.: Pinhole imaging in Legg-Perthes disease: further observations. Semin. Nucl. Med. 6: 69–82, 1976.
8. Dorr, U., Zieger, M., and Hauke, H.: Ultrasonography of the painful hip: Prospective studies in 204 patients. Pediatr. Radiol. 19: 36–40, 1988.
9. Erken, E.H.W., and Katz, K.: Irritable hip and Perthes' disease. J. Pediatr. Orthop. 10: 322–326, 1990.
10. Frazier, J.K., and Anzel, S.H.: Osteomyelitis of the greater trochanter in children. J. Bone Joint Surg. 63A: 833–836, 1981.
11. Galbraith, R.T., Gelberman, R.H., Hajek, P.C., Baker L.A., Sartoris, D.J., Rab, G.T., Cohen, M.S., and Griffin, P.P.: Obesity and decreased

femoral anteversion in adolescence. J. Orthop. Res. 5: 523–528, 1987.

12. Gelberman, R.H., Cohen, M.S., Shaw, B.A., Kasser, J.R., Griffin, T.T., and Wilkinson, R.H.: The association of femoral retroversion with slipped capital femoral epiphysis. J. Bone Joint Surg. 68A: 100–107, 1986.

13. Hardinge, K.: The etiology of transient synovitis of the hip in childhood. J. Bone Joint Surg. 52B: 100–107, 1970.

14. Hirano, T., Stamelos, S., Harris, V., and Dumbovic, N.: Association of primary hypothyroidism and slipped capital femoral epiphysis. J. Pediatr. 93: 262–264, 1978.

15. Illingworth, C.M.: Recurrences of transient synovitis of the hip. Arch. Dis. Child. 58: 620–623, 1983.

16. Ingram, A.J., and Bachynski, B.: Fractures of the hip in children. J. Bone Joint Surg. 35A: 867–887, 1953.

17. Jacobs, B.: Diagnosis and natural history of slipped femoral capital epiphysis. Instruct. Course Lect. Am. Acad. Orthop. Surg. 21: 167–173, 1972.

18. Jacobs, B.W.: Synovitis of the hip in children and its significance. Pediatrics 47: 558–566, 1971.

19. Kay, S.P., and Hall, J.E.: Fracture of the femoral neck in children and its complications. Clin. Orthop. 80: 53–71, 1971.

20. Kaye, J.J.: Bacterial infections of the hips in infancy and childhood. Curr. Probl. Radiol. 3: 17–29, 1973.

21. Klein, A., Joplin, R.J., Reidy, J.A., and Hanelin, J.: Roentgenographic features of slipped capital femoral epiphyses. A.J.R. 66: 361–374, 1951.

22. Lam, S.F.: Fractures of the neck of the femur in children. J. Bone Joint Surg. 53A: 1165–1179, 1971.

23. Ledwith, C.A., and Fleisher, G.R.: Slipped capital femoral epiphysis without hip pain. Pediatrics 89: 660–662, 1992.

24. Meyer, J.: Dysplasia epiphysealis capitis femoris. Acta Orthop. Scand. 34: 183–197, 1964.

25. Miller, W.E.: Fractures of the hip in children from birth to adolescence. Clin. Orthop. 92: 155–188, 1973.

26. Mitchell, M.D., Kundel, H.L., Steinberg, M.E., Kressel, H.Y., Alavi, A., and Axel, L.: Avascular necrosis of the hip: Comparison of MR, CT and scintigraphy. A.J.R. 147: 67–71, 1986.

27. Mirkopulos, N., Weiner, D.S., and Askew, M.: The evolving slope of the proximal femoral growth plate relationship to slipped capital femoral epiphysis. J. Pediatr. Orthop. 8: 268–273, 1888.

28. Morrey, B.F., Bianco, A.J., and Rhodes, K.H.: Suppurative arthritis of the hip in children. J. Bone Joint Surg. 58A: 388–392, 1976.

29. Neuhauser, E.B.D., and Wittenborg, M.H.: Synovitis of the hip in infancy and childhood. Radiol. Clin. North Am. 1: 13–16, 1963.

30. Nixon, G.W.: Hematogous osteomyelitis of metaphyseal-equivalent locations. A.J.R. 130: 123–129, 1978.

31. Norman, A., and Bullough, P.: The radiolucent crescent line—an early diagnostic sign of avascular necrosis of the femoral head. Bull. Hosp. Joint Dis. 24: 99–104, 1963.

32. Offerski, C.M.: Traumatic dislocation of the hip in children. J. Bone Joint Surg. 63B: 194–197, 1981.

33. Pearson, D.E., and Mann, R.J.: Traumatic hip dislocation in children. Clin. Orthop. 92: 189–194, 1973.

34. Pinto, M.R., Peterson, H.A., and Berquist, T.H.: Magnetic resonance imaging in early diagnosis of Legg-Calve-Perthes disease. J. Pediatr. Orthop. 9: 19–22, 1989.

35. Ponseti, I.V., and McClintock, R.: Pathology of slipping of the upper femoral epiphysis. J. Bone Joint Surg. 38A: 71–83, 1956.

36. Pritchett, J.W., and Perdue, K.D.: Mechanical factors in slipped capital femoral epiphysis. J. Pediatr. Orthop. 8: 385–388, 1988.

37. Rappaport, E.B., and Fife, D.: Slipped capital femoral epiphysis in growth hormone-deficient patients. Am. J. Dis. Child. 139: 396–399, 1985.

38. Ratliff, A.H.C.: Traumatic separation of the upper femoral epiphysis in young children. J. Bone Joint Surg. 50B: 757–770, 1968.

39. Royle, S.G.: Investigation of the irritable hip. J. Pediatr. Orthop. 12: 396–397, 1992.

40. Schlonsky, J., and Miller, P.R.: Traumatic hip dislocations in children. J. Bone Joint Surg. 55A: 1056–1063, 1973.

41. Smith, S.R., Ions, G.K., and Gregg, P.J.: The radiological features of the metaphysis in Perthes disease. J. Pediatr. Orthop. 2: 401–404, 1982.

42. Spock, H.: Transient synovitis of the hip joint in children. Pediatrics 24: 1042–1049, 1959.

43. Stansberry, S.D., Swischuk, L.E., and Barr, L.L.: Legg-Perthes disease: Incidence of the subchondral fracture. Appl. Radiol. 19: 30–33, 1990.

44. Sutherland, A.D., Savage, J.P., Paterson, D.C., et al.: The nuclide bone-scan in the diagnosis and management of Perthes disease. J. Bone Joint Surg. 61B: 300–306, 1980.

45. Swischuk, L.E.: Childhood limp: Early diagnosis of his problem. In A.R. Margulis and C.A. Gooding (eds.): Diagnostic Radiology, pp. 61–80. University of California Press, San Francisco, 1975.

46. Terjesen, T., and Osthus, P.: Ultrasound in the diagnosis and followup of transient synovitis of the hip. J. Pediatr. Orthop. 11: 608–613, 1991.

47. Volberg, F.M., Sumner, T.E., Abramson, J.S., and Winchester, P.H.: Unreliability of radiographic diagnosis of septic hip in children. Pediatrics 74: 118–120, 1984.

48. Wilcox, P.G., Weiner, D.S., and Leighley, B.: Maturation factors in slipped capital femoral epiphysis. J. Pediatr. Orthop. 8: 196–200, 1988.
49. Wingstrand, H., Egund, N., Lidgren, L., and Sahlstrand, T.: Sonography in septic arthritis of the hip in the child: Report of four cases. J. Pediatr. Orthop. 7: 206–209, 1987.

FEMORAL SHAFT

Fractures of the femoral shaft are common in childhood, but generally not difficult to detect. Usually they result from serious, known injuries and are of the transverse, spiral, or oblique variety. It is important to note that with femoral shaft fractures a small degree of overriding of the fracture fragments is desirable (Fig. 4.143). Furthermore, healing with abundant callus formation is the rule. The reason overriding is desirable is that the hyperemia associated with the fracture leads to accelerated growth of the femur. The fact that the femur is the fastest growing long bone in the body, especially at its distal end, causes this combination of factors to lead to overgrowth and excessive length of the femur. Initial overriding protects against this.

Greenstick, buckle (torus), and plastic

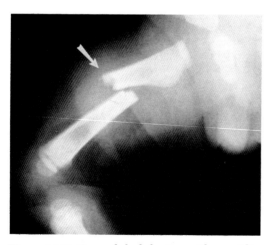

Figure 4.143. *Femoral shaft fracture with overriding fragments.* Note the overriding femoral fracture *(arrow).* This is desirable to prevent overgrowth of the femur during the healing phase. This infant was a battered child.

bending fractures are distinctly uncommon in the femur in any age group. However, they can occur (3). Stress fractures of the midshaft of the femur can occasionally be encountered in children (2), but more often they occur in the femoral neck (see Fig. 4.132).

Recently, some note has been made of the fact that many times what appears to be an ordinary fractured femur in an infant is actually part of the battered child syndrome (1, 4). The main theme of these reports is that in young infants, where one might not expect to see femoral shaft fractures with any degree of frequency, if any suspicion regarding the fracture arises, the possibility of the infant being battered should be entertained, and the yield, indeed, is relatively high. This problem is discussed in more detail later in the section dealing with infant abuse (see p. 561.)

REFERENCES

1. Beals, R.K., Tufts, E.: Fractured femur in infancy: The role of child abuse. J. Pediatr. Orthop. 3: 583–586, 1983.
2. Burks, R.T., and Sutherland, D.H.: Stress fracture of the femoral shaft in children: Report of two cases and discussion. J. Pediatr. Orthop. 4: 614–616, 1984.
3. Cail, S.S., Keats, T.E., and Sussman, M.D.: Plastic bowing fracture of the femur in a child. A.J.R. 130: 780–782, 1978.
4. Gross, R.H., and Stranger, M.: Causative factors responsible for femoral fractures in infants and young children. J. Pediatr. Orthop. 3: 341–343, 1983.

KNEE

Normal Fat Pads and Soft Tissues. There are numerous normal fat pads around the knee, and all can be useful. However, those demonstrable on lateral view are the most beneficial (Fig. 4.144). Indeed, one of the best ways to determine whether fluid is present in the knee joint is to assess the soft tissues and fat pads on the lateral view of the knee (see next section).

Detection of Fluid in the Knee Joint. The knee joint does not widen significantly

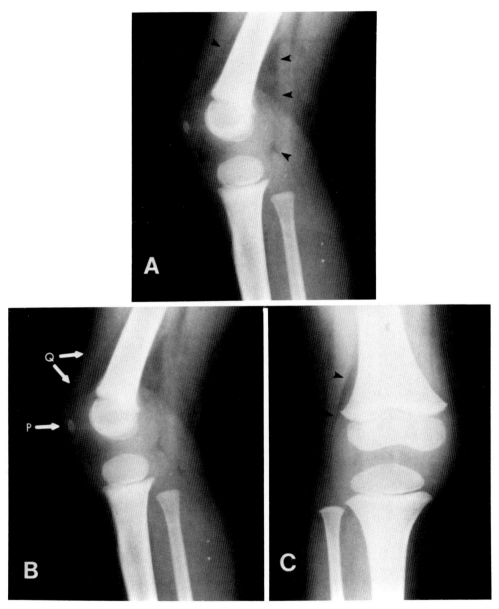

Figure 4.144. *Normal soft tissues and fat pads of the knee.* (**A**) Lateral view; the most useful view for evaluation of the joint space and fat pads. The anterior *upper arrows* delineate the prefemoral fat pad, while the fat pad posterior to the distal femur is outlined by the posterior *upper arrows.* The *lower anterior arrow* delineates the infrapatellar fat pad, while the fat pad over the cartilaginous tibial epiphysis is outlined by the *posterior lower arrow.* (**B**) Same knee; other findings. Note the small ossification center of the basically cartilaginous patella (*P*) and the easily visualized quadriceps tendon (*Q*), just anterior to the prefemoral fat pad. (**C**) Frontal view demonstrating the most frequently visible fat pad *(arrows).*

with accumulations of fluid, and thus one must depend on soft tissue and fat pad changes for the detection of fluid in the knee joint (23, 25). In this regard, it is the lateral view of the knee that is most useful. On this view, fluid almost always first accumulates in the suprapatellar bursa, which lies behind the quadriceps tendon and in front of the prefemoral fat pad. When this occurs, the quadriceps tendon is displaced anteriorly and the fat pad posteriorly. Early on, just the neck of the suprapatellar bursa may be distended (Fig. 4.145A), but this finding, almost always, is seen in older children and not in infants.

With greater fluid accumulations, the bursa itself can be identified as a discrete structure (Fig. 4.145B), and once again, this most often occurs in older children after trauma. In infants and young children, especially if the fluid is pus, the discrete nature of the distended suprapatellar bursa may be lost and the confluent soft tissue density of the quadriceps tendon and distended bursa erroneously suggests that the entire tendon is thickened (Fig. 4.145C and D). In addition to these findings it should be noted that while fluid first accumulates in the suprapatellar bursa, it thereafter also begins to accumulate in the

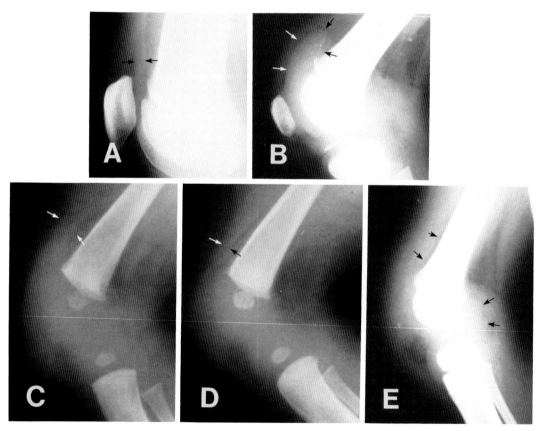

Figure 4.145. *Detecting fluid in the knee joint.* (A) Lateral view. Early findings consisting of distension of the neck *(arrows)* of the suprapatellar bursa. (B) Another patient with discrete distension of the suprapatellar bursa *(arrows).* (C) In this case, fluid in the suprapatellar bursa blends in with the quadriceps tendon and causes subtle pseudothickening of the tendon *(arrows).* (D) Normal side for comparison. Note normal quadriceps tendon *(arrows).* (E) More extensive fluid collection in the suprapatellar bursa leads to marked pseudothickening of the quadriceps tendon. Also note that the prefemoral fat pad is compressed against the femur *(upper arrows)*, and that there is early accumulation of fluid in the posterior popliteal bursa *(posterior arrows).*

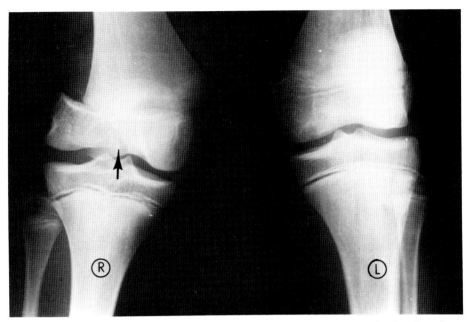

Figure 4.146. *Salter-Harris type III epiphyseal-metaphyseal injury.* Note the grossly displaced epiphysis and the fracture through the middle of the epiphysis *(arrow)* of the distal right femur.

posterior popliteal bursa (Fig. 4.145C), but one always should look at the suprapatellar bursa first, for fluid accumulates here before it does so in the posterior popliteal bursa. Seldom, then, will one use the posterior popliteal bursa for fluid detection.

Injuries of the Distal Femur and Proximal Tibia. Cortical buckle (torus) fractures around the knee are uncommon, for the cortex in both the distal femur and proximal tibia is sturdy. On the other hand, epiphyseal-metaphyseal injuries, transverse fractures of the upper tibia, patellar fractures, and cruciate ligament avulsions are quite common. Meniscal injuries also occur, but more frequently in the older child and, in any event, they usually produce normal roentgenograms. Other injuries sustained around the knee include acute and chronic tibial tubercle and inferior patellar avulsions.

Epiphyseal-metaphyseal injuries are common about the knee and in gross form are not difficult to detect (Fig. 4.146). The more subtle, nondisplaced Salter-Harris type I or II injuries, on the other hand, frequently elude initial observation. In these cases, one must, once again, learn to study the soft tissues first, and then to suspect the slightest degree of widening of the epiphyseal line (Fig. 4.147). In other cases, additional oblique (Fig. 4.148) or stress views may be required to confirm or further delineate the injury. Epiphyseal-metaphyseal injuries of the knee can be sustained in a number of ways but usually trauma is not minor: i.e., automobile accidents, athletic injuries (47, 48), etc., and most often the stresses applied to the knee are dissipated through the epiphyseal-metaphyseal junctions. However, in some cases, rather than the forces being dissipated through this area, collateral ligament strains cause small, marginal avulsions of either the epiphysis or metaphysis (Fig. 4.149).

Cruciate ligament avulsions most often involve the anterior cruciate ligament at its bony insertion onto the anterior tibial spine of the tibial epiphysis (22). With large fragment avulsions, the findings are

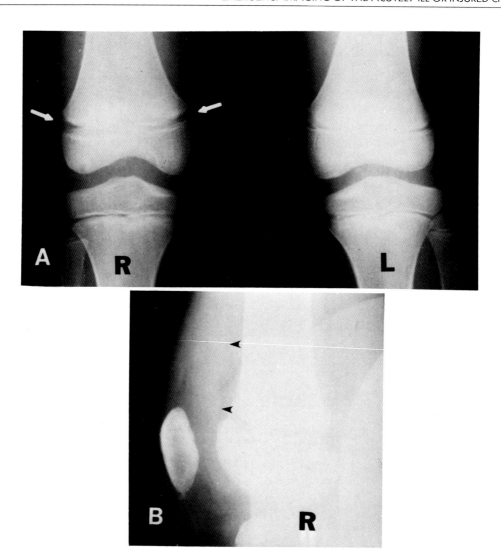

Figure 4.147. *Subtle Salter-Harris type I epiphyseal-metaphyseal injury.* (*A*) First, note that the soft tissues are more opaque around the right knee. This indicates the presence of edema. In addition, however, note that the epiphyseal line of the distal right femur is wider *(arrows)* than its counterpart on the normal left side. The findings represent a nondisplaced epiphyseal-metaphyseal separation. (*B*) Lateral view showing associated hemarthrosis manifesting in distension of the suprapatellar bursa *(arrows)*.

Figure 4.148. *Multiple, subtle, Salter-Harris type I epiphyseal-metaphyseal injuries.* (*A*) Note widening of the epiphyseal line of the distal right femur and proximal left tibia *(arrows)*. Compare these epiphyseal lines with their normal counterparts on the other side. Also note a fracture in the upper left fibula. (*B*) Oblique view demonstrating widening of the right distal femoral and left proximal tibial epiphyseal lines *(arrows)*. The left fibular fracture is noted again. (*C*) Two weeks later note evidence of healing of the previously noted epiphyseal-metaphyseal fractures. There is irregular sclerosis along the distal right femoral epiphyseal-metaphyseal junction *(right arrows)* and along the upper left tibial epiphyseal-metaphyseal line *(left arrows)*. The fibular fracture is noted again.

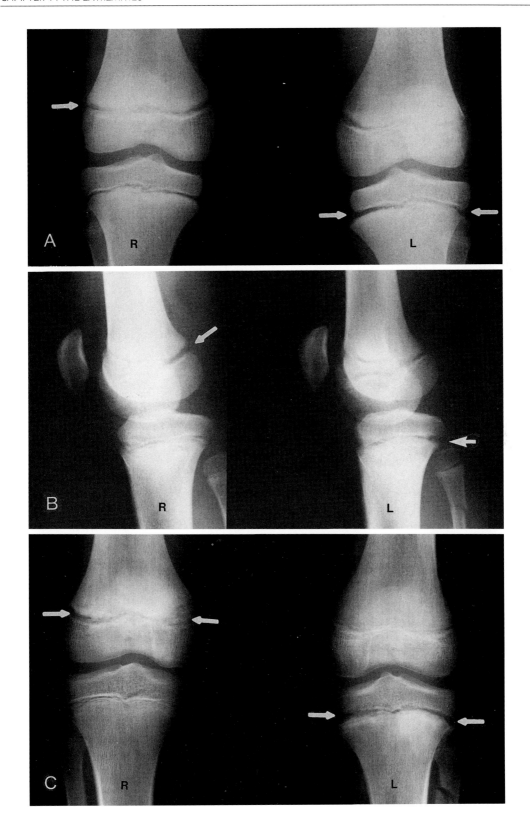

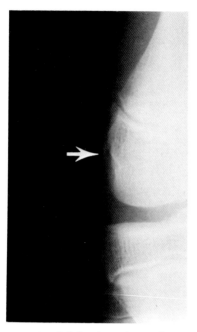

Figure 4.149. *Subtle lateral epiphyseal avulsion.* Note the barely visible avulsed bony epiphyseal fragment *(arrow)*. This patient sustained a lateral knee strain injury.

straightforward and it is difficult to miss the fragment (Fig. 4.150). With smaller avulsions, however, it is easy to miss the fragment on initial studies (Fig. 4.151A). A similar problem can arise, although less commonly, with cruciate ligament avulsions involving the femoral condyle (Fig. 4.151B). In either case, tunnel views of the knee usually more clearly delineate the avulsed fragment (Fig. 4.151C).

Cruciate ligament injuries currently are best assessed with MRI (32, 54). Occult associated fractures also can be detected with MRI (30). The latter show focal decrease in the normal high signal of bone marrow on T_1-weighted images, while ligament injuries manifest in distortion of the cruciate ligament (Fig. 4.152).

Supracondylar fractures of the distal femur are not difficult to identify for most often they are gross. However, seldom do they occur in healthy bones, for in such bones the weakest area is the epiphyseal-metaphyseal junction and fractures occur here. On the other hand, in a severely demineralized or otherwise weakened bone, this is not true, and consequently it is in this type of bone that supracondylar fractures occur. Contrarily, in the *proximal tibia* one commonly sees *transverse metaphyseal fractures* in normal individuals (Fig. 4.153), and when these fractures are hairline, they are difficult to detect (see Fig. 4.3A). Another interesting feature of these fractures is that there is a tendency for valgus (knock-knee) deformity to develop, especially if there is an associated inbending deformity (9, 30, 51). When an initial valgus deformity is present it is easy to see why it might persist (Fig. 4.154), but in other cases another, probably more important, factor is involved. This deals with the fact that there is overgrowth of the tibia, during healing, through the medial portion of the epiphyseal-metaphyseal junction (19, 31, 47, 59). This probably is related to the hyperemia associated with the fracture which in the end causes accelerated growth of the medial aspect of the proximal tibia which then results in a knock-knee deformity. In this regard it has been noted that normally there is a greater blood supply to the upper medial tibia, and that with trauma this is exaggerated (57).

Compression fractures of the tibial plateau are less common in children than in adults, but upper fibular fractures occur rather frequently, both with knee injuries (see Fig. 4.148), and ankle injuries. Compression fractures of the proximal tibia also occur with trampoline injuries and may be related to chronic stress factors (3).

In terms of stress fractures around the knee they most commonly occur in the upper tibia. Although some can be seen in the distal femur, most occur in the proximal tibia. In the acute phase, the fracture line usually is not visible, and it is only after healing begins that the fracture and typical sclerosis and periosteal new bone deposition are seen (Fig. 4.155). In the early stages, these changes can be quite subtle, but later periosteal new bone deposition is profound and often a more serious lesion such as a bone tumor erroneously is suggested (11). Periosteal newbone typically is deposited most abundantly posteriorly. The findings also can be demonstrated with CT, and are especially well seen in the early stages with MRI. In these cases the occult fracture line becomes visible as a line of decreased signal on T_1-weighted images.

Patellar Fractures and Dislocations. Fractures of the patella usually occur with direct blows to the patella or with injuries producing quadriceps tendon stresses. When these fractures are gross, they are not difficult to detect (Fig. 4.156), but with lesser injuries the fracture may be difficult

to visualize, and one may be left with soft tissue and joint effusion changes only (Fig. 4.157). This is especially true of small avulsion injuries of the patella (see Fig. 4.159). In interpreting these chip fractures, the greatest pitfall lies in the misinterpretation of the so-called "bipartite" or "tripartite" patella, or a normal irregularly ossified patella, as a fracture (see Figs. 4.178 and 4.179). Avulsion fractures can involve the superior pole (quadriceps tendon), inferior pole (infrapatellar tendon), or medial edge (18, 21). The latter is associated with acute patellar dislocation (see Fig. 4.159).

Both acute and chronic, recurrent, dislocation of the patella is reasonably common in childhood (Fig. 4.158), but in most cases the patella relocates before roentgenograms are obtained. In some cases, a

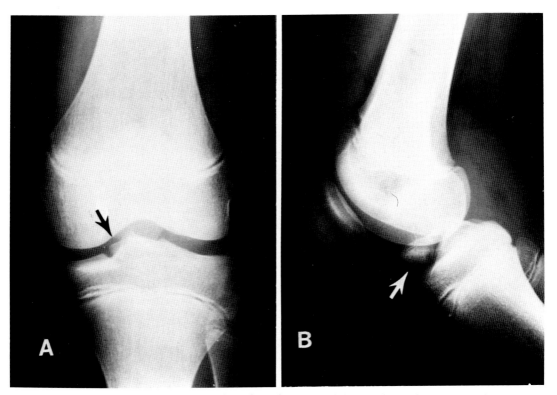

Figure 4.150. *Anterior cruciate ligament avulsion; large fragment.* (**A**) Frontal view demonstrating large avulsed bony fragment *(arrow)*. (**B**) Lateral view demonstrating the same avulsed bony fragment *(arrow)*. Also note distension of the suprapatellar bursa (hemarthrosis).

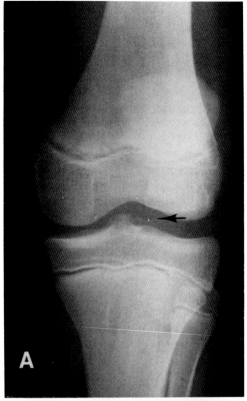

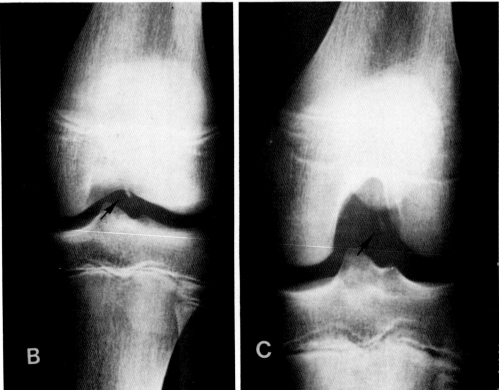

Figure 4.151. *Cruciate ligament avulsions; more subtle changes.* (**A**) Note the thin, sliver-like avulsed bony fragment *(arrow)* in this patient with an anterior cruciate ligament avulsion. (**B**) Another patient with a small avulsed bony fragment *(arrow)* from the lateral femoral condyle. (**C**) Tunnel view in same patient demonstrating the avulsed bony fragment *(arrow)* to greater advantage.

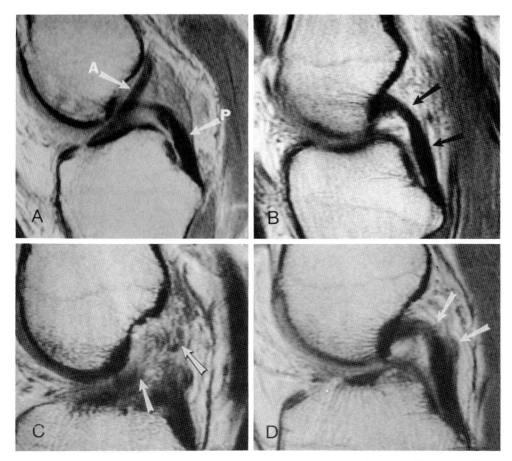

Figure 4.152. *Anterior cruciate ligament tear.* (*A*) Normal anterior cruciate ligament (*A*) and partially visible, normal posterior cruciate ligament (*P*). (*B*) Another patient with a normal posterior cruciate ligament *(arrows)*. (*C*) Anterior cruciate ligament tear completely disrupts the normal architecture of the anterior cruciate ligament *(arrows)*. (*D*) Concomitantly, there is laxity and buckling of the posterior cruciate ligament *(arrows)*.

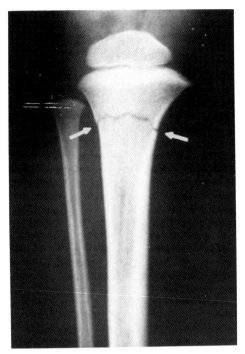

Figure 4.153. *Transverse fracture, upper tibia.* Note the clearly visible transverse fracture through the upper left tibia *(arrow).* There is no angulation through the fracture site.

residual telltale sign consisting of a medial avulsion fracture of the patella can be seen (18, 21) (Fig. 4.159), but most often bony changes are absent. If the fracture is present, it is best demonstrated on tangential or so-called "skyline" views of the patella. Patients with chronic recurrent dislocation often have associated patella alta, a condition where the patella is higher in position than normal (28, 34, 41). Abnormal tracking of the patella results and the patellofemoral groove becomes shallow (38). Patella alta is best seen on lateral view, while the shallow groove and associated flattening of the lateral condyle are best seen on skyline views (30% flexion) of the patella. Most dislocations, whether acute or chronic, are lateral dislocations.

Chondromalacia of the patella is a difficult diagnosis to make with certainty. It is not particularly common in children and

currently is best evaluated with MRI (40). In these cases there will be abnormal signal and variable degrees of deficiency of the cartilage on the posterior aspect of the patella. Stress fractures of the patella are uncommon, but linear, lateral stress fractures have been identified (29).

Miscellaneous Knee Problems. Miscellaneous knee problems include acute and chronic tibial tubercle and inferior patellar avulsions, osteochondritis dissecans, and meniscus injuries. *Acute total tibial tubercle avulsions* are relatively uncommon but tend to occur in athletes (6, 7, 17, 24, 36, 39, 43). Clinically and roentgenographically, these fractures are not difficult to detect (Fig. 4.160A–C), but the more subtle minimal avulsion can pose a greater problem (Fig. 4.160D). *Osgood-Schlatter's disease* results from repeated, subclinical avulsions of the tibial tubercle (8, 17, 35, 37, 55, 57), and the findings consist of pretubercular swelling and tubercular fragmentation (Fig. 4.161). With healing, considerable hypertrophic bone can be seen at the site of avulsion (Fig. 4.161C). All of these configurations are virtually pathognomonic of the condition, but occasionally Osgood-Schlatter's disease can be mimicked by the very rare periosteal chondroma of the tibial tubercle (33). This lesion is more bulky, mostly lytic, and is associated with destruction of the upper tibia under the tibial tubercle. Osteomyelitis of the tibial tubercle is very rare, if it occurs at all.

A lesion similar to Osgood-Schlatter's disease occurring along the inferior aspect of the patella (Fig. 4.162) is termed *Sinding-Larsen-Johansson* disease (27, 53, 56). It should be noted that both Osgood-Schlatter's disease and Sinding-Larsen-Johansson disease are chronic manifestations of acute avulsion injuries at these sites. They are more tendinous than bony in nature and both now can be demonstrated with ultrasound, CT, and MR (35, 49). However, plain films usually suffice. Fi-

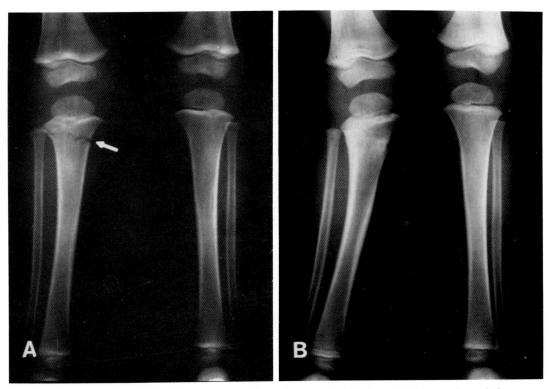

Figure 4.154. *Upper tibial fracture with inward bending.* (*A*) Note the clearly visible fracture through the upper right tibia (*arrow*). Also note that the fracture line is wider medially and that there is slight inward angulation of the tibia. (*B*) Late healing phase demonstrating pronounced knockknee deformity.

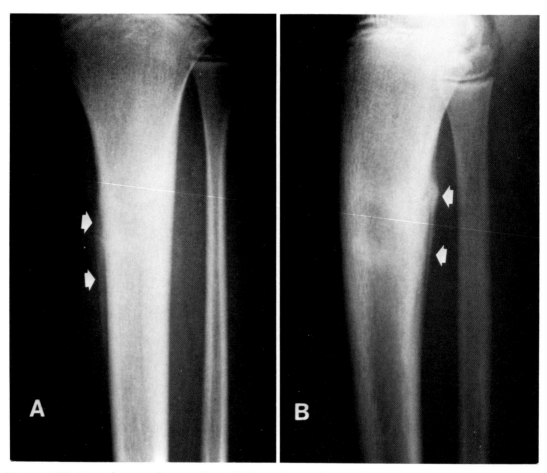

Figure 4.155. *Stress fracture of upper tibia.* (**A**) Frontal view demonstrating periosteal deposition along the upper inner aspect of the tibia *(arrows)*. (**B**) Lateral view demonstrating typical posterior deposition of periosteal new bone around the fracture site *(arrows)*. In addition, note sclerosis through the medullary cavity indicating the location of the healing stress fracture.

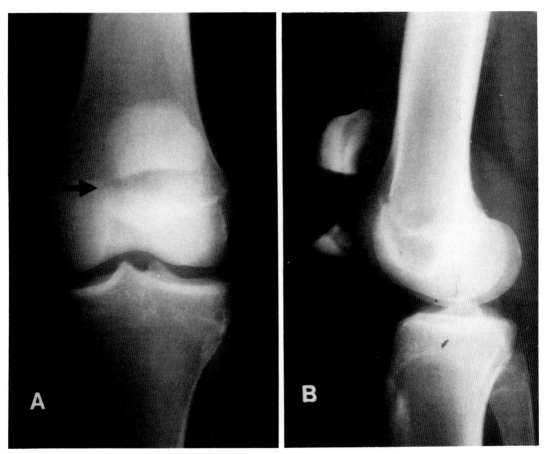

Figure 4.156. *Overt patellar fracture.* (*A*) Note the clear-cut patellar fracture *(arrow)*. (*B*) Lateral view demonstrating marked separation of the bony fragments.

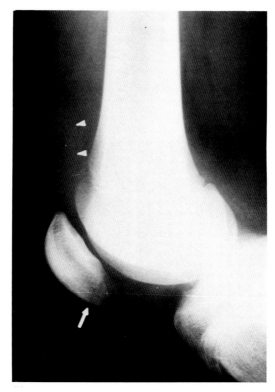

Figure 4.157. *Subtle patellar fracture.* First, note the presence of fluid in the suprapatellar bursa *(upper arrows).* Then note the barely detectible transverse fracture through the inferior aspect of the patella *(lower arrow).*

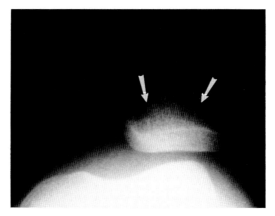

Figure 4.158. *Acute dislocation of the patella.* Note the lateral displacement of the patella *(arrows)* as it has been dislocated out of the patellofemoral groove.

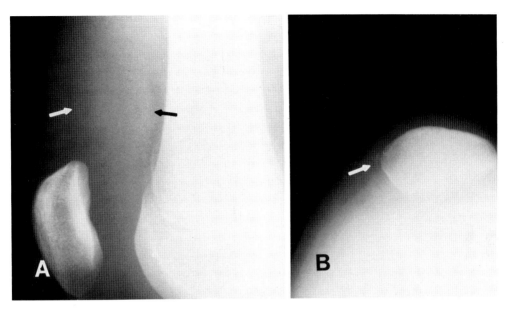

Figure 4.159. *Acute dislocation of patella with fracture fragments.* (**A**) Note only fluid in the suprapatellar bursa *(arrows)*. (**B**) Two weeks later, note small fracture fragment *(arrow)* attesting to the previous dislocation.

nally, it might be noted that both conditions tend to be self-limiting, although they may leave a residual lump in the area. This is especially prone to occur with Osgood-Schlatter's disease. Only rarely will significant complications result, but in this regard, tibia recurvatum has been noted to develop as a complication of Osgood-Schlatter's disease (37). This, however, is quite uncommon.

Another cause of knee pain in childhood is *osteochondritis dissecans* of the distal femoral epiphysis and, less often, the patella. Most often, these lesions occur in older children and adolescents (20), and while many cases are symptomatic, other individuals are asymptomatic. Roentgenographically, typical findings are those of a bony defect along the anteromedial aspect of the medial femoral condyle (Fig. 4.163). This should be differentiated from normal irregularity which often occurs along the posterior aspect of the lateral femoral condyle. In the patella, osteochondritis dissecans produces an irregular defect on the posterior aspect of the patella (Fig. 4.164).

All of these lesions probably represent subchondral fractures, and now are assessed with MRI if there is question of instability (13, 42, 44). MRI clearly demonstrates whether the fragment is displaced and extends beyond the articular surface of the involved bone (Fig. 4.165*B*).

Meniscus injuries are not as common in childhood as in the young adult, but they do occur. Plain film findings usually are absent and most cases are subsequently diagnosed by MRI (Fig. 4.165*A*). However, this study generally is not performed on an acute basis. In terms of meniscal injuries in childhood, a note about the lateral meniscus in children is in order. Often this meniscus is very large, and rather than being disk-shaped, assumes a semi-circular shape. Consequently, the medial aspect extends almost to the intercondylar notch (10, 26) and, because of this, the cartilage is very prone to tearing. It is termed the discoid lateral meniscus and is best demonstrated with double-contrast arthrography or, currently, MRI. A detailed dissertation of all of the findings associated with

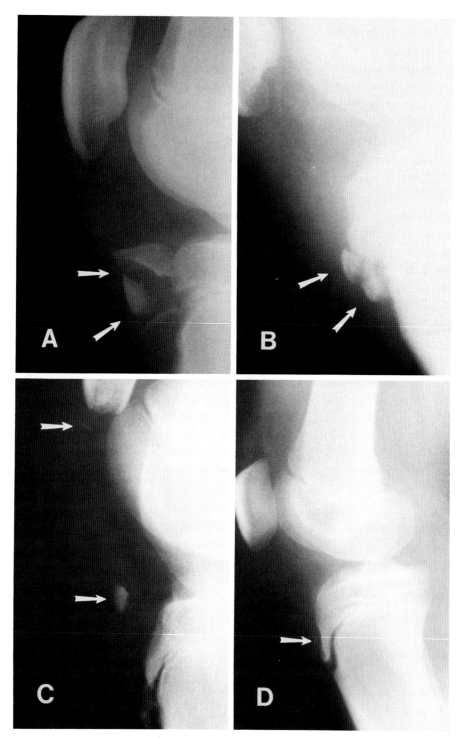

Figure 4.160. *Acute tibial tubercle avulsions.* (**A**) Note the grossly disorganized, avulsed, tibial tubercle; basketball injury. (**B**) Another patient with a more subtle tibial tubercle avulsion *(arrow)*. Also note soft tissue edema extending into and obliterating the infrapatellar fat pad. (**C**) Note the avulsed tibial tubercle fragment *(lower arrow)* and the small sliver of avulsed bone from the patella *(upper arrow)*. (**D**) Very subtle tibial tubercle avulsion consisting of a small sliver of bone *(arrow)*. Note again that the infrapatellar fat pad is obliterated.

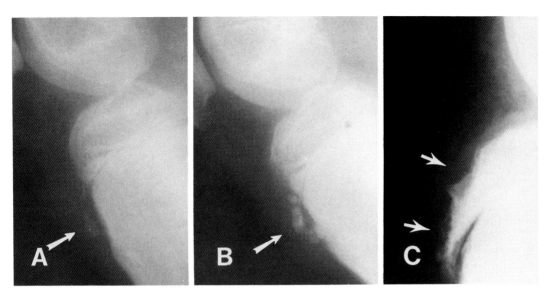

Figure 4.161. *Osgood-Schlatter's disease.* (**A**) Minimal changes consisting of slight irregularity of the tibial tubercle and a little overlying edema *(arrow)*. (**B**) More pronounced changes in the same patient, in the other knee *(arrow)*. (**C**) Another patient with very gross irregularity of the tibial tubercle *(arrows)*.

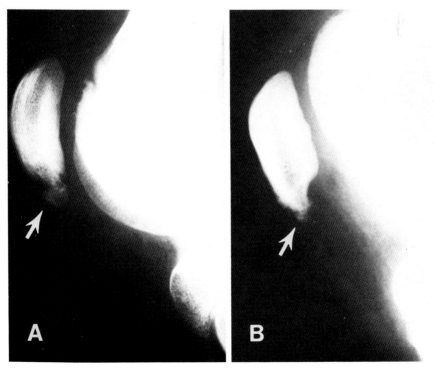

Figure 4.162. *Sinding-Larsen-Johansson disease of the patella.* (**A**) Note the large bony fragment just below the inferior aspect of the patella *(arrow)*. (**B**) Less pronounced changes in another patient *(arrow)*.

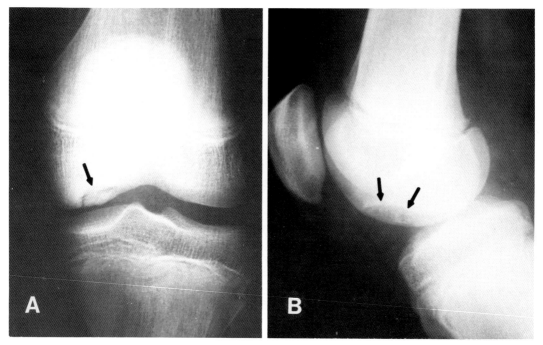

Figure 4.163. *Osteochondritis dissecans.* (*A*) Typical condylar defect in the medial femoral condyle *(arrow)*. (*B*) Characteristic location and appearance on lateral view *(arrows)*.

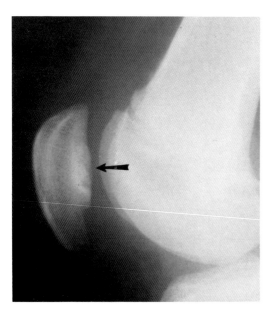

Figure 4.164. *Osteochondritis dissecans of patella.* Note irregularity with surrounding sclerosis along the posterior aspect of the patella *(arrow)*. Also note distension of the suprapatellar bursa and its neck due to an associated effusion.

meniscal tears and other meniscal abnormalities is beyond the scope of this book.

An uncommon problem related to trauma around the knee is rupture of the synovium of the knee joint (50). In such cases, chronic extrasynovial fluid collections can extend deep into the calf and the clinical findings can be confused with deep vein thrombosis (50). Ultrasonography is invaluable in these cases as it will demonstrate the fluid collection due to synovial rupture. By the same token, it is also useful in the detection of deep vein thrombosis.

Septic Arthritis, Osteomyelitis, and Cellulitis of the Knee. In the knee, one of the more common clinical problems is that of differentiating septic arthritis from simple cellulitis. Indeed, this comes up far more often than does the differentiation of septic arthritis from osteomyelitis, for soft tissue infections (cellulitis) are especially prone to develop over the patella, and many times it is difficult to clinically determine whether the joint space is involved. This is especially true in the young child and infant. However, the problem must be resolved, for with septic arthritis, arthrocentesis is required, while with cellulitis it is contraindicated. Although not well appreciated, the lateral view of the knee can solve this dilemma in almost every instance.

With septic arthritis, fluid (pus) accumulates in the various bursae, but it first always accumulates in the suprapatellar bursa (Fig. 4.166A). When it does so, it displaces the quadriceps tendon anteriorly and the prefemoral fat pad posteriorly. As a result, the soft tissue space between the quadriceps tendon and the prefemoral fat pad becomes thickened (Fig. 4.166B). At first the findings might suggest that the entire quadriceps tendon is thickened, but actually they represent the confluent images of the normal quadriceps tendon and abnormal, pus-filled suprapatellar bursa. In addition to this finding, sooner or later there is bulging of the posterior popliteal bursa, and the greater the accumulation of pus, the greater the bulging (Fig. 4.166). With more extensive collections, the suprapatellar and posterior popliteal bursae

can show enormous bulging and, indeed, even the infrapatellar fat pad can become obliterated. However, no matter how extensive the accumulation of pus in the joint, the soft tissues anterior to the patella usually remain normal and distinct. They do not become edematous, and this is most important in differentiating septic arthritis from prepatellar cellulitis. In advanced cases, however, the deep soft tissues around the knee may become edematous, but distension of the suprapatellar bursa should identify the problem as septic arthritis or septic arthritis with osteomyelitis (Fig. 4.166B).

With prepatellar cellulitis, as opposed to septic arthritis, the suprapatellar bursa does not become distended, but rather the soft tissues anterior to the quadriceps tendon and patella become thickened and/or edematous (Fig. 4.167). Of course, if soft tissue edema is extensive, the suprapatellar and infrapatellar fat pads may become hazy and the soft tissues behind the femur also may become indistinct (Fig. 4.167B). Such extensive edema also can be seen with severe septic arthritis or osteomyelitis, but with septic arthritis bursal distention occurs and prepatellar edema gener-

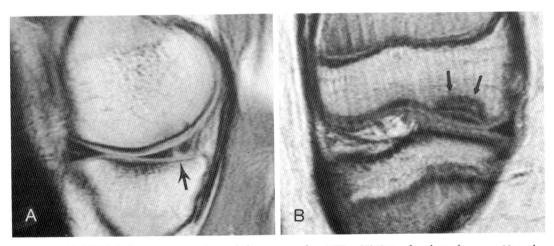

Figure 4.165. (A) Medial meniscus tear (arrow) demonstrated on MRI.   (B) Osteochondritis dissecans. Note the low signal area (arrows) in the medial condyle due to an area of osteochondritis dissecans. Note that the cartilage over it is intact and that the segment is not free-floating.

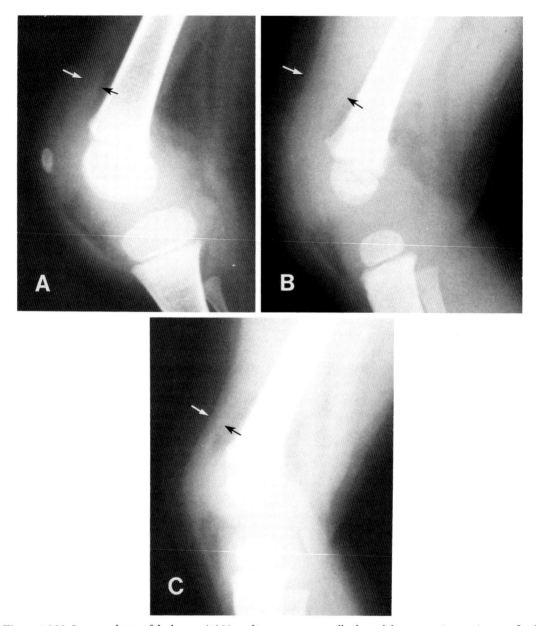

Figure 4.166. *Septic arthritis of the knee.* (**A**) Note discrete suprapatellar bursal distension *(arrows)*. Some fluid also is present in the posterior popliteal bursa. (**B**) The distended suprapatellar bursa blends with the quadriceps tendon to produce subtle pseudothickening of the tendon *(arrows)*. Associated soft tissue swelling also has extended behind the knee. (**C**) Normal side for comparison. Note normal thickness of quadriceps tendon *(arrows)*.

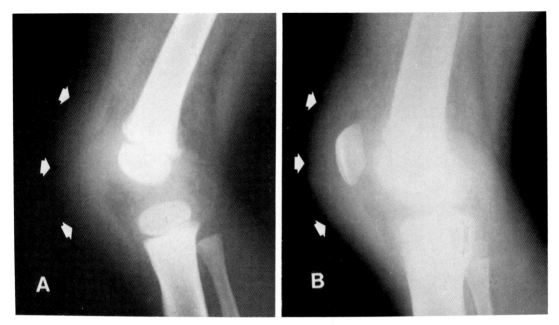

Figure 4.167. *Cellulitis of the knee.* (A) First, note that swelling is present in the soft tissues anterior to the quadriceps tendon and unossified cartilaginous patella only *(arrows)*. The quadriceps tendon is still clearly visible, and there is no evidence of accumulation of fluid in the suprapatellar bursa. (B) Another patient demonstrating extensive swelling of the soft tissues anterior to the patella and quadriceps tendon *(arrows)*. In this case, soft tissue swelling is so pronounced that there is associated obliteration of the quadriceps tendon and suprapatellar fat pad. The findings, however, are not those of septic arthritis, for edema of the soft tissues anterior to the patella and quadriceps tendon generally does not occur with septic arthritis. Also note edema posterior to the femur.

ally is not seen with either septic arthritis or osteomyelitis (see Figs. 4.166B and 4.168B).

With osteomyelitis of the distal femur, early stage findings consist only of soft tissue edema and obliteration or displacement of the fat pads (5, 25) around the distal femur (Figs. 4.168 and 4.169). Unlike septic arthritis, there is no filling of the suprapatellar bursa with pus, and unlike prepatellar cellulitis, prepatellar edema is absent (Fig. 4.168). Of course, once again one must make an exception in the young child or infant, for in this age group osteomyelitis and septic arthritis often occur together and present features of both conditions.

In more advanced cases of osteomyelitis, frank bony destruction and periosteal new bone deposition are seen, and then the diagnosis is no problem. In early cases,

however, the area of bone destruction may be small and subtle, and may cause confusion with a benign cortical defect (Fig. 4.170). Of course, as with osteomyelitis anywhere, one should turn to nuclear scintigraphy or MRI for further delineation if there is doubt on the basis of the plain films.

Tendonitis. Tendonitis can occur anywhere in the body but it most commonly occurs around the shoulder and knee. Even then, it is more common around the knee than around the shoulder in children. Both the infra- and suprapatellar tendons can be involved, and the findings on plain films are simply those of thickening and indistinctness of the tendon (Fig. 4.171A). These findings also can be demonstrated with ultrasound (12) and with MRI (12, 15). With both of these modalities, the findings are those of a thickened, swollen,

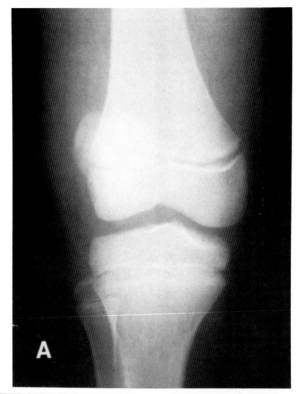

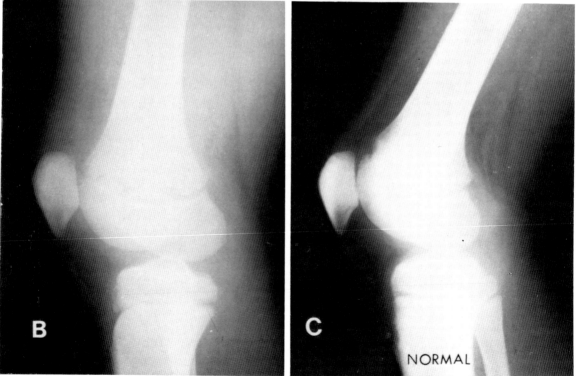

Figure 4.168. *Osteomyelitis—deep soft tissue changes.* (*A*) Note extensive swelling of all the soft tissues around the distal femur. No normal fat-muscle interfaces remain. (*B*) Lateral view demonstrating similar findings. Note that the suprapatellar fat pads and the fat pads posterior to the distal femur have been totally obliterated. Obliteration of these fat pads, especially the ones posterior to the distal femur, is a most important finding, for it is not seen with septic arthritis. (*C*) Normal knee of the same patient for comparison. Note the clearly identified fat-muscle interfaces and the various normal fat pads, both anterior and posterior to the distal femur.

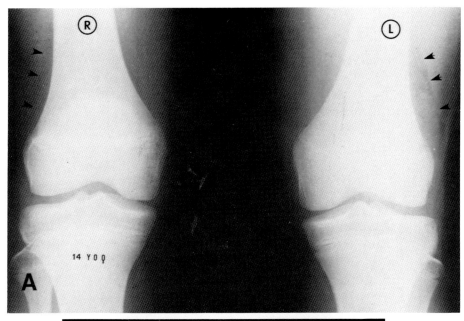

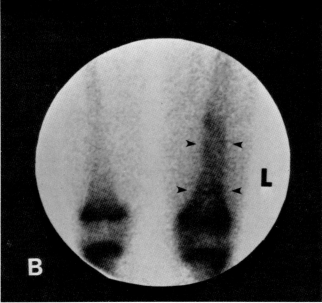

Figure 4.169. *Osteomyelitis—early displacement of the fat pads.* (*A*) First note the generalized increase in soft tissue density and thickness around the distal left femur. Then note displacement of the lateral fat pad outwardly *(arrows)*. Compare this with the same fat pad on the normal right side *(arrows)*. (*B*) Bone scan demonstrating increased uptake of isotope in the distal left femur *(arrows)*, characteristic of osteomyelitis. (Courtesy of M. Capitanio, M.D.)

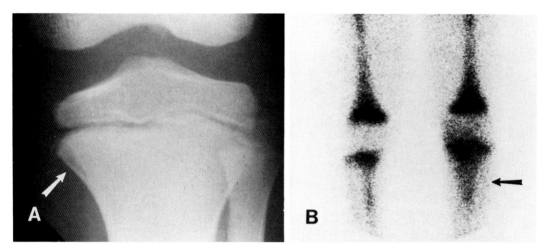

Figure 4.170. *Osteomyelitis—subtle findings.* (**A**) Note the subtle lytic lesion in the upper tibia *(arrow).* This could be confused with a benign cortical defect. (**B**) Bone scan, however, demonstrates increased isotope activity in the upper tibia *(arrow).* This does not occur with benign cortical defects. The patient had surgically proven osteomyelitis.

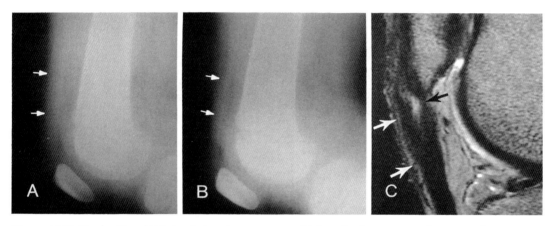

Figure 4.171. *Tendonitis.* (**A**) Lateral view demonstrates a thickened, edematous quadriceps tendon *(arrows).* (**B**) Contralateral, normal side for comparison. Note the normal width of the quadriceps tendon *(arrows).* (**C**) MR evaluation of tendonitis. Note the thickened infrapatellar tendon *(white arrows)* and the area of high signal at the patellar insertion *(black arrow)* due to bleeding.

edematous tendon, but MR can also show focal areas of high signal representing foci of inflammation or bleeding (Fig. 4.171*C*).

Normal Findings Causing Problems. One of the more common normal findings around the knee is *irregularity of the distal femur,* just along the *medial supracondylar ridge.* It occurs most commonly in older children and adolescents and should not be misinterpreted for an area of osteomyelitis or a bone tumor (2, 52, 58). The irregular-

ity occurs along the line of muscle insertion, recently suggested to be that of the adductor magnus (46). In terms of etiology, there is histologic support for the concept that this lesion results from chronic avulsion (14, 46) and, depending on the degree of healing, the lesion can appear quite ragged or somewhat scalloped (Fig. 4.172). Unfortunately, however, benign cortical defects also occur here and can appear somewhat similar. Technetium-99 pyrophosphate bone scanning shows no increased isotope activity in most of these lesions (4, 16). This attests to the low-grade activity of these lesions. They are not a serious finding, but yet it is very tempting to assign a causative, often serious, role to them in patients with nonspecific knee pain.

Benign cortical (fibrous) defects can be found in any of the long bones and frequently are multiple. However, they most commonly occur in the distal femur and proximal tibia, and characteristically are eccentric and very peripheral (cortical) in location. They seldom extend beyond a half-centimeter or so into the medullary cavity of the bone (Fig. 4.173). When seen *en face*, they can resemble a lytic lesion of the bone, and should not be mistaken for low-grade osteomyelitis (i.e., Brodie's abscess) or a bone tumor (Fig. 4.174). Benign cortical defects are related to the somewhat larger benign nonossifying fibroma. This latter lesion also is eccentric but often more definitely corticated and larger than a benign cortical defect (Fig. 4.173*B*). Be-

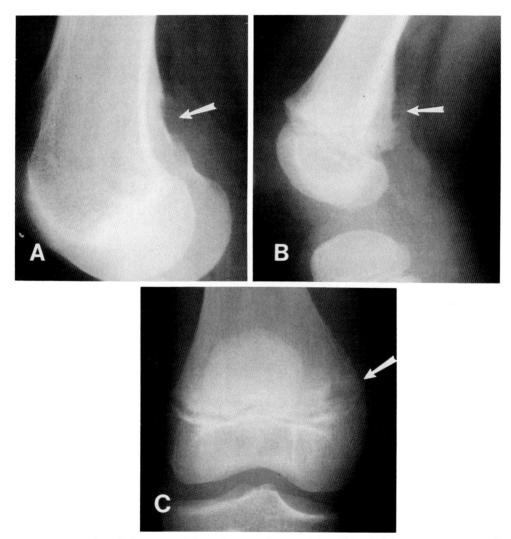

Figure 4.172. *Normal medial supracondylar ridge irregularity.* (**A**) Well-healed, benign appearing scalloped out area *(arrow).* (**B**) Another patient with more worrisome irregularity *(arrow).* (**C**) Another patient demonstrating similar, worrisome findings on frontal view *(arrow).*

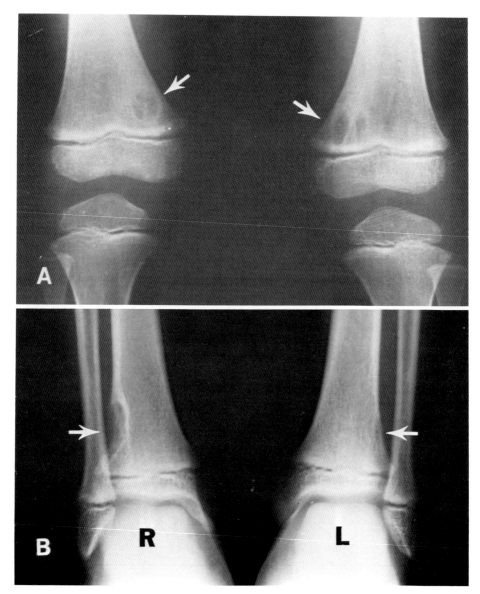

Figure 4.173. *Benign cortical defects, classic appearance.* (**A**) Note typical oval or round, slightly sclerotic, benign cortical defects in both distal femurs *(arrows)*. (**B**) Large benign cortical defect in distal right tibia *(arrow)*. This lesion is large enough to be considered a small nonossifying fibroma. The two lesions probably are related. On the left, a very small benign cortical defect is noted in the distal tibia *(arrow)*.

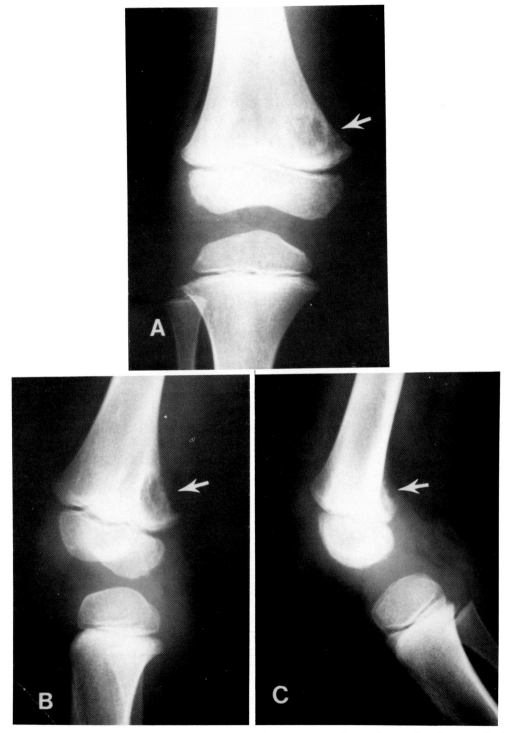

Figure 4.174. *Benign cortical defect mimicking osteomyelitis.* (**A**) Frontal view showing lytic lesion in the distal femur *(arrow)*. This patient presented with a swollen, hot knee. (**B**) Oblique view demonstrates the "pseudo" lytic, destructive appearance of this lesion *(arrow)*. (**C**) Lateral view demonstrating the irregular lesion *(arrow)*. This was misinterpreted as osteomyelitis, although, in fact, it was a benign cortical defect. The knee was swollen because of cellulitis of the soft tissues anterior to the patella.

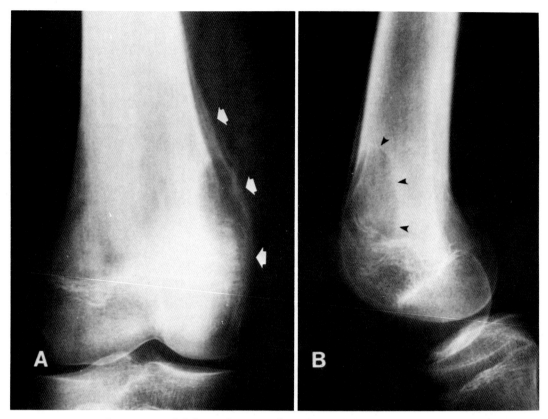

Figure 4.175. *Cystic benign cortical defect with periosteal new bone.* (**A**) Note the layered periosteal new bone over the cystic lesion of the distal femur *(arrows)*. This young boy presented with recent onset of knee pain. (**B**) Lateral view demonstrating lytic nature of the lesion and periosteal new bone anterior to it. The findings represent avulsion of the thin cortex of this benign cortical defect with subsequent periosteal new bone formation (histologically proven). (Reprinted with permission from Kumar, R., Swischuk, L.E., and Madewell, J.E.: Benign cortical defect: Site for an avulsion injury. Skeletal Radiol. 15: 553–555, 1986.)

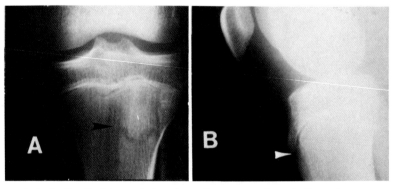

Figure 4.176. *Normal tibial tubercle defect.* (**A**) On frontal view, note the radiolucent line *(arrow)* just beneath an area of transverse sclerosis. The area of sclerosis represents the inferior aspect of the tibial tubercle, while the radiolucent line is the normal defect just beneath it. (**B**) Lateral view demonstrating the site of the radiolucent defect *(arrow)* under the normal tibial tubercle.

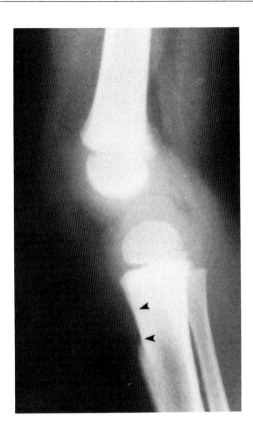

Figure 4.177. *Normal upper tibial notch.* In young infants, the tibial tubercle does not ossify and a normal notch is noted at its site *(arrows)*. This notch should not be misinterpreted for a destructive lesion.

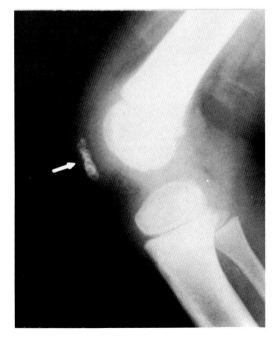

Figure 4.178. *Normal irregular patellar ossification.* Note the normal, irregularly ossified patella *(arrow)*. The patella usually begins to ossify at about 5 years of age.

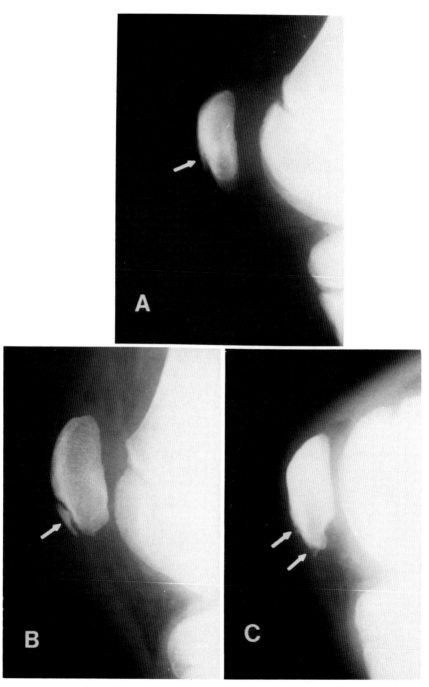

Figure 4.179. *Various normal patellar ossification patterns.* (*A*) Sliver-like normal ossicle *(arrow)*. In some cases, this thin sliver-like piece of bone can appear completely detached from the patella. (*B*) Larger accessory ossification center of the patella *(arrow)*. (*C*) Normal irregular ossification of the anterior-inferior aspect of the patella *(arrows)*. This should not be confused with Sinding-Larsen-Johansson disease where similar fragmentation associated with pain and local swelling can be seen.

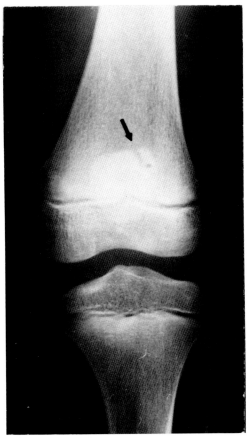

Figure 4.180. *Bipartite patella.* Note typical appearance and location of a bipartite patella *(arrow)*.

The *patella is very prone to irregular ossification* (Fig. 4.178). Furthermore, when it finally does ossify, a number of peculiar irregularities and deformities can persist. Some of these are so fracture-like in appearance that it is almost impossible to differentiate them from a true fracture (Fig. 4.179). However, very often the same configuration is present on the other side, and this solves the problem. Another common normal ossification anomaly of the patella is the bipartite or tripartite patella. In these cases, the extra portion of the patella usually lies in the upper outer quadrant (Fig. 4.180), and very often the anomaly is bilateral. There has been a suggestion that occasionally the bipartite patella can be painful (45). In such cases it has been suggested that the bipartite patella actually represents an incompletely united stress

nign cortical defects proper have variably sclerotic margins. In a few cases, *benign cortical defects appear very cystic* and possess a thin cortex. In such cases, normal muscle pull on the cortex can cause acute avulsion and fragmentation. In these patients, the roentgenographic findings often first suggest malignancy (Fig. 4.175).

In older children, the *tibial tubercle has a normal defect along its inferior aspect.* On lateral view, this defect is not difficult to interpret, but on frontal view, it can be taken for a lytic lesion of the knee (Fig. 4.176). In young infants, the tibial tubercle is not ossified at all, and a scoop-like bony defect in the area can present a problem (Fig. 4.177).

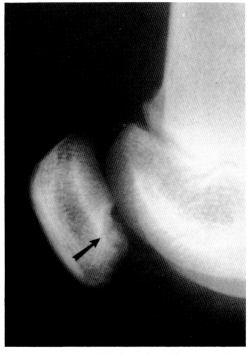

Figure 4.181. *Dorsal defect of patella.* Note the irregular dorsal defect *(arrow)*. This patient was entirely asymptomatic. The finding can be confused with osteochondritis dessicans.

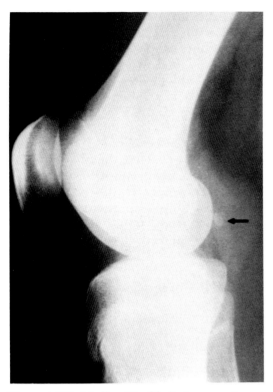

Figure 4.182. *Fabella.* The fabella is a normal sesamoid bone occurring in the gastrocnemius tendon *(arrow).*

fracture, and that it is positive on isotope bone scanning (45). However, most bipartite patellae are asymptomatic. Finally a normal dorsal fibrous defect of the patella (1) should not be confused with a lesion such as osteomyelitis or osteochondritis dessicans (Fig. 4.181).

The fabella is a normal ossicle occurring in the lateral limb of the gastrocnemius tendon and is best visualized on lateral view (Fig. 4.182). The *distal femoral epiphysis frequently ossifies irregularly* and can appear very disturbing to the uninitiated (Fig. 4.183). However, these irregularities are common, especially in infants and young children where the epiphysis may appear irregular, all around its periphery. In older children, normal irregularities tend to occur in the lateral condyle, posteriorly (Fig. 4.184).

REFERENCES

1. Alexander, J.E., Seibert, J.J., Aronson, J.: Dorsal defect of the patella and infection. Pediatr. Radiol. 17: 325–327, 1987.
2. Barnes, G.R., Jr., and Gwinn, J.L.: Distal irregularities of the femur simulating malignancy. A.J.R. 122: 180–185, 1974.
3. Boyer, R.S., Jaffe, R.B., Nixon, G.W., and Condon, V.R.: Trampoline fracture of the proximal tibia in children. A.J.R. 1467: 83–85, 1986.
4. Burrows, P.E., Greenberg, I.D., and Reed, M.H.: The distal femoral defect: Technetium-99m pyrophosphate bone scan results. J. Can. Assoc. Radiol. 33: 91–93, 1982.
5. Capitanio, M.A., and Kirkpatrick, J.A.: Early roentgen observation in acute osteomyelitis. A.J.R. 108: 488–497, 1970.
6. Chow, S.P., Lam, J.J., and Leong, J.C.Y.: Fracture of the tibial tubercle in the adolescent. J. Bone Joint Surg. 71B: 231–234, 1990.
7. Christie, M.J., and Dvonch, V.M.: Tibial tuberosity avulsion fracture in adolescents. J. Pediatr. Orthop. 1: 391–394, 1981.
8. Cohen, B., and Wilkinson, R.W.: The Osgood-Schlatter lesion: A radiological and histological study. Am. J. Surg. 95: 731, 1958.
9. Currarino, G., and Pinckney, L.E.: Genu valgum after proximal tibial fractures in children. A.J.R. 136: 915–918, 1981.
10. Dashefsky, J.H.: Discoid lateral meniscus in three members of family. J. Bone Joint Surg. 53A: 1208–1210, 1971.
11. Davies, A.M., Evans, N., and Grimer, R.J.: Fatigue fractures of the proximal tibia simulating malignancy. Br. J. Radiol. 61: 903–908, 1988.
12. Davies, S.G., Baudouin, C.J., King, J.B., and Perry, J.D.: Ultrasound, computed tomography and magnetic resonance imaging in patellar tendonitis. Clin. Radiol. 43: 52–56, 1991.
13. DeSmet, A.A., Fisher, D.R., Graf, B.K., and Lange, R.H.: Osteochondritis dissecans of the knee: Value of MR imaging in determining lesion stability and the presence of articular cartilage defects. A.J.R. 155: 549–553, 1990.
14. Dunham, W.K., Marcus, N.W., Enneking, W.F., and Haun, C.: Developmental defects of the distal femoral metaphysis. J. Bone Joint Surg. 62A: 801–806, 1980.
15. El-Khoury, G.Y., Wira, R.L., Berbaum, K.S., Pope, T.L., Jr., and Monu, J.U.V.: MR imaging of patellar tendonitis. Radiology 184: 849–854, 1992.
16. Feine, U., and Ahlemann, L.M.: Differentiation of the periosteal desmoid of the metaphysis from malignant tumors using bone scanning. R.O.F.O. 135: 193–196, 1981.
17. Fitch, R.D.: Tibial tubercle avulsions. J. Pediatr. Orthop. 6: 186–192, 1986.

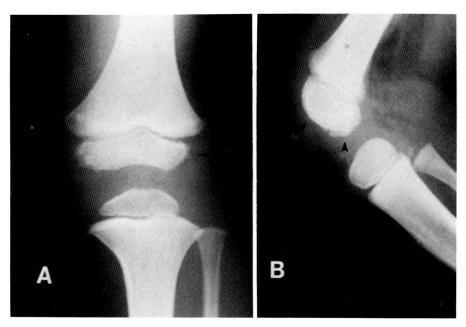

Figure 4.183. *Normal distal femoral epiphyseal irregularities.* (**A**) Frontal view showing normal irregularity of the distal femoral epiphysis *(arrows).* Radiolucencies in the metaphyseal corners also are normal. (**B**) Lateral view showing normal irregular ossification pattern of distal femoral epiphysis *(arrows).*

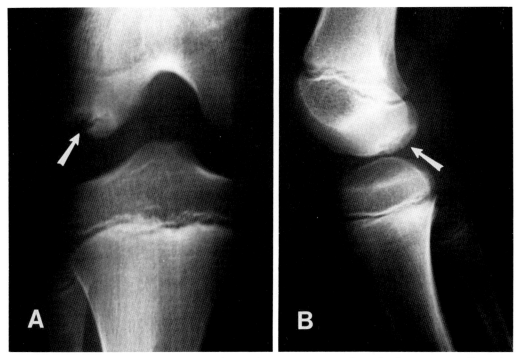

Figure 4.184. *Normal distal femoral epiphyseal irregularities.* (**A**) Note deep, focal irregularity of lateral condyle *(arrow).* (**B**) Lateral view demonstrating the irregularity to be posterior *(arrow).* This patient was asymptomatic. (Courtesy of Virgil Graves, M.D.)

18. Freiberg, R.H., and Kotzen, L.M.: Fracture of the medial margin of the patella, a finding diagnostic of lateral dislocation. Radiology 88: 902, 1967.

19. Green, N.E.: Tibia valga caused by asymmetrical overgrowth following a nondisplaced fracture of the proximal tibial metaphysis. J. Pediatr. Orthop. 3: 235–237, 1983.

20. Green, W.T., and Banks, H.H.: Osteochondritis dissecans in children. J. Bone Joint Surg. 35A: 26, 1953.

21. Grogan, D.P., Carey, T.P., Leffers, D., and Ogden, J.A.: Avulsion fractures of the patella. J. Pediatr. Orthop. 10: 721–730, 1990.

22. Gronkvist, H., Hirsch, G., and Johansson, L.: Fracture of the anterior tibial spine in children. J. Pediatr. Orthop. 4: 465–468, 1984.

23. Hall, F.: Radiographic diagnosis and accuracy in knee joint effusions. Radiology 115: 49–54, 1975.

24. Hand, W.L., Hand, C.R., and Dunn, A.N.: Avulsion fractures of the tibial tubercle. J. Bone Joint Surg. 53A: 1579, 1971.

25. Hayden, C.K., Jr., and Swischuk, L.E.: Para-articular soft tissue changes in infants and trauma of the lower extremity in children. A.J.R. 134: 307–311, 1980.

26. Haverson, S.B., and Rein, B.J.: Lateral discoid meniscus of knee: Arthrographic diagnosis. A.J.R. 109: 581–586, 1970.

27. Holstein, E.R., Lewis, G.B., and Schulze, E.R.: Heterotopic ossification of patella tendon. J. Bone Joint Surg. 45A: 656, 1963.

28. Insall, J., and Salvati, E.: Patella position in the normal knee joint. Radiology 101: 101–104, 1971.

29. Iwaya, T., and Takatori, Y.: Lateral longitudinal stress fracture of the patella: Report of three cases. J. Pediatr. Orthop. 5: 73–75, 1985.

30. Jackson, D.W., and Cozen, L.: Genu valgum as a complication of proximal tibial metaphyseal fractures in children. J. Bone Joint Surg. 53A: 1571, 1971.

31. Jordan, S.E., Alonson, J.E., and Cook, F.F.: The etiology of valgus angulation after metaphyseal fractures of the tibia in children. J. Pediatr. Orthop. 7: 450–457, 1987.

32. Kaplan, P.A., Walker, C.W., Kilcoyne, R.F., Brown, D.E., Tusek, D., and Dussault, R.G.: Occult fracture patterns of the knee associated with anterior cruciate ligament tears: Assessment with magnetic resonance imaging. Radiology 183: 835–838, 1992.

33. Kirchner, S.G., Pavlov, H., Heller, R.M., and Kay, J.J.: Periosteal chondromas of the anterior tibial tubercle: Two cases. A.J.R. 131: 1088–1089, 1978.

34. Lancourt, J.E., and Cristini, J.A.: Patella alta and patella infera: Their etiologic role in patellar dislocation, chondromalacia and apophysitis of the tibial tubercle. J. Bone Joint Surg. 57: 1112–1115, 1975.

35. Lanning, P., and Heikkinen, E.: Ultrasonic features of the Osgood-Schlatter lesions. J. Pediatr. Orthop 11: 538–540, 1991.

36. Levi, J.H., and Coleman, C.R.: Fracture of the tibial tubercle. Am. J. Sports Med. 4: 254–263, 1976.

37. Lynch, M.C., and Walsh, H.P.J.: Tibia recurvatum as a complication of Osgood-Schlatter's disease: A report of two cases. J. Pediatr. Orthop. 11: 543–544, 1991.

38. Malghem, J., Maldague, B.: Depth insufficiency of the proximal trochlear groove on lateral radiographs of the knee: Relation to patellar dislocation. Radiology 170: 507–510, 1989.

39. Mayba, I.I.: Avulsion fracture of the tibial tubercle apophysis with avulsion of patellar ligament. J. Pediatr. Orthop. 2: 303–305, 1982.

40. McCauley, T.R., Kier, r., Lynch, K.J., and Jokl, P.: Chondromalacia patallae: Diagnosis with MR imaging. A.J.R. 158: 101–105, 1992.

41. McNab, I.: Recurrent dislocation of the patella. J. Bone Joint Surg. 34A: 957–967, 1952.

42. Mesgarzadeh, M., Sapega, A.A., Bonakdarpour, A., Revesz, G., Moyer, R.A., Maurer, A.H., and Alburger, P.D.: Osteochondritis dissecans: Analysis of mechanical stability with radiography, scintigraphy, and MR imaging. Radiology 165: 775–780, 1987.

43. Mirby, J., Besancenot, J., Chambers, R.T., Durey, A., and Vichard, P.: Avulsion fractures of the tibial tuberosity in the adolescent athlete: Risk factors, mechanism of injury and treatment. Am. J. Sports Med. 16: 336–340, 1988.

44. Nelson, D.W., DiPaola, J., Colville, M., and Schmidgall, J.: Osteochondritis dissecans of the talus and knee: Prospective comparison of MR and arthroscopic classifications. J. Comp. Assist. Tomogr. 14: 804–808, 1990.

45. Ogden, J.A., McCarthy, S.M., and Jokl, P.: The painful bipartite patella. J. Pediatr. Orthop. 2: 263–269, 1982.

46. Resnick, D., and Greenway, G.: Distal femoral cortical defects, irregularities and excavations: A critical review of the literature with the addition of histologic and paleopathologic data. Radiology 143: 345–354, 1982.

47. Robert, M., Khouri, N., Carlioz, H., and Alain, J.L.: Fractures of the proximal tibial metaphysis in children: Review of a series of 25 cases. J. Pediatr. Orthop. 7: 444–449, 1987.

48. Rogers, L.F., Jones, S., Davis, A.R., and Dietz, G.: "Clipping injury" fracture of the epiphysis in the adolescent football player: An occult lesion of the knee. A.J.R. 121: 69–78, 1974.

49. Rosenberg, Z.S., Kawelblum, M., Cheung, Y.Y., Beltran, J., Lehman, W.B., and Grant, A.D.: Osgood-Schlatter lesion: fracture of tendonitis: Scintigraphic, CT, and MR imaging features. Radiology 185: 853–858, 1992.

50. Rosewarne, M.D.: Synovial rupture of the knee joint: Confusion with deep vein thrombosis. Clin. Radiol. 29: 417–420, 1978.

51. Salter, R.B., and Best, T.: The pathogenesis and prevention of valgus deformity following fractures of the proximal metaphyseal region of the tibia in children. J. Bone Joint Surg. 55A: 1324, 1973.

52. Simon, H.: Medial distal metaphyseal femoral irregularity in children. Radiology 90: 258–260, 1968.

53. Sinding-Larson, M.F.: A hitherto unknown affection of the patella in children. Acta Radiol. [Diagn.] (Stockh.) 1: 171–173, 1921.

54. Vahey, T.N., Broome, D.R., Kayes, K.J., and Shelbourne, K.D.: Acute and chronic tears of the anterior cruciate ligament: Differential features at MR imaging. Radiology 81: 251–253, 1991.

55. Willner, P.: Osgood-Schlatter's disease: Etiology and treatment. Clin. Orthop. 62: 178–179, 1969.

56. Wolf, J.: Larsen-Johansson disease of patella: 7 new case records. Br. J. Radiol. 23: 335–347, 1950.

57. Woolfrey, B.F., and Chandler, E.F.: Manifestations of Osgood-Schlatter's disease in late teenage and early adulthood. J. Bone Joint Surg. 42A: 327–332, 1960.

58. Young, D.W., Nogardy, M.B., Dunbar, J.S., and Wiglesworth, F.W.: Benign cortical irregularities in the distal femur of children. J. Can. Assoc. Radiol. 23: 107–115, 1972.

59. Zionts, L.E., Harcke, T., Brooks, K.M., and MacEwen, G.D.: Posttraumatic tibia valga: A case demonstrating asymmetric activity at the proximal growth plate on technetium bone scan. J. Pediatr. Orthop. 7: 458–462, 1987.

LOWER LEG (MIDSHAFTS OF THE TIBIA AND FIBULA)

Injuries of the Lower Leg. Overt fractures of the midshafts of the tibia and fibula are not difficult to recognize. However, it might be noted that such fractures show a distinct tendency to occur in the tibia, but not in the fibula. In some of these cases, even though this might be one's initial impression, with closer perusal of the films, often it will be noted that the fibula actually is bent (Fig. 4.185). In other words, the overt fracture of the tibia is accompa-

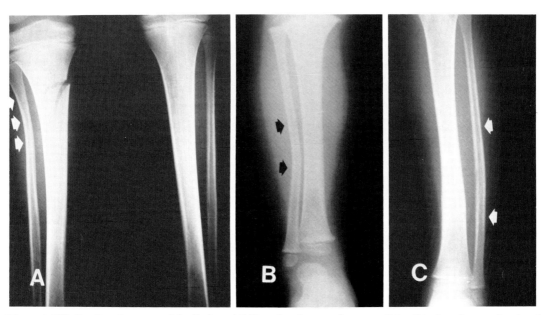

Figure 4.185. *Bending fractures of the fibula.* (**A**) Note the clear-cut fracture of the tibia, but also note localized bending of the upper fibula *(arrows)*. (**B**) Marked inward bending of the right fibula *(arrows)*. This is the common direction of bending. (**C**) Unusual outward bending of the fibula *(arrows)*. (Part **A** courtesy of J. Bjelland, M.D.)

nied by an associated acute, bending, plastic fracture of the fibula which occurs at the same level as the transverse fracture of the tibia. These plastic bending fractures of the fibula probably are more common than generally appreciated (7), and in some cases the fibula may be bent outward, rather than inward (Fig. 4.185C).

In young infants, a very common fracture of the tibia is the so-called *"toddler's fracture"* (1, 5, 6). This fracture characteristically is a spiral, hairline fracture and often is invisible, or nearly invisible, on initial roentgenograms. It almost behaves like a stress fracture and even in those cases where it is visible, it often appears clearer on one view than the other (Fig. 4.186). In other cases, soft tissue swelling of the muscles around the tibia can bring attention to the fracture, but it cannot be overstressed that many of these children present with normal or very subtle findings (Fig. 4.187). Because of this, the situation can become quite puzzling (i.e., these children will not walk, or if they walk they do so with a limp, and yet on physical examination the findings are relatively negative [6]). When this is coupled with the fact that no fracture is visible roentgenographically, one has a definite diagnostic puzzle. *However, if torque stress is placed on the tibia (one hand on the knee and one on the ankle and twisting in opposite directions), pain will be evoked and the diagnosis clarified.*

A somewhat similar fracture has been recorded in ballet dancers. These individuals, in general, are prone to stress injuries of the lower extremities (2–5). Of course,

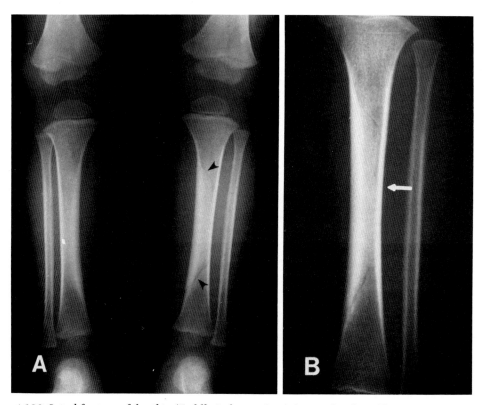

Figure 4.186. *Spiral fracture of the tibia (Toddler's fracture).* (A) Note that the calf *on the left* is a little bigger and slightly more opaque than that *on the right*. This is due to edema. Then note the two limbs of the typical spiral fracture of the tibia *(arrows)*. (B) Follow-up film 2 weeks later again demonstrates the fracture line, but this time early periosteal new bone is visible *(arrow)*.

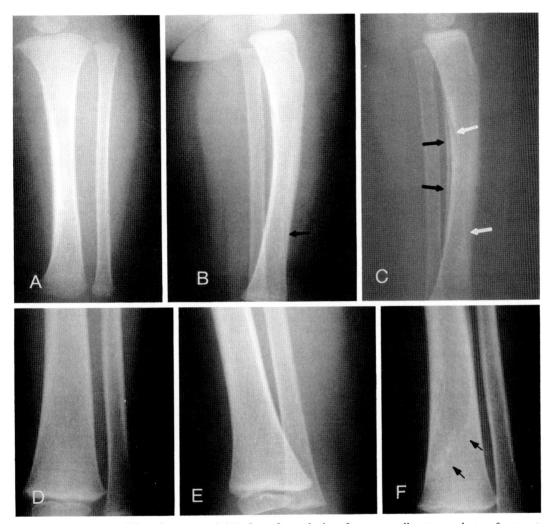

Figure 4.187. *Occult toddler's fractures.* (**A**) In this infant, a little soft tissue swelling is seen but no fracture is noted. (**B**) On lateral view there is subtle suggestion of a fracture line *(arrow)*. (**C**) Two weeks later, periosteal new bone is seen along the posterior aspect *(black arrows)*. The fracture line still is difficult to visualize *(white arrows)*. (**D**) Another patient in whom no fracture is seen on the frontal view. (**E**) On the lateral view no fracture is seen. (**F**) Two weeks later, there is evidence of a healing fracture with a fine, white sclerotic fracture line *(black arrows)* now visible.

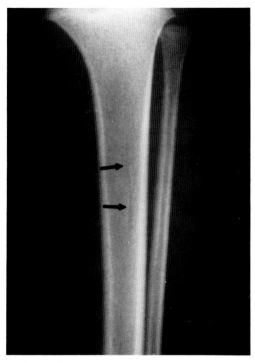

Figure 4.188. *Tibial vascular groove; pseudofracture.* Note the vascular groove *(arrows)* in the upper tibia. This vascular groove is quite common and should not be misinterpreted as a spiral fracture of the tibia.

as with any stress fracture, if these fractures are identified in their advanced healing phase, profound periosteal new bone deposition may erroneously suggest the presence of a bone tumor. Stress fractures of the fibula also occur (2), and all of these fractures are readily discovered with bone scintigraphy.

Normal Findings Causing Problems. About the only normal finding in the midshaft of the tibia or fibula that can be confused with an underlying lesion is a normal vascular groove (Fig. 4.188). These vascular grooves appear no different from those in other long bones, but in the tibia can be misinterpreted as a spiral, toddler's type fracture.

REFERENCES

1. Dunbar, J.S., Owen, H.F., Nogrady, M.B., and McLeese, R.: Obscure tibial fracture of infants—
the toddler's fracture. J. Can. Assoc. Radiol. 15: 136–144, 1964.
2. Kozlowski, K., Azouz, M., and Hoff, D.: Stress fracture of the fibula in the first decade of life: Report of eight cases. Pediatr. Radiol. 21: 381–383, 1991.
3. Miniaci, A., McLaren, A.C., and Haddad, R.G.: Longitudinal stress fracture of the tibia: Case report. Can. Assoc. Radiol. 39: 221–223, 1988.
4. Nussbaum, A.R., Treves, S.T., and Micheli, L.: Bone stress lesions in ballet dancers: Scintigraphic assessment. A.J.R. 150: 851–855, 1988.
5. Schneider, H.J., King, A.Y., Bronson, J.L., and Miller, E.H.: Stress injuries and developmental change of lower extremities in ballet dancers. Radiology 113: 627–632, 1974.
6. Singer, J., and Towbin, R.: Occult fractures in production of gait disturbances in childhood. Pediatrics 64: 192–196, 1979.
7. Stenstrom, R., Gripenberg, L., and Bergius, A.R.: Traumatic bowing of forearm and lower leg in children. Acta Radiol. 19: 243–249, 1978.

ANKLE

Normal Soft Tissues and Fat Pads of the Ankle. In the infant and child, three fat pads around the ankle usually are visualized on lateral view. The largest is the pre-Achilles fat pad, located just anterior to the Achilles tendon, but this fat pad is not utilized for the detection of joint fluid. Rather, the anterior and posterior fat pads lying against the joint capsule are the ones to be assessed for joint fluid detection (Fig. 4.189). In the older child, the anterior fat pad may be comprised of two fat pads, but it is the inner one that should be assessed. With soft tissue edema, both the anterior and posterior fat pads are obliterated, while with joint fluid accumulations they are displaced outwardly (4).

Detecting Fluid in the Ankle Joint. In determining whether fluid is present in the ankle joint, it is best to study the lateral view (4, 17). On frontal view, only soft tissue swelling around the ankle is seen, but on lateral view outward displacement of the anterior or posterior fat pads is seen (Fig. 4.190). In older children, bulging of the capsule, in more discrete fashion, has led to the "teardrop" sign (15) (Fig. 4.191). No joint space widening is seen, for the ligaments around the ankle joint are very sturdy and usually do not allow for much in the way of joint distraction.

Injuries of the Distal Tibia and Fibula. A variety of injuries can be sustained in the distal tibia and fibula, and most often these result from a combination of inversion, eversion, and rotational forces. In the young infant, *cortical buckle (torus)* fractures through the distal tibia and fibula are very common (Fig. 4.192). In the older child, however, the more common injury is some type of Salter-Harris *epiphyseal-metaphyseal fracture.* In the ankle, all of the Salter-Harris type injuries, with the exception of the type V injury, are common. Salter-Harris type III and IV injuries often are associated with some degree of epiphyseal displacement and generally are not difficult to identify (Fig. 4.193), but if dis-

placement of the epiphysis is not present, they may be just as difficult to identify as Salter-Harris type I and II injuries. In this regard, the key to detecting these more subtle fractures lies in comparing the width of the epiphyseal lines in the injured ankle to those on the normal side and in assessing the soft tissues for evidence of swelling (Fig. 4.194). The Salter-Harris type III injury is quite common in the distal tibia and often is missed on initial inspection. Indeed, oblique views may be required for its delineation (7). The reason for this is that the distal tibial epiphysis fuses earlier medially than it does laterally. Consequently, with an inversion injury of the ankle there is separation of the epiphysis laterally but not medially (Fig. 4.195*B*). These fractures, the equivalent of the Tillaux fracture (3), are best assessed with CT (Fig. 4.195). This is required to define the degree of fracture fragment displacement and whether internal fixation is required.

Inversion-rotation injuries of the ankle are very common, and while in most cases they result only in a sprained ankle, in other instances Salter-Harris injuries result. In still other instances, one may encounter an epiphyseal-metaphyseal separation of the distal fibular epiphysis and an associated fracture through the medial malleolus of the distal tibial epiphysis (Fig. 4.196*A*). In these cases, the distal fibular fracture is a Salter-Harris type I or II injury, while the medial malleolar fracture is a type III injury. Less commonly, one may encounter only a small sliver-like cortical avulsion of the distal fibular metaphysis or epiphysis (Fig. 4.196*B*). These latter fractures must be differentiated from normal accessory ossicles occurring in this area (see Fig. 4.208). In all of these injuries, there will be a certain degree of soft tissue swelling over the lateral malleolus. Obviously, if an underlying fracture is visualized, the soft tissue thickening is of lesser consequence, but many times there is nothing more to see than soft tissue thick-

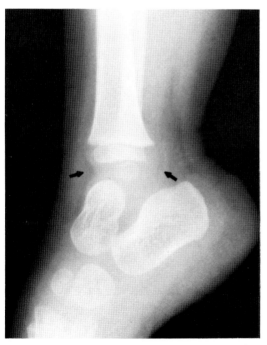

Figure 4.189. *Normal soft tissues and fat pads of the ankle.* The pre-Achilles fat pad is clearly visible but not utilized for joint fluid detection. The anterior *(anterior arrow)* and posterior *(posterior arrow)* fat pads are readily visualized and, as seen, normally are tucked tightly against the joint capsule. With joint fluid, they are displaced outwardly (see Fig. 4.190).

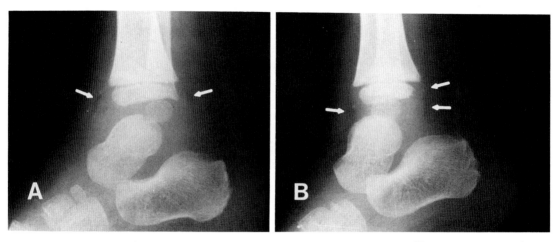

Figure 4.190. *Detecting fluid in the ankle joint.* (**A**) Note outward displacement of both the anterior and posterior fat pads *(arrows)*. (**B**) Normal side for comparison. Note normal position of the fat pads *(arrows)*.

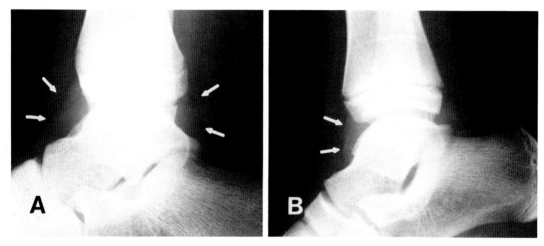

Figure 4.191. *Teardrop configuration of ankle fluid.* (**A**) Note typical teardrop sign anteriorly *(anterior arrows)*. A similar configuration exists posteriorly *(posterior arrows)*. (**B**) Another patient with a less pronounced teardrop sign anteriorly *(arrows)*. Similar, subtle findings are present posteriorly.

ening. In such cases, I have found it useful to assume that an occult Salter-Harris epiphyseal-metaphyseal injury has been sustained if soft tissue thickening is greater than 1 cm.

With eversion injuries, the ankle mortise often is seriously disturbed and a wide range of relatively severe injuries can be encountered (Fig. 4.197). So-called *"posterior malleolar fractures"* actually are Salter-Harris type II epiphyseal-metaphy-

seal fractures (Fig. 4.198), and many times the fracture is visible only on lateral view. When these fractures occur with fractures through the medial and lateral maleoli, the term "trimalleolar fracture" is applied. These posterior malleolar fractures often are associated with a type III epiphyseal-metaphyseal fracture as part of a Tillaux fracture.

Injuries of the Tarsal Bones. Fractures and dislocations of the tarsal bones

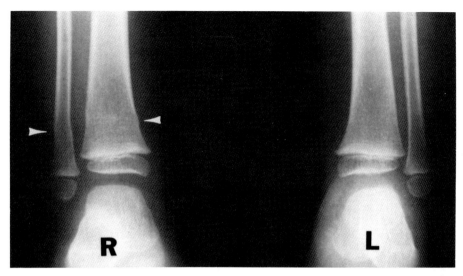

Figure 4.192. *Cortical buckle (torus) fractures of distal tibia.* Note the cortical buckle fracture along the inner aspect of the distal right tibia *(arrow)*. A more subtle cortical buckle fracture is present on the opposite side of the tibia. Also note the acute bending fracture of the distal fibula at the same level *(arrow)*.

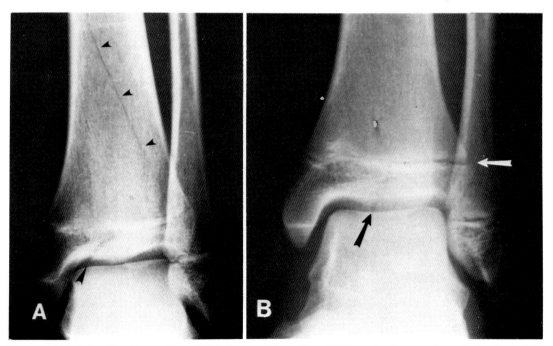

Figure 4.193. *Salter-Harris type III and IV injuries of the ankle.* (**A**) Note the fracture through the distal tibial epiphysis *(lower arrow)* and the fracture through the metaphysis *(upper arrows)*. This is a Salter-Harris type IV injury. (**B**) Note the fracture through the distal tibial epiphysis *(lower arrow)*. Also note slight separation of the lateral epiphyseal fragment from the metaphysis *(lateral arrow)*. This is a Salter-Harris type III injury.

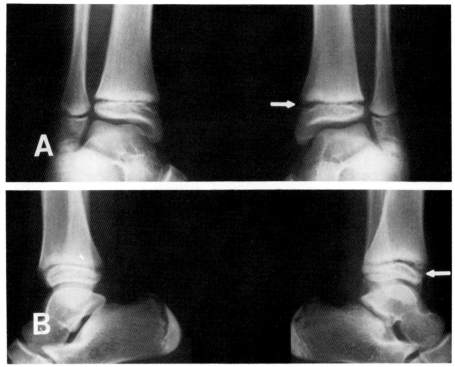

Figure 4.194. *Salter-Harris type I injury of the ankle.* (**A**) Note that the epiphyseal line through the distal tibia is wider *on the left (arrow)* than *on the right*. (**B**) Lateral view confirms *widening of the epiphyseal line on the left (arrow)*. These findings are those of a Salter-Harris type I injury.

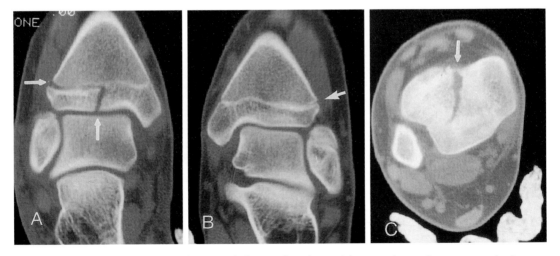

Figure 4.195. *Salter-Harris type III fracture of tibia—value of CT.* (**A**) Coronal view demonstrates the fracture *(lower arrow)*. Note that the epiphyseal line is widened laterally *(upper arrow)*. Also note that the epiphyseal line through the medial aspect has closed. (**B**) On the normal side, note that, while medially the epiphyseal line is completely closed, it is still a little open on the lateral side. This leads to the common occurrence of a type III Salter-Harris fracture with an inversion injury. (**C**) Axial CT scan demonstrates the fracture through the epiphysis *(arrow)*.

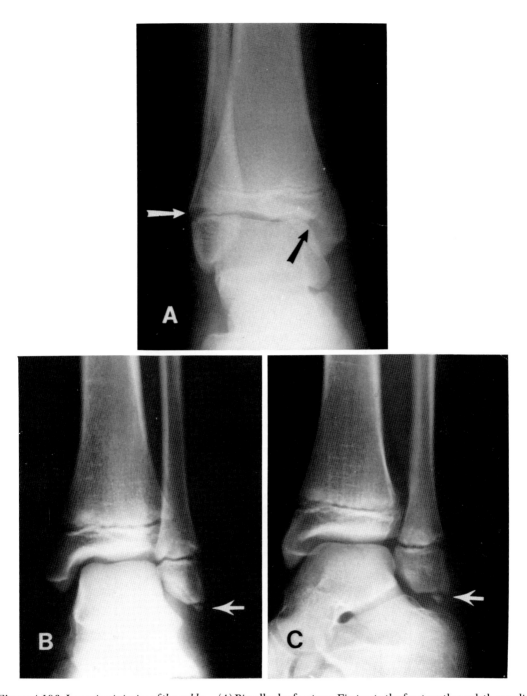

Figure 4.196. *Inversion injuries of the ankle.* (**A**) Bimalleolar fracture. First note the fracture through the medial malleolus *(black arrow)*, and then note that the distal fibular epiphysis has been separated from the metaphysis (i.e., there is widening of the epiphyseal line and a small metaphyseal avulsion fracture [white arrow]). The fibular fracture is a Salter-Harris type II injury, while the medial malleolar fracture is a Salter-Harris type III injury. (**B**) Small avulsion fracture of the distal fibula. Note the small avulsed distal fibular bony fragment *(arrow)*. (**C**) Oblique view demonstrates the fragment *(arrow)* to better advantage. There is no epiphyseal-metaphyseal injury of either the tibia or fibula in this patient. The small avulsion fracture should be differentiated from the normal ossicle (os subfibulare) commonly occurring in this area (Fig. 4.209).

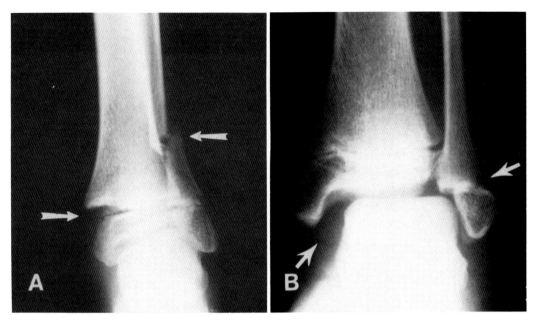

Figure 4.197. *Eversion injuries of the ankle.* (**A**) Note the displaced fracture of the distal fibula *(upper arrow)* and the displaced Salter-Harris type II epiphyseal-metaphyseal fracture of the distal tibia *(lower arrow)*. The ankle mortise is not disturbed. (**B**) Note the displaced Salter-Harris type I injury of the distal fibula *(lateral arrow)* and the widely opened joint space medially *(medial arrow)*. The ankle is dislocated and the ankle mortise grossly disturbed. Note, however, that there is no epiphyseal-metaphyseal fracture of the distal tibia.

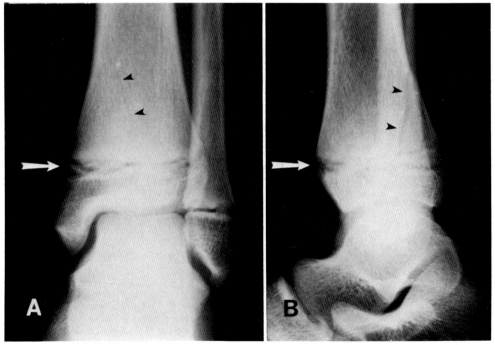

Figure 4.198. *Posterior malleolar fracture.* (**A**) On frontal view, the fracture line is just barely visible *(upper arrows)*. However, note that the epiphyseal line is a little wider medially *(lower arrow)* than laterally. (**B**) Lateral view demonstrating the posterior malleolar metaphyseal fracture with greater clarity *(upper arrows)*. The epiphyseal line is slightly wider than normal anteriorly *(lower arrow)*, and overall the findings constitute a Salter-Harris type II epiphyseal-metaphyseal injury.

534

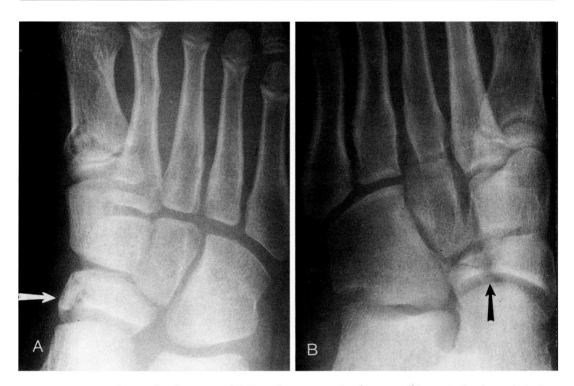

Figure 4.199. *Tarsal navicular fractures.* (**A**) Note the compression fracture of the navicular *(arrow)*. An impaction-compression fracture of the base of the first metatarsal also is present, and there is an angulated cortical fracture through the midshaft of the second metatarsal. (**B**) Another patient with a compression fracture of the navicular *(arrow)*.

are generally less common in childhood than in adulthood. This is especially true in the infant and young child. In the older child, one can encounter fractures of bones such as the navicular and talus (Figs. 4.199 and 4.200), but the most commonly fractured bone is the calcaneus (Fig. 4.201). With fractures through the talus, dislocation of one of the fragments can occur and, in addition, subsequent aseptic necrosis is a known complication. Cuboid fractures are rare, but may present the same as a toddler's tibial fracture (1).

Fractures of the calcaneus usually result from patients jumping or falling on their heels, and because one often is not thinking of these fractures, they may remain occult (8, 14). Nuclear scintigraphy is helpful in detecting some of these fractures, but in other cases a clear-cut fracture line may be visible (Fig. 4.200*B*). Otherwise, one may have to look for indirect findings such as soft tissue swelling, loss of Boehler's angle, decreased height of the calcaneus, or increased density (impaction) of the calcaneus (Fig. 4.201). In addition, when a calcaneal fracture is suspected, it is mandatory that tangential views of the calcaneus be obtained. On this view, the most productive in calcaneal injuries, compression fractures almost always are visualized with clarity and, indeed, previously unsuspected fractures also may become visible (Fig. 4.201). Finally, with calcaneal fractures, it is most important that the normally sclerotic and irregular calcaneal apophysis not be misinterpreted for such fractures (Fig. 4.210*A*).

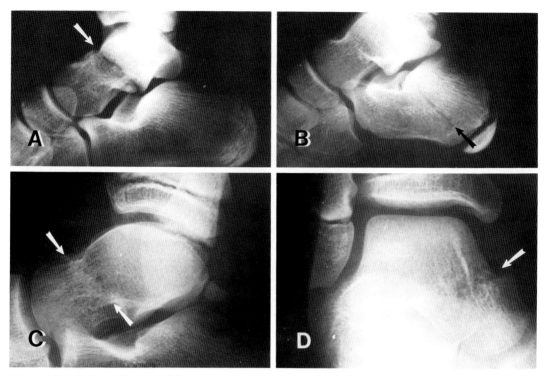

Figure 4.200. *Talar and calcaneal fractures.* (*A*) Note the clear-cut talar fracture *(arrow)*. (*B*) Linear fracture through the calcaneus *(arrow)*. (*C*) Subtle fracture through the neck of the talus *(arrows)*. (*D*) Oblique view demonstrates offsetting of the fracture *(arrow)*.

Small avulsion fractures of the various tarsal bones and other bones around the ankle also can be encountered. These are more common than generally appreciated, and while they may be visible on standard views, very often oblique views first bring these fractures to light (Fig. 4.202). Indeed, in some cases visualization of these fractures is strictly fortuitous, and all of them must be differentiated from normal accessory ossification centers of the various bones around the ankle (see Fig. 4.208).

Sprained Ankle. *As compared to the sprained wrist, a sprained ankle most often turns out to be nothing more than a sprained ankle.* Of course, this is not to say that fractures never occur, but only to point out that the high incidence of underlying fracture that accompanies wrist sprains is not present with ankle sprains. Another important aspect of a sprained ankle due to an inversion injury, is that *very often there is an associated fracture of the base of the fifth metatarsal.* The peroneus brevis muscle inserts onto this bone, and with inversion injuries, an avulsion fracture frequently occurs. This fracture usually is overlooked clinically, but almost always is detectable roentgenographically (see Fig. 4.221).

Achilles Tendonitis. Children very commonly develop acute or chronic pain over the insertion of the Achilles tendon onto the calcaneus. Actually, the condition represents a bursitis or tenosynovitis and usually is considered to be the result of subclinical tendon injury in the active child (2, 5, 6, 9, 12). Some children are more prone to develop this problem than

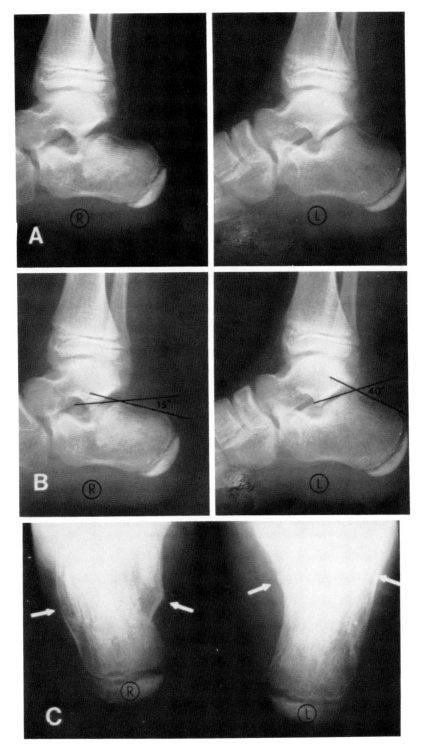

Figure 4.201. *Calcaneal fracture; indirect signs.* (*A*) *On the right,* note that the calcaneus has lost considerable height, and that there is an area of central sclerosis due to impaction. The left ankle appears normal. (*B*) Boehler's angle *on the right* has been markedly reduced, while *on the left* it is within normal range. Normally, it measures between 30 and 40°. Anything <28° is considered abnormal. (*C*) Tangential view of the calcanei demonstrates the previously documented compression fracture of the calcaneus *on the right (arrows),* but in addition detects the presence of a previously unsuspected, noncompressed, subtle calcaneal fracture *on the left (arrows).*

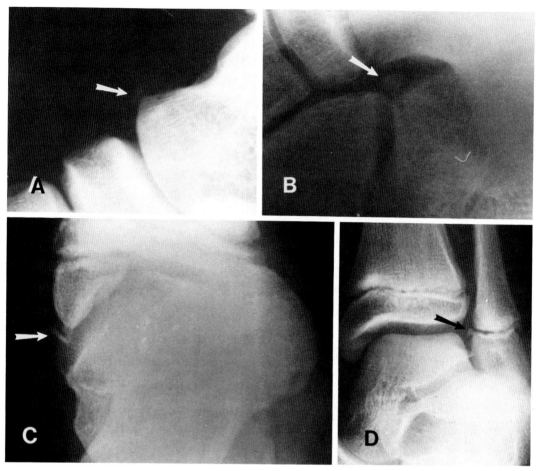

Figure 4.202. *Avulsion fractures around the ankle.* (*A*) Note small avulsion of the talus *(arrow)*. This is a common fracture. (*B*) Small corner avulsion of the calcaneus *(arrow)*, seen only on oblique view. (*C*) Avulsion fracture of the distal fibular epiphysis *(arrow)*. (*D*) Another avulsion fracture of the fibula *(arrow)*, seen only on oblique view.

others, and frequently it is recurrent. It is similar to Osgood-Schlatter's disease of the knee, and conservative measures are in order. There are no roentgenographic findings except, perhaps, localized swelling over the area. However, there is a great temptation to erroneously attribute the problem to the nearby, normally sclerotic and irregular, but abnormal-appearing calcaneal apophysis. Such a diagnosis should be avoided, for this is the expected appearance of the normal calcaneus (see Fig. 4.210), and never is it involved in Achilles tendonitis. Ultrasonography and MRI can be used to detect the thickened tendon or associated fluid collection (6) but generally are superfluous.

Osteochondritis Dissecans of the Tarsal Bones. Osteochondritis of the tarsal bones is not particularly common in childhood, but does occur and most often involves the talus (10). The findings are similar to those of osteochondritis dissecans elsewhere in that there is a bony defect with slight peripheral sclerosis (Fig. 4.203). An intra-articular piece of bone may or may not be visualized. It might be noted, however, that as with osteochondritis dissecans elsewhere, the lesion may or may not be symptomatic at the time of detection. MRI can be utilized to detect the degree of fragment displacement.

Aseptic Necrosis of the Tarsal Bones. Aseptic necrosis of the various tarsal bones can be a cause of foot pain, and in this regard, the tarsal navicular is the most commonly involved bone. Köhler's disease (16) is the term applied to aseptic necrosis of the navicular. The roentgenographic features consist of irregularity and sclerosis of the bone (Fig. 4.204A and B). In addition, one can utilize the soft tissues (18) for detection of less than classic Köhler's disease. The soft tissues over the aseptically necrotic bone are edematous (Fig. 4.204C), whereas when normal irregular ossification mimics Köhler's disease, the soft tissues are normal.

Septic Arthritis, Osteomyelitis, and Cellulitis. Septic arthritis of the ankle

manifests primarily in joint space distension, causing outward displacement of the fat pads (Fig. 4.205). Cellulitis around the ankle manifests primarily in edema of the soft tissues and obliteration of the various fat pads. The fat pads are not displaced outwardly unless there is pus in the joint (i.e., septic arthritis). With osteomyelitis of the distal tibia and fibula, similar deep soft tissue swelling and obliteration of fat muscle interfaces occur, but no joint space distension is seen. Of course, if septic arthritis accompanies the problem, fluid will be present in the joint.

Unfortunately, the deep soft tissue changes of osteomyelitis around the ankle are not particularly different from those seen with cellulitis. To be sure, in the ankle, differentiation of superficial, from deep, edema is more difficult than around the other large joints of the body. However, whatever the cause of edema, the anterior and posterior fat pads remain in normal position unless joint fluid (pus) is present (Fig. 4.206).

Eventually, with osteomyelitis, bone destruction is seen (Fig. 4.207), but the disease may be present for some time before this becomes evident. This is especially true of the tarsal bones and, consequently, bone scans are indispensable when looking for early osteomyelitis in and around the ankle (Fig. 4.207).

Normal Variations Causing Problems. Numerous accessory ossicles occur in the ankle and to illustrate all of them would be excessive. The most common are those occurring at the distal ends of the lateral and medial malleoli and the posterior aspect of the talus (Fig. 4.208). However, many more commonly occur in the ankle, and a diagrammatic representation of these accessory ossicles is presented in Fig. 4.209. It is most important not to misinterpret these secondary ossification centers and accessory ossicles as avulsion fractures, even though avulsion of the secondary centers themselves can occur (11).

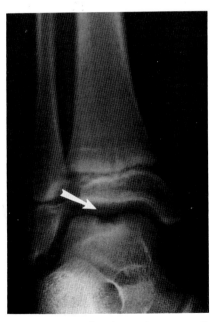

Figure 4.203. *Osteochondritis dissecans of talus.* Note the characteristic defect *(arrow)* in the articular surface of the talus.

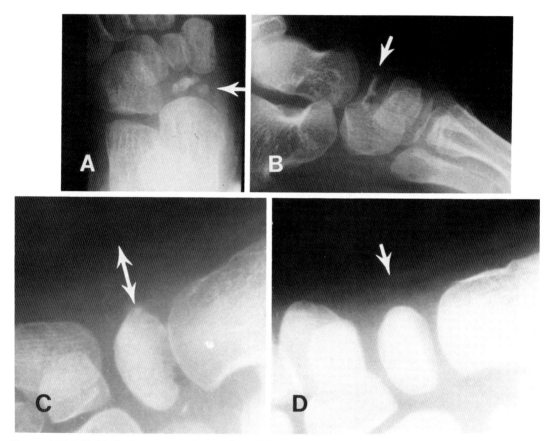

Figure 4.204. *Köhler's disease; tarsal navicular.* (A) Note the small, irregular, fragmented navicular bone *(arrow)*. (B) Lateral view showing similar fragmentation. (C) In this case the navicular bone is a little sclerotic, but note mostly that the soft tissues over the bone are thickened because of edema *(arrows)*. (D) Normal side for comparison. Note the normal appearance of the navicular bone and lack of swelling of the soft tissues.

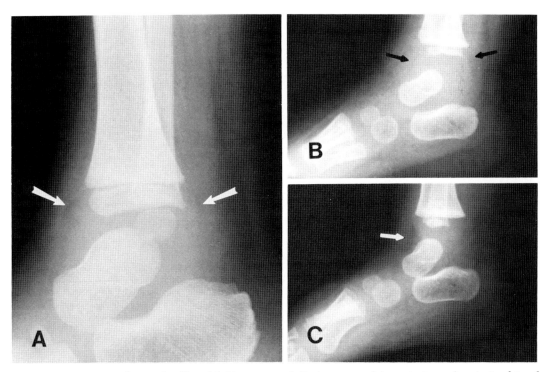

Figure 4.205. *Septic arthritis of ankle.* (**A**) Note outward displacement of the anterior and posterior fat pads *(arrows)*. (**B**) Another patient with just barely visible outwardly displaced fat pads *(arrows)*. The reason for poor visualization of the fat pads is that there is marked associated edema of the soft tissues. Note also that the pre-Achilles fat pad, behind the posterior fat pad, is outwardly displaced and curved. (**C**) Normal side for comparison. Note especially the normal anterior fat pad *(arrow)*.

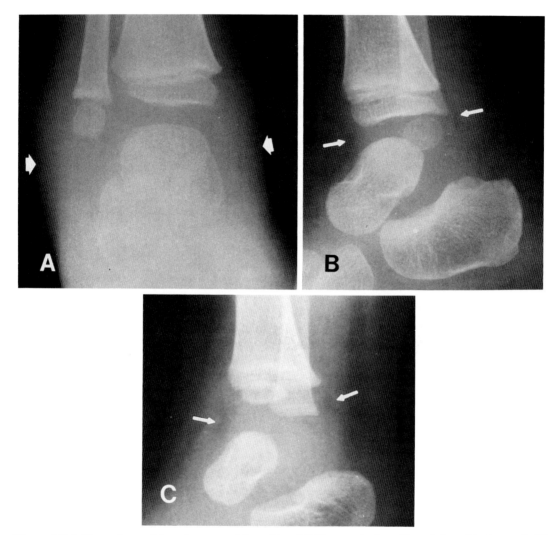

Figure 4.206. *Deep edema of the soft tissues of the ankle.* (**A**) Note marked swelling of the ankle *(arrows)*. (**B**) Lateral view, however, demonstrates normal position of the anterior and posterior fat pads *(arrows)*. This excludes fluid in the joint and suggests that the findings are due to soft tissue edema alone. (**C**) Another patient with edema around the ankle and persistent visualization of the anterior and posterior fat pads in their normal location *(arrows)*. It is important in these cases to note that the fat pads are in normal position. If they were outwardly displaced, fluid (pus) in the joints should be suspected.

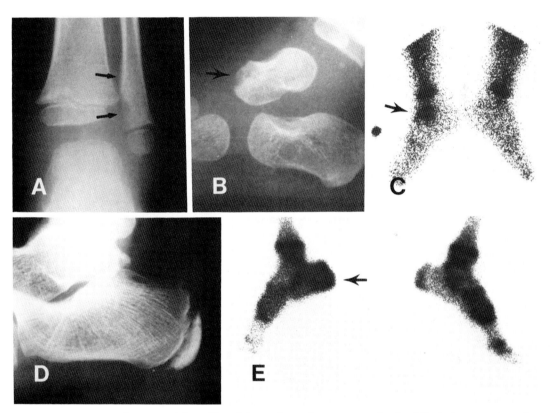

Figure 4.207. *Osteomyelitis around the ankle.* (*A*) Note bone destruction in the distal fibula *(arrows)*. (*B*) Subtle destruction of the talus *(arrow)* in an infant. (*C*) Bone scan in same patient shows clear-cut hot area in right talus *(arrow)*. (*D*) Patient with calcaneal pain. The x-ray is normal. (*E*) Bone scan, however, shows clear-cut increased uptake in the calcaneus *(arrow)*.

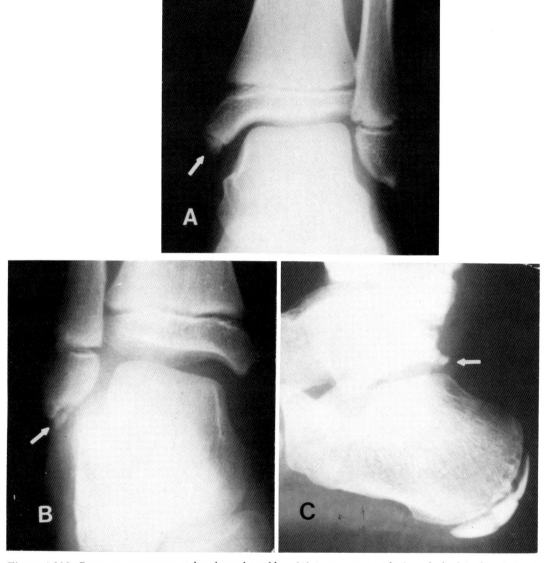

Figure 4.208. *Common accessory ossicles about the ankle.* (**A**) Accessory ossicle (os subtibiale) of medial malleolus *(arrow)*. (**B**) Accessory ossicles (os subfibulare) of the distal fibular epiphysis *(arrow)*. (**C**) Os trigonum *(arrow)* of talus.

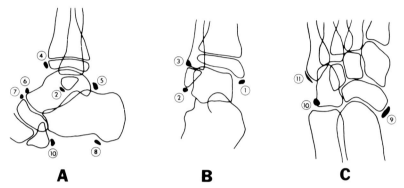

Figure 4.209. *(A–C) Accessory ossicles about the ankle; diagrammatic representation.*   *(1)* Accessory center of medial malleolus or os subtibiale; *(2)* accessory center of distal fibular epiphysis or os subfibulare; *(3)* accessory metaphyseal fibular ossicle; *(4)* os talotibale; *(5)* os trigonum; *(6)* os supratalare; *(7)* os supranaviculare; *(8)* os subcalcis; *(9)* os subtibiale externum; *(10)* os peroneum; *(11)* os vesalianum.

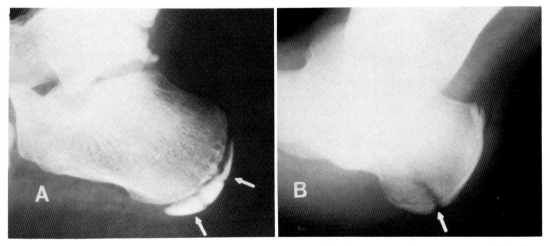

Figure 4.210. *Normal calcaneal apophysis.*   (**A**) Note the typical sclerotic, irregular appearance of the fragmented calcaneal apophysis *(arrows)*. (**B**) With obliquity, the normal defects through the calcaneal apophysis can suggest a calcaneal fracture *(arrow)*.

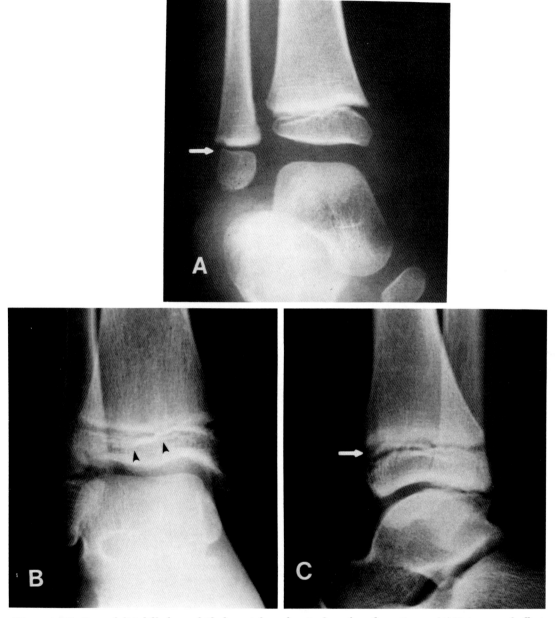

Figure 4.211. *Normal distal fibular and tibular epiphyseal-metaphyseal configurations.* (A) Note normal offsetting of the distal fibular epiphysis *(arrow)*. This is a common finding on oblique views of the normal ankle. It should not be misinterpreted for a displaced epiphyseal fracture. *Also note slight irregularity along the inner aspect of the fibula. This also is normal.* (B) Note the typically irregular appearance of the epiphyseal-metaphyseal junction of the normal distal tibia *(arrows)*. This should not be misinterpreted for a Salter-Harris epiphyseal-metaphyseal fractures. (C) Lateral view of another ankle demonstrating what appears to be a metaphyseal avulsion *(arrow)*. However, the finding is normal. Of all the epiphyseal-metaphyseal junctions in the body, the one through the distal tibia is most prone to such normal variations.

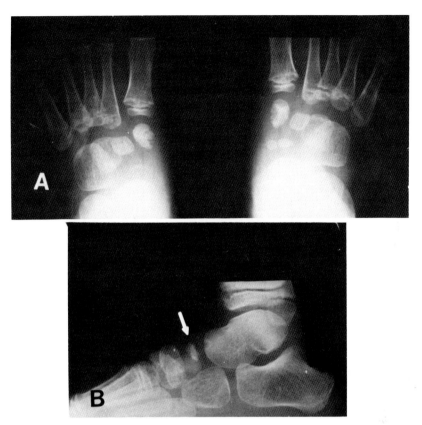

Figure 4.212. *Normal irregular ossification of various tarsal bones and pseudoepiphyses of the metatarsals.* (A) Note the various irregular configurations of the tarsal bones and pseudoepiphyses of the third through fifth metatarsals. (B) Lateral view demonstrating underossification and irregular sclerosis of the normal navicular bone *(arrow)*. The findings should not be misinterpreted for those of aseptic necrosis. (See Fig. 4.204.)

The normal, sclerotic, irregular calcaneal apophysis (13) notoriously is misinterpreted as being due to aseptic necrosis of the calcaneus. *Indeed, its normal appearance is often so frightening that is it almost impossible not to assign some type of pathologic condition to the bone* (Fig. 4.210A). *This is especially true in cases of Achilles tendonitis.* Another problem with the calcaneal apophysis is that with certain degrees of obliquity its fragmented appearance can suggest a calcaneal fracture (Fig. 4.210B).

Another normal finding frequently misinterpreted for abnormality is the apparently offset distal fibular epiphysis on oblique views of the ankle (Fig. 4.211). This is a normal finding on this view. In addition, the distal tibial epiphyseal-metaphyseal junction tends to be very irregular in normal children, and can suggest a fracture (Fig. 4.211). Finally, it should be noted that tarsal bones are especially prone to irregular ossification which should not be misinterpreted for fracturing or aseptic necrosis (Fig. 4.212).

REFERENCES

1. Blumberg, K., and Patterson, R.J.: The toddler's cuboid fracture. Radiology 179: 93–94, 1991.
2. Dickinson, P.H., Coutts, M.B., Woodward, E.P.,

et al.: Tendo achilli bursitis. J. Bone Joint Surg. 48A: 77–81, 1966.

3. Felman, A.H.: Tillaux fractures of the tibia in adolescents. Pediatr. Radiol. 20: 87–89, 1989.

4. Hayden, C.K., Jr., and Swischuk, L.E.: Para-articular soft tissue changes in infections and trauma of the lower extremity in children. A.J.R. 134: 307–311, 1980.

5. Heneghan, M.A., and Wallace, T.: Heel pain due to retrocalcaneal bursitis-radiographic diagnosis. Pediatr. Radiol. 15: 119–122, 1985.

6. Kainberger, F.M., Engel, A., Barton, P., Huebsch, P., Neuhold, A., and Salomonowitz, E.: Injury of the Achilles tendon: Diagnosis with sonography. A.J.R. 155: 1031–1036, 1990.

7. Letts, R.M.: The hidden adolescent ankle fracture. J. Pediatr. Orthop. 2: 161–164, 1982.

8. Matteri, R.E., and Frymoier, J.W.: Fracture of the calcaneus in three children. J. Bone Joint Surg. 55A: 1091–1094, 1973.

9. Micheli, L.J., and Ireland, M.L.: Prevention and management of calcaneal apophysitis in children: An overuse syndrome. J. Pediatr. Orthop. 7: 34–38, 1987.

10. Newberg, A.H.: Osteochondral fractures of the dome of the talus. Br. J. Radiol. 52: 105–109, 1979.

11. Ogden, J.A., and Lee, J.: Accessory ossification patterns and injuries of the malleoli. J. Pediatr. Orthop. 10: 306–316, 1990.

12. Shapiro, J.R., Fallat, R.W., Tsang, R.C., and Glueck, C.J.: Achilles tendinitis and tenosynovitis. Am. J. Dis. Child. 128: 486–490, 1974.

13. Shopfner, C.E., and Coin, C.G.: Effect of weight-bearing on the appearance and development of the secondary calcaneal epiphysis. Radiology 86: 201–206, 1966.

14. Starshak, R.J., Simons, G.W., and Sty, J.R.: Occult fracture of the calcaneus—another toddler's fracture. Pediatr. Radiol. 14: 37–40, 1984.

15. Towbin, R., Dunbar, J.S., Towbin, J., and Clark, R.: Teardrop sign: Plain film recognition of ankle effusion. A.J.R. 134: 985–990, 1980.

16. Waught, W.: The ossification and vascularization of the tarsal-navicular and a relation to Köhler's disease. J. Bone Joint Surg. 40B: 765, 1958.

17. Weston, W.J.: Traumatic effusions of the ankle and posterior subtaloid joints. Br. J. Radiol. 31: 445–447, 1958.

18. Weston, W.J.: Köhler's disease of the tarsal scaphoid. Australas. Radiol. 12: 332–337, 1978.

FOOT

Normal Soft Tissues and Fat Pads. As in the hand, there are no particularly valuable fat pads to evaluate in the foot. Con-sequently, except for localized edema, there is little else to analyze.

Detecting Fluid in the Small Joints of the Foot. The detection of fluid in the small joints of the foot rests with noting soft tissue swelling around the involved joint. Occasionally, the joint space can be widened due to distension, but this is not a common finding (see Fig. 4.225).

Injuries of the Metatarsals and Phalanges. Dislocation of the various joints of the foot is uncommon except perhaps for dislocation of the great toe. *Cortical, buckle, or torus fractures,* on the other hand, are quite common and, as in the hand, often require oblique views for adequate visualization (Fig. 4.213). However, some of these fractures still can be quite subtle, and only telltale soft tissue edema (Fig. 4.214) or meticulous inspection of the films will aid one in detecting them (Fig. 4.215). The buckle fracture through the first metatarsal demonstrated in Fig. 4.214 also is considered by some a form of toddler's fracture.

Another more recently documented injury commonly seen in young infants is the bunkbed or Lisfranc fracture (2, 3). This fracture is believed to be a fracture dislocation of the first metatarsal and cuneiform bone (2, 3), and in subtle cases may be missed. Comparative views are important here except when the avulsed fracture fragment is clearly visible (Fig. 4.216A). When these fractures heal they may leave an exostotic-like bony bulge (Fig. 4.216B). This fracture also is at times considered a toddler's fracture.

Epiphyseal-metaphyseal injuries are much less common in the foot than in the hand and, similarly, fractures of the various epiphyses themselves are less common. A problem, however, can arise in the great toe, where the occasional type III Salter-Harris fracture (Fig. 4.217) is confused with the more common normal bipartite epiphysis (Fig. 4.218).

Salter-Harris type I, and even type II, epiphyseal-metaphyseal injuries also can

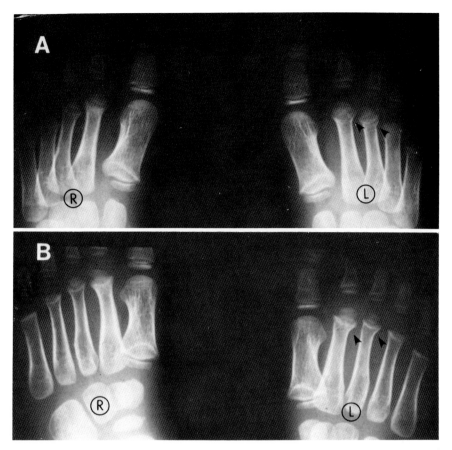

Figure 4.213. *Subtle cortical fractures of metatarsals.* (*A*) *On the left*, note subtle cortical buckling of the second and third metatarsals *(arrows)*. Also note that the soft tissues in the area are a little more opaque because of underlying edema. (*B*) Oblique view more clearly demonstrates the cortical buckles *(arrows)*. Compare these findings with the corresponding cortices on the normal right side.

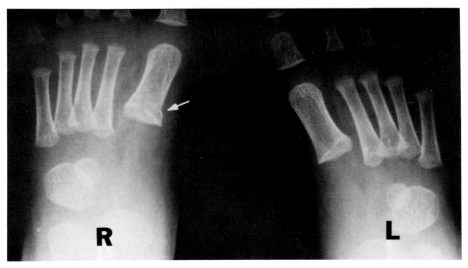

Figure 4.214. *Cortical fracture of first metatarsal.* First, note extensive edema of the soft tissues of the right forefoot. Then note the cortical buckle fracture at the base of the first metatarsal *(arrow)*.

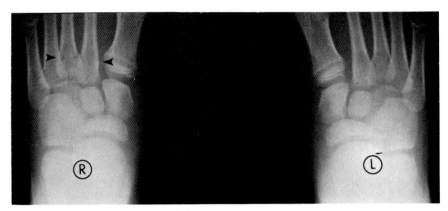

Figure 4.215. *Metatarsal fractures, subtle findings.* *On the right,* note subtle fractures through the base of the second and third metatarsals *(arrows).* These fractures easily could be missed unless the findings are compared with those in the normal bones *on the left side.*

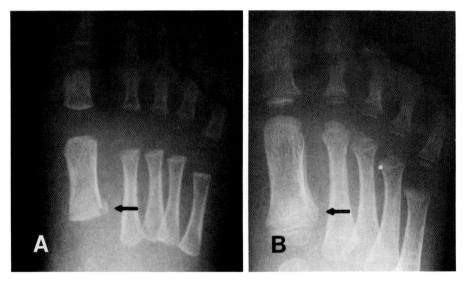

Figure 4.216. *"Bunkbed" fracture of first metatarsal.* **(A)** Note typical location of this dislocation-avulsion fracture *(arrow).* **(B)** Healing phase demonstrates an exostotic-like hump *(arrows).*

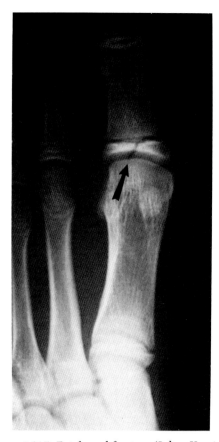

Figure 4.217. *Epiphyseal fracture (Salter-Harris type III injury).* Note the fracture through the epiphysis *(arrow)* of the proximal phalanx of the great toe. Also note that the epiphyseal line is a little wider medially, giving further support to the presence of this Salter-Harris type III injury.

occur in the small bones of the feet, especially in the great toe. Indeed, these fractures have a propensity to becoming infected, because there often is a break through the nail bed (4). These fractures usually can be suspected when there is excessive widening of the epiphyseal line and, once again, comparative views are indispensable here (Fig. 4.219).

Other fractures of the small bones of the foot include a variety of spiral and transverse fractures, many of which are hairline (Fig. 4.220), and the *avulsion fracture of the base of the fifth metatarsal.* Actually,

this latter injury is common, and usually is sustained with inversion sprains of the ankle. Also called the Jones fracture, it results from pulling on the base of the fifth metatarsal by the peroneus brevis muscle. However, many times swelling around the ankle diverts attention from this fracture, and it is not until the fracture is detected roentgenographically that the injury comes to light. In this regard, it is most fortunate that on almost any roentgenogram of the ankle the base of the fifth metatarsal is included, *and thus if one always looks at this area in patients with a sprained ankle, one will be the first to detect a good many of these fractures.*

In *differentiating base of the fifth metatarsal fractures from the normal os vesalianum,* it should be noted that the fractures almost always are transverse or near transverse (Fig. 4.221), while the os vesalianum usually is a longitudinal structure (Fig. 4.222). If avulsion of the os vesalianum occurs, a variable degree of separation from the base of the fifth metatarsal is seen and, clinically, the findings are accompanied by local tenderness (Fig. 4.223). Occasionally, the os vasalianum can be fractured as part of the Jones fracture.

Miscellaneous Injuries of the Foot. Stress fractures in the foot are reasonably common in the older child but not in the infant. Of these, the best known is the stress fracture of the second metatarsal, the so-called "march" fracture. As with any stress fracture, the fracture line may be difficult to detect in its early stages, but later on the fracture becomes evident because it causes abundant periosteal new bone deposition (Fig. 4.224). Stress fractures of the proximal phalanx of the great toe also have been described (5).

Another lesion in the foot causing pain is aseptic necrosis of the second metatarsal head or Freiberg's disease. Roentgenographically, the findings range from increased sclerosis to sclerosis interspersed

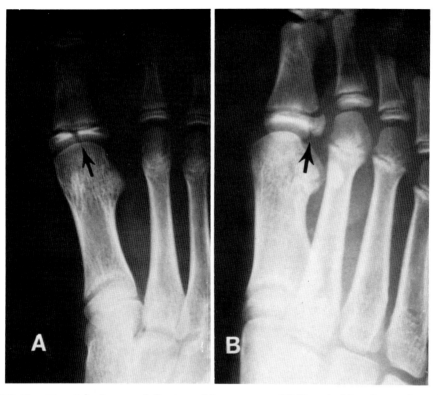

Figure 4.218. *Bipartite epiphysis—pseudofracture of the great toe.* (**A**) Note the bipartite epiphysis *(arrow)* of the great toe. The findings are virtually indistinguishable from the fracture demonstrated in Figure 4.217. (**B**) Another example of an eccentric bipartite epiphysis mimicking a fracture *(arrow).*

with focal bony resorption of the second metatarsal head. Osteochondritis dissecans elsewhere in the foot is rare but has been documented in the epiphysis of the first metatarsal (1).

Septic Arthritis, Osteomyelitis, and Cellulitis of the Foot. Septic arthritis is manifest by swelling around the joint space and, occasionally, distension of the joint space (Fig. 4.225). Osteomyelitis and cellulitis, on the other hand, usually present with soft tissue swelling only. Indeed, they are difficult to differentiate from one another, but eventually osteomyelitis results in bony destruction (Fig. 4.226). Finally, it should be noted that patients with sickle cell disease can present with extensive soft tissue swelling, bony destruction, and periosteal new bone deposition as part

of the hand-foot syndrome. The findings are no different from those seen in the hand (see Fig. 4.104), and are difficult to differentiate from osteomyelitis.

Normal Findings Causing Problems. The os vesalianum, or accessory ossification center at the base of the fifth metatarsal, has been dealt with earlier and is a common normal finding misinterpreted as a base of the fifth metatarsal fracture (see Fig. 4.222). Irregular ossifications of the epiphyses or pseudoepiphyses of the metatarsals and phalanges are less commonly misinterpreted as fractures but can be misinterpreted as areas of aseptic necrosis (Fig. 4.227).

The bipartite epiphysis of the great toe, a common normal variation, also has been dealt with earlier (Fig. 4.218), and is a nor-

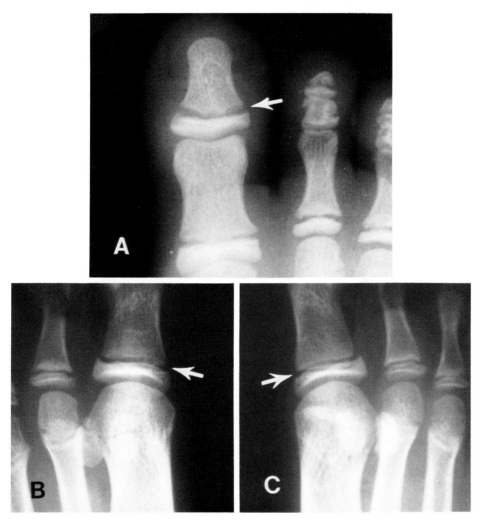

Figure 4.219. *Epiphyseal-metaphyseal fractures of the great toe.* (**A**) Note widening of the epiphyseal line of the distal phalanx *(arrow)*. Compare it with the width of the other lines. (**B**) Another patient with somewhat subtle widening of the epiphyseal line *(arrow)*. (**C**) Compare with the same epiphyseal line on the normal side.

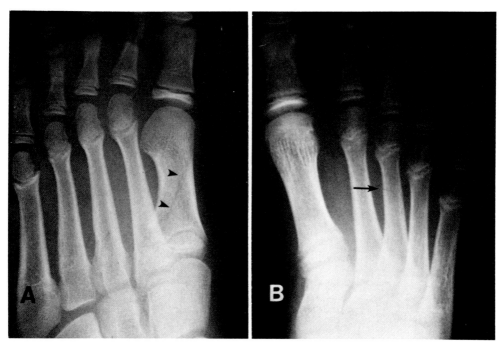

Figure 4.220. *Hairline fractures of the metatarsals.* (*A*) Note the oblique hairline fracture of the first metatarsal *(arrows)*. (*B*) Very subtle transverse, hairline fracture of the third metatarsal *(arrow)*.

Figure 4.221. *Base of the fifth metatarsal fracture.* (*A*) Typical transverse fracture *(arrow)* through the base of the fifth metatarsal. (*B*) Same fracture *(arrow)* on anteroposterior view. (*C*) Oblique view of the fracture *(arrow)*. Typically, this fracture occurs in the transverse plane.

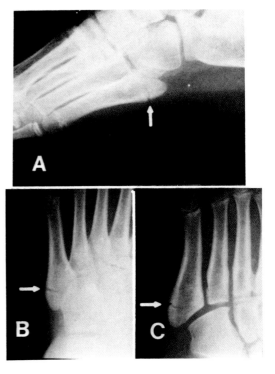

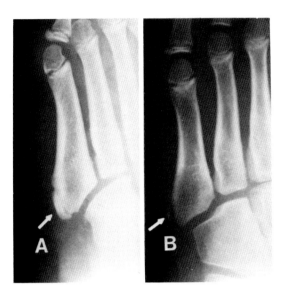

Figure 4.222. *Os vesalianum—base of fifth metatarsal accessory center.* (**A**) Large os vesalianum *(arrow).* (**B**) Thin sliver-like os vesalianum *(arrow).* As opposed to a fracture through the base of the fifth metatarsal, the os vesalianum always lies in the longitudinal plane.

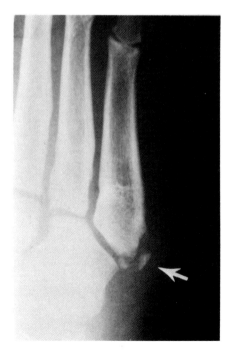

Figure 4.223. *Avulsion of the os vesalianum.* Note the fragmented, partially avulsed os vesalianum *(arrow).* Not visible on this reproduction is localized soft tissue swelling over the avulsed bony fragment. Clinically, point tenderness over the area was present.

Figure 4.224. *Stress fracture of second metatarsal.* Note extensive periosteal new bone deposition along the second metatarsal *(arrows)*. This is a healing stress fracture.

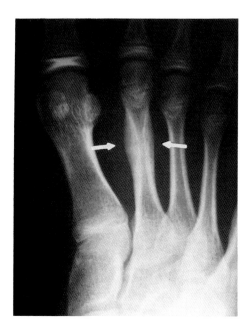

Figure 4.225. *Septic arthritis of the small joints of the foot.* Note the widened joint space between the fourth metatarsal and the adjacent proximal phalanx *(arrows)*. Also note that the joint is dislocated and that the epiphysis of the phalanx has been partially destroyed.

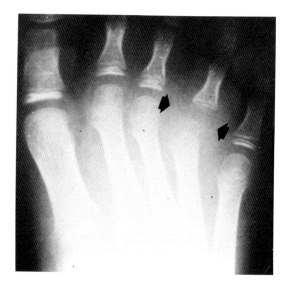

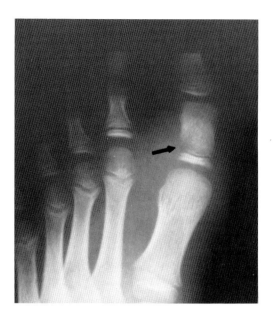

Figure 4.226. *Osteomyelitis—small bones of the foot.* Note swelling around the great toe and early bone destruction *(arrow)*.

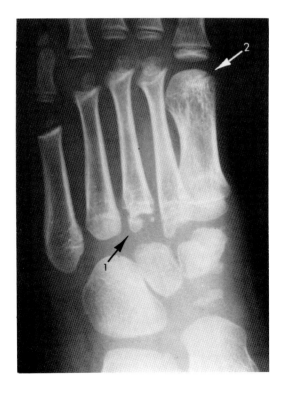

Figure 4.227. *Normal irregular ossification of the metatarsal apophyses.* Note the irregular ossification pattern of the apophysis (pseudoepiphysis) of the third metatarsal *(1)*. Also note irregular ossification of some of the tarsal bones. The radiolucent defect through the head of the first metatarsal *(2)* should not be misinterpreted as a fracture. It is a residual defect caused by the apophysis (pseudoepiphysis) of the first metatarsal.

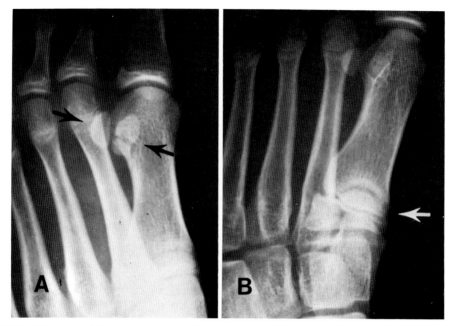

Figure 4.228. *Other normal findings causing problems.* (*A*) Note the sesamoid bones of the great toes *(arrows)*. One of the bones is bipartite and should not be misinterpreted as a fracture of the sesamoid bone. (*B*) Irregular appearance of the epiphysis of the first metatarsal *(arrow)*. The finding should not be misinterpreted as a fracture.

mal finding commonly misinterpreted as a fracture. In addition, bipartite or even tripartite sesamoid bones over the head of the first metatarsal are common and frequently misinterpreted as fractures of these bones (Fig. 4.228A). Finally, it should be noted that the normal proximal epiphysis of the first metatarsal, when seen in oblique projection, can have a very bizarre appearance. In many of these cases, a fracture is suggested (Fig. 4.228B), but knowlege of this phenomenon should enable one to avoid such a misinterpretation.

REFERENCES

1. Falkenberg, M.P., Dickens, D.R.V., and Menelaus, M.B.: Osteochondritis of the first metatarsal epiphysis. J. Pediatr. Orthop. 10: 797–799, 1990.
2. Foster, S.C., and Foster, R.R.: Lisfranc's tarsometatarsal fracture-dislocation. Radiology 120: 79–83, 1976.
3. Johnson, G.F.: Pediatric Lisfranc injury: "Bunkbed" fracture. A.J.R. 137: 1041–1044, 1981.
4. Pinckney, L.E., Currarino, G., and Kennedy, L.A.: The stubbed great toe: A cause of occult compound fracture and infection. Radiology 138: 375–377, 1981.
5. Yokoe, K., and Mannoji, T.: Stress fracture of the proximal phalanx of the great toe: A report of three cases. Am J. Sports Med. 14: 240–242, 1986.

MISCELLANEOUS EXTREMITY PROBLEMS

Battered Child Syndrome. A complete discussion of the battered child syndrome is beyond the scope of this book, but one or two pertinent observations are in order. First, it is not uncommon for a battered infant to first present as an emergency patient, and one should be suspicious if: (a) roentgenographic evidence of trauma is greater than the clinical history would suggest, (b) roentgenographic evidence of trauma is poorly correlated with clinical history, and (c) unsuspected fractures are detected. The main job of the emergency room physician is to be suspicious and know when to proceed with further investigation. *In this regard the importance of taking an accurate history in these patients cannot be overstated.* One needs to know the distance of a fall, the surface involved in the fall, the leading part of the body in the fall, etc. The more detailed history one takes, the more likely one is to uncover discrepancies. In this regard, often the individuals bringing the infant to the emergency room will say that the infant fell out of bed. It recently has been demonstrated (21) that it is unlikely that an infant would sustain an extremity fracture from such a fall. Injuries from such a fall are minimal and usually involve the scalp and face (21). In addition, retinal hemorrhages, due to shaking, are an important finding in the battered child syndrome (7), and this becomes important since many of these patients arrive at the trauma center or emergency room unconscious and have received cardiopulmonary resuscitation. The question then often arises as to whether resuscitation could have caused the retinal hemorrhages. Once again, a recent study (12) has demonstrated that retinal hemorrhages after cardiopulmonary resuscitation alone are uncommon. Finally it should be noted that battered infants arriving dead can erroneously be considered as having died from sudden infant death syndrome (25).

Another group of patients who are maltreated are those who sustain burns, and the most suspicious burn is the circumferential immersion burn. However, the frequency of fractures in these children is relatively low (27). Other infants, namely those who present in an unconscious state often are subject to CT studies. If the patient has been asphyxiated, there will be little to see except for findings secondary to anoxia. On the other hand, if a shaking-type injury has occurred, one can see small cerebral bleeds or contusions, so-called "shearing" tears, at the junction of the white and gray matter. These contusions or small hemorrhages can be identified with ultrasound (11), but are more clearly identified with CT (Fig. 4.229).

In terms of skeletal injury, it first should be noted that many battered children present with calvarial injuries and underlying subdural hematomas. Consequently, any unexplained skull fracture or subdural hematoma should be treated with a great deal of suspicion. However, the most characteristic lesion in the battered child syndrome is the epiphyseal-metaphyseal fracture (5, 6, 13, 17, 30). These fractures usually are Salter-Harris type I and II fractures, and their multiplicity along with their different stages of healing are characteristic of this syndrome (Fig. 4.230). Some of these fractures are more subtle than others, and when healing occurs they become more obvious (Fig. 4.231). They result from violent shaking of the infant as do most of the intracranial injuries and retinal hemor-

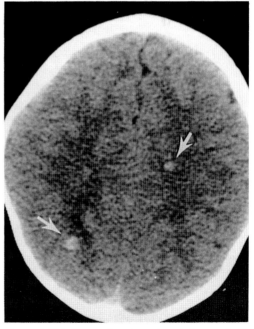

Figure 4.229. *Brain-shearing injury in battered child syndrome.* Note small areas of hemorrhage along the white-gray matter junction.

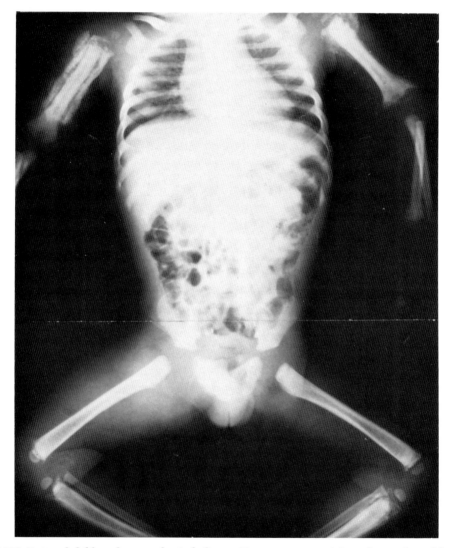

Figure 4.230. *Battered child syndrome—classic findings.*   Note numerous epiphyseal-metaphyseal fractures in numerous stages of healing in the shoulders, elbows, and knees. Periosteal new bone deposition at certain sites is profound. Also note that the right hip joint is distended and that the femur is displaced laterally. This represents an acute hemarthrosis due to an occult hip fracture. On later films, a healing Salter-Harris epiphyseal-metaphyseal injury became evident.

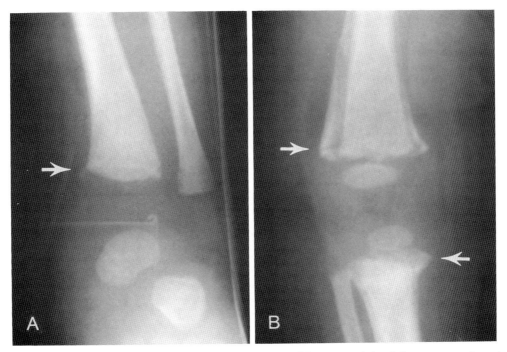

Figure 4.231. *Battered child syndrome—epiphyseal-metaphyseal fractures.* (**A**) Subtle, corner epiphyseal-metaphyseal fracture of distal tibia *(arrow)*. Note the almost ring-like configuration of the fracture fragment. (**B**) Typical healing epiphyseal-metaphyseal fractures of all bones.

rhages. However, although this fracture is most pathognomonic of the battered child syndrome, it is not the most common to be seen. Many fractures result from direct blows and often only a single fracture is present (14). Furthermore, this fracture often is an ordinary transverse spiral or oblique long bone fracture.

It has become increasingly apparent that many infants, perhaps as many as 50%, present with injuries other than those involving the epiphyseal-metaphyseal junction (2, 4, 14, 19, 21, 23). These injuries may be soft tissue injuries, unremarkable appearing spiral or transverse fractures of the extremity, or no bony injury at all. Consequently, in the emergency room, any injury that does not seem to fit with the clinical history should be treated with suspicion and if necessary a bone survey should be obtained at the time (Fig. 4.232).

In terms of long bone injuries, the fem-

oral fracture has received a great deal of attention in recent years (3, 8, 20, 26, 33). All of these communications agree on the fact that an ordinary-appearing fracture through the femur or any other long bone in a young infant should be treated with suspicion if there is no correlation with clinical history. *In this regard, in a child <1 year of age, an isolated, unexplained femoral or other long bone fracture should be considered highly suspicious of the battered child syndrome* (Fig. 4.233). One should remain suspicious of isolated femoral and other long bone fractures after 1 year of age, but at the same time one should be aware of the fact that these papers also have demonstrated that legitimate, accidental trauma was shown to be more common after 1 year of age. Therefore greater caution is required in the evaluation of these fractures after one year of age; many, if not most, are legitimate.

Finally, it should be remembered that

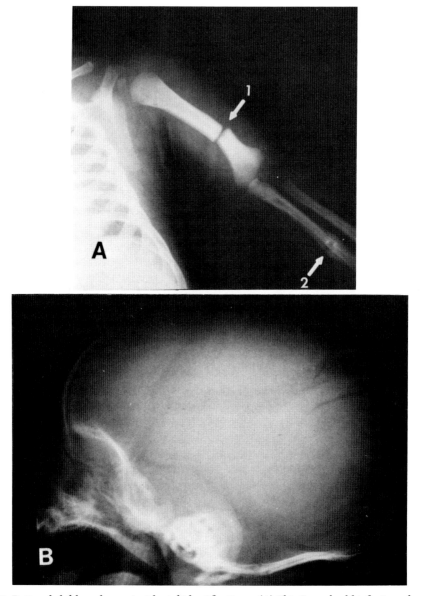

Figure 4.232. *Battered child syndrome; incidental identification.*   (*A*) This 6-week-old infant was brought to the emergency room by the mother because she thought the infant's arm was broken. A clear-cut fracture through the humerus is visible (*1*), but also note periosteal new bone deposition around an old distal ulnar fracture (*2*). This latter fracture was unexpected and unexplained. Consequently, a bone survey was obtained. (*B*) Skull film obtained as part of the bone survey demonstrates a number of totally unsuspected calvarial fractures. In addition, this patient demonstrated fractures of the lower extremities and ribs.

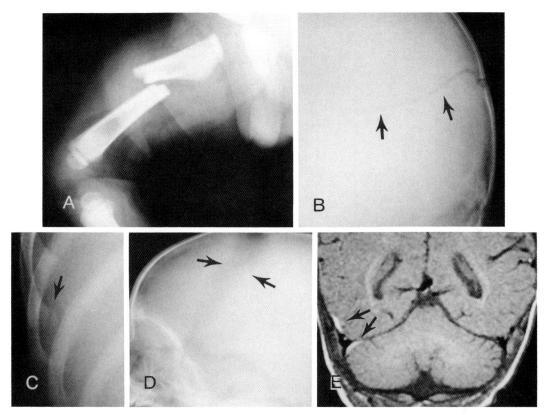

Figure 2.233. *Battered child syndrome—various presentations.* (*A*) Note the transverse fracture through the femur of this 4-month-old infant. This was the only fracture present at the time of this admission. (*B*) Two weeks later, the patient returned with an unexplained skull fracture *(arrows)*. The skull fracture was not present on the previous bone survey. (*C*) Note the anterior rib fracture *(arrow)*. This was the only other bony injury in this child. (*D*) Skull film demonstrates spread coronal sutures *(arrows)*. This indicates increased intracranial pressure. (*E*) MR scan, coronal view, demonstrates subdural bleeding at two sites *(arrows)*.

while the classic epiphyseal-metaphyseal fracture, and now the ordinary long bone fracture, are given most attention in the battered child syndrome, almost any other bone can be fractured. Certainly all are aware of calvarial fractures, but rib fractures, clavicular fractures, spinal fractures, and pelvic fractures all occur in the battered child syndrome (1, 18, 19, 28). Indeed rib, clavicular, and scapular fractures can be treated just as suspiciously as the classic epiphyseal-metaphyseal fractures (Fig. 4.234). Distal clavicular and acromial fractures usually result from shaking injuries, although midshaft clavicular fractures usually result from direct blows. Rib fractures are believed to result from squeezing and characteristically occur posteriorly, laterally, and anteriorly along the costochondral junctions (16, 19). Often they are multiple and detected when callus formation is profound. Anterior healing produces excessive cupping of the costochondral junctions (Fig. 4.234). These rib fractures are important for they are not the type seen with legitimate trauma or cardiopulmonary resuscitation (7). To be sure rib fractures are rare in infants.

A number of reviews on imaging of infant abuse are available (15, 24, 29) and, in addition, it has been suggested by some that initial screening for injury be accomplished with nuclear scintigraphy (10, 32). There is no question that the isotope bone

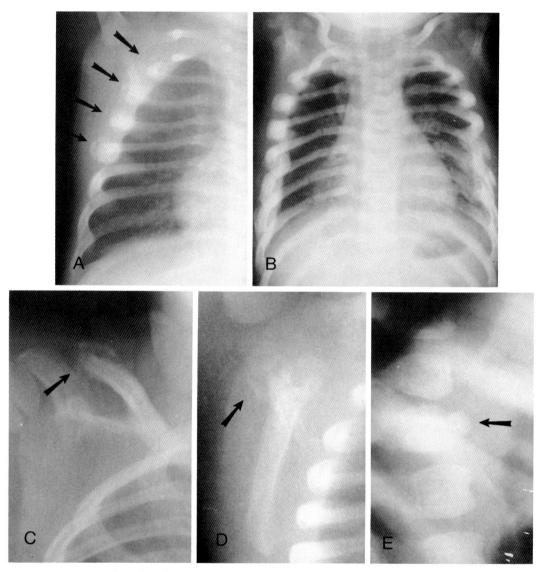

Figure 4.234. *Battered child syndrome—other fractures.* (*A*) Note healing fractures *(arrows)*, with abundant callus formation, of numerous ribs, laterally. (*B*) Another patient with numerous similar fractures on both sides. In addition, note a number of transverse fractures of the posterior ribs on both sides. (*C*) Epiphyseal-metaphyseal equivalent fracture of the distal clavicle *(arrow)*. (*D*) Fragmented acromial fracture *(arrow)*. (*E*) Compression fracture with notched vertebra *(arrow)* in another infant. (Parts *A* and *C–E* from M. Kogutt, L.E. Swischuk, and C.J. Fagan: Patterns of injury and significance of uncommon fractures in the battered child syndrome. A.J.R. 121: 143–149, 1974.)

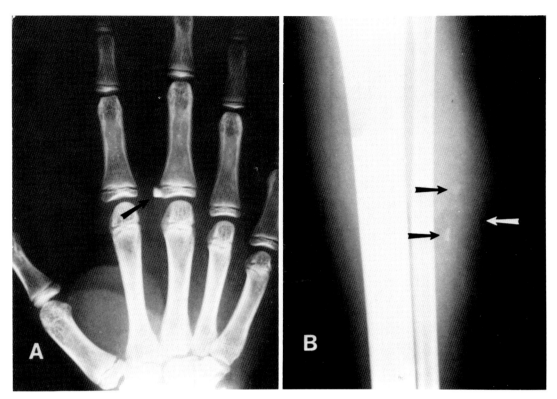

Figure 4.235. *Glass in the soft tissues.* (*A*) Clearly visible glass fragment *(arrow)* in the soft tissues of the third digit. (*B*) Less clearly visualized fragments of glass *(black arrows)* in the soft tissues of the leg. Also note edema in the leg and air in the soft tissues *(white arrow).*

scan can detect areas of injury, but the findings are nonspecific. There are, however, two opinions regarding this matter, but most institutions still perform the roentgenographic bone survey. In this regard, it has been suggested that the bone survey be quite detailed (29), but actually most institutions settle on an adequate, more abbreviated screening study. In our institution, we obtain anteroposterior views of the upper extremities and chest and of the pelvis and lower extremities. We also obtain a lateral view of the complete spine and an anteroposterior and lateral view of the skull. If there are any areas of suspicion on these studies whatsoever, whether soft tissue or bony, focused studies on those areas are then obtained. The detailed bone survey suggested (29) is

very time consuming, and one must remain somewhat practical about the whole problem. With a good screening sequence, it is doubtful that one would miss any injuries. The key to all of this is to be very astute in one's observations and follow any suspicious finding with focused films.

Visceral injury (31) is becoming more common in the battered child syndrome as is sexual abuse (31). Visceral injury most commonly involves the pancreas and duodenum but involvement of other intra-abdominal organs also is seen. These are best studied with CT scanning. Similarly, brain injuries are extremely common and a wide variety of traumatic lesions ranging from simple bleeds to completely destroyed brains can be seen. In addition, one should appreciate that some patients are asphyxi-

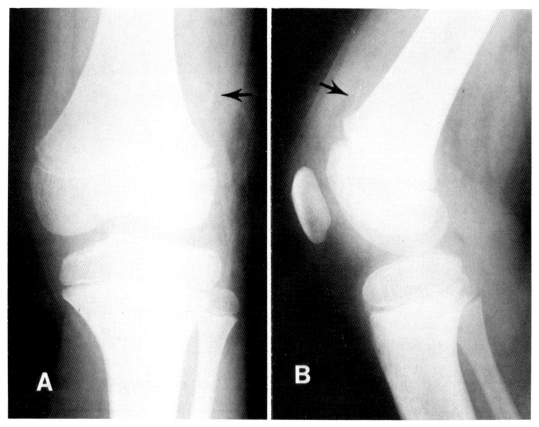

Figure 4.236. *Pencil lead in soft tissues.*   (**A**) Note the barely visible lead pencil fragment in the soft tissues of the knee *(arrow)*. (**B**) Lateral view demonstrating the same lead pencil fragment *(arrow)*.

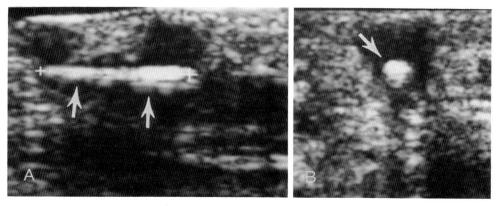

Figure 4.237. *Foreign body; ultrasound detection.*   (**A**) Note the echogenic palm thorn *(arrows)*. (**B**) Transverse image also demonstrates the thorn *(arrow)*. There is a surrounding collar of hypoechoic fluid.

ated and nothing more than brain edema is visualized. On a practical basis, CT is the most readily available imaging modality with which to assess brain injury although MRI often produces more detailed information.

Foreign Bodies in the Soft Tissues. Soft tissue foreign bodies are a common problem in childhood. Metallic foreign bodies and pebbles or dirt, of course, are readily demonstrable, but less opaque or totally nonopaque foreign bodies present more of a problem. In this regard, pieces of glass may or may not be visible, but overall, most are visible (1, 7, 14), and visibility depends entirely upon the amount of lead in the glass. In some of these cases the glass fragment is readily demonstrable, while in other cases it is more difficult to see (Fig. 4.235). Lead from a lead pencil is another foreign body commonly embedded in the soft tissues, and in some cases may be demonstrable roentgenographically (Fig. 4.236). Plastic generally is invisible (7), but all foreign bodies now readily can be identified, if needed, with ultrasound (5, 8, 10, 12) and CT (3, 5) (Figs. 4.237 and 4.238).

Of special interest is the *thorn or wooden or other organic foreign body* that can become embedded in the soft tissues on a chronic basis (2–6, 9, 11, 13, 15, 16). In such instances, most often one is dealing with a toothpick, although thorns and tree twigs, etc., also have been encountered. Most of these foreign bodies, of course, are not visible roentgenographically, but now usually are readily detected with ultrasound. Until then one must rely on secondary findings consisting of widening of the soft tissues between the adjacent bones and, eventually, periosteal new bone deposition, i.e., reactive periostitis (Fig. 4.239). In some cases, the resulting periosteal new bone and adjacent demineralization of the bones can lead to a pseudoosteomyelitis or tumor-like appearance.

Soft Tissue Infections, Edema, and Air in the Soft Tissues. Many times, children

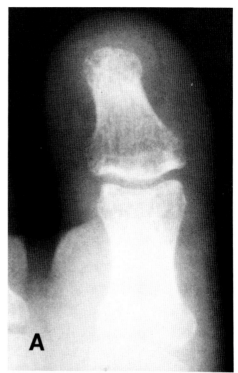

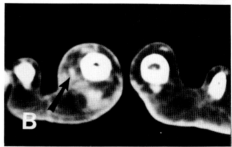

Figure 4.238. *Soft tissue foreign body; CT scan.* (*A*) This big toe was swollen for a prolonged period of time. No clear-cut foreign body is seen but one was suspected medially. (*B*) CT scan clearly demonstrates the foreign body *(arrow)* and the swollen soft tissues around the big toe.

come to the emergency room with extensive soft tissue swelling secondary to trauma or infection. Roentgenographically, the findings in both cases consist of thickening of the soft tissues, obliteration of the fat-muscle interfaces, and a characteristic reticulation of the fatty tissues. Reticulation is caused by the accumulation of fluid within the fibrous septae of the fatty

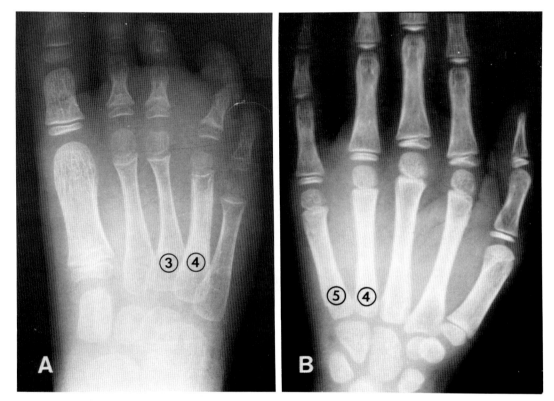

Figure 4.239. *Chronically embedded toothpick.* (*A*) Note widening of the soft tissues between the third (3) and fourth (4) digits, and periosteal new bone deposition along the fourth metatarsal. This patient presented with a chronically draining lesion between the third and fourth toes. A toothpick was extracted. (*B*) Note increased density of the soft tissues around the fourth (4) and fifth (5) metacarpals, and that the soft tissue space between the fourth and fifth metacarpals is widened. Also note periosteal new bone deposition along the shaft of the fourth metacarpal. This patient had a toothpick embedded between these bones.

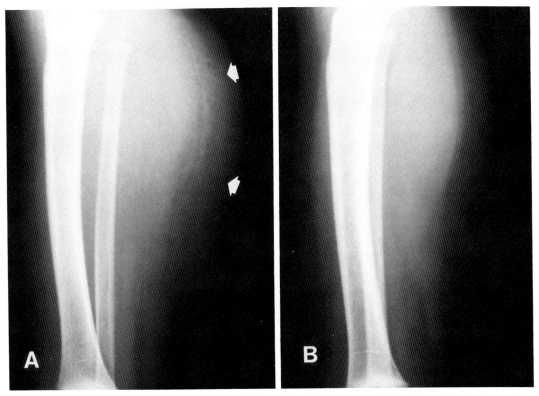

Figure 4.240. *Superficial cellulitis.* (**A**) Note typical reticulated appearance of the edematous soft tissues of the posterior aspect of the calf *(arrows)*. (**B**) Compare with normal side.

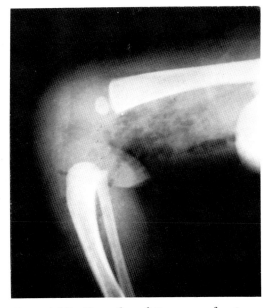

Figure 4.241. *Air on the soft tissues; gas forming organism.* Young infant with cellulitis of the thigh. Note numerous air bubbles and linear collections of air in the soft tissues of the thigh.

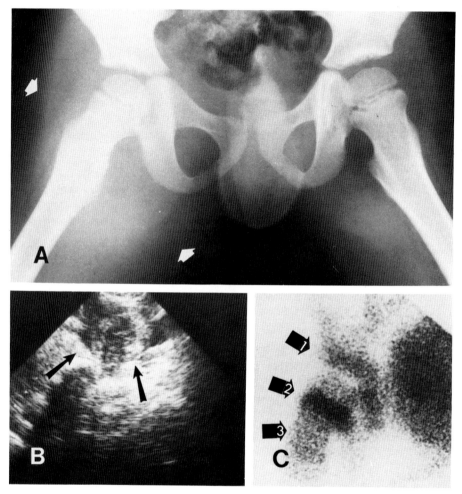

Figure 4.242. *Soft tissue abscess—value of ultrasound.* (*A*) Note extensive soft tissue swelling around the upper femur *(arrows)*. (*B*) Ultrasound study clearly identifies an abscess in the medial soft tissues of the thigh *(arrows)*. (*C*) Isotope study performed previously is normal. Normal uptake in acetabular roof (*1*), epiphyseal-metaphyseal junction (*2*), and upper femur (*3*). There is no increased uptake at any of these sites.

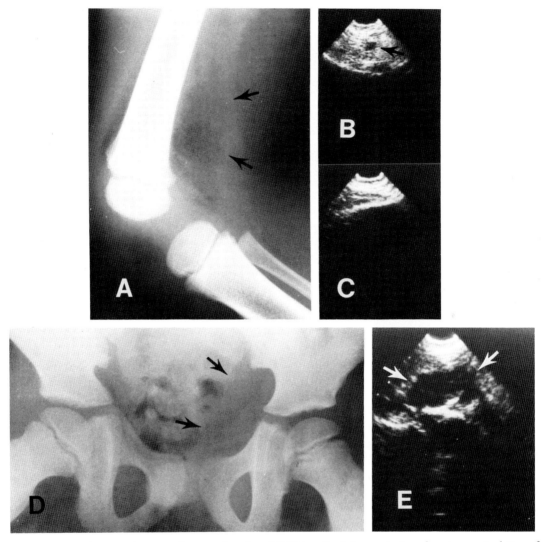

Figure 4.243. *Soft tissue abscess—ultrasound study.* (*A*) This patient demonstrates edematous reticulation of the soft tissues posterior to the knee *(arrows)*. (*B*) Ultrasound study demonstrates a sonolucent abscess in the area *(arrow)*. (*C*) Normal side for comparison. (*D*) Another patient with deep soft tissue swelling in the pelvis *(arrows)*. (*E*) Ultrasonography over the buttocks demonstrates a large abscess *(arrows)*.

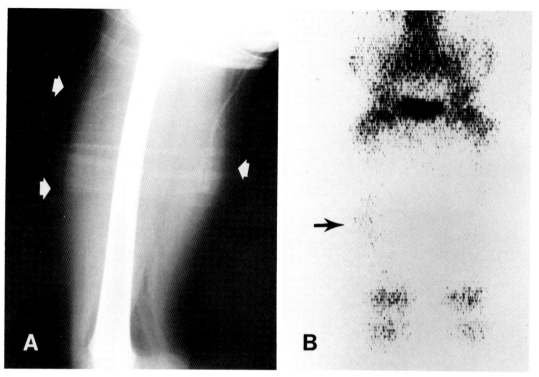

Figure 4.244. *Pyomyositis.* (*A*) Note thickening of the soft tissues of the thigh *(arrows).* (*B*) Nuclear scintigraphy demonstrates increased, albeit vague, tracer accumulation in the area of muscle inflammation *(arrow).*

tissues, and is seen primarily with cellulitis and superficial contusions (Fig. 4.240). In other instances, deep soft tissue infections are associated with gas-producing organisms and gas will be seen in the soft tissues (Fig. 4.241). Air also can be seen in the soft tissues in association with extensive lacerations and with blast injuries.

As noted in the preceding paragraph, superficial edema produces reticulation of the subcutaneous fatty tissue. When edema is deeper, however, a problem arises as to whether it is due to osteomyelitis or to soft tissue infection (i.e., pyomyositis, abscess, etc.). In the past, often it was difficult to make this determination, but with ultrasound, CT, and MRI (2, 3, 5, 10, 12) it has become increasingly easier. Ultrasound can clearly identify soft tissue abscesses (11) and should be used whenever soft tissue infection is suspected. The findings are not difficult to define or inter-

pret (Figs. 4.242 and 4.243). Such soft tissue abscesses, often involving the muscles, are more common than generally appreciated. The term "pyomyositis" (1, 3, 4, 6, 7, 11) is applied to the condition. Isotope studies frequently are helpful in identifying these sites of infection (Fig. 4.244), but, as already noted, ultrasonography is the most valuable study.

Inflammatory adenopathy often can be a presenting problem in the emergency room. In the past, it was difficult to document but currently ultrasonography can readily document the presence of enlarged, inflamed lymph nodes (Fig. 4.245). These lymph nodes can suppurate or become necrotic (8), and this also can readily be identified with ultrasonography. Color flow Doppler frequently demonstrates increased blood flow to inflamed lymph nodes (Fig. 4.245*B*). Such increased blood flow to lymph nodes is a nonspecific phe-

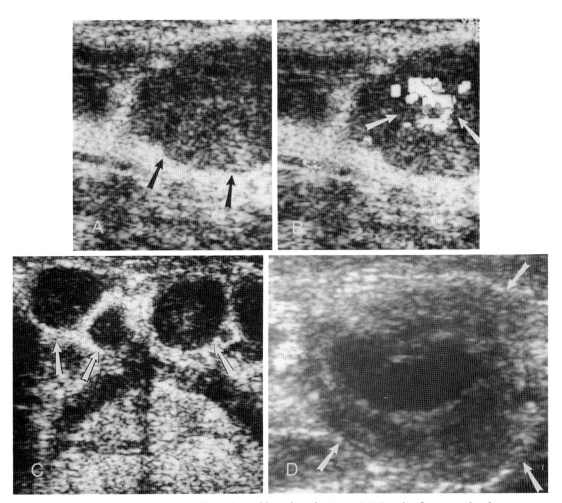

Figure 4.245. *Adenopathy.* (*A*) Note the enlarged lymph node *(arrow)*. (*B*) Color flow Doppler demonstrates exuberant blood flow *(arrow)* within the lymph node. (*C*) Another patient with multiple enlarged, relatively hypoechoic lymph nodes *(arrows)*. (*D*) Enlarged lymph node *(arrows)* with central hypoechoic suppuration. (Parts *A* and *B* from L.E. Swischuk, et al: Exuberant blood flow in enlarged lymph nodes: Findings on color flow Doppler. Pediatr. Radiol. 22: 419–421, 1992.

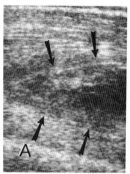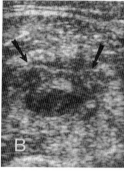

Figure 4.246. *Soft tissue hematoma.* (*A*) Note the heterogeneous texture of the hematoma *(arrows)* dissecting in between muscle planes. (*B*) Cross-sectional view demonstrates the hematoma *(arrows)* with a liquifying relatively hypoechoic center.

nomenon and occurs both with inflammatory and tumoral adenopathy (9). Ultrasonographically, lymph nodes appear as oval to round, relatively hypoechoic structures. With suppuration, their centers become relatively hypoechoic (Fig. 4.245*D*).

Soft tissue hematomas also can be demonstrated with ultrasound. Initially, they produce an area of vague echogenicity, but later, as liquefaction of the hematoma occurs, central fluid collections can be seen (Fig. 4.246). Hematomas also can be demonstrated with CT and MR, but MR is more exquisite and informative.

REFERENCES

Battered Child Syndrome

1. Ablin, D.S., Greenspan, A., and Reinhart, M.A.: Pelvic injuries in child abuse. Pediatr. Radiol. 22: 454–457, 1992.
2. Akbarnia, B., Torg, J.S., Kirkpatrick, J., and Sussman, S.: Manifestations of the battered child syndrome. J. Bone Joint Surg. 56A: 1159–1166, 1974.
3. Beals, R.K., Tufts, E.: Fractured femur in infancy: The role of child abuse. J. Pediatr. Orthop. 3: 583–586, 1983.
4. Bergman, A.B., Larsen, R.M., and Mueller, B.A.: Changing spectrum of serious child abuse. Pediatrics 77: 113–116, 1986.
5. Caffey, J.: Multiple fractures in long bones of children suffering from chronic subdural hematoma. A.J.R. 56: 163–173, 1946.
6. Caffey, J.: Parent-infant traumatic stress syndrome (Caffey-Kempe syndrome, battered baby syndrome). First Annual Neuhauser Presidential Address of the Society for Pediatric Radiology. A.J.R. 114: 217–229, 1972.
7. Caffey, J.: The whiplash shaken infant syndrome: manual shaking by the extremities with whiplash-induced intracranial and intraocular bleedings, linked with residual permanent brain damage and mental retardation. Pediatrics 54: 396–403, 1974.
8. Dalton, H.J., Slovis, T., Helfer, R.E., Comstock, J., Schuerer, S., and Riolo, S.: Undiagnosed abuse in children younger than 3 years with femoral fracture. Am. J. Dis. Child. 144: 875–878, 1990.
9. Feldman, K.W., Brewer, D.K.: Child abuse, cardiopulmonary resuscitation and rib fractures. Pediatrics 73:339, 1984.
10. Haase, G.M., Ortiz, V.N., Sfakianakis, G.N., and Morse, T.S.: Value of radionuclide bone scanning in the early recognition of deliberate child abuse. J. Trauma 20: 873–875, 1980.
11. Jaspan, T., Narborough G., Punt, J.A.G., and Lowe, J.: Cerebral contusional tears as a marker of child abuse: Detection by cranial sonography. Pediatr. Radiol. 22: 237–245, 1992.
12. Kanter, R.K.: Retinal hemorrhage after cardiopulmonary resuscitation or child abuse. J. Pediatr. 108: 430–432, 1986.
13. Kempe, C.H., Silverman, F.N., Steel, B.F., Droegenmueller, W., and Silver, H.K.: Battered child syndrome. J.A.M.A. 181: 17–24, 1962.
14. King, J., Diefendorf, D., Apthorp, J., Negrete, V.F., and Carlson, M.: Analysis of 429 fractures in 189 battered children. J. Pediatr. Orthop. 8: 585–589, 1988.
15. Kleinman, P.K.: Diagnostic imaging in infant abuse. A.J.R. 155: 703–712, 1990.
16. Kleinman, P.K., Marks, S.C., Adams, V.: Factors affecting the visualization of anterior rib fractures in abused infants. Am. J. Roentgenol. 150: 635, 1987.
17. Kleinman, P.K., Marks, S.C., and Blackbourne, B.: The metaphyseal lesion in abused infants: A radiologic-histopathologic study. A.J.R. 146: 895–905, 1986.
18. Kleinman, P.K., and Zito, J.L.: Avulsion of the spinous processes caused by infant abuse. Radiology 151: 389–392, 1984.
19. Kogutt, M.S., Swischuk, L.E., and Fagan, C.J.: Patterns of injury and significance of uncommon fractures in the battered child syndrome. A.J.R. 121: 143–149, 1974.
20. Leventhal, J.M., Thomas, S.A., Rosenfield, N.S., and Markowitz, R.I.: Fractures in young children: Distinguishing child abuse from unintentional injuries. Am. J. Dis. Child. 147: 87–92, 1993.
21. Merten, D.F., Radkowski, M.A., and Leonidas, J.C.: The abused child: A radiological reappraisal. Radiology 146: 377–381, 1983.

22. Nimityongskul, P., and Anderson, L.D.: The likelihood of injuries when children fall out of bed. J. Pediatr. Orthop. 7: 184–186, 1987.
23. O'Neill, J., Jr., Meacham, W., Griffin, P., and Sawyers, J.: Patterns of injury in the battered child syndrome. J. Trauma 13: 332–339, 1973.
24. Radkowski, M.A., Merten, D.F., and Leonidas, J.C.: The abused child: Criteria for radiologic diagnosis. Radiographics 3: 262–297, 1983.
25. Reece, R.M.: Fatal child abuse and sudden infant death syndrome: A critical diagnostic decision. Pediatrics 91: 423–429, Feb. 1993.
26. Rivera, F.P., Kamitsuka, M.D., and Quan, L.: Injuries to children younger than one year of age. Pediatrics 81: 93–97, 1988.
27. Rosenberg, N.M., and Marino, D.: Frequency of suspected abuse/neglect in burn patients. Pediatr. Emerg. Care 5: 219–221, 1989.
28. Schweich, P., and Fleisher, G.: Rib fractures in children. Pediatr. Emerg. Care 1: 187–189, 1985.
29. Section on Radiology: Diagnostic imaging of child abuse. Pediatrics 87: 262–264, 1991.
30. Silverman, F.N.: Roentgen manifestations of unrecognized skeletal trauma in infants. A.J.R. 69: 413–427, 1953.
31. Sivit, C.J., Taylor, G.A., and Eichelberger, M.R.: Visceral injury in battered children: A changing perspective. Radiology 173: 659–661, 1989.
32. Sty, J.R., and Starshak, R.J.: The role of bone scintigraphy in the evaluation of the suspected abused child. Radiology 146: 369–375, 1983.
33. Thomas, S.A., Rosenfield, N.S., Leventhal, J.M., and Markowitz, R.I.: Long-bone fractures in young children: Distinguishing accidental injuries from child abuse. Pediatrics 88: 471–476, 1991.

Foreign Bodies in the Soft Tissues

1. Avner, J.R., and Baker, D.: Lacerations involving glass: The role of routine roentgenograms. Am. J. Dis. Child. 146: 600–602, 1992.
2. Barton, L.L., and Saied, K.R.: Thorn-induced arthritis. J. Pediatrics 93: 322–323, 1978.
3. Bauer, A.R., Jr., and Yutani, D.: Computed tomographic localization of wooden foreign bodies in children's extremities. Arch. Surg. 118: 1084–1086, 1983.
4. Borgia, C.A.: Unusual bone reaction to organic foreign body in hand. Clin. Orthop. 30: 188–192, 1963.
5. Bray, H., Stringer, D.A., Poskitt, K., Newman, D.E., and MacKenzie, W.G.: Maple tree knee: A unique foreign body—value of ultrasound and CT examination. Pediatr. Radiol. 21: 457–458, 1991.
6. Cahill, N., and King, J.D.: Palm thorn synovitis. J. Pediatr. Orthop. 4: 175–179, 1984.
7. deLacey, G., Evans, R., and Sandin, B.: How easy is it to see glass (and plastic) on radiographs? Br. J. Radiol. 58: 27–30, 1985.
8. Fornage, B.D., and Schernberg, F.L.: Sonographic diagnosis of foreign bodies of the distal extremities. A.J.R. 147: 567–569, 1986.
9. Gerle, R.D.: Thorn-induced pseudo-tumors of bone. Br. J. Radiol. 44: 642–645, 1971.
10. Gooding, G.A.W., Hardiman, T., Sumers, M., Stess, R., Graf, P., and Grunfeld, C.: Sonography of the hand and foot in foreign body detection. J. Ultrasound Med. 6: 441–447, 1987.
11. Maylahn, D.J.: Thorn-induced "tumors" of bone. J. Bone Joint Surg. 34A: 386–388, 1952.
12. Shiels, W.E.II, Babcock, D.S., Wilson, J.L., and Burch, R.A.: Localization and guided removal of soft-tissue foreign bodies with sonography. A.J.R. 155: 1277–1281, 1990.
13. Swischuk, L.E., Jorgenson, F., Jorgenson, A., and Capen, D.: Wooden splinter induced "pseudo-tumors" and "osteomyelitis-like lesions" of bone and soft tissue. A.J.R. 122: 176–179, 1974.
14. Tandberg, D.: Glass in hand and foot: Will X-ray film show it? J.A.M.A. 248: 1872–1874, 1982.
15. Weston, W.J.: Thorn and twig-induced pseudo-tumors of bone and soft tissues. Br. J. Radiol. 36: 323–326, 1963.
16. Yousefzadeh, D.K., and Jackson, J.R., Jr.: Organic foreign body reaction: Report of two cases of thorn-induced "granuloma" and review of literature. Skeletal Radiol. 3: 167–176, 1978.

Soft Tissue Infection

1. Broadfoot, E., and Chaitow, J.: Primary suppurative myositis. Australas. Radiol. 25: 175–176, 1981.
2. Fornage, B.D., Touche, D.H., Segal, P., and Rifkin, M.D.: Ultrasonography in the evaluation of muscular trauma. J. Ultrasound Med. 2: 549–554, 1983.
3. Gibson, R.K., Rosenthal, S.J., and Lukert, B.P.: Pyomyositis: Increasing recognition in temperate climates. Am. J. Med. 77: 768–772, 1984.
4. Grose, C.: Staphylococcal pyomyositis in south Texas. J. Pediatr. 93: 457–458, 1978.
5. Hernandez, R.J., Leim, D.R., Chenevert, T.L., Sullivan, D.B., and Aisen, A.M.: Fat-suppressed MR imaging of myositis. Radiology 182: 217–219, 1992.
6. Hirano, T., Srinivasan, G., Jamakiraman, N., Pleviak, D., and Mukhopadhyay, D.: Gallium-67 citrate scintigraphy in pyomyositis. J. Pediatr. 97: 596–598, 1980.
7. Sirinavin, S. and McCraken, G.H., Jr.: Primary supurative myositis in children. Am. J. Dis. Child. 133: 263–265, 1979.
8. Smith, H.L., II: Necrotizing lymphadenitis (Kikuchi's disease). Pediatrics 91: 152, 1993.

9. Swischuk, L.E., Desai, P.B., and John, S.D.: Exuberant blood flow in enlarged lymph nodes: Findings on color flow Doppler. Pediatr. Radiol. 22: 419–421, 1992.

10. Tang, J.S.H., Gold, R.H., Bassett, L.W., and Seeger, L.L.: Musculoskeletal infection of the extremities: Evaluation with MR imaging. Radiology 166: 205–209, 1988.

11. van Sonnenberg, E., Wittich, G.R., Casola, G., Cabrera, O.A., Gosink, B.B., and Resnick, D.L.: Sonography of thigh abscess: Detection, diagnosis, and drainage. A.J.R. 149: 769–772, 1987.

12. Yousefzadeh, D.K., Schumann, E.M., Mulligan, G.M., Bosworth, E.E., Young, C.S., and Pringle, K.C.: The role of imaging modalities in diagnosis and management of pyomyositis. Skeletal Radiol. 8: 285–289, 1982.

CHAPTER 5

The Head

HEAD TRAUMA

Trauma to the calvarium and intracranial structures is common in childhood, but roentgenographic examination of the skull in most cases is relatively unrewarding (1–5, 7, 12–15, 19). Indeed, it has been demonstrated that at most only about 25% of patients demonstrate skull fractures (7, 8, 11), and that most injuries are minor (6). For these reasons, the use of skull roentgenograms has decreased and has remained low for over a decade. This is, of course, appropriate, for it is intracranial injury and not the skull fracture per se that is most important. CT scans are best for demonstrating such injury, but at the same time are less effective in demonstrating overall fracture patterns (Fig. 5.1). This, however, is not so great a problem as most of these fractures usually can be seen on the preliminary topogram (Fig. 5.1*B*).

MR imaging also can be used to image intracranial problems (10, 17), but it is not as easily obtained and is not dependable in detecting fresh bleeding. It is most rewarding with chronic or subacute bleeds that are >3 days old (10, 17).

Indications for obtaining CT scans in patients with head injury, interestingly enough, are really no different from those utilized for obtaining skull films in the past (Table 5.1). These criteria parallel the Glasgow coma scale where a score of 12 or greater signifies the presence of a minor injury (9, 16, 18). However, some studies have demonstrated that even in cases where the Glasgow score is 12 or more, significant intracranial injury can still be present (16, 18). Therefore, final decisions will be individual and generally guided by the criteria outlined in Table 5.1. Suspected battered children are the one exception, where skull films for the detection of fractures still are important (Fig. 5.1*C* and *D*).

REFERENCES

1. Bell, R.S., and Loop, J.W.: The utility and futility of radiographic skull examination for trauma. N. Engl. J. Med. 284: 236–239, 1971.
2. Boulis, Z.F., Dick, R., and Barnes, N.R.: Head injuries in children—aetiology, symptoms, physical findings and x-ray wastage. Br. J. Radiol. 51: 851–845, 1978.
3. Cummins, R.O.: Clinician's reasons for overuse of skull radiographs. A.J.R. 135: 549–552, 1980.
4. de Lacey, G., Guilding, A., Wignall, B., Reidy, J., and Bradbrook, S.: Mild head injuries: A source of excessive radiography? Clin. Radiol. 31: 457–462, 1980.
5. DeSmet, A.A., Fryback, D.G., and Thornbury, J.R.: A second look at the utility of radiographic skull examination for trauma. A.J.R. 132: 95–97, 1979.
6. Duhaime, A.C., Alario, A.I., Lewander, W.J., Schut, L., Sutton, L.N., Seidel, T.S., Nudelman, S., Budenz, D., Hertle, R., Tsiaras, W., and Loporcio, S.: Head injury in very young children: Mechanisms, injury types, and ophthalmologic findings in 100 hospitalized patients younger than 2 years of age. Pediatrics 90: 179–185, 1992.
7. Harwood-Nash, D.C., Hendrick, E.B., and Hudson, A.R.: The significance of skull fractures in children: A study of 1,187 patients. Radiology 101: 151–155, 1971.
8. Hendrick, E.B., Harwood-Nash, D.C., and Hudson, A.R.: Head injuries in children: A survey of 4,465 consecutive cases at the Hospital for Sick Children, Toronto, Canada. Clin. Neurosurg. 11: 46–65, 1974.
9. Hennes, H., Lee, M., Smith, D., Sty, J.R., and Losek, J.: clinical predictors of severe head trauma in children. Am. J. Dis. Child. 142: 1045–1047, 1988.
10. Hesselink, J.R., Dowd, C.F., Healy, M.E., Hajek, P., Baker, L.L., and Luerssen, T.G.: MR imaging

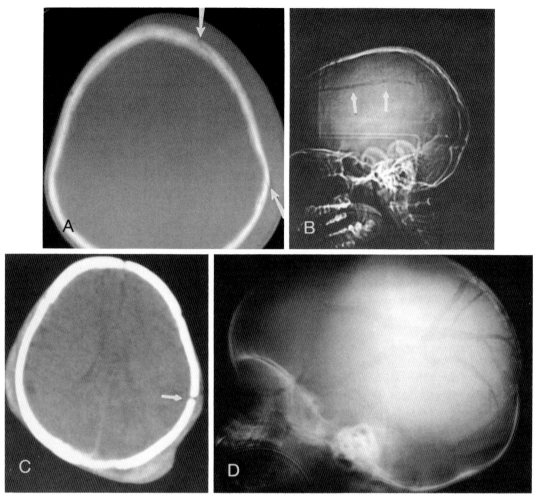

Figure 5.1. *Skull films and CT scans.* (*A*) On this CT scan, note subtle suggestion of a left parietal fracture (*arrows*). (*B*) Topogram more clearly delineates the fracture (*arrows*). (*C*) Another patient with brain edema and a left parietal fracture (*arrow*). Note extensive subcutaneous thickening due to numerous hematomas. This was a battered child. (*D*) Lateral view of the skull reveals the extensive degree of fracturing present. This is an eggshell fracture. In the battered child syndrome especially, it is important to obtain a combination of the two studies, that is, plain films and CT scan.

of brain contusions: A comparative study with CT. A.J.R. 150: 1133–1142, 1988.

11. Jamison, D.L., and Kay, H.H.: Accidental head injury in childhood. Arch. Dis. Child. 49: 376–381, 1974.

12. Jennett, B.: Skull x-rays after recent head injury. Clin. Radiol. 31: 463–469, 1980.

13. Leonidas, J.C., Ting, W., Binkiewiez, A., Vas, R., Scott, R.M., and Pauker, S.G.: Mild head trauma in children: When is a roentgenogram necessary? Pediatrics 69: 139–143, 1982.

14. Masters, S.J.: Evaluation of head trauma: Efficacy of skull films. A.J.R. 135: 539–547, 1980.

15. Newman, D.E.: Routine skull radiographs in children with seizures or head trauma. J. Can. Assoc. Radiol. 23: 234–235, 1977.

16. Rivara, F., Tanaguchi, D., Parish, R.A., Stimac, G.K., and Mueller, B.: Poor prediction of positive computed tomographic scans by clinical criteria in symptomatic pediatric head trauma. Pediatrics 80: 579–584, 1987.

17. Snow, R.B., Zimmerman, R.D., Gandy, S.E., and Deck, M.D.F.: Comparison of magnetic resonance imaging and computed tomography in the evaluation of head injury. Neurosurgery 18: 45–52, 1986.

Table 5.1
Clinical Findings Predisposing to CT Examination

History

- Age less than 1 year[a]
- Unconsciousness or amnesia of greater than 5-min duration
- Gunshot wound or skull penetration
- Focal neurologic symptoms

Physical Examination

- Focal neurologic or ocular signs
- Skull depression
- CSF discharge from ear or nose
- Blood in middle ear
- Battle's sign
- Blackeye (hematoma)
- Lethargy, coma, or stupor

[a]With more severe trauma only.

18. Stein, S.C., and Ross, S.E.: The value of computed tomographic scans in patients with low-risk head injuries. Neurosurgery 26: 638–640, 1990.

19. Thornbury, J.R., Campbell, J.A., Masters, S.J., and Fryback, D.G.: Skull fracture and the low risk of intracranial sequelae in minor head trauma. A.J.R. 143: 661–664, 1984.

Which Skull Views Should Be Obtained? Skull films certainly are not obtained as often as they were in the past, but still it is important to know which ones to obtain when they are necessary. Generally speaking, both lateral, a posteroanterior, and Towne's views suffice. In addition, if facial injuries are being assessed, the Water's view should be included. In most instances, there is little reason to obtain a base of the skull view, but in some cases special tangential or oblique views may be necessary to fully visualize a suspected fracture. *In the patient who is not alert or in the patient in whom a neck injury also is suspected, one should confine the initial calvarial study to cross-table lateral, anteroposterior, and Towne's views; all should be obtained without moving the patient.*

Importance of Site and Type of Fracture. Much more important than the mere detection of a fracture is the determination of the type and site of the fracture. For example, compound skull fractures and fractures through air-filled structures such as the paranasal sinuses and mastoid air cells are important because they can lead to complications such as meningitis, pneumocephalus (1, 3), and cerebrospinal fluid leaks. Depressed fractures are clearly important and place the patient into a markedly higher risk category. Most of these fractures require elevation and repair of underlying dural tears, and associated brain damage and long-lasting complications such as focal seizures are a definite additional problem. Multiple calvarial fractures (eggshell fractures) such as might be sustained in automobile accidents or from falls on the head from great heights are of obvious significance and, likewise, linear fractures traversing vascular structures such as the middle meningeal artery and deep venous sinuses are more significant than the same linear fractures not traversing these sites. Base of skull fractures also are generally considered more significant fractures, for they tend to extend into the mastoid air cells, sphenoid sinus, cribriform plate, ethmoid sinuses, nasal cavity, or foramen magnum.

Can One Predict the Site and Type of Fracture from the Site and Type of Injury? There is usually good correlation of the site of fracture with the site of injury, for the contrecoup phenomenon associated with brain injury is not applicable to calvarial fractures. To restate this: if trauma occurs over the forehead, then the fracture is most likely to be in this location. Furthermore, if the blow is delivered with a small, high-velocity object such as a baseball bat, hammer, or dashboard knob, the fracture usually lies immediately below the point of impact (Fig. 5.2A). On the other hand, if the blow is delivered by a broad surface, high-velocity object such as the flat surface of a door, floor, or windshield, the fracture may be somewhat removed from the center of impact (Fig. 5.2B). The same general information is useful in predicting the actual type of fracture present. For example,

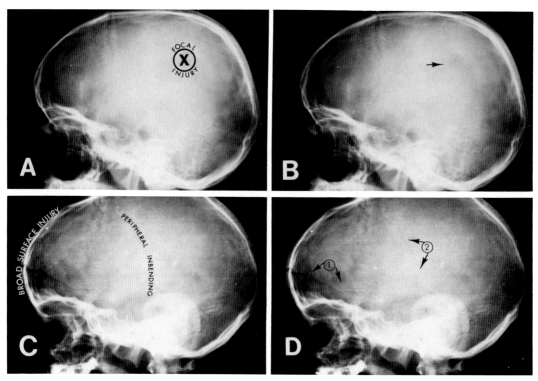

Figure 5.2. *Fracture mechanics.* (*A* and *B*) Focal injury. High velocity focal injury results in dissipation of forces over a small area (*X*). The resulting fracture is a small, stellate depressed fracture (*arrow*). (*C* and *D*) Broad surface injury. High-velocity broad surface injury results in a central, diastatic, V-shaped fracture (*1*), and a more peripheral curvilinear arc-like fracture at the zone of peripheral inbending (*2*).

in the first instance, when a small, high-velocity object delivers the blow, the fracture often is focally depressed, while in the other instance, linear or broad curvilinear fractures result (Fig. 5.2*C* and *D*). All of these considerations are important in the assessment of calvarial fractures, and the specific types of fractures produced are dealt with in later sections.

How Important Is the Mode of Injury? The mode of injury is most important, especially in the battered child syndrome, for often it leads to information regarding severity of injury. For example, an infant falling backward and striking his occiput on a well-cushioned floor represents a problem very different from that of an infant falling backward on a concrete floor, sidewalk, or the edge of a sink or bathtub. Clearly, one would not expect a fracture in

the first instance, but in the latter case, the possibility of calvarial fracturing is much greater. Consequently, it is most important to determine just how the patient was injured, for it may foretell the type and site of fracture.

Types of Fractures Seen. As stated earlier, the type of fracture depends on the mode of injury, but generally speaking, one can encounter linear, curvilinear, stellate, eggshell, depressed, and diastatic sutural fractures. *Linear fractures* are perhaps the most common type of fracture encountered. Many of these are hairline fractures (Fig. 5.3*A*), and some may be more difficult to see on one view than another. When linear fractures result from greater forces, they often spread at the end closest to the point of impact, and the fracture assumes a V-shaped configuration

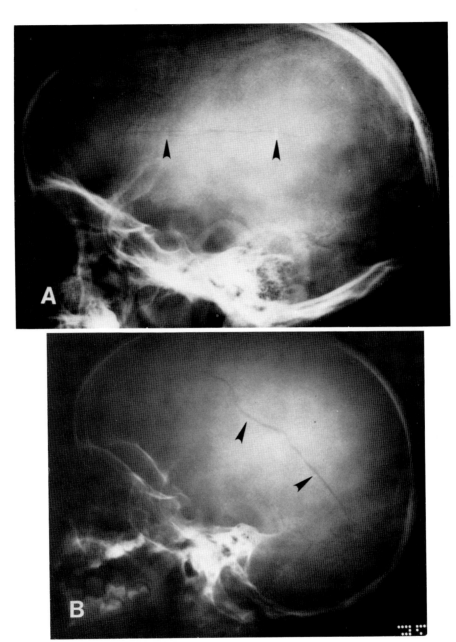

Figure 5.3. *Linear fractures.* (**A**) Hairline linear fracture (*arrows*) crossing middle meningeal artery area anteriorly. (**B**) Slightly diastatic linear fracture (*arrows*). Note that the fracture is wider in the center than at either end, and note that the fracture stops at the coronal and lambdoid sutures.

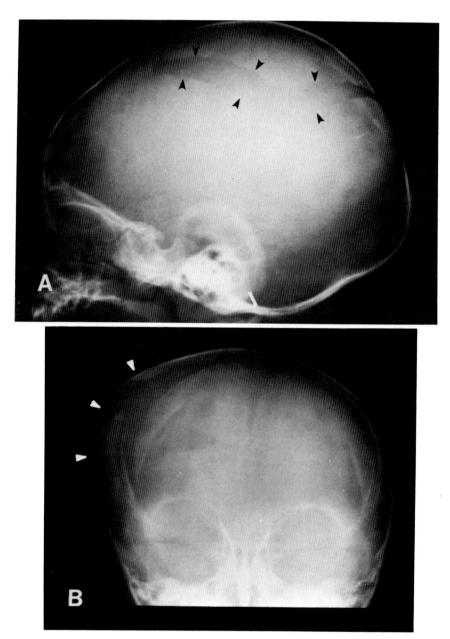

Figure 5.4. *Widely diastatic linear fracture.*   (*A*) Note the widely diastatic fracture (*arrows*) on this lateral view. (*B*) Frontal view demonstrating how the bone edges have been displaced outwardly and how the cranial contents bulge outward (*arrows*).

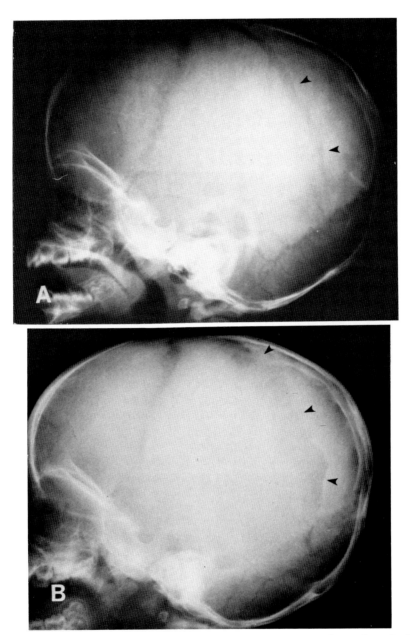

Figure 5.5. *Diastatic fracture with subsequent leptomeningeal cyst.* (*A*) Note the moderately diastatic linear fracture of the parietal bone (*arrows*). (*B*) Months later note how the fracture has grown, and how its edges have become scalloped (*arrows*). These findings are characteristic of a leptomeningeal cyst.

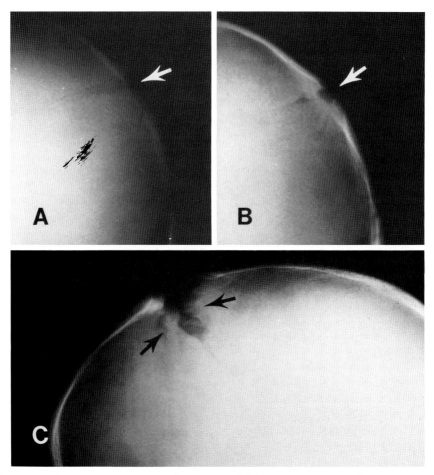

Figure 5.6. *Leptomeningeal cysts, varying configurations.* (*A*) Note initial fracture (*arrow*). (*B*) Months later, note a small leptomeningeal cyst (*arrow*). (*C*) Large leptomeningeal cyst (*arrows*). (Part *C* courtesy of Virgil Graves, M.D.)

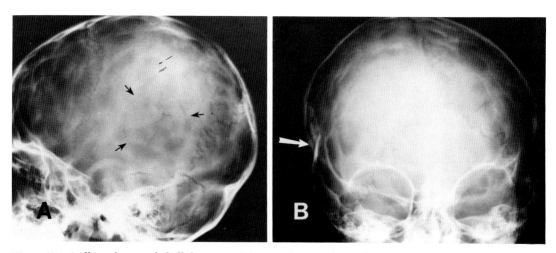

Figure 5.7. *Stellate, depressed skull fracture.* (*A*) Note the round peripheral zone of inbending producing a complete circle (*arrows*). Also note stellate fractures radiating outward from the center of the circle. (*B*) Frontal view. Note degree of depression of the central fragments (*arrow*).

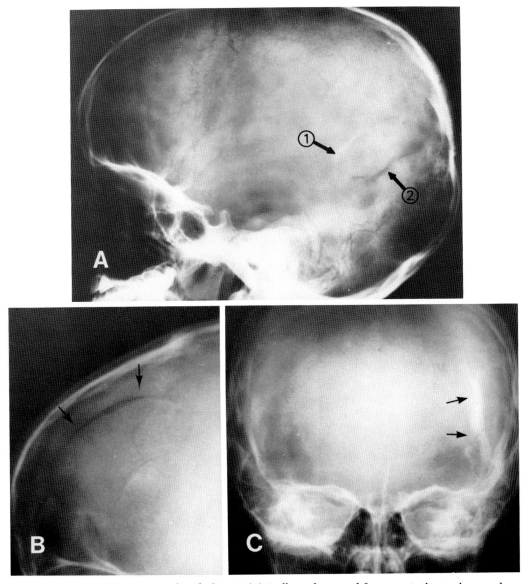

Figure 5.8. *Depressed fractures—other findings.* (*A*) Stellate, depressed fracture similar to the one demonstrated in Figure 5.7. Note the area of increased sclerosis due to overlapping of the bony fragments (*1*), and the radiolucent, diastatic portion (*2*) of this circular, depressed fracture. Also note the typical, diastatic, central stellate limbs of the fracture. (*B*) Note the curvilinear frontal bone fracture (*arrows*) and that it is wider in the center than at either end. This denotes depression. (*C*) Frontal view demonstrating the profound degree of depression of the central fragment (*arrows*). The degree of depression is not suspected from the lateral view in *B*.

(Fig. 5.3*B*). Another interesting feature of these fractures is that they usually do not cross sutures (Fig. 5.3*B*).

Linear fractures that are not widely diastatic are not a cause for alarm unless they: (a) cross a critical area such as the middle meningeal artery groove or the deep venous sinuses, or (b) extend into the paranasal sinuses or mastoid air cells. When they cross a vascular structure, intracranial bleeding can be a problem, and when they extend into the paranasal sinuses or mastoid air cells, meningitis can be a complication. If linear fractures are widely diastatic (Fig. 5.4), they often are associated with underlying dural or meningeal tears, subdural hematomas, or cerebral injury. In those cases where a dural tear only occurs, the leptomeninges may herniate through the tear and cause the fracture to become progressively wider. This often is termed the *growing fracture* and eventually the bulging, pulsating leptomeningeal sac causes calvarial erosion and a round or oval, scalloped calvarial defect around a *leptomeningeal cyst* (2) (Figs. 5.5 and 5.6).

Broad, curvilinear fractures, that is, fractures with a broad, peripheral arc, usually result from high-velocity, broad surface injuries, and the curvilinear arc-like portion of the fracture outlines the peripheral-most points of bony inbending. In many cases, these peripheral curvilinear fractures are associated with linear fractures originating from the point of impact (see Fig. 5.2*B*). *Stellate fractures* are classic examples of such a fracture in that the fracture lines radiate from the center of impact, and circumferentially a peripheral arc demarcates the zones of maximal inbending. Stellate fractures usually are depressed (Fig. 5.7).

With *depressed fractures*, the injury usually results from: (a) high velocity impacts dissipating their forces over a relatively small area of the skull (i.e., injuries sustained from baseball bats, hammers, dashboard knobs, etc.), and (b) high-velocity broad surface blows. In those cases where the impact site is over a small area, a relatively small stellate-peripheral arc type of fracture results (Fig. 5.7*A*). Very often these fractures are visualized better on one view than the other, and tangential views are required for adequate evaluation of the degree of depression (Fig. 5.7*B*). When seen *en face*, sclerosis along the edge of one of the fracture fragments, undue widening of the space between two fracture fragments or disproportionate widening of the peripheral arc portion of the fracture can serve to alert one to the presence of the depressed element of these fractures (Fig. 5.8). Nonetheless, it cannot be overstated that depressed fractures can be most elusive on the *en face* view, and in such cases, one must learn to suspect the slightest degree of sclerosis, disproportionate radiolucency, etc., and then to pursue these findings with tangential views (Fig. 5.9). Of course, currently CT scans usually are obtained for the delineation of these fractures (Fig. 5.10) and tangential views then become superfluous.

With depressed fractures resulting from broad area injuries, the stellate peripheral arc appearance is replaced by irregular rectangular- or triangular-shaped bony fragments seen at various angles (Fig. 5.11). Because these fragments are rotated and titled, one or more may appear unduly sclerotic, or, once again, one side of a fragment will be sclerotic (overlap) while the other is wide and radiolucent (diastasis). The most common normal finding to be misinterpreted as a depressed fracture is a normal inner table convolutional marking. This can occur anywhere over the calvarium (Fig. 5.12).

Diastatic Sutural Fractures. Diastatic sutural fractures can occur in isolated form or in association with a linear fracture. In these latter cases, the fracture often runs directly into the suture (Fig. 5.13). Diastatic sutural fractures can involve any suture but are especially prone to occur in the posterior fossa where unilateral sutural

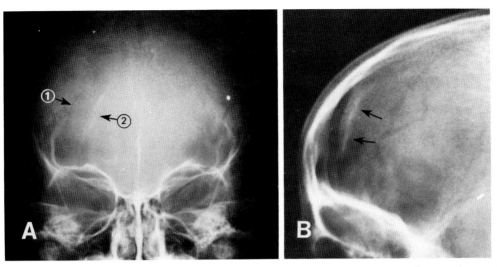

Figure 5.9. *Depressed fracture—subtle findings.* (**A**) Once again, note the combination of a central vertical radiolucent line (*1*) and a vertical area of increased sclerosis just medial to it (*2*). These findings represent a depressed fracture. (**B**) Lateral, tangential view more clearly demonstrates the depressed fracture fragment (*arrows*).

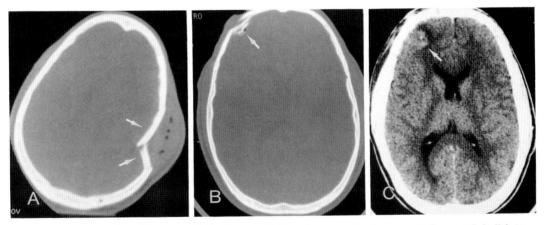

Figure 5.10. *Depressed skull fracture: CT findings.* (**A**) Note the markedly depressed left parietal skull fracture (*arrows*). There is a subcutaneous hematoma present with a few bubbles of air within it. (**B**) Another patient with a focally depressed right frontal fracture (*arrow*). There is a small bubble of air along the inner table representing a mild degree of pneumocephalus. (**C**) Same patient demonstrating an underlying contusion (*arrow*).

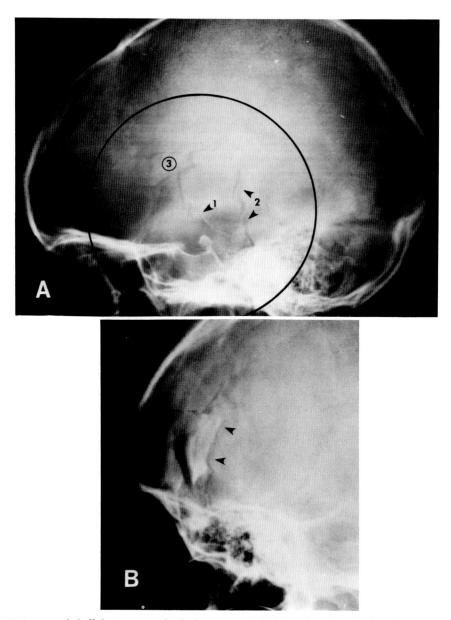

Figure 5.11. *Depressed skull fracture—multiple fragments.* (**A**) **A** broad surface, high-velocity injury has resulted in a mosaic pattern of depressed fracture fragments (*large circle*). Note linear sclerosis due to overlapping (*1*), diastasis due to depression (*2*), and a generalized increase in density of one of the fragments due to depression and tangential positioning (*3*). (**B**) Tangential view demonstrating the degree of depression of one of the fragments (*arrows*). Depression of this fragment causes the fracture to appear wide and radiolucent.

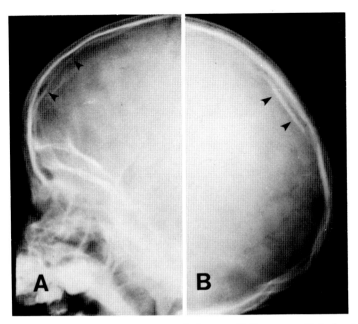

Figure 5.12. (*A* and *B*) *Inner table convolutions—"pseudodepressed" fractures.* Note frontal and posterior parietal inner table sclerosis mimicking fracture fragment depression (*arrows*).

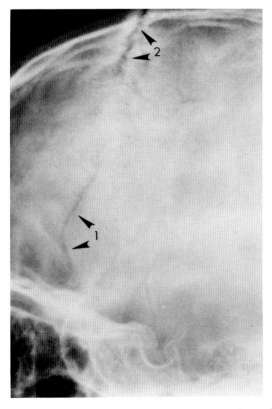

Figure 5.13. *Fracture causing diastasis of suture.* Note the fracture (*1*) in the lower frontal parietal region. Then note the associated spread (diastasis) of the ipsilateral coronal suture (*2*). The radiolucent line above the sella is the normal groove of the middle meningeal artery.

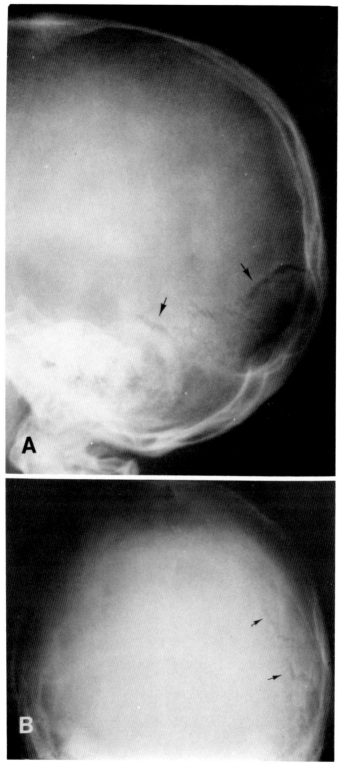

Figure 5.14. *Unilateral posterior fossa suture diastasis.* (A) Note unilateral diastasis of the lambdoid and parietomastoid sutures (*arrows*). (B) Towne's projection confirms unilateral spreading of these sutures (*arrows*). No fracture, however, is present.

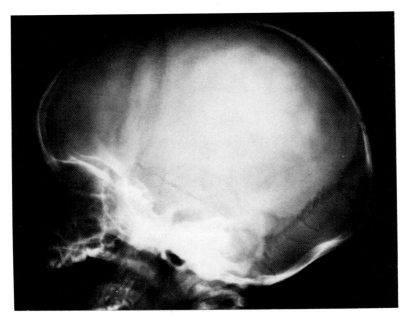

Figure 5.15. *Generalized suture diastasis.*   This infant suffered a blow to the head. No fractures were detected, but all of the sutures showed moderate spreading. The linear lines extending posteriorly from the lambdoid and occipitomastoid sutures are normal Mendosal and other accessory sutures. They are not fractures.

spread can serve to alert one to the presence of underlying intracranial injury (Fig. 5.14). *Generalized sutural diastasis* in the young infant or child with a closed head injury is a common problem and can occur with or without associated fracturing of the calvarium (Fig. 5.15). In explaining this phenomenon, it is most likely that the sutures spread because of an associated acute increase in cerebral mass due to post-traumatic hyperemia. Indeed, this has been shown to be the most common intracranial manifestation of head trauma in childhood (4). Of course, generalized sutural diastasis also can be seen with other intracranial space-occupying problems such as subdural or epidural hematomas, but spread because of post-traumatic hyperemia alone is more common.

Finally, a few comments on the so-called *"eggshell fracture" of the calvarium* are in order. This fracture presents a startling roentgenographic picture (Fig. 5.16A and B) and, obviously, in most of these cases the fracture is not a surprise.

However, there is one practical aspect to these fractures, and that is that they should not be confused with similar roentgenographic findings in normal infants with numerous intraparietal accessory sutures (Fig. 5.16C and D). With these latter patients, there often is discrepancy between the clinical history and the apparent extent of calvarial fracturing. However, roentgenographic differentiation often still is a problem, but it is of some assistance to note that multiple intraparietal accessory sutures usually are very symmetric (Fig. 5.16D).

When Should Follow-up Films be Obtained?   Generally speaking, the mere presence of a linear fracture does not mandate a follow-up roentgenogram. However, widely diastatic fractures or even mildly diastatic fractures should be followed up with repeat roentgenograms a few weeks or months later. The reason for this is to check for the development of a post-traumatic leptomeningeal cyst (see Fig. 5.6). Of course, these cysts often are

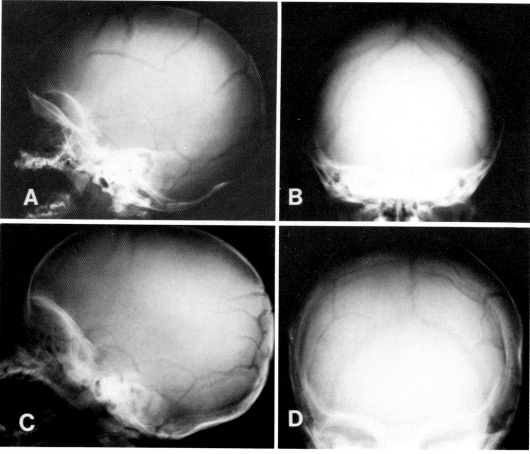

Figure 5.16. *Eggshell fracture versus multiple intraparietal fissures.* (*A* and *B*) Eggshell fracture. On the lateral view, note the numerous, moderately diastatic fractures and generalized spreading of the sutures. On frontal view, note asymmetry of the fractures. (*C* and *D*) Multiple intraparietal fissures. Note fracture-like appearance of the numerous intraparietal fissures on lateral view. On frontal view, note how symmetric these accessory fissures are.

first suspected clinically (i.e., soft, pulsatile, bulge is palpable), but before such a cyst becomes palpable, the radiologist often will be able to detect that the fracture is spreading.

REFERENCES

1. Bhimani, S., Virapongse, C., Sabshin, J.K., Sarwar, M., and Paterson, R.H., Jr.: Intracerebral pneumatocele: CT findings. Radiology 154: 111–114, 1985.
2. Genieser, N., and Becker, M.: Head trauma in children. Radiol. Clin. North Am. 12: 333 342, 1974.
3. Mendelsohn, D.B., and Hertzanu, Y.: Intracere-

bral pneumatoceles following facial trauma: CT findings. Radiology 154: 115 118, 1985.
4. Zimmerman, R.A., Bilaniuk, L.T., Bruce, D., Dolinskas, C., Obrist, W., and Kuhl, D.: Computed tomography of pediatric head trauma: Acute general cerebral swelling. Radiology 126: 403–408, 1978.

Intracranial Manifestations of Head Injuries. Intracranial manifestations of head injuries are numerous and consist of acute epidural hematomas, acute subdural hematomas, vascular lacerations and aneurysms, cerebral contusions, intracere-

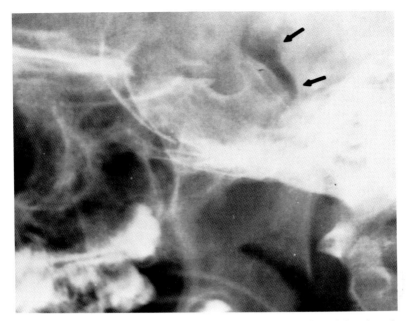

Figure 5.17. *Traumatic pneumocephalus.* Note air in the basal cistern (*arrows*), and that the sphenoid sinus has been obliterated by blood. Also note disruption of the base of the skull just anterior to the anterior clinoids and unilateral depression of one of the anterior fossa floors.

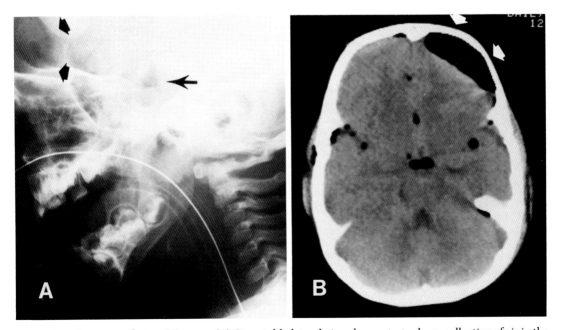

Figure 5.18. *Intracranial air—CT scan.* (*A*) Cross-table lateral view demonstrates large collection of air in the frontal region (*anterior arrows*). Air also is seen in the middle fossa (*single arrow*). (*B*) CT scan study more vividly demonstrates the large collection of air over the frontal region (*arrows*) and scattered throughout the ealvarium.

bral bleeds, focal or generalized cerebral edema, and traumatic pneumocephalus (1, 9, 13). Traumatic pneumocephalus can be seen on plain films (Fig. 5.17), but is more clearly visualized on CT scans (Fig. 5.18). Indeed, CT scanning is the main imaging modality for the evaluation of any intracranial injury (2, 4, 6, 14, 15, 20). MRI also can be used but is not as useful in the early stages, because it does not detect fresh blood (11). Overall, CT scanning is the preferred modality, and it also is excellent for detecting occult intracranial damage in the battered child syndrome (3, 7, 8, 18, 19). In addition, it is very useful in demonstrating the phenomenon of the contrecoup injury. In these cases, while the blow to the head is sustained on one side, cerebral contusion and hemorrhage occur on the side directly opposite (Fig. 5.19). CT scanning, of course, also is excellent in delineating subdural, epidural, intracerebral, and subarachnoid bleeding (Fig. 5.20). Subarachnoid bleeding is characterized by an increase in density along the falx and tentorium (5). A similar appearance can be seen with the normal falx if there is pronounced cerebral edema. In these cases

the brain becomes hypodense and the falx is seen in relief. With subarachnoid bleeding the cerebral tissue usually has normal density and it is important to appreciate a subtle scalloped appearance of the dense falx (Fig. 5.21). Scalloping results from blood creeping into the neighboring sulci. Similar collections of blood can be seen in the sylvian fissures and occasionally around the brainstem.

Brain edema, with resultant intracranial pressure, manifests in loss of the sulci and decrease in ventricular size (Fig. 5.22). However, it is decrease in third ventricular size and obliteration of the basal cisterns (Fig. 5.22) which is most important in detecting early brain edema (17). It is important to appreciate these early findings of brain edema, for they may be the first findings to herald impending brainstem herniation (17).

In terms of *subdural hematomas, it should be remembered that midway through their course they may appear isodense on CT studies,* and under such circumstances may be missed unless one notices other findings such as ipsilateral ventricular compression and shift of the

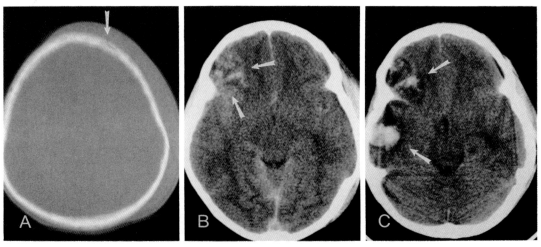

Figure 5.19. *Contrecoup injury.* (**A**) Note extensive edema of the scalp on the left and an underlying fracture (*arrow*). (**B**) Focal area of contusion and bleeding in the right frontal region (*arrows*). There is slight contralateral midline shift, representing a contrecoup injury. (**C**) The next day evidence that bleeding and edema are more extensive is apparent throughout the frontal and temporal lobes (*arrows*).

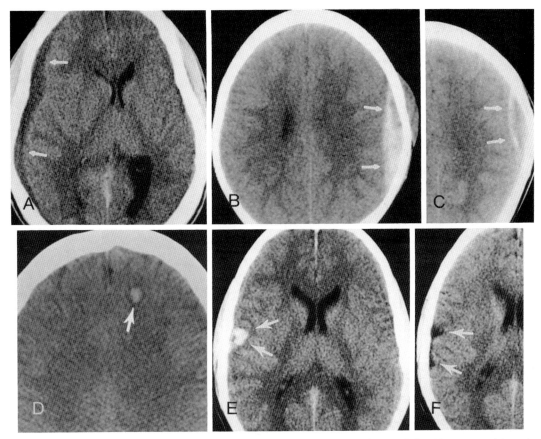

Figure 5.20. *Intracranial manifestations of head injury.*   (*A*) Note the hypodense subdural hematoma (*arrows*). There is ipsilateral compression of the ventricles and contralateral midline shift. (*B*) Epidural bleed (*arrows*) with some soft tissue swelling of the scalp. (*C*) A slightly higher cut demonstrates the more characteristic elliptical appearance of the epidural bleed. (*D*) Focal small parenchymal bleed (*arrow*). (*E*) Another patient with a focal parenchymal bleed (*arrows*). (*F*) Later gliosis is seen in the region (*arrows*).

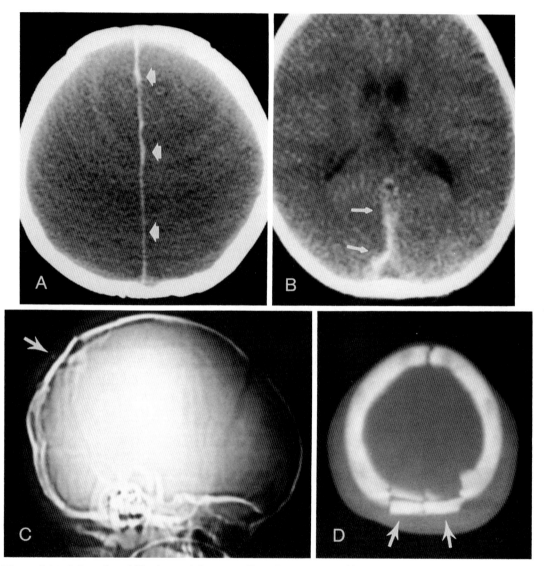

Figure 5.21. *Subarachnoid bleeding.* (*A*) Note scalloped appearance of blood along the falx (*arrows*). (*B*) Another patient with bleeding along the posterior falx. Brain edema also is present. (*C*) Same patient demonstrating a fracture fragment over the posterior parietal occipital region (*arrow*). (*D*) CT scan through the upper calvarium demonstrates the comminuted posterior parietal fracture (*arrows*).

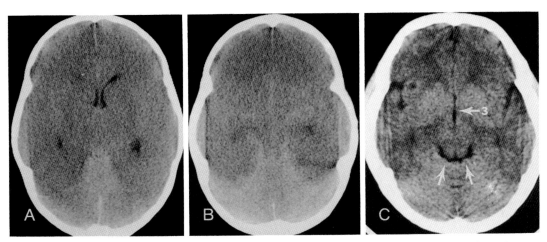

Figure 5.22. *Brain edema.* (*A*) Pronounced cerebral edema in this patient results in the absence of visualization of the various gyri and sulci. Furthermore, the lateral ventricles are markedly compressed and there is no visualization of the third ventricle. The posterior fossa contents remain opaque, while the supratentorial portion of the brain is hypodense (edema). This is characteristic of cerebral edema. (*B*) A slightly lower slice demonstrates the same findings. There is no visualization of the third ventricle or of the quadrigeminal plate cistern. (*C*) Normal patient for comparison with a CT slice at about the same level as that demonstrated in *B* demonstrates the normal appearance of the third ventricle (3) and the quadrigeminal plate cistern (*lower arrows*).

midline structures. Of course, if the subdurals are bilateral, such shift may not be present. Rapid, high-dose contrast CT scanning has been suggested as a method useful in circumventing this problem (10). Isodense subdural hematomas also are a problem in anemic patients, in whom the decreased iron content of the blood is the cause of the problem (16).

Finally, as has been noted earlier, the CT scan is excellent in detecting intracranial injury in the battered child syndrome. Such injury may be massive or may appear much the same as intracranial injuries sustained in other ways. However, it has come to light that when so-called "white-gray matter interface tears," resulting in small foci of increased density (12), are seen, they should be considered highly suspicious for the battered child syndrome (see Fig. 4.228). It is believed that such tears are sustained from violent shaking of the child, much as are subdural hematomas and retinal hemorrhages.

REFERENCES

1. Arkins, T.J., McLennan, J.E., Winston, K.R., Strand, R.D., and Suzuki, Y.: Acute posterior fossa epidural hematomas in children. Am. J. Dis. Child. 131: 690–692, 1977.
2. Bruce, D.A., and Schut, L.: The value of CT scanning following pediatric head injury. Clin. Pediatr. 19: 719–725, 1980.
3. Caffey, J.: The whiplash shaken infant syndrome: Manual shaking by the extremities with whiplash-induced intracranial and intraocular bleedings, linked with residual permanent brain damage and mental retardation. Pediatrics 54: 396–403, 1974.
4. Cohen, R.A., Kaufman, R.A., Myers, P.A., and Towbin, R.B.: Cranial computed tomography in the abused child with head injury. A.J.R. 146: 97–102, 1986.
5. Dolinskas, C.A., Zimmerman, R.A., and Bilaniuk, L.T.: A sign of subarachnoid bleeding on cranial computed tomograms of pediatric head trauma patients. Radiology, 126: 409–411, 1978.
6. Dublin, A.B., French, B.N., and Rennick, J.M.: Computed tomography in head trauma. Radiology 122: 365–370, 1977.
7. Ellison, P.H., Tsai, F.Y., and Largent, J.A.: Computed tomography in child abuse and cerebral contusion. Pediatrics 62: 151–154, 1978.
8. Guthkelch, A.N.: Infantile subdural hematoma and its relationship to whiplash injuries. Br. Med. J. 2: 430–431, 1971.
9. Harwood-Nash, D.C.: Craniocerebral trauma in children. Curr. Probl. Radiol. 3: 3–24, 1973.
10. Hayman, L.A., Evans, R.A., and Hinck, V.C.: Rapid-high-dose contrast computed tomography

of isodense subdural hematoma and cerebral swelling. Radiology 131: 381–383, 1979.

11. Hayman, L.A., Pagani, J.J., Kirkpatrick, J.B., and Hinck, V.C.: Pathophysiology of acute intracerebral and subarachnoid hemorrhage: Applications to MR imaging. A.J.R. 153: 135–139, 1989.

12. Jaspan, T., Narborough, G., Punt, J.A.G., and Lowe, J.: Cerebral contusional tears as a marker of child abuse-detection by cranial sonography. Pediatr. Radiol. 22: 237–245, 1992.

13. Kahn, R.J., and Daywitt, A.L.: Traumatic pneumocephalus. A.J.R. 90: 1171–1175, 1963.

14. Koo, A.H., and LaRoque, R.L.: Evaluation of the head trauma by computed tomography. Radiology 123: 345–350, 1977.

15. Merino-deVillasante, J., and Taveras, J.M.: Computerized tomography (CT) in acute head trauma. A.J.R. 126: 765 778, 1976.

16. Smith, W.P., Jr., Batnitzky, S., and Rengachary, S.S.: Acute isodense subdural hematomas: A problem in anemic patients. A.J.R. 136: 543–546, 1981.

17. Teasdale, E., Cardoso, E., and Galbraith, S.: CT scan in severe diffuse head injury: Physiological and clinical correlations. J. Neurol. Neurosurg. Psychiatry 47: 600–603, 1984.

18. Touddry, M., LeFrancois, M.C., LeMarc, B., Gandon, Y., Carsin, M., and Senecal, J.: Computed tomography of the skull on the battered child. Ann. Radiol. 25: 237–243, 1982.

19. Tsai, F.Y., Zee, C.-S., Apthrop, J.S., and Dixon, G.H.: Computed tomography in child abuse head trauma. Comput. Tomogr. 4: 277–286, 1980.

20. Zimmerman, R.A., Bilaniuk, L.T., Gennarelli, T., Bruce, D., Dolinskas, C., and Uzzell, B.: Cranial computed tomography in diagnosis and management of acute head trauma. A.J.R. 131: 27–34, 1978.

BASAL SKULL FRACTURES

Fractures through the base of the skull often are most difficult to detect roentgenographically. Clinically, they can be suspected when nasal discharge of cerebral spinal fluid is present, when there is bleeding from the ear, or when there is blood behind the eardrum. Roentgenographically, when looking for these fractures it is best to divide the skull into three zones: (a) the anterior fossa, (b) the middle fossa, and (c) the posterior fossa. Fractures through the *floor of the anterior fossa* frequently involve the orbital roof and are best visualized on frontal views. In such cases, discontinuity of the cortex of the roof of the orbit, a clearly visible fracture line, or a depressed orbital fracture fragment usually alerts one to the problem (Fig. 5.23). CT scans, in some cases, can considerably augment the data obtained regarding these fractures (Fig. 5.24). In other instances, air may be present in the orbit (i.e., from the

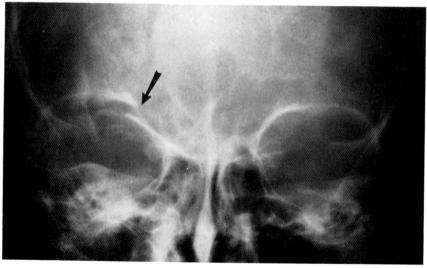

Figure 5.23. *Anterior fossa floor fracture—frontal view.* Note depressed supraorbital (anterior fossa floor) fracture (*arrow*).

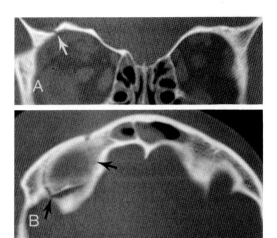

Figure 5.24. *Anterior fossa floor fracture—CT visualization.* (**A**) Note the supraorbital rim fracture (*arrow*). (**B**) Axial view demonstrates the fracture fragment (*arrows*) as it involves the upper wall of the orbit. Blood is seen in the frontal sinuses.

adjacent paranasal sinuses), or opacification of, or an air-fluid level in the adjacent paranasal sinuses may be noted. On lateral view, these fractures can be seen to extend through the cribriform plate into the ethmoid sinuses (Fig. 5.25*A* and *B*), but they are not always easy to detect. Furthermore, they must be differentiated from the normal, unfused planum sphenoidal (4), a commonly occurring "pseudofracture" in this area (Fig. 5.25*C*).

Fractures through the *floor of the middle fossa* also frequently are best visualized on frontal projection, but of course also are visible on lateral view. Many of these fractures also extend into the region of the sella turcica (1, 2), and one may see complete disruption of the sella, fracturing through the various sellar structures, or an

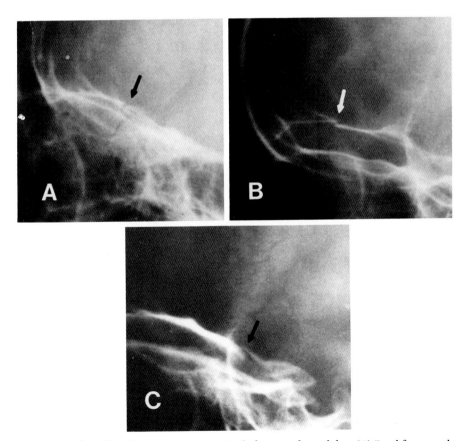

Figure 5.25. *Anterior fossa floor fracture versus ununited planum sphenoidale.* (**A**) Basal fracture through anterior fossa floor. Note the irregular radiolucent fracture (*arrow*) extending into the ethmoid sinus. (**B**) Another basal fracture (*arrow*). (**C**) Normal defect (*arrow*) due to unfused planum sphenoidale.

Figure 5.26. *Middle fossa basal fractures.* (**A**) Injured patient demonstrating a barely discernable fracture extending to the base of the skull (*arrow*). (**B**) Indirect evidence of a basal fracture extending into the sphenoid sinus is present in this patient in the form of an air-fluid level in the sphenoid sinus (*arrows*). This was a cross-table lateral view with the face pointing upward.

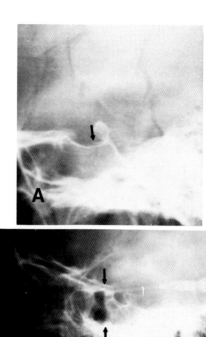

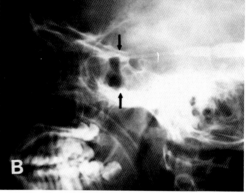

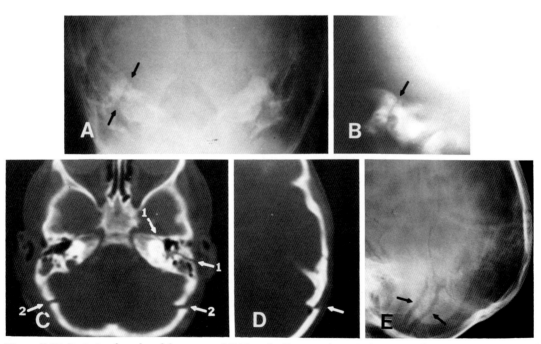

Figure 5.27. *Posterior fossa basal fractures.* (**A**) Note the fracture through the petrous bone on the right. Note also that the mastoid air cells are hazy due to bleeding. (**B**) Tomogram demonstrates the fracture to better advantage (*arrow*). (**C**) CT study in another patient demonstrates a basal fracture (*1*) and bilateral occipitomastoid sutural diastatic fractures (*2*). The one on the right is offset. Also note that both mastoid air cells are hazy due to bleeding. Another fracture was present on the other side, on another cut. (**D**) Slightly higher cut demonstrates a small bubble of air under the right occipitomastoid fracture (*arrow*). (**E**) X-ray demonstrates numerous occipital fractures and the bilateral occipitomastoid suture diastatic fractures (*arrows*).

air-fluid level in the sphenoid sinus (Fig. 5.26). The air-fluid levels, of course, usually are visualized on cross-table lateral views of the skull or axial CT scans, and the fluid represents blood in the sphenoid sinuses. If air from the sphenoid sinuses escapes into the calvarium, one may see air in the basal cisterns (see Fig. 5.17).

Fractures through the *posterior fossa floor* involve the temporal bone and may be associated with hearing and equilibrium problems (3). In some cases one can clearly see the linear fracture extending through the temporal bone (Fig. 5.27), but in other cases one first is alerted to the problem by the presence of unilateral opacification of the mastoid air cells only. Obliteration of the mastoid air cells is due to bleeding, and even if a fracture is not visible, the presence of such obliteration should cause one to assume that an occult fracture is present. Thereafter, clinical correlation will determine whether opacification is in fact due to acute bleeding or to the inflammatory changes of coincidental mastoid and middle ear infection. This, of course, is very important, for middle ear infections, with mastoid involvement, are common in children. Consequently, if one does not take the time to determine whether opacification of the air cells truly is due to bleeding, one could overdiagnose these injuries. Fractures through the tympanic portion of the temporal bone or, for that matter, any fracture through the temporal bone, usually are best detected with CT scanning (Fig. 5.27C and D).

The other common fracture of the base of the skull in the posterior fossa is the vertical occipital bone fracture. Most often these fractures are midline, but they may be set off to one side or the other (Fig. 5.28). The midline fracture must be differentiated from the fortuitous superimposition of the normally open metopic suture. In the latter instance, of course, the apparent fracture line will cross the foramen magnum, while with a true occipital bone fracture the fracture line stops at the pos-

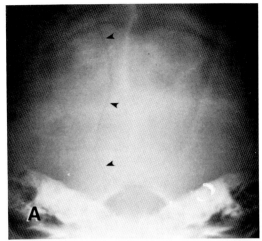

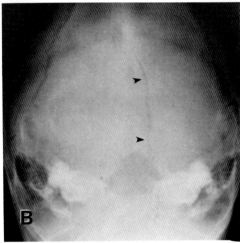

Figure 5.28. *Posterior occipital basal skull fractures.* (A) Note the typical appearance of a slightly diastatic occipital fracture (*arrows*). (B) Another patient demonstrating a thin linear posterior occipital fracture (*arrows*).

terior lip of the foramen magnum (Fig. 5.29). These fractures also must be differentiated from the infrequently occurring, unusually prominent median occipital bone fissure. Normally, these fissures are short and extend upward from the lip of the foramen magnum or downward from the region of the posterior fontanel. However, in some cases these fissures are unusually long and are misinterpreted as occipital bone fractures (see Fig. 5.49).

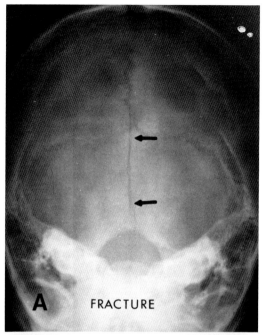

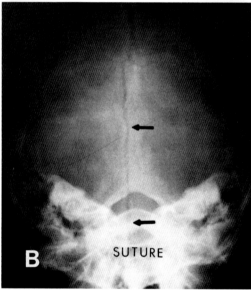

Figure 5.29. *Midline occipital fracture versus metopic suture.* (*A*) Note the typical appearance of a midline occipital fracture (*arrows*). Note that it stops at the posterior lip of the foramen magnum. (*B*) Metopic suture mimicking occipital fracture (*arrows*). Note that the metopic suture crosses the foramen magnum.

REFERENCES

1. Archer, C.R., and Sundaram, M.: Uncommon sphenoidal fractures and their sequelae. Radiology 122: 157–161, 1977.

2. Dublin, A.B., and Poirier, V.C.: Fracture of the sella turcica. A.J.R. 127: 969–972, 1976.
3. Harwood-Nash, D.C.: Fractures of the petrous and tympanic parts of the temporal bone in children. A.J.R. 110: 598–607, 1970.
4. Smith, T.R., and Kier, E.L.: The unfused planum sphenoidal: Differentiation from fracture. Radiology 98: 305–309, 1971.

FRACTURES VERSUS NORMAL SUTURES, FISSURES, AND VASCULAR GROOVES

So common is the problem of a normal suture, fissure, or vascular groove mimicking a fracture, that it is just as important to be familiar with these structures as with the fractures themselves. In this regard, it is best to become familiar with the direction in which these normal sutures, fissures, and vascular grooves travel (1, 8–10). The sutures and fissures more than the vascular grooves are remarkably consistent from patient to patient, and almost always appear in the same place. Consequently, if one sees a radiolucent line that does not conform to the site and location of one of these structures, then one should consider it to represent a fracture. These normal variations are considered in three general areas: (a) the frontal region, (b) the temporoparietal region, and (c) the occipital region.

Frontal Region Fractures and Pseudofractures. One of the most common structures misinterpreted for a fracture in the frontal bone is the vascular groove produced by the supraorbital branch of the ophthalmic artery. The problem is not so great on frontal view (Fig. 5.30), but on lateral view, often it is almost impossible to differentiate the two (Figs. 5.31 and 5.32). However, a few general rules can be applied: (a) most vascular grooves are located in the anterior third of the frontal bone, (b) most vascular grooves run in a vertical fashion with a gentle, posterior curve, (c) vascular grooves tend to have sclerotic edges while fractures have sharp nonsclerotic edges, and (d) vascular grooves seldom run in a horizontal or anteriorly sloping direction.

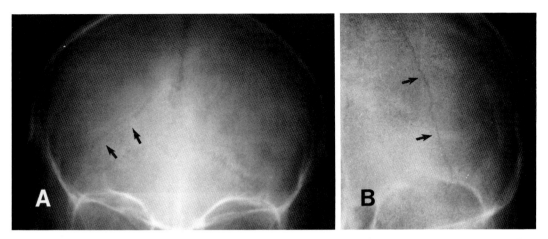

Figure 5.30. *Frontal vascular groove versus fracture.* (*A*) Note the radiolucent line resulting from a normal frontal vascular groove (*arrows*). (*B*) Thin, long radiolucent line representing a frontal fracture extending into the left orbital roof (*arrows*). Distinction between a vascular groove and fracture on frontal view usually is not difficult.

Another problem arising in the anterior fossa, but this time on frontal view, is the misinterpretation of a persistently open metopic suture (11) for a fracture. This suture commonly is open in children, and to the unwary will suggest a midline frontal bone fracture (Fig. 5.33A). This is an even greater problem if the suture is partially closed (Fig. 5.33B). The metopic suture also is notorious for mimicking an occipital bone fracture on Towne's projection (see Fig. 5.29B). On lateral view, a less common problem in the frontal region is the misinterpretation of the fissure representing the unfused planum sphenoidal (7) for a basal, anterior fossa floor skull fracture (see Fig. 5.25C).

Temporoparietal Region Fractures and Pseudofractures. In terms of vascular grooves in this portion of the skull, it is the outer table groove of one of the branches of the superficial temporal artery that causes most problems (Fig. 5.34B). In some of these cases, these vascular grooves virtually defy distinction from fractures except perhaps that often the grooves show sclerosis along their edges. These grooves can be seen projected over the entire sellar region and, in addition, one also can encounter similar problems with the posterior branch of the middle meningeal artery (Fig. 5.34A). Parietal diploic vascular grooves are not easily confused with calvarial fractures nor are the inner table vascular grooves produced by the main branches of the middle meningeal artery (Fig. 5.35). It is only when either of these vascular grooves is very thin that confusion with calvarial fractures can occur (Fig. 5.35).

As far as sutures in this area are concerned, although a number exist (Fig. 5.36), it is the squamosal suture that causes most difficulty. Indeed, with slight degrees of rotation of the calvarium, either from front to back or top to bottom, these sutures can appear so like a fracture that it is impossible to convince one that they simply represent a normal suture (Fig. 5.37). This is less of a problem with the other sutures in the area (Fig. 5.37C). On frontal view, the squamosal suture also is a problem and commonly mimics a fracture (Fig. 5.38). Fortunately, however, almost always the sclerotic line along either side of the suture identifies it as such. Either the posterior or anterior limbs of the squamosal suture can present in this fashion.

In the young infant, accessory fissures along the posterior parietal bone can

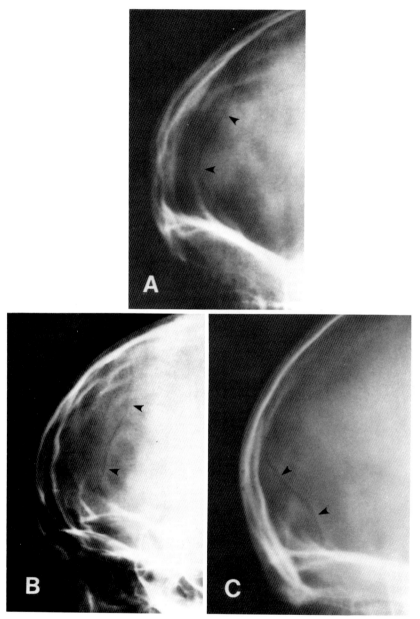

Figure 5.31. *Frontal vascular grooves—lateral view.* (*A*) Note typical appearance of a vascular groove in the frontal region (*arrows*). Characteristically it assumes a gentle posteriorly curving course. (*B*) Another vascular groove, somewhat less typical (*arrows*), and one that might easily be misinterpreted for a frontal bone fracture. (*C*) Unusual direction of another normal vascular groove (*arrows*). However, in this case the slight sclerosis along the edge of the groove identifies it as a vascular groove.

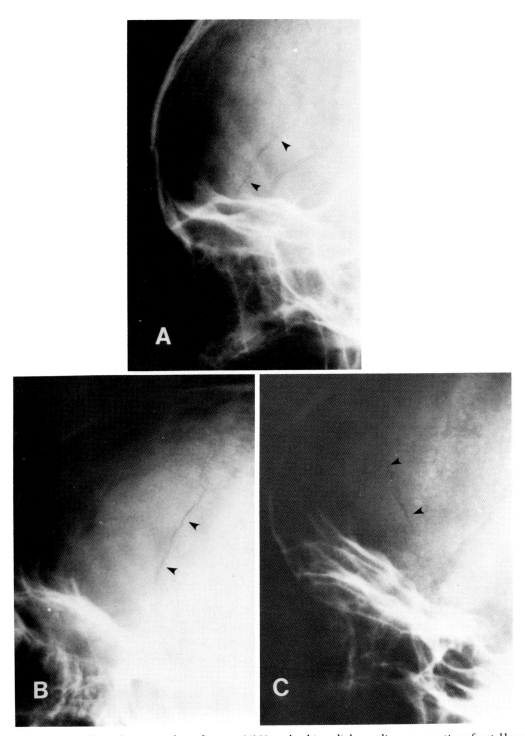

Figure 5.32. *Frontal bone fractures—lateral view.* (*A*) Note the thin radiolucent line representing a frontal bone fracture (*arrows*). Its gentle posterior curving course could cause one to misinterpret it for a vascular groove. A true vascular groove of the middle meningeal artery lies just posterior to the fracture. (*B*) Frontal bone fracture located in the posterior third of the frontal bone (*arrows*). Frontal vascular grooves are quite uncommon in this area and fracture identification is easier. (*C*) Anteriorly sloping frontal fracture (*arrows*). Vascular grooves usually do not head in this direction.

Figure 5.33. *Metopic suture—pseudofracture.* (*A*) Note the typical location of the metopic suture (*arrows*). (*B*) Partially obliterated metopic suture (*arrows*) extending from the anterior aspect of the anterior fontanel. The fontanel is not visualized on this reproduction. Note slight sclerosis along the suture edge, identifying it as a normal suture and not a fracture.

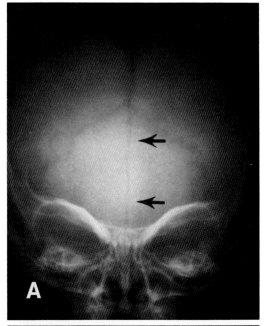

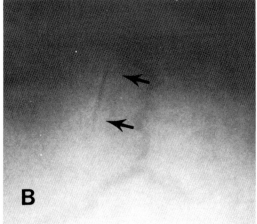

mimic small wedge-like linear fractures. Generally speaking, these fissures occur in the lower two-thirds of the parietal bone and often are multiple. In some cases, they are associated with a posterior parietal bony defect, the so-called "third fontanel" (2). If these fissures occur over the lower two-thirds of the parietal bone and if no soft tissue swelling overlies them, then they most likely are normal fissures. However, if they lie in the upper third of the posterior parietal bone and soft tissue

swelling overlies them, then a fracture is most likely (Fig. 5.39). This rule, of course, is not 100% foolproof, for obviously one can encounter fractures in the lower two-thirds of the parietal bone and normal fissures in the upper third, but still it is useful in a most cases.

Another problem with accessory sutures in the parietal bone is the one concerned with the so-called "intraparietal" sutures or fissures (5). The fissures have a great propensity to mimic parietal bone

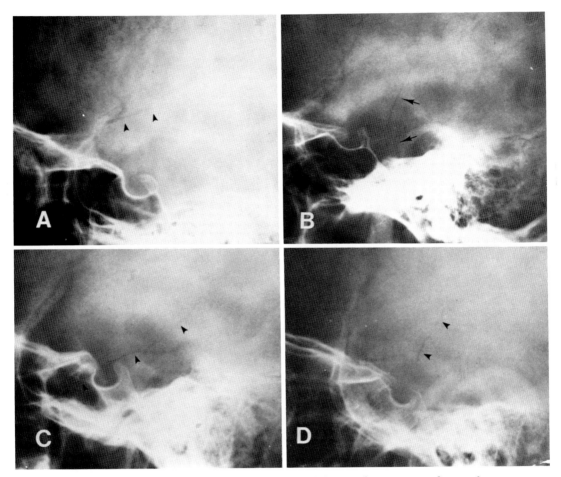

Figure 5.34. *Middle fossa vascular grooves versus fracture.* (**A**) Typical appearance of a vascular groove produced by the posterior branch of the middle meningeal artery (*arrows*). (**B**) Fracture-like appearance of a vascular groove produced by one of the branches of the superficial temporal artery (*arrows*). It would be difficult
to differentiate this groove from a fracture. (**C**) True fracture (*arrows*) of the middle fossa. The fracture line is
somewhat sharper than the vascular groove in **B** but still the two might be confused. (**D**) Small linear fracture in
the lower parietal bone (*arrows*). Irregularity of the bone edges suggests a fracture.

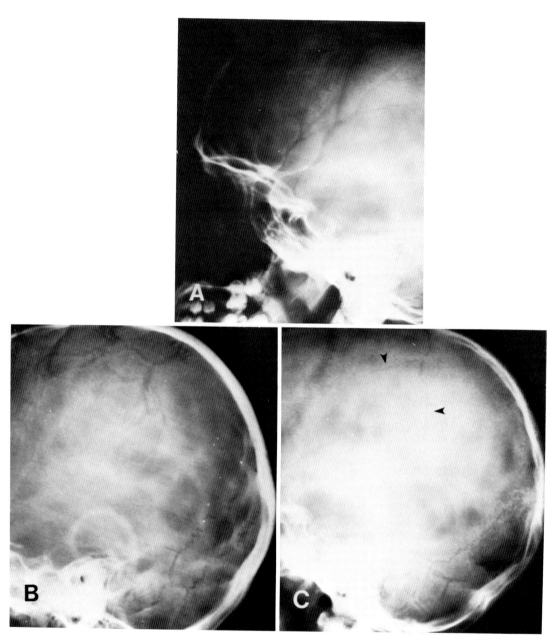

Figure 5.35. *Normal parietal vascular patterns.*   (*A*) Typical vascular grooves produced by the middle meningeal arteries and their branches. (*B*) Typical diploic venous vascularity in the upper parietal bone. (*C*) Small diploic venous channels in the upper parietal bone, some of which (*arrows*) could be misinterpreted for a fracture.

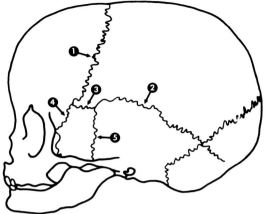

Figure 5.36. *Normal anterior and middle fossa sutures—diagrammatic representation.* Coronal suture (*1*), squamosal suture (*2*), sphenoparietal suture (*3*), sphenofrontal suture (*4*), and sphenosquamosal suture (*5*).

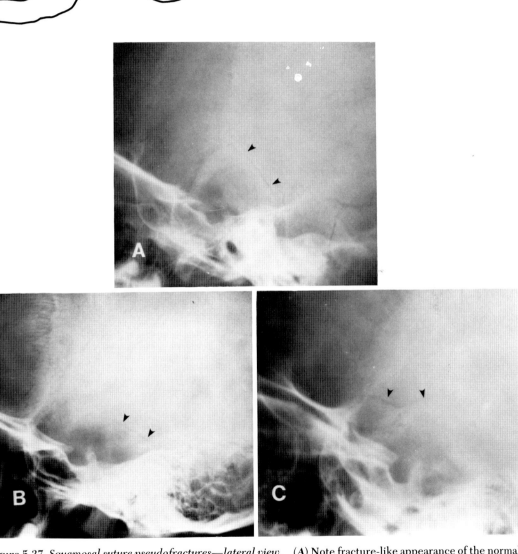

Figure 5.37. *Squamosal suture pseudofractures—lateral view.* (**A**) Note fracture-like appearance of the normal squamosal suture (*arrows*). The near-vertical radiolucent line about an inch posteroinferior to it is the occipitomastoid suture which also appears fracture-like because of rotation of the skull. (**B**) Another normal squamosal suture (*arrows*) that is virtually indistinguishable from a fracture. (**C**) Normal sphenoparietal suture (*arrows*) mimicking a fracture. Compare these findings with true fractures in this area demonstrated in Figure 5.34C and **D**.

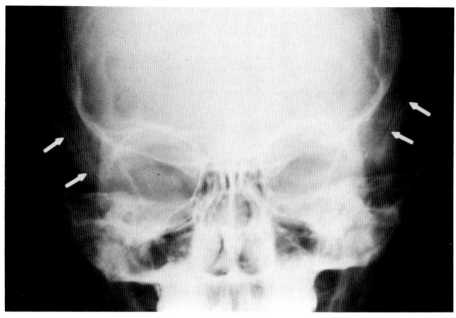

Figure 5.38. *Squamosal suture pseudofractures—frontal view.* In certain patients, the anterior or posterior limbs of the squamosal suture can appear slit-like on frontal projection (*arrows*) and suggest a fracture. In this case, note typical sclerosis on either side of the radiolucent lines identifying them as normal squamosal sutures. *On the left,* both anterior and posterior limbs of the squamosal suture are demonstrated.

fractures, especially if they are unilateral (Fig. 5.40). However, it is of some value to note that these fissures usually are relatively horizontal in position, and because of this if a vertical, radiolucent line is encountered, it should represent a fracture. In addition, if the radiolucent line truly represents a fracture, overlying soft tissue edema usually is present (Fig. 5.41). Of course, if the fissures are bilateral, and they commonly are, their remarkable symmetry usually serves to identify them correctly (Fig. 5.42). Nonetheless, when multiple, these sutures still can mimic multiple, eggshell calvarial fractures.

Along the base of the skull in the middle fossa, the only normal structures to be misinterpreted as fractures are the spheno-occipital and intersphenoid synchondrosis (Fig. 5.43). The intersphenoid synchondrosis usually disappears by the age of 2 years (6), but the spheno-occipital synchondrosis remains open until the late teens and early adulthood (4).

Occipital Region Fractures and Pseudofractures. The only vascular groove that can cause confusion in the occipital region of the skull is the groove for the mastoid emissary vein, but usually it is so tortuous that it offers no real problem. Sutures, on the other hand, are a significant problem in this area, for the occipital region of the skull is virtually cluttered with normal and accessory sutures and synchondroses (Fig. 5.44). *Familiarity with all of them is mandatory, for otherwise one is sure to misinterpret one of them as a fracture.*

On lateral view, the sutures most commonly visible are the lambdoid, parietomastoid, occipitomastoid, and Mendosal, while the visible synchondrosis is the innominate synchondrosis. The four sutures radiate outward from the region of the posterior-lateral fontanel, but the Mendosal suture usually is visible more in infancy. The problem with these sutures is not that they are difficult to identify in the average patient, but rather that with slight degrees

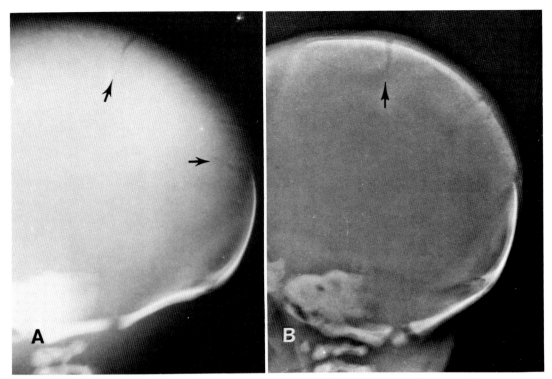

Figure 5.39. *Posterior parietal fissures versus fracture.*   (**A**) Typical posterior parietal fissuring. This is a normal. Two of the fissures stand out more prominently (*arrows*), and either one could be misinterpreted as a fracture. (**B**) True parietal bone fracture (*arrow*). Note slight degree of soft tissue swelling over the fracture site. (Reproduction enhanced to bring out soft tissues.)

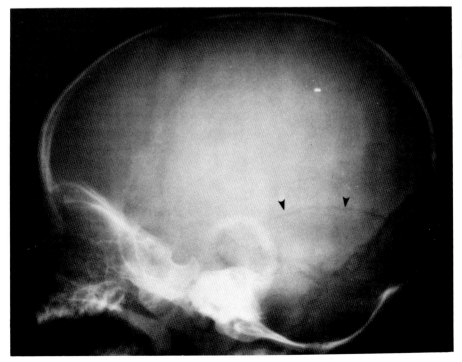

Figure 5.40. *Unilateral intraparietal fissure mimicking fracture.*   Note the fracture-like appearance of this normal intraparietal fissure (*arrows*). All of the sutures in the occipital bone also are normal.

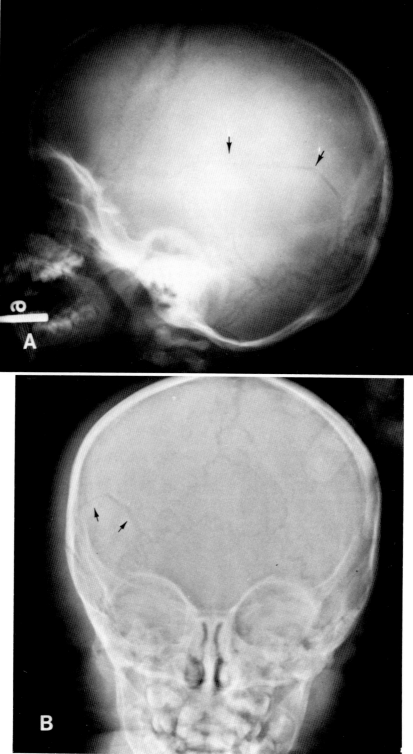

Figure 5.41. *Transverse parietal fracture.* (**A**) Note the transverse parietal bone fracture (*arrows*). Also note that all of the sutures show minimal diastasis. (**B**) Frontal view demonstrating the fracture (*arrows*). Also note extensive soft tissue edema over the right side of the calvarium. Such edema is not present with normal intraparietal accessory fissures. (Frontal view altered to bring out soft tissues.)

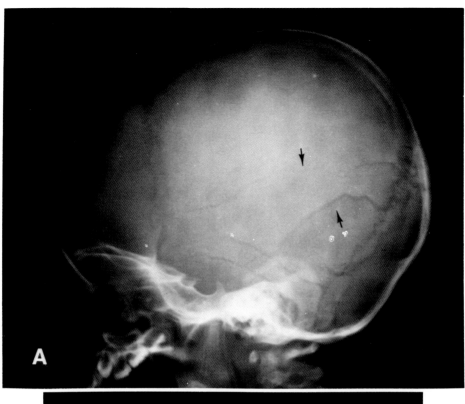

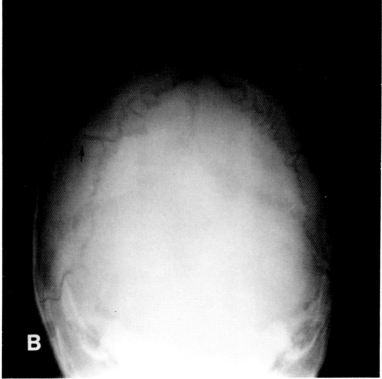

Figure 5.42. *Bilateral intraparietal accessory fissures.* (**A**) Either one of these normal fissures can be misinterpreted as a fracture (*arrows*). (**B**) Frontal view demonstrating characteristic symmetry of these normal fissures (*arrows*).

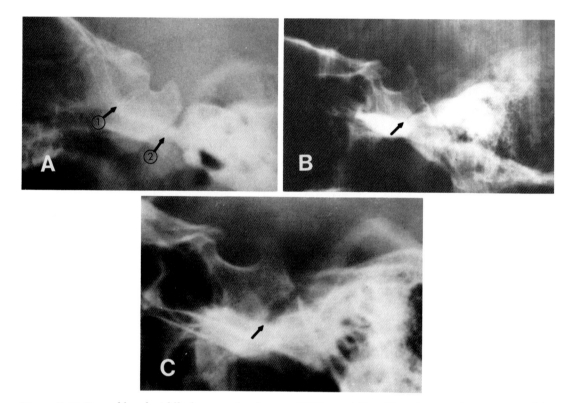

Figure 5.43. *Normal basal middle fossa synchondroses.* (*A*) Young infant. Note the typical appearance of the intersphenoid synchondrosis (*1*) and the wider spheno-occipital synchondrosis (*2*). (*B*) Older child demonstrating a residual spheno-occipital synchondrosis (*arrow*) easily misinterpreted as a basal skull fracture. (*C*) Another patient with a very wide but normal spheno-occipital synchondrosis (*arrow*). (Part *C* courtesy of M. Kogutt, M.D., New Orleans.)

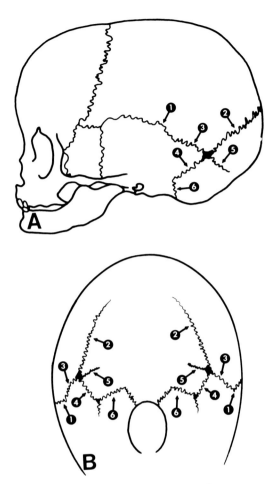

Figure 5.44. *Posterior fossa sutures—diagrammatic representation.* Lateral (A) and Towne's (B) projections. Squamosal suture (1), lambdoid suture (2), parietomastoid suture (3), occipitomastoid suture (4), Mendosal suture (5), and innominate synchondrosis complex (6).

lines heading in the same direction are identified, then one can be confident that the fracture-like appearing line is simply a normal suture. However, when an extra line exists (i.e., a third radiolucent line) or when one finds these radiolucent lines to be traveling in unusual directions, then one should consider them to be fractures (Figs. 5.46 and 5.47). These sutures also are a problem on frontal and Towne's projections where slight degrees of rotation also can cause them to appear absolutely fracture-like (Fig. 5.48).

In the posterior fossa, if one remembers that most of the sutures are paired, a third radiolucent line, even though heading in a direction suggestive of a normal suture, should be considered a fracture. In addition, of course, if a radiolucent line is located in a totally unexpected place, a fracture should be considered.

In addition to these problems, the occipital bone also is prone to irregular ossification over the posterior lip of the foramen magnum. Furthermore, the median occipital fissure (3) visualized just below the posterior fontanel commonly is misinterpreted as a fracture. This fissure usually is seen in young infants only and is not more than 1 to 2 cm in length (Fig. 5.49A). Very rarely it is longer, and then it is more likely to suggest a midline occipital fracture (Fig. 5.49B). A similar problem can occur with an abnormally long but normal fissure extending upward from the posterior lip of the foramen magnum (Fig. 5.49C).

Finally, one should note that a number of interparietal accessory bones can be seen in the occipital bone, just at the junction of the lambdoid and sagittal sutures. On frontal view, this bone (inca bone), or bones, is of characteristic appearance and location, and usually not misinterpreted for fractures (Fig. 5.50). On lateral view, however, they often appear very sclerotic and frequently are misinterpreted for a depressed fracture (Fig. 5.50).

of rotation any one of them can appear absolutely fracture-like (Fig. 5.45). This is not to say that true fractures in this area do not occur, for indeed they do (Fig. 5.46), and because of this one must be able to differentiate a fracture from a suture. In this regard, when one believes that a radiolucent line represents a normal suture, one should look for its mate on the other side. Whether this contralateral suture appears fracture-like or not, if only two radiolucent

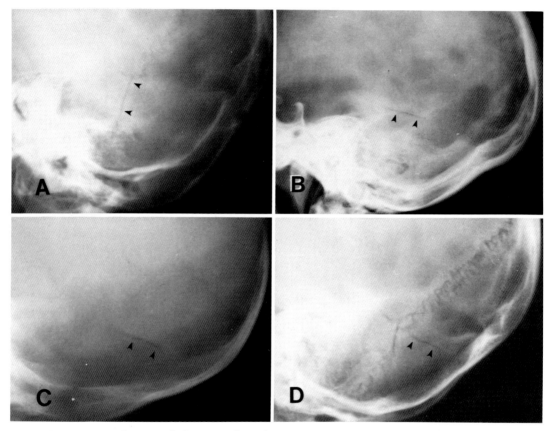

Figure 5.45. *Posterior fossa pseudofractures—lateral view.* (**A**) Note fracture-like appearance of the normal occipitomastoid suture (*arrows*). (**B**) Fracture-like appearance of the normal parietomastoid suture (*arrows*). (**C**) Isolated visualization of one Mendosal suture (*arrows*) in a young infant. To the uninitiated, this is virtually indistinguishable from a fracture. (**D**) Mendosal suture pseudofracture (*arrows*) in an older child.

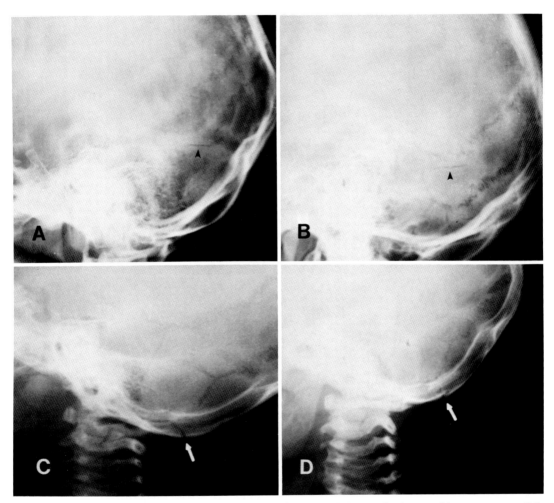

Figure 5.46. *Posterior fossa pseudofractures versus true fracture.* (**A**) Note the fracture-like appearance of the normal parietomastoid suture (*arrow*). (**B**) Fracture of the posterior fossa (*arrow*) mimicking a parietomastoid suture. However, when one lines this radiolucent line up with the two, true parietomastoid sutures, one finds that it represents an extra radiolucent line and hence should be a fracture. (**C**) Normal innominate synchondrosis (*arrow*). (**D**) Diastatic, slightly offset fracture of innominate synchondrosis (*arrow*). Normal fissures and synchondroses are not offset, and, thus, this should be a fracture.

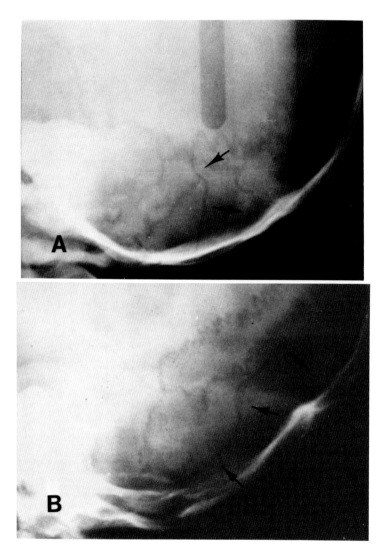

Figure 5.47. *True occipital fractures—lateral view.*   (*A*) Note the fracture in the occipital bone (*arrows*). There are no normal sutures in this area. (*B*) Another patient demonstrating a long linear fracture of the occipital bone (*arrows*). All of the normal sutures are identified, and this represents an extra radiolucent line, or in other words, a fracture.

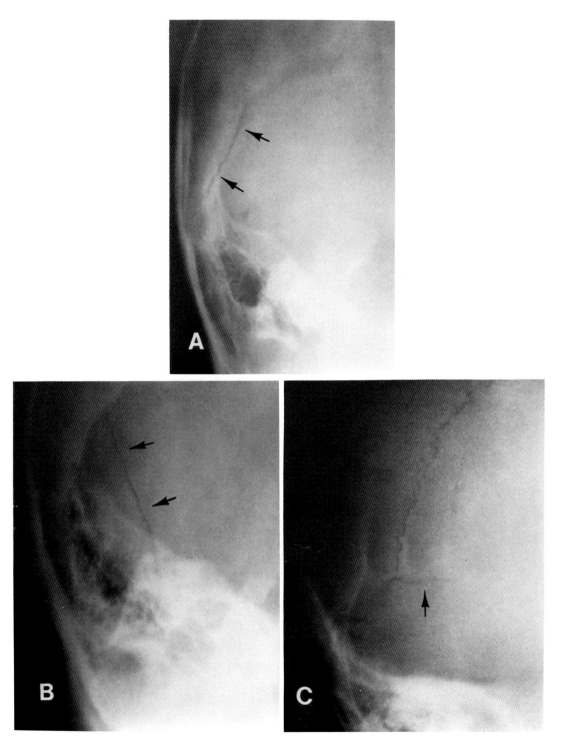

Figure 5.48. *Occipital suture pseudofractures—Towne's view.*   (**A**) Note fracture-like appearance and characteristic slope of the normal parietomastoid suture (*arrows*). (**B**) Pseudofracture appearance and characteristic slope of the occipitomastoid suture (*arrows*). (**C**) Small residual Mendosal suture (*arrow*) mimicking a fracture.

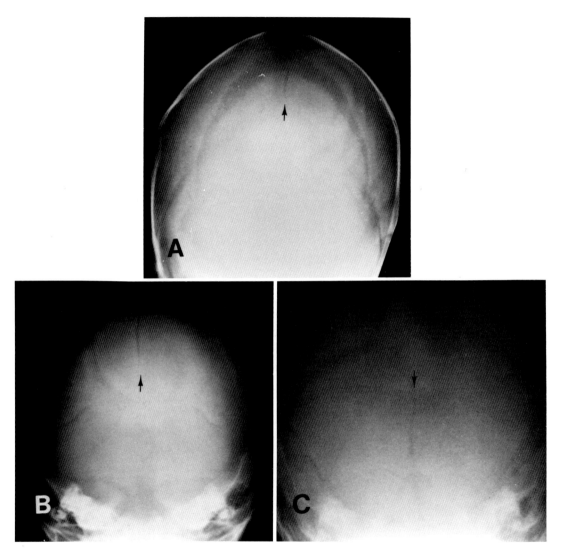

Figure 5.49. *Midline occipital fissures—pseudofractures.*   (*A*) Note typical appearance and length of the median occipital fissure (*arrow*) visualized on Towne's projection in young infants. (*B*) Unusually long but normal median occipital fissure (*arrow*) in another infant. Also, note residual Mendosal sutures on both sides. (*C*) Unusually long occipital fissure (*arrow*) arising from the posterior lip of the foramen magnum.

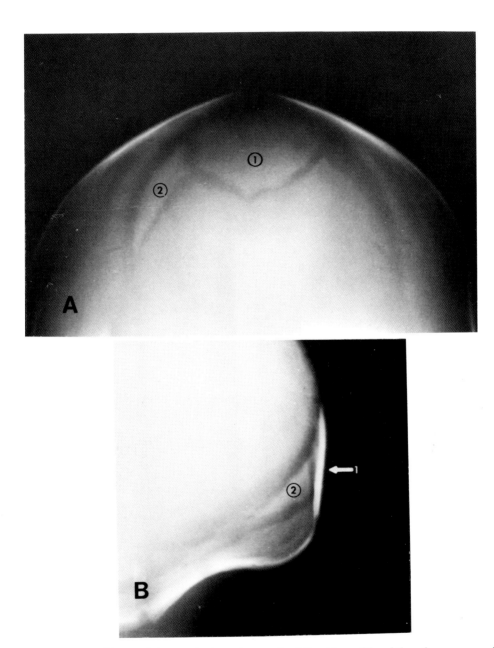

Figure 5.50. *Interparietal bone.* (*A*) Note the large interparietal (inca) bone (*1*) and the other accessory bone (*2*). These usually are not misinterpreted as fractures on this view. (*B*) On lateral view, however, their extremely sclerotic appearance (*arrows*) can strongly suggest a depressed fracture, especially if the skull is slightly obliqued.

Figure 5.51. *Sutural pseudofractures on basal views.* (*A*) Note the coronal suture crossing the base of the skull (*arrows*). (*B*) Occipitomastoid suture (*arrows*) appearing as though it were a fracture on basal view.

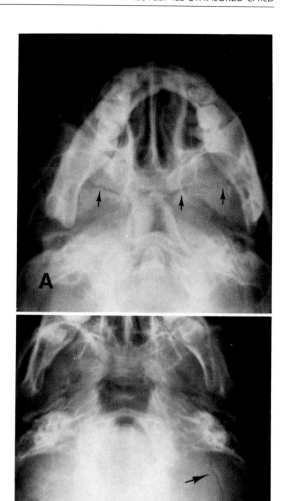

Base of Skull Pseudofractures. On basal skull views, almost any of the normal sutures mentioned, with certain degrees of obliquity, can be projected so as to mimic a fracture. Most often, this occurs with the coronal suture or one of the posterior fossa sutures (Fig. 5.51). The various sutures and synchondroses posing problems on plain films are not nearly the same problem on CT scans. However, they still can be a problem, and most of these are demonstrated in Figure 5.52.

REFERENCES

1. Allen, W., Kier, E., and Rothman, S.: Pitfalls in the evaluation of skull trauma: A review. Radiol. Clin. North Am. 11: 479–503, 1973.
2. Chemke, J., and Robinson, A.: Third fontanelle. J. Pediatr. 75: 617–622, 1969.
3. Franken, E.A., Jr.: The midline occipital fissure: Diagnosis of a fracture versus anatomic variants. Radiology 93: 1043–1046, 1969.

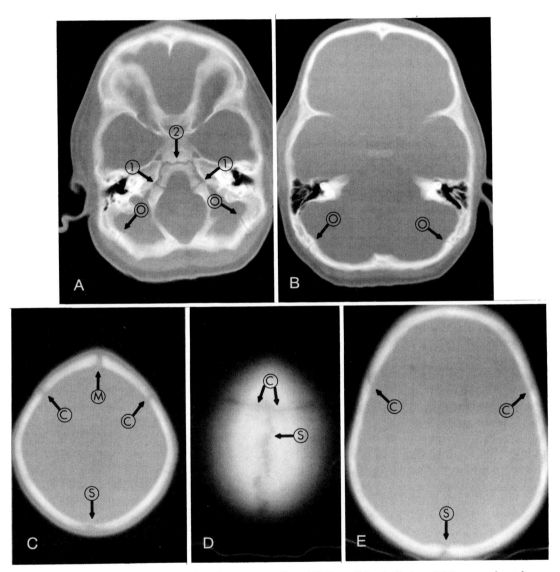

Figure 5.52. *Normal sutures, and synchondroses: CT study.*   (*A*) Base of the skull view. (*B*) Lower calvarial posterior fossa view. (*C*) Upper calvarial view. (*D*) Another upper calvarial view. (*E*) Midcalvarial view. Coronal suture (*C*), sagittal suture (*S*), metopic suture (*M*), occipito mastoid suture (*O*), innominate synchondrosis (*1*), and spheno-occipital synchondrosis (*2*).

4. Irwin, A.L.: Roentgen demonstration of the time of closure of the spheno-occipital synchondrosis. Radiology 75: 451–452, 1960.

5. Shapiro, R.: Anomalous parietal sutures and the bipartite parietal bone. A.J.R. 115: 569–577, 1972.

6. Shopfner, C.E., Wolfe, T.W., and O'Kell, R.T.: The intersphenoid synchondrosis. A.J.R. 104: 184–193, 1968.

7. Smith, T.R., and Kier, E.L.: The unfused planum sphenoidal: Differentiation from fracture. Radiology 98: 305–309, 1971.

8. Swischuk, L.E.: The normal pediatric skull: Variations and artifacts. Radiol. Clin. North Am. 10: 277–290, 1972.

9. Swischuk, L.E.: The growing skull. Semin. Roentgenol. 9: 115–124, 1974.

10. Swischuk, L.E.: The normal newborn skull. Semin. Roentgenol. 9: 101–113, 1974.

11. Torgerson, J.: A roentgenologic study of the metopic suture. Acta Radiol. 33: 1–11, 1950.

ARTIFACTS MIMICKING CALVARIAL FRACTURES

A number of artifacts can be mistaken for calvarial abnormalities (1). However, one of the most common is the laceration that projects as a radiolucent defect or pseudofracture of the calvarium (Fig. 5.53A). Clinical correlation is the rule here, and it is most important that such correlation be accomplished, for if the laceration suggests a fracture, it often suggests a depressed one. Other artifacts that can cause problems in the interpretation of skull roentgenograms include dirt and pebbles over the scalp and in the hair (Fig. 5.53B), hair soaked with water or blood (Fig. 5.54C), hair braids, air trapped in the pinna of the ear so as to suggest pneumocephalus, and abnormal shadows produced by the pinna and earlobe itself (Fig. 5.54).

REFERENCE

1. Swischuk, L.E.: The normal pediatric skull: Variations and artifacts. Radiol. Clin. North Am. 10: 277–290, 1972.

FACIAL, ORBITAL, AND MANDIBULAR FRACTURES

Fractures of the face, orbit, and mandible are certainly not as common in the infant and young child as they are in the adult. Nasal fractures might be considered an exception, but generally speaking, facial fractures do not become a major problem until the child is older, and at this age, the considerations are not different from those in the adult. In this regard, the presence or absence of symmetry is the key to the assessment of facial bone fractures. Most faces are very symmetrical, and thus, if one encounters any asymmetry of cortical continuity or contour, one should suspect a fracture. In terms of *which views to obtain,* one usually obtains frontal, posteroanterior, lateral, and Waters' views. *The Waters' view, however, is the most productive* and the single most important view in the assessment of facial injuries. Thereafter, one might require special orbital, zygomatic arch, or mandibular views for complete assessment. These views now often are supplanted by CT scans (5, 21), but still, in most cases of facial trauma, standard plain films are the starting point and thus require significant expertise in assessment.

TYPES OF FRACTURES

Facial fractures generally can be divided into: (a) nasal fractures, (b) orbital fractures, (c) zygomatic-maxillary fractures, and (d) mandibular fractures (3–6).

Nasal Bone Fractures. These fractures usually are best demonstrated with moderately penetrated lateral views of the nasal bone and a Waters' view for assessment of nasal septal deviation. Fractures of the nasal bone can be simple linear fractures, depressed fractures, or comminuted fractures, and all can be associated with other facial fractures or fractures of the spine of the maxillary bone (Fig. 5.55). Linear fractures must be differentiated from three normal radiolucent lines commonly seen around the nose; the nasomaxillary suture, the groove for the nasociliary nerve, and the nasofrontal suture (Fig. 5.56). The lines produced by the nasomax-

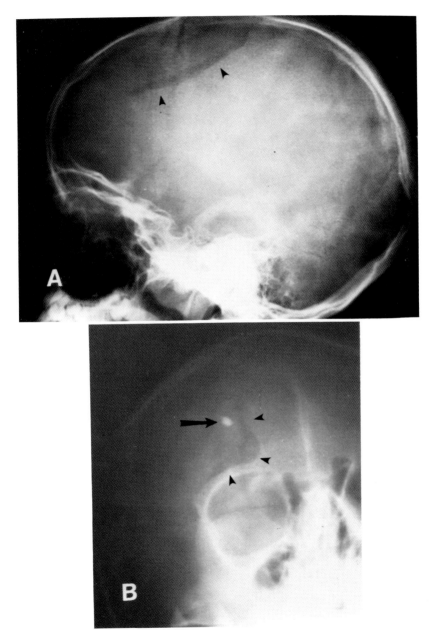

Figure 5.53. *Scalp laceration and pebble artifacts.* (*A*) Note the radiolucency secondary to a deep laceration over the calvarium (*arrows*). (*B*) Another patient with a laceration over the forehead (*small arrows*) and a pebble embedded in the laceration (*large arrow*). Such a laceration should not be misinterpreted as a depressed skull fracture.

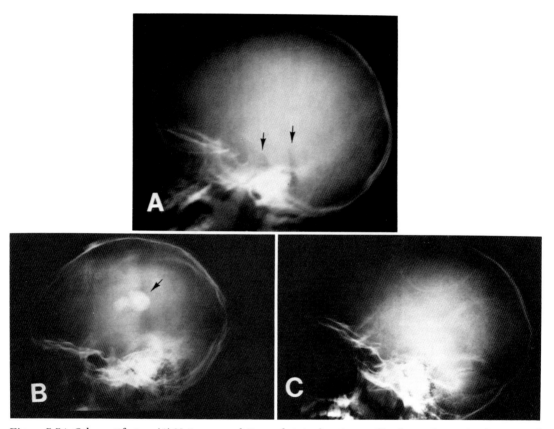

Figure 5.54. *Other artifacts.* (**A**) Note accumulations of air in the pinnae of both ears (*arrows*). These air collections should not be misinterpreted for pneumocephalus. (**B**) Tightly braided hair mimicking an intracranial calcification (*arrow*). (**C**) Whorl-like configurations of strands of wet hair.

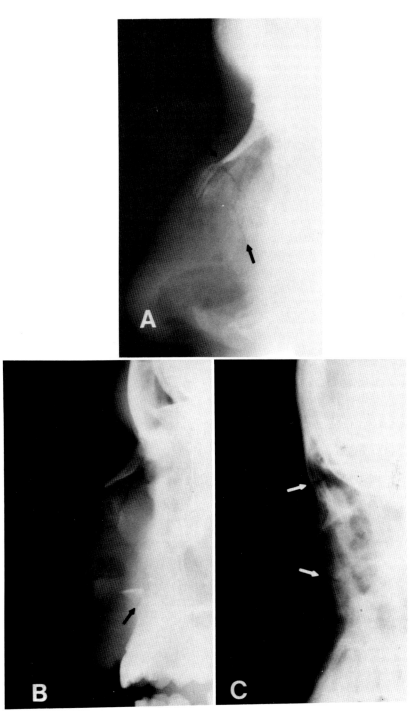

Figure 5.55. *Nasal fractures.* (**A**) Note the comminuted nasal fracture. Two of the fracture lines are identified with *arrows.*(**B**) Note the comminuted fracture of the nasal bone. The vertical radiolucent line is a fracture. It is too far anterior to be the nasomaxillary suture and too sharp and radiolucent to be the nasociliary groove. Both of these normal structures are shown in Figure 5.56. Also note the fracture through the spinous process of the maxillary bone (*arrow*). (**C**) This patient was hit in the nose and face. Note fractures through the anterior wall of the frontal sinus (*upper arrow*) and the maxillary bone below the nose (*lower arrow*).

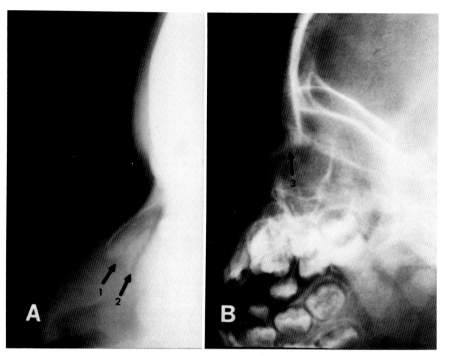

Figure 5.56. *Pseudofractures of nasal bone.* Note the barely visible groove for the nasociliary nerve (*1*) and the more prominent vertical radiolucent line representing the nasomaxillary suture (*2*). Both of these structures can be misinterpreted as fractures. (*B*) Normal nasofrontal suture (*3*).

illary suture and groove for the nasociliary nerve are straight, and more or less parallel the anterior aspect of the nasal bone. This is not to say that fractures do not occur in this plane, but only to indicate that if one sees a radiolucent line traveling in the opposite direction or, even better, in the horizontal plane, then one should assume the line to represent a fracture (12).

Orbital Fractures. Fractures of the orbits can be linear or depressed, and often occur in conjunction with frontal bone or other facial fractures. However, they also occur alone (9, 17), and Caldwell, Waters, lateral, or oblique (optic foramen) views may be required for their complete demonstration (Fig. 5.57). However, CT scans eventually will be obtained and will more precisely demonstrate these fractures (Fig. 5.58).

A special type of fracture of the orbit is the *blowout fracture.* This fracture occurs through the floor of the orbit and results from blunt trauma to the eye (2, 4, 5, 15,

19, 22). Usually it occurs in isolated form but it can be associated with other facial fractures, especially the tripod fracture of the maxillary bone. In the blowout fracture, the hydrostatic pressure produced within the globe blows out, or displaces, the orbital wall at its weakest point. This point is along its inferior aspect, or floor, of the orbit and the orbital contents decompress through it. Because of this, the globe becomes partially fixed and cannot move in all directions. Typically, diplopia secondary to lack of upward gaze is present in these patients.

Roentgenographically, the best view for detecting blowout fractures is the Waters' view. On this view, one should look for asymmetry of the floors of the orbits and, in some cases, one may see actual downward displacement of the bony fragments. In other cases, one will note only that a soft tissue mass (usually just intraorbital fat) has prolapsed into the maxillary antrum (Fig. 5.59). The prolapsed soft tissue mass

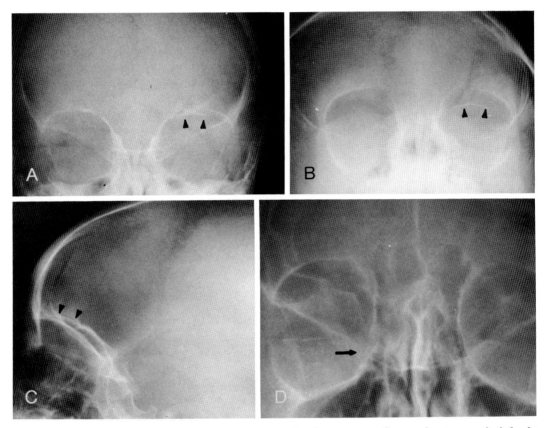

Figure 5.57. *Superior orbital rim fracture.* (**A**) Note generalized increase in soft tissue density over the left orbit and also note discontinuity of the left orbital roof (*arrows*). A depressed fracture fragment and a fracture extending into the frontal bone above the orbit are suggested. (**B**) Waters' view more clearly demonstrates the depressed fragment (*arrows*) and clearly demonstrates the fracture extending into the frontal bone. (**C**) Lateral view demonstrating the fracture of the frontal bone and the malaligned left anterior orbital roof (*arrows*). Compare the configuration of the left orbital roof with the normal right orbital roof beneath it. (**D**) Medial orbital wall fracture. Note suble discontinuity of the cortex of the medial orbital wall on the right (*arrow*). Also note that the ethmoid air sinuses are obliterated because of associated bleeding.

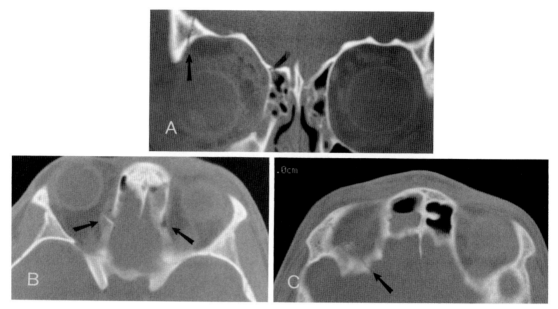

Figure 5.58. *Orbital fractures: CT findings.* (*A*) Note the fracture through the lateral aspect of the superior orbital rim (*arrow*). (*B*) Another patient with extensive facial fractures demonstrating bilateral fractures of the medial walls of the orbits (*arrows*). The fracture fragment on the right is displaced. (*C*) Another patient demonstrating an irregular fracture (*arrow*) through the right orbital roof.

has been referred to as the "teardrop" sign, while the depressed bony fragments have been referred to as the "open bombbay" door sign. The maxillary sinus may be totally clear or obliterated by blood, and, once again, this fracture is best demonstrated with CT scanning (10, 20) (Fig. 5.59). However, plain films (Waters' and Caldwell views) still are quite reliable in initially detecting this fracture (11).

Most often blowout fractures occur through the floor of the orbit, but occasionally they can occur medially and extend into the ethmoid sinus cavities. They also have been reported to extend into the frontal sinuses (3), and fractures in all of these latter sites are more difficult to detect. Indeed, this is precisely the time to use CT scanning.

Fractures of the Zygomatic and Maxillary Bones. These include solitary zygomatic arch fractures, tripod fractures of the zygomaticomaxillary bone complex, isolated maxillary fractures, and Le Fort fractures of the face. Of course, many times

these fractures occur in conjunction with one another, but they also occur in isolated form. Of all the fractures of the maxillary bone, the most common is the *tripod fracture.* This fracture results from a direct blow to the cheek (7, 8, 18) and characteristically, fracturing occurs at three sites: (a) the zygomatic-frontal suture, (b) the inferior orbital rim and maxillary bone (i.e., junction of the zygoma and maxillary bone), and (c) the zygomatic arch (Fig. 5.60). Depending on the severity of the injury and the extent of the fracture through the inferior orbital rim and maxillary sinus, more or less lateral and downward displacement of the fracture fragment occurs. In actual fact, this fracture fragment is the entire zygoma and roentgenographically its depression results in a variable degree of asymmetry of the lower orbital rims (Fig. 5.61). In children, it is important not to misinterpret the normal zygomaticfrontal suture for the superiormost fracture of the tripod fracture complex.

Other fractures of the maxillary bone

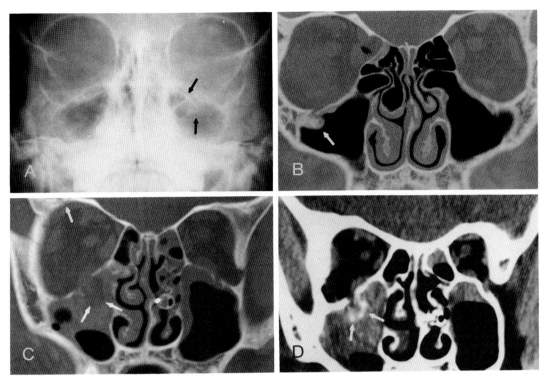

Figure 5.59. *Blowout fracture.* (*A*) Suspicious plain film findings. Note an indistinct mass (*lower arrow*) in the roof of the left maxillary sinus. In addition, there is a depressed fracture fragment involving the floor (*upper arrow*). (*B*) Coronal CT study in another patient demonstrates a small blowout fracture (*arrow*) *on the right.* (*C*) Another patient with a blowout fracture on the right demonstrating fat (*arrows*) herniating into the blood-filled maxillary sinus. The floor of the orbit is disrupted. The *upper arrow* points to an associated superorbital fracture (*arrow*). (*D*) Soft tissue windows in the same patient demonstrate the blowout fracture (*arrows*) with fragments of bone displaced into the blood-filled sinus. Some fluid is also present in the other maxillary sinus cavity and the ethmoid sinuses *on the left.*

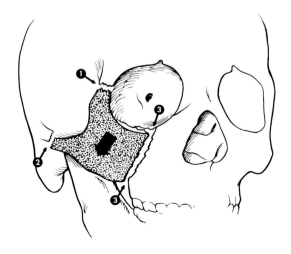

Figure 5.60. *Tripod fracture—diagrammatic representation.* Characteristically, fractures occur through the zygomatico-frontal suture (*1*), zygomatic arch (*2*), and the junction of the zygoma and maxillary bone (*3*). In addition, the fracture fragment is displaced downward and outward (*large arrow*).

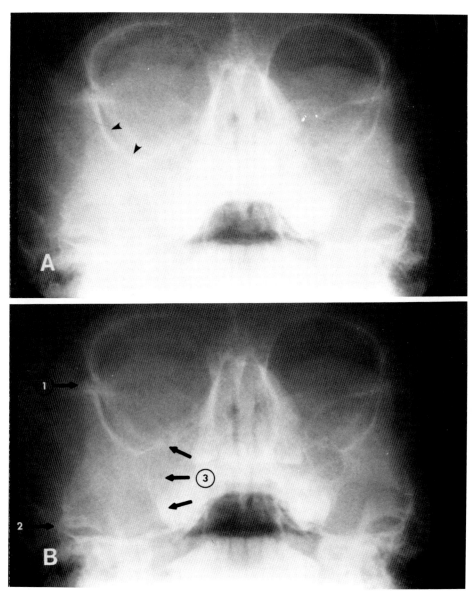

Figure 5.61. *Tripod fracture in infant—subtle findings.* (A) First, note a generalized increase in soft tissue density over the right orbit and maxillary sinus region. Then note asymmetry of the inferior aspects of the orbits. *On the right,* there is downward and outward orbital floor displacement (*arrows*). (B) Same patient demonstrating bony detail. Note the fracture through the zygomaticofrontal suture (*1*), a distorted, fractured zygomatic arch (*2*), and a poorly defined, although obligatorily present fracture through the orbital floor and maxillary sinus (*3*). Very often, in young infants, these fractures are difficult to define on plain films.

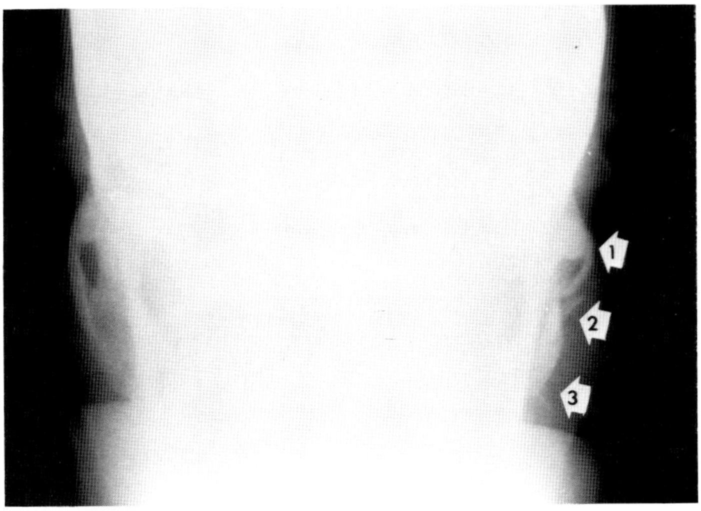

Figure 5.62. *Zygomatic arch fracture.* Note the typical configuration of the fractured zygomatic arch (*arrow*). The fracture occurs at three sites (*1–3*) and is depressed in the middle site (*2*). Other zygomatic arch fractures are demonstrated in Figures 5.61*B* and 5.65*B*.

are less common but also result from direct blows to the cheek. Many of these fractures extend into the alveolar process of the maxilla, and in so doing produce a loose fragment with separation of the teeth.

Fractures isolated to the *zygomatic arch* usually result from direct blows to the side of the face. These fractures can be depressed or nondepressed, and in those cases where depression occurs, the zygomatic arch fractures at three sites. Depression occurs at the middle site (Fig. 5.62). Zygomatic arches can be visualized on Towne's projections (see Fig. 5.65), Waters' projection, and posteroanterior projections with the chin tucked tightly against the neck. If these views do not suffice, special tangential views or base of the skull views can be obtained.

One of the more serious facial injuries is the *Le Forte fracture.* This fracture is a transverse maxillary fracture extending across the face (4, 5, 14, 15, 18), and often is associated with a fracture of the pterygoid process (16). Le Fort fractures usually are classified into three types, depending on the level of fracture (Fig. 5.63). The lowermost of these fractures is the Le Fort

I or transverse maxillary fracture, and the fracture line is located above the level of the teeth but below the nose. There is separation of the teeth and the hard palate from the upper portions of the maxilla. In the Le Fort II fracture, the fracture line is located at a higher level and generally runs along the upper aspect of the maxillary bones and nose. Laterally, it may extend along the infraorbital ridge. This fracture often is referred to as the pyramidal fracture because of the shape of the main fracture fragment. In Le Fort III injuries, there is craniofacial separation. The fracture is high in position and is located somewhere upward of the bridge of the nose. It usually extends into the orbits, and to a varying degree separates the face from the base of the skull. The main fracture fragment is the entire face. Le Fort fractures usually are complex and serious injuries, and are sustained from head-on blows to the face such as those sustained in automobile accidents. All of these and other facial fractures, once suspected, require further delineation with CT scanning (Fig. 5.64).

Mandibular Fractures. These fractures usually result from direct blows to

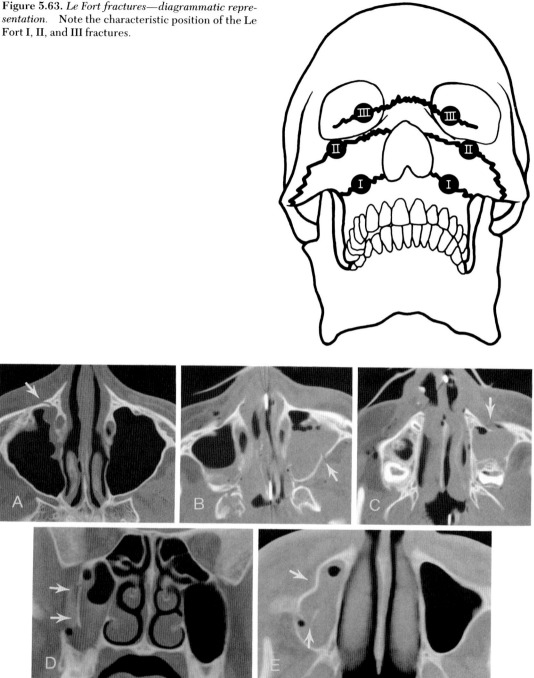

Figure 5.63. *Le Fort fractures—diagrammatic representation.* Note the characteristic position of the Le Fort I, II, and III fractures.

Figure 5.64. *Maxillary fractures: CT scan appearance.* (**A**) Note the nondisplaced fracture (*arrow*) through the maxillary bone *on the right*. There is some underlying mucosal edema in the sinus cavity. (**B**) Another patient with extensive facial injuries demonstrates a slightly displaced fracture (*arrow*) through the posterior wall of the left maxillary sinus. Air and fluid are seen in the sinus cavity. A fluid level is seen in the contralateral maxillary sinus, and a few air bubbles are seen in the soft tissues overlying the left maxillary sinus. (**C**) An adjacent cut demonstrates a markedly displaced anterior maxillary fracture (*arrow*). Again, air and fluid are seen in the maxillary sinus and air bubbles are scattered in the soft tissues on the right side of the face. (**D**) Another patient whose coronal CT scan demonstrates an inwardly displaced lateral maxillary wall fracture (*arrows*). Blood is present in the sinus cavity. (**E**) Axial view demonstrates the depressed lateral wall (*upper arrow*). In addition, there are one or two displaced bony fragments lying in the sinus cavity (*lower arrow*). Blood virtually fills the sinus cavity. Note the normal sinus on the other side.

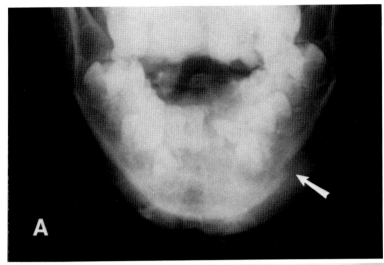

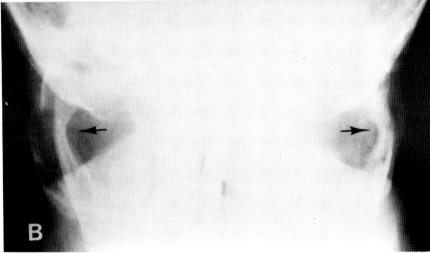

Figure 5.65. *Fractures of the mandible.* (*A*) Note the displaced fracture through the body of the mandible (*arrow*). Alignment of the teeth is disrupted. This patient did not have any other mandibular fractures. (*B*) Bilateral greenstick (bending) fractures of the mandibular condyles (*arrows*) in a young infant. The zygomatic arch, *on the right,* also is fractured but not depressed. It merely is separated at the zygomatic frontal suture.

the lower jaw and, often, because of the ring-like configuration of the mandible, fractures occur at two sites. However, single fractures also commonly occur and usually are not too difficult to detect (Fig. 5.65A). In other cases, fractures can occur through the condylar processes of the mandible. These fractures can be unilateral or bilateral, and in young infants often are of the greenstick or bending (1, 13) variety (Fig. 5.65B). Usually, these fractures

are best demonstrated on Towne's or Caldwell views of the head. On this latter view, if one has the patient tuck the chin tightly against his or her chest, the mandibular condyles become readily visible. With more extensive fractures of the mandible, that is, where fracturing might occur at three sites, the mandible often is noted to be wider than it should be: in other words, the mandible appears magnified on the frontal view and too large for the remain-

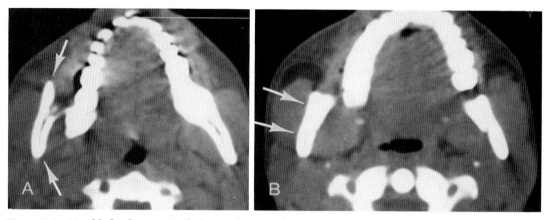

Figure 5.66. *Mandibular fracture: CT findings.* (*A*) Note the comminuted fracture through the right mandibular angle (*arrow*). The mandibular ramus is displaced outwardly. (*B*) Another cut demonstrates the same displaced fracture (*arrow*).

der of the face (17). Mandibular fractures, of course, also are readily demonstrable with CT scanning and the study is obtained in virtually all cases. It is much easier to assess bone alignment with CT (Fig. 5.66).

Dislocation of the mandible is not particularly common but can occur. Of course, clinically it should be readily apparent, for the patient will be unable to open and close the mouth. On Law's projection and subsequent regular or computerized tomography, the condyles are visualized with considerable clarity, and it can be determined that in the dislocated joint the condyle lies anterior to the articular fossa.

Soft Tissue Changes with Facial Injury. Very often the soft tissues are swollen and distorted with facial injury. This can occur with or without underlying bony abnormality, and it is important to appreciate these changes. In some instances, considerable edema and swelling are present and can distract one from a more serious underlying problem (Fig. 5.67). In this regard, one of the more distracting soft tissue changes is that produced when air is trapped between the palpebral fissures. In such cases, air within the orbit might erroneously be suggested (Fig. 5.67*B*).

Normal Findings Causing Problems. The facial bones are so complexly constructed and united by so many sutures that it is no surprise that many normal structures are misinterpreted as fractures. This can occur both on plain films and CT scans. The most common of these have been dealt with at appropriate places in earlier paragraphs, and perhaps at this point *it is best merely to underscore the value of assessing symmetry in the face.* If one notes a finding which suggests that a fracture might be present, then one should immediately compare this area with the same one on the other side. If the finding is normal, chances are that it will be seen, and appear the same, on the other side. Of course, this is with the understanding that the examination is performed with proper positioning, that is, without rotation, obliquity, etc.

In the mandible, the most commonly misinterpreted normal structure is the synchondrosis of the symphysis menti. This is a radiolucent, vertical line in the middle of the mandible and usually is seen in infants and young children. Knowledge of its midline position should avoid its misinterpretation as a fracture. The groove for the mandibular branch of the trigeminal nerve also can be misinterpreted as a fracture of the body of the mandible.

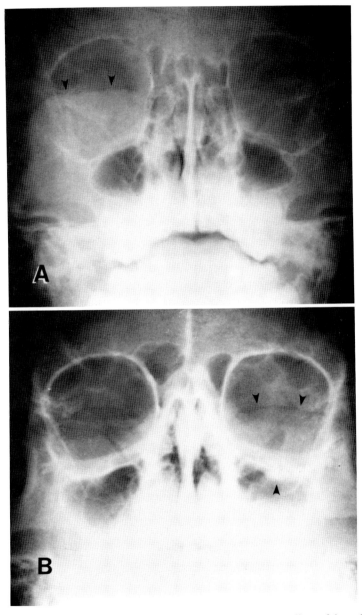

Figure 5.67. *Soft tissue abnormalities in facial trauma.* (*A*) Note extensive swelling of the soft tissues above the right maxillary sinus (*arrows*). All of the bony structures, however, are normal. (*B*) Another patient sustaining a blow to the left orbit. Note some generalized increase in soft tissue density over the lower left orbit and the slit-like transverse radiolucency caused by air being trapped in the palpebral fissure (*upper arrows*). Swelling of the lower eyelid causes the trapped air to appear slit-like. Note its normal appearance *on the right* side. In addition, note a minimal blowout fracture *on the left* (*lower arrow*).

REFERENCES

1. Ahrendt, D., Swischuk, L.E., and Hayden, C.K., Jr.: Incomplete (bending?) fractures of the mandibular condyle in children. Pediatr. Radiol. 14: 140–141, 1984.

2. Brown, O.L., Longacre, J.J., DeStefano, G.A., Wood, R.W., and Kahl, J.B.: Roentgen manifestations of blowout fracture of the orbit. Radiology 85: 908–913, 1965.

3. Curtin, H.D., Wolfe, P., and Schramm, V.: Orbital roof blow-out fractures. A.J.R. 139: 969–972, 1982.

4. Dolan, K.D., and Jacoby, C.G.: Facial fractures. Semin. Roentgenol. 13: 37–51, 1978.

5. Dolan, K.D., Jacoby, C., and Smoker, W.: The radiology of facial fractures. Radiographics 4: 577–663, 1984.

6. Freimanis, A.K.: Fractures of the facial bones. Radiol. Clin. North Am. 4: 341–363, 1966.

7. Fueger, G.F., Milauskas, A.T., and Britton, W.: The roentgenologic evaluation of orbital blow-out injuries. A.J.R. 97: 614–617, 1966.

8. Gerlock, A.J., and Sinn, D.P.: Anatomic clinical, surgical, and radiographic correlation of zygomatic complex fracture. A.J.R. 128: 235–248, 1977.

9. Gould, H.R., and Titus, C.O.: Internal orbital fractures: The value of laminography in diagnosis. A.J.R. 97: 618–623, 1966.

10. Hammerschlag, S.B., Hughes, S., O'Reilly, G.V., Naheedy, M.H., and Rumbaugh, C.L.: Blow-out fractures of the orbit: A comparison of computed tomography and conventional radiography with anatomical correlation. Radiology 143: 487–492, 1982.

11. Hammerschlag, S.B., Hughes, S., O'Reilly, G.V., and Weber, A.L.: Another look at blow-out fractures of the orbit. A.J.R. 139: 133–137, 1982.

12. Lacey, G.F., Wignall, B.K., Hussain, S., and Reidy, J.R.: The radiology of nasal injuries: Problems of interpretation and clinical relevance. Br. J. Radiol. 50: 412–414, 1977.

13. Lee, C.Y.S., McCullom, C., III, and Blaustein, D.I.: Pediatric chin injury: Occult condylar fractures of the mandible. Pediatr. Emerg. Care 7: 160–162, 1991.

14. Le Fort, R.: Fracture de la machoire superieure. Congr. Internat. Med. Paris, Sect. Chir. Gen. 1900, pp. 275–278.

15. Le Fort, R.: Etude experimentale sur les fractures de la machoire superieure. Rev. Chir. 23: 208–209, 1901.

16. Lewin, J.R., Rhodes, D.H., Jr., and Pasek, E.J.: Roentgenologic manifestations of fracture of orbital floor (blow-out fracture). A.J.R. 83: 628–632, 1960.

17. Trapnell, D.H.: The "magnification sign" of triple mandibular fracture. Br. J. Radiol. 50: 97–100, 1977.

18. Unger, J.D., and Unger, F.G.: Fracture of the pterygoid processes accompanying severe facial bone injury. Radiology 98: 311–316, 1971.

19. Vinik, M., and Gargano, F.P.: Orbital fractures. A.J.R. 97: 607–613, 1966.

20. Zilkha, A.: Computed tomography of blow-out fracture of medial orbital wall. A.J.R. 137: 963–965, 1981.

21. Zilkha, A.: Computed tomography in facial trauma. Radiology 144: 545–548, 1982.

22. Zismor, J., Smith, B., Fasano, C., and Converse, J.M.: Roentgen diagnosis of blow-out fractures of orbit. A.J.R. 87: 1009–1018, 1962.

DETECTING INCREASED INTRACRANIAL PRESSURE (SPREAD SUTURES)

In infancy and early childhood, increased intracranial pressure is manifest primarily in widening or spreading of the calvarial sutures. The coronal suture usually is the first to spread, and in the infant < 3 months of age no valid measurements are available. Consequently, one must rely on one's objective observation that the coronal suture is wider and more V-shaped than normal (4). In addition to this finding, one may well note that the anterior fontanel is bulging (Fig. 5.68). In the older infant and child, it has been suggested that if the coronal suture measures >3 mm at its uppermost aspect, then spread should be present (2). This measurement is the most useful one available, but in some cases borderline measurements still cause uncertainty. It is in such cases that I have found it worthwhile to examine the sagittal suture as well (3). The reason for this is that while the normal coronal suture often appears spread when, in truth, it is not, seldom

Figure 5.68. *Spread sutures in infancy.* (A) Normal infant demonstrating upper limits of normal of the coronal suture (*arrows*). Note that the coronal suture is slightly V-shaped. (B) Exaggerated V-shaped configuration of the coronal suture (*arrows*) due to markedly increased intracranial pressure. Also note that the anterior fontanel is bulging. In A the anterior fontanel is not bulging.

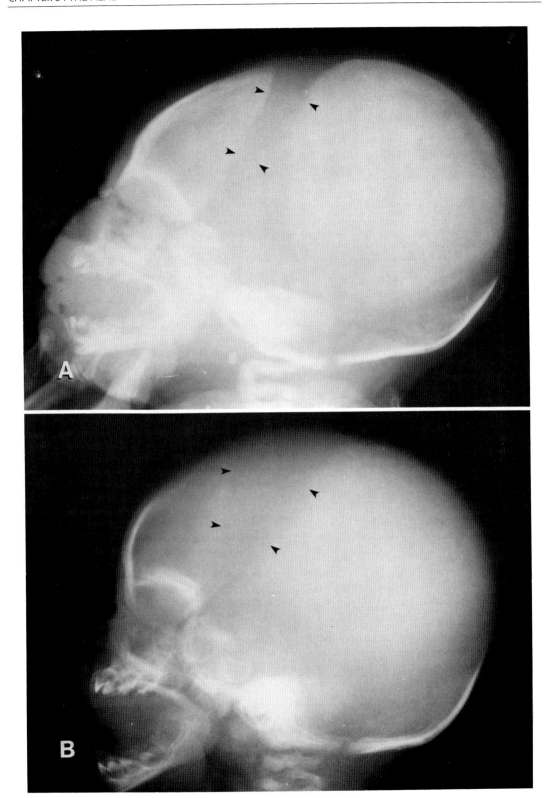

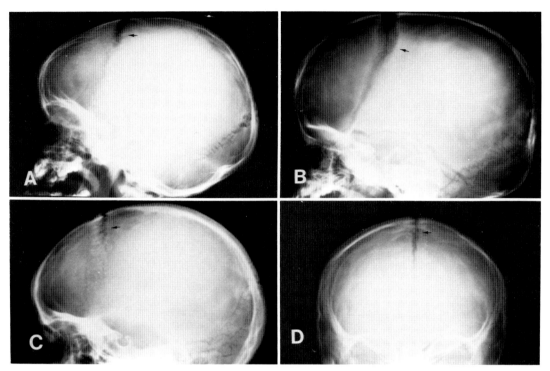

Figure 5.69. *Spread sutures in older infants and children.* (*A*) Note clearly spread coronal suture (*arrow*). (*B*) Gross spreading with an exaggerated V-shaped configuration of the coronal suture (*arrow*) in an infant with meningitis. All of the other sutures also are spread. (*C*) Questionably spread coronal suture (*arrow*). Such a configuration often is difficult to differentiate from normal. (*D*) Frontal view demonstrating definite spread of the sagittal suture (*arrow*). This should suggest that the coronal suture in (*C*) truly is spread. This patient had an intracranial bleed.

does this occur with the sagittal suture. Consequently, if the sagittal suture is judged to be spread, then increased intracranial pressure is likely (Fig. 5.69).

Spread of the cranial sutures is a nonspecific finding and can be seen with increased intracranial pressure secondary to cerebral edema, subdural hematomas, cerebral hematomas, meningitis (1), and brain tumors. In the emergency setting, however, one usually is confronted with sutural spread secondary to calvarial injury with intracranial bleeding, cerebral edema, or meningitis.

REFERENCES

1. Holmes, R.D., Kuhns, L.R., and Oliver, W.J.: Widened sutures in childhood meningitis: Unrecognized sign of an acute illness. A.J.R. 128: 977–979, 1977.
2. Segal, H.D., Mikity, V.G., Rumbaugh, C.L., et al.: Cranial sutures in the first year of life: Limits of normal and the "sprung suture." Presented at the 57th annual meeting of the Radiological Society of North America, Chicago, 1971.
3. Swischuk, L.E.: The growing skull. Semin. Roentgenol. 9: 115–124, 1974.
4. Swischuk, L.E.: The normal newborn skull. Semin. Roentgenol. 9: 101–113, 1974.

MISCELLANEOUS SKULL AND FACE PROBLEMS

Ocular Foreign Body Localization. Ocular foreign bodies are a common problem in the emergency room. Nonopaque ones pose obvious problems, but most opaque foreign bodies are relatively easily localized with plain films and CT scans (2) (Fig. 5.70). Orbital ultrasonography also is useful in detecting ocular foreign bodies (1).

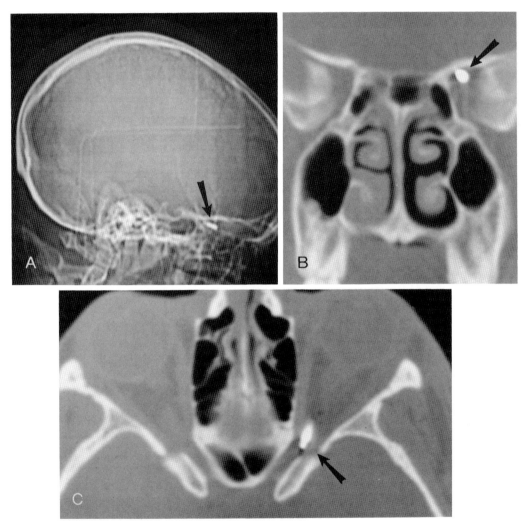

Figure 5.70. *Ocular foreign body: CT scan.*   (**A**) Topogram demonstrates the opaque foreign body (*arrow*). (**B**) Axial CT cut demonstrates the metallic pellet (*arrow*) embedded deep in the orbit just next to the optic nerve. (**C**) Coronal CT cut demonstrates the foreign body (*arrow*) again.

REFERENCES
1. Coleman, D.J., and Trokel, S.L.: A protocol for B-scan and radiographic foreign body localization. Am. J. Ophthalmol. 71: 84–89, 1971.
2. Tate, E., and Cupples, H.: Detection of orbital foreign bodies with computed tomography: Current limits. A.J.R. 137: 493–495, 1981.

Proptosis and Orbital Cellulitis. Proptosis can result from a number of causes, but in the child, acute unilateral proptosis usually is secondary to trauma or orbital inflammatory disease. Trauma, of course, is self-evident, and with orbital inflammatory disease, most often the problem is preorbital cellulitis (1). Thereafter, one should consider orbital inflammation secondary to sinusitis (3, 7, 8, 10). In most of these cases, there is no true osteomyelitis of the bones of the orbit, but rather adjacent, sympathetic soft tissue, intraorbital inflam-

mation. Less common causes of proptosis associated with orbital swelling include orbital bone infarction in sickle cell disease (2, 12, 14), pseudotumor of the orbit (11), and nonspecific orbital cellulitis.

In the past, periorbital and intraorbital inflammatory diseases often were difficult to differentiate clinically (5), but now they are readily differentiated with CT scanning (4, 6, 9). On CT scanning, preorbital cellulitis presents with normal intraorbital contents and swelling over the front of the eye. Intraorbital inflammatory disease associated with sinusitis usually presents with displacement of the medial rectus muscle and adjacent collections of intraorbital fluid or an actual abscess. In addition, bone destruction may be seen, but the commonest findings are displacement of the medial rectus muscle and adjacent

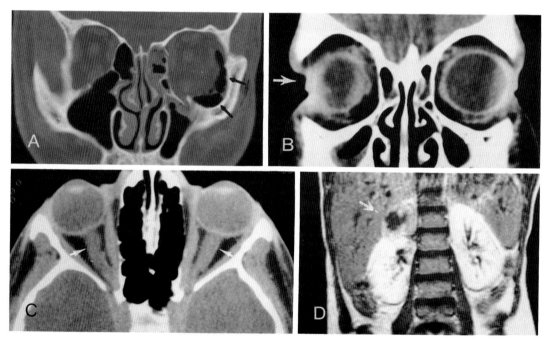

Figure 5.71. *CT of orbital disease.* (*A*) Intraorbital air (*arrows*) resulting from facial trauma. Note the associated blowout fracture through the floor of the orbit. (*B*) Penetrating injury to the right globe has resulted in its decompression (*arrow*). (*C*) Bilateral thickened optic nerves in a patient with acute systemic hypertension. This patient had papilledema and such optic nerve thickening (*arrows*) is commonly seen with papilledema. (*D*) Same patient demonstrating a super-renal mass (*arrow*) that turned out to be a pheochromocytoma presenting with acute systemic hypertension. (Parts *C* and *D* courtesy of C. Keith Hayden, Jr., M.D., Fort Worth, Texas.) For inflammatory orbital disease associated with sinusitis, see Figure 2.28.

edema. All of these findings are demonstrated in Figure 2.28.

Other Intraorbital Problems. Bleeding into the globe can occur with trauma (13) and is readily demonstrable with CT scanning. Similarly, retinal hemorrhages, characteristic of the battered child syndrome, also can be identified with CT scans. Thick optic nerves are seen with optic neuritis and also with papilledema (Fig. 5.71C and D). Penetrating injuries to the globe may result in decompression of the globe (Fig. 5.71B) and, in addition, air in the orbit also is readily demonstrable with CT scanning (Fig. 5.71A).

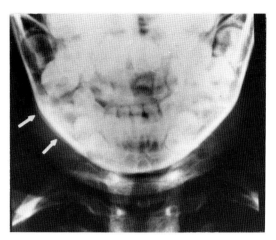

Figure 5.72. *Mandibular periostitis.* Note early deposition of periosteal new bone *on the right* (*arrows*). This patient presented with soft tissue swelling of the mandible in this area. No osteomyelitis is present. (Courtesy of V. Mikity, M.D.)

REFERENCES

1. Barkin, R.M., Todd, J.K., and Amer, J.: Periorbital cellulitis in children. Pediatrics 62: 390–392, 1978.
2. Blank, J.P., and Gill, F.M.: Orbital infarction in sickle cell disease. Pediatric 67: 879–881, 1981.
3. Chandler, J.R., Langenbrunner, D.J., and Stevens, E.R.: The pathogenesis of orbital complications in acute sinusitis. Laryngoscope 80: 1414, 1970.
4. DeSilva, M., Lam, V., and Broadfoot, J.: CT findings of orbital inflammation in children. Australas. Radiol. 31: 241–245, 1987.
5. Gellady, A.M., Shulman, S.T., and Ayoub, E.M.: Periorbital and orbital cellulitis in children. Pediatrics 61: 272–277, 1978.
6. Goldberg, F., Berne, A.S., and Oski, F.A.: Differentiation of orbital cellulitis from preseptal cellulitis by computed tomography. Pediatrics 62: 1000–1005, 1978.
7. Hawkins, D.B., and Clark, R.W.: Orbital involvement in acute sinusitits: Lessons from 24 childhood patients. Clin. Pediatr. 16: 464–471, 1977.
8. Haynes, R.E., and Crambleth, H.G.: Acute ethmoiditis, its relationship to orbital cellulitis. Am. J. Dis. Child. 114: 261, 1967.
9. Hirsch, M., and Lifshitz, T.: Computerized tomography in the diagnosis and treatment of orbital cellulitis. Pediatr. Radiol. 18: 302–305, 1988.
10. Jarret, W.H., II, and Gutman, F.A.: Ocular complication of infection in the paranasal sinuses. Arch. Ophthalmol. 81: 83, 1969.
11. Nugent, R.A., Rootman, J., Robertson, W.D., Lapointe, J.S. and Harrison, P.B.: Acute orbital pseudotumors: Classification and CT features. A.J.R. 137: 957–962, 1981.
12. Seeler, R.A.: Exophthalmos in hemoglobin SC disease. J. Pediatr. 102: 90–91, 1983.
13. Tomasi, L.G., and Rosman, N.P.: Purtscher's retinopathy in the battered child syndrome. Am. J. Dis. Child. 129: 1335–1337, 1975.
14. Wolff, M.H., and Sty, J.R.: Orbital infarction in sickle cell disease. Pediatr. Radiol. 15: 50–52, 1985.

Swollen Jaw. Very often, children presenting with a "swollen jaw" have, as their underlying problem, submandibular adenopathy, and in some of these cases periosteal new bone deposition along the body of the mandible can be seen (Fig. 5.72). These findings, however, do not represent osteomyelitis but rather a reactive periostitis secondary to the soft tissue inflammation (1). Other causes of swelling of the mandible include Caffey's disease, submandibular salivary gland inflammations, and primary bone tumors and infections. However, the most common cause is submandibular adenopathy. Currently, such adenopathy is most expediently confirmed with ultrasonography.

REFERENCE

1. Suydam, M.J., and Mikity, V.C.: Cellulitis with underlying inflammatory periostitis of the mandible. A.J.R. 56: 133–135, 1969.

Seizures. Seizures are a common problem in the pediatric population, and while the occasional seizure can herald the presence of an intracranial tumor, most are idiopathic or febrile seizures. In either case, skull roentgenograms are most unproductive (1, 3–6). In addition, although transient postictal edema can be seen on CT scanning (7), CT scans for childhood seizures also are relatively unproductive (2). MR scanning, however, is becoming more helpful, but generally is not obtained on an emergent basis.

REFERENCES

1. Committee on Radiology: Skull roentgenography of infants and children with convulsive disorders. Pediatrics 62: 835–837, 1978.
2. Harwood-Nash, D.C.: Computed tomography and seizures in children. J. Neuroradiol. 10: 130–136, 1983.
3. Hayes, W.G., and Shopfner, C.E.: Plain skull roentgenographic findings in infants and children with convulsions. Am. J. Dis. Child. 126: 785–787, 1973.
4. Nealis, J.G.T., McFadden, S.W., Asnes, R.A., and Ouellette, E.M.: Routine skull roentgenograms in the management of simple febrile seizures or head trauma. J. Can. Assoc. Radiol. 23: 234–235, 1977.
5. Newman, D.E.: Routine skull radiographs in children with seizures or head trauma. J. Can. Assoc. Radiol. 23: 234–235, 1977.
6. Ogunmekan, A.O.: Routine skull roentgenography in the clinical evaluation of children with febrile convulsions. Br. J. Radiol. 53: 815, 1980.
7. Rumack, C.M., Guggenheim, M.A., Fasules, J.W., and Burdick, D.: Transient positive postictal computed tomographic scan. J. Pediatr. 97: 263–264, 1980.

ACUTE INTRACRANIAL VASCULAR AND INFLAMMATORY DISEASES

In the past, the diagnosis of meningitis, for the most part, was nonradiologic. However, with CT scanning, one now can see early brain edema and, later, with contrast enhancement, increased definition (enhancement) of the meninges or areas of associated cerebritis (Fig. 5.73). Enhancement of the meninges is especially profound with tuberculous and fungal meningitis. Brain abscess characteristically produces an area of hypodensity on plain CT scans and a ring of enhancement on contrast studies (Fig. 5.74). Epidural abscesses also can be identified with CT and, as with parenchymal abscesses, demonstrate a hyperemic rim (Fig. 5.74). A similar hyperemic rim with surrounding edema can be seen with cysticercosis in its active stages (Fig. 5.75). Later, as the lesion heals, a punctate calcification remains.

As far as acute vascular problems are concerned, spontaneous intracranial bleeding in children is quite uncommon. Nonetheless, it does occur, either with angiomas, aneurysms, or blood dyscrasias (Fig. 5.76). Deep venous thrombosis is readily identified with CT scanning. On contrast-enhanced studies, a radiolucent, triangular defect is seen at the confluence of the straight and transverse sinuses (1, 3). Stroke due to vascular occlusive disease also is uncommon in children, but with CT scanning produces an area of hypodensity (infarction-edema) which is later followed by luxury perfusion around the infarcted area on contrast-enhanced scans (Fig. 5.77). Such infarcts can occur spontaneously (infantile hemiplegia) or as a complication of trauma or intracranial infection such as meningitis. Brain death resulting from acute hypoxia to the brain is usually best defined with nuclear scintigraphy or angiography (Fig. 5.78). Nuclear scintigraphy is preferred, however, because it is easier to obtain.

With the battered child syndrome, CT of the brain is invaluable (2). The findings are quite variable and may be very extensive. On the other hand, they may consist of nothing more than brain edema or subtle evidence of a shearing injury between the white and gray matter (see Fig. 4.228). When more profound injury occurs, the findings are not difficult to identify (Fig. 5.79). In addition to intracranial hemorrhage and other abnormalities, retinal

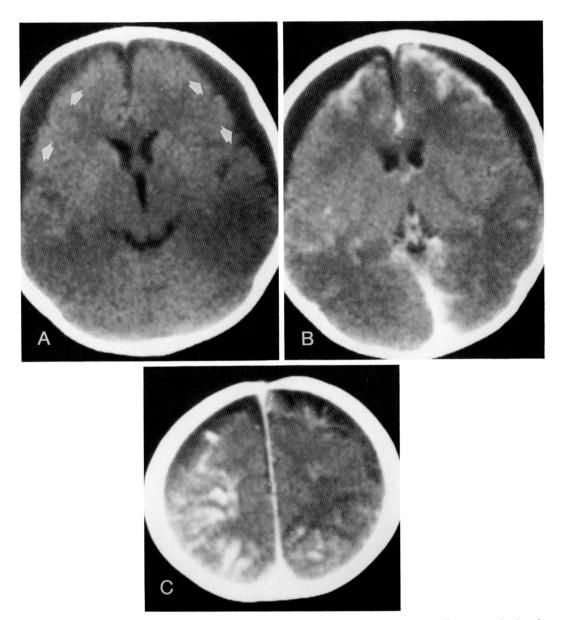

Figure 5.73. *Meningitis—cerebritis.* (**A**) Nonenhanced scan demonstrates subdural effusions on both sides (*arrows*). (**B**) Contrast study demonstrates diffuse enhancement of the meninges over the frontal regions and along the falx. (**C**) A higher cut demonstrates diffuse enhancement of the meninges over the various sulci of the brain.

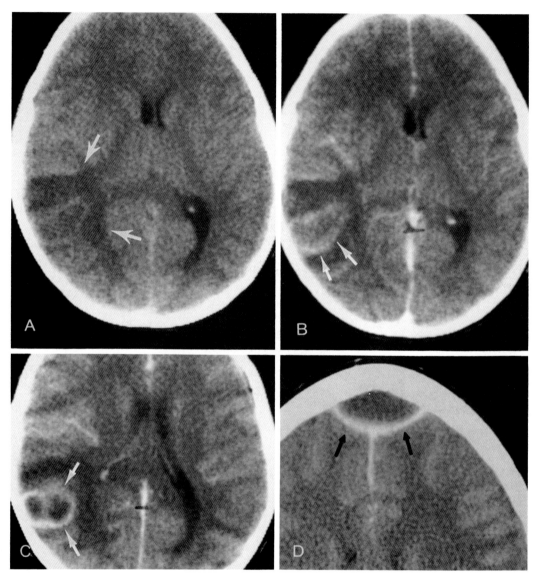

Figure 5.74. *Intracranial inflammatory disease: CT finding.* (*A*) Brain abscess. Nonenhanced CT scan demonstrates an area of hypodensity in the right posterior parietal-occipital region (*arrows*). There is some contralateral midline shift, and the occipital horn of the right lateral ventricle has been compressed and is not visible. (*B*) After administration of contrast, a brain abscess with an enhancing rim (*arrows*) is seen. (*C*) A slightly higher slice demonstrates the characteristic ring-like appearance of the enhancing rim of the brain abscess (*arrows*). (*D*) Enhancing rim (*arrow*) of a frontal epidural abscess secondary to sinus disease.

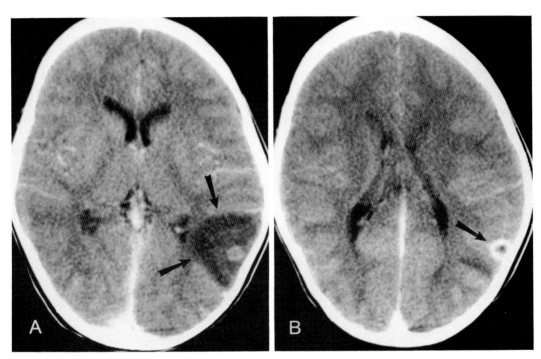

Figure 5.75. *Cysticercosis.*   (*A*) Note the focal area of edema (*arrows*) in the posterior parietal region *on the left.*
A central enhancing ring-like lesion is visible. (*B*) Slightly higher cut demonstrates the enhancing ring to better
advantage. Later, as these lesions heal, a small focus of calcification will remain.

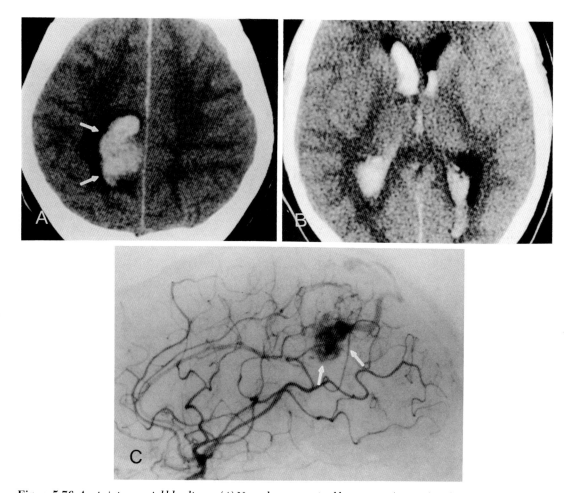

Figure 5.76. *Acute intracranial bleeding.* (*A*) Note the parasagittal hematoma (*arrows*) in this patient with acute apoplexy. (*B*) Another CT scan demonstrates widespread blood in both ventricles. (*C*) Angiogram demonstrates an arteriovenous malformation (*arrows*) with early filling of the veins.

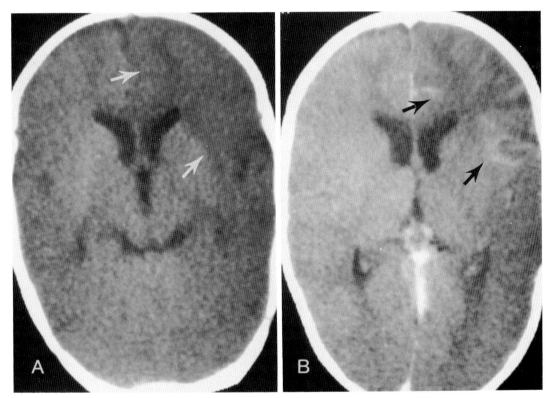

Figure 5.77. *Cerebral infarction.* (*A*) Note area of hypodensity in the left frontal lobe (*arrows*). (*B*) Contrast enhancement shows luxury perfusion in the area of the infarction (*arrows*).

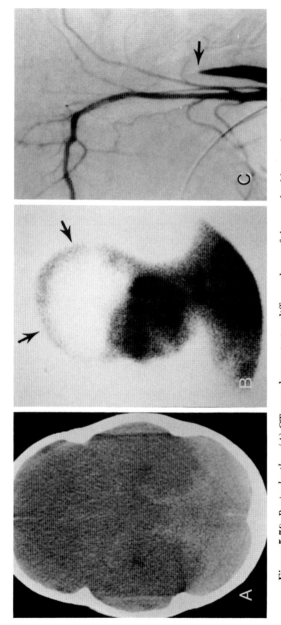

Figure 5.78. *Brain death.* (*A*) CT scan demonstrates diffuse edema of the cerebral hemispheres. There are no sulci, gyri, or ventricles visible. (*B*) Nuclear scintigraphy demonstrates normal distribution of isotope over the face and scalp (*arrows*) but no evidence of distribution to the brain. (*C*) Another patient with an arteriogram demonstrating no flow in the internal carotid artery (*arrow*).

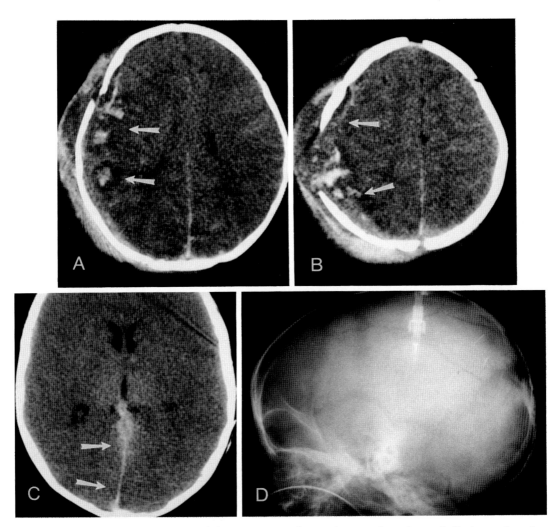

Figure 5.79. *Battered child syndrome.* (**A**) Note extensive hemorrhages in the right cerebellar hemisphere (*arrows*). There is midline shift of the falx and evidence of subarachnoid bleeding along it. There is also extensive scalp edema and bleeding and an underlying fracture. (**B**) A slightly higher cut demonstrates the extensive nature of the intracranial bleed (*arrow*), the diastatic fracture, and the associated subgaleal hematoma. (**C**) Another patient demonstrating diffuse edema of the brain and bleeding along the falx (*arrows*). (**D**) Skull film demonstrates the numerous fractures and spread sutures.

hemorrhages also can be demonstrated with CT.

REFERENCES

1. Eick, J.J., Miller, K.D., Bell, K.A., and Tutton, R.H.: Computed tomography of deep cerebral venous thrombosis in children. Radiology 140: 399–402, 1981.

2. Merten, D.F., Osborne, D.R.S., Radkowski, M.A., and Leonidas, J.C.: Craniocerebral trauma in the child abuse syndrome: Radiological observations. Pediatr. Radiol. 14: 272–277, 1984.

3. Rao, K.C.V.G., Knipp, H.C., and Wagner, E.J.: Computed tomographic findings in cerebral sinus and venous thrombosis. Radiology 140: 391–398, 1981.

CHAPTER 6

The Spine and Spinal Cord

CERVICAL SPINE INJURIES

Injuries of the cervical spine are less common in the infant and young child than in the older child and adult but, when they occur, injuries involving C_1, C_2, and C_3 are more common (2–5, 7, 14). In the end, however, one's approach to the analysis of the roentgenograms is the same whatever the age. *In this regard, one's most important job is to determine whether the cervical spine is stable or unstable.* To do this, one must understand all of the mechanisms of cervical spine injury and the abnormal findings they produce. It is to this end that this chapter is primarily devoted.

There is no question that the evaluation of the cervical spine in trauma, be it overt or subtle, is a problem. In this regard, it has been demonstrated that delay in adequate diagnosis often stems from not obtaining a flexion view, not having an experienced radiologist review the x-ray, and, of course, the inherent difficulty in obtaining adequate films in many of these patients (12). In addition, it has been demonstrated that protocol- driven imaging regimens for suspected cervical spine injuries are generally unrewarding (9, 11). In other words, *there should be some attempt at evaluating the patient clinically before he is automatically sent to the radiography suite to be examined. Certainly this has become a great problem in terms of the so-called "EMI collar." Most emergency ambulance operators are instructed to place a collar on a patient at the slightest indication of a neck injury and, indeed, even if there is no such indication. These patients should be clinically evaluated before they are sent to the radiography suite, for many will not require x-ray examination. A carefully executed physical examination is easy to accomplish in the patient who is coherent, and if it is negative, it can save enormous amounts of time and dollars in the evaluation of these patients. This seems such a practical approach, and yet it is ignored over and over again.*

What Views Are Necessary? Patients with cervical spine injuries fall into two groups: (a) those who are freely coherent and can move their necks, and (b) those who are not coherent or unconscious. In the latter group, one should confine the examination to cross-table lateral, frontal, and open-mouth odontoid views, and all should be obtained without moving the patient. In the coherent patient, lateral, frontal, open-mouth odontoid, and oblique views usually are obtained. *However, for years I have omitted the oblique views, unless lateral views detect some finding requiring further investigation. For the most part, routine oblique views of the cervical spine are not required in the pediatric age group. On the other hand, flexion views are indispensable* (3, 12). I have maintained for years that an alert, coherent patient should not be allowed to leave the emergency room before a flexion view of the cervical spine is obtained. Flexion views are indispensable in detecting occult posterior ligamentous injuries sustained from hyperflexion forces (see Fig. 6.23).

Once one adopts the attitude that a flexion view should be obtained, then one must develop some type of protocol for obtaining these views. *Obviously the views are not obtained in patients who are incoherent or comatosed.* Flexion views require that the patient be communicative and alert. Under these circumstances it is best for the patients to perform the flexion maneuver themselves. In this way, it is highly unlikely that they will sustain any significant neurologic injury. If they have a fracture or, indeed, if they have a neck sprain, they will not flex their neck to the point where neurologic injury will result. *On the other hand, forced flexion of the spine in a patient who is incoherent or unconscious can lead to such a problem and certainly one would not even think of obtaining a flexion view in such a patient. However, all of this has been overexuberantly transferred to the patient who is coherent and who simply has been placed in a collar because emergency medicine ambulance services require it.* All of this is understandable, but one must decide where to abort this sequence of events: in the initial examining room or the x-ray suite. Ideally this should be accomplished with physical examination, during the initial encounter with the patient. On a practical basis, this is how one might approach the problem.

First, it must be underscored that the patient must be coherent. If the patient is coherent, one should ask if he or she has any pain. If the answer is "no" one can remove the collar and if motion is normal no x-rays are necessary. If pain is present, one still should remove the collar and see what spontaneous movements occur. Thereafter, the patient should be asked to move the neck through a full range of motion, knowing that being able to fully flex the neck is the most important maneuver. With significant underlying injury the patient will not move the neck freely, if at all, and certainly will not want to flex the neck. At this point one should make a judgment as to whether the patient really has pain or is merely frightened. If one suspects that the patient is frightened, then he or she should be asked to flex his or her neck further. Usually this requires some gentle but positive and judicious encouragement. This can be done by placement of the examiner's hand on the occiput and gently urging flexion of the neck. It is important to remember that *flexion should be encouraged, not forced.* If this is adhered to there is little chance that a patient will get into trouble. Indeed, if a patient can fully flex his or her neck spontaneously or with encouragement, it is unlikely that a significant injury is present. Certainly an unstable fracture would be unlikely. Patients with these latter lesions usually have so much pain that they will not flex their neck even with encouragement. These latter patients obviously constitute a different group than the former. With the former group, once flexion of the neck has been accomplished clinically, the patient should be examined roentgenographically just to make sure that a subtle, nondisplaced fracture is not present. These patients can be subject to all of the views, including the flexion view.

With the latter group of patients, that is, those with pain and an inability to flex the neck fully, one should replace the collar and proceed with the roentgenographic examination. This examination should include the lateral, anteroposterior, and open mouth odontoid views, but not the flexion view. The flexion view should be obtained after the first views are reviewed and the spine judged to be stable. Then the flexion views should be obtained with as much flexion as the patient permits. No forced flexion should be utilized.

With the foregoing protocol, only those patients with pain would require x-rays and no patient should get into trouble. Of course, if a patient is incoherent, unconscious, or uncooperative, then one should obtain all views with the collar in place. This also pertains to patients who are too young to be reliable or cooperative patients.

Visualize All of the Cervical Spine. Visualization of the cervical spine is necessary, for if the cervical spine is not fully visualized, that is, if the shoulder covers the lower cervical spine, one can miss significant lesions in that area. Consequently, it is most important to count the vertebral bodies to ensure that all of them are included on any given film. *Always count seven vertebrae.* If seven vertebrae cannot be visualized, one can use special views such as the swimmer's view, but eventually one may have to resort to CT with sagittal and/or coronal reconstruction.

It is also important to remember that spinal injuries may occur at multiple levels. They can occur in the cervical spine alone, or throughout the entire vertebral column (1, 6, 15). *In addition, it might also be recalled that facial injuries often are associated with hyperextension spinal injuries, and that blows to the back of the head can induce concomitant flexion injuries of the cervical spine.*

CT and MR Scanning. Generally speaking, CT (10, 13) is now a standard method for evaluating suspected vertebral injury. *However, as opposed to cranial and intracranial injury, the plain film still remains the most important initial study in the assessment of spinal trauma.* MRI, for the most part, is reserved for evaluation of complicating soft tissue, spinal canal, and spinal cord injury (8). It is especially useful when neurologic findings are present but no bony abnormality is seen on the preliminary roentgenograms.

REFERENCES

1. Calenoff, L., Chessar, J.W., Rogers, L.F., Toerge, J., and Rosen, J.S.: Multiple level spinal injuries: Importance of early recognition. A.J.R. 130: 665–669, 1978.
2. Dietrich, A.M., Ginn-Pease, M.E., Barkowski, H.M., and King, D.R.: Pediatric cervical spine fractures: Predominantly subtle presentation. J. Pediatr. Surg. 26: 995–1000, 1991.
3. Dunlap, J.P., Morris, M., and Thompson, R.G.: Cervical spine injuries in children. J. Bone Joint Surg. 40A: 681–686, 1958.
4. Evans, D.L., and Bethem, D.: Cervical spine injuries in children. J. Pediatr. Orthop. 9: 563–568, 1989.
5. Ehara, S., El-Khoury, G.Y., and Sato, Y.: Pictorial essay. Cervical spine injury in children: Radiologic manifestations. A.J.R. 151: 1175–1178, 1988.
6. Gehweiler, J.A., Jr., Clark, W.M., Schaaf, R.E., Powers, B., and Miller, M.D.: Cervical spine

trauma: The common combined conditions. Radiology 130: 77–86, 1979.
7. Hadley, M.N., Zabramski, J.M., Browner, C.M., Rekate, H., and Sonntag, V.K.H.: Pediatric spinal trauma: Review of 122 cases of spinal cord and vertebral column injuries. J. Neurosurg. 68: 18–24, 1988.
8. Kalfas, I., Wilberger, J., Goldberg, A., and Prostko, E.R.: Magnetic resonance imaging in acute spinal cord trauma. Neurosurgery 23: 295–299, 1988.
9. Kreipke, D.L., Gillespie, K.R., McCarthy, M.C., Mail, J.T., Lappas, J.C., and Broadie, T.A.: Reliability of indications for cervical spine films in trauma patients. J. Trauma 29: 1438–1439, 1989.
10. McInerney, D.P., and Sage, M.R.: Computer assisted tomography in the assessment of cervical spine trauma. Clin. Radiol. 30: 203–206, 1979.
11. Mirvis, S.E., Diaconis, J.N., Chirico, P.A., Reiner, B.I., Joslyn, J.N., and Militello, P.: Protocol-driven radiologic evaluation of suspected cervical spine injury: Efficacy study. Radiol. 170: 831–834, 1989.
12. Orenstein, J.B., Klein, B.L., and Ochsenschlager, D.W.: Delayed diagnosis of pediatric cervical spine injury. Pediatrics 89: 1185–1188, 1992.
13. Radmor, R., Davis, K.R., Roberson, G.H., New, P.F.J., and Taveras, J.M.: Computed tomographic evaluation of traumatic spinal injuries. Radiology 127: 825–827, 1978.
14. Ruge, J.R., Sinson, G.P., McLone, D.G., and Cerullo, L.J.: Pediatric spinal injury: The very young. J. Neurosurg. 68: 25–30, 1988.
15. Scher, A.T.: Double fractures of the spine—an indication for routine radiographic examination of the entire spine after injury. S. Afr. Med. J. 53: 411–413, 1978.

WHAT TO LOOK FOR IN CERVICAL SPINE INJURIES

One should have some system for analyzing the cervical spine and, in this regard, I have found it best to start with the lateral view. This view is the most informative one, and a number of assessments should be accomplished before turning to the frontal and oblique views. First, one should note the general curvature of the spine, and then one should assess the individual structures from front to back. These structures include the prevertebral soft tissues, predental space (C_1 to dens distance), odontoid process, individual vertebral bodies, disc spaces, apophyseal joints, neural arches, and spinous tips.

Loss of Normal Cervical Spine Curvature. On lateral view, the cervical spine in the normal, neutral position assumes a gentle lordotic curve (Fig. 6.1), and on frontal view, it is straight. Deviation from these normal alignments usually reflects the presence of underlying muscle spasm and/or bony/ligament injury. Spasm usually produces a straight spine on lateral view, but in many children may lead to a mild to striking anterior, kyphotic angulation of C_2 on C_3 (Fig. 6.2). In such cases, there is no associated anterior displacement of the body of C_2 on the body of C_3,

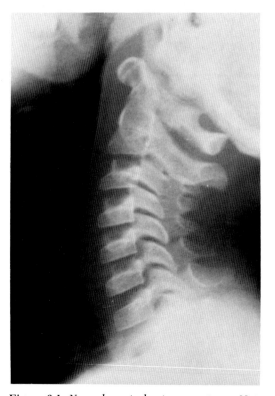

Figure 6.1. *Normal cervical spine curvature.* Note the gentle lordosis of the cervical spine. Also note the normal predental distance, the normal synchondrosis (horizontal radiolucent line) between the dens and body of C_2, and the normal prevertebral soft tissues. In addition, note the high position of the anterior arch of C_1. This occurs during extension and is normal.

and although the overall configuration may appear worrisome, it is quite reversible and not representative of a fracture or dislocation. Localized kyphosis at lower levels, on the other hand, is significant and usually indicates the presence of ligamentous laxity secondary to a hyperflexion injury.

Prevertebral Soft Tissue Thickening. Prevertebral soft tissue swelling or thickening due to edema or hematoma formation is an important ancillary finding in cervical spine injuries. *However, it should be noted from the outset that it is not present in all cases (2).* There is good reason for this, for in those cases where no significant anterior spinal ligament or vertebral body injury occurs, there is no reason for the prevertebral soft tissues to become widened. *Consequently, in a good many significant cervical spine injuries, the prevertebral soft tissues are normal.* This lack of prevertebral soft tissue thickening frequently occurs with minimal fractures of the dens (2).

Another problem with the assessment of the prevertebral soft tissues in the infant and young child is that, if the airway is not fully distended, or the spine not fully extended, pseudothickening can be suggested (Fig. 6.2). True soft tissue swelling should be reproducible from film to film, and also should cause "smooth" anterior displacement of the airway (Fig. 6.3). In the upper cervical spine, however, even these considerations may not solve the problem, for normal adenoidal lymphoid tissue extending into the retropharyngeal space can significantly interfere with interpretation (Fig. 6.4). Over the lower cervical spine, in those cases where soft tissue thickening is borderline, it may be helpful to note whether the prevertebral fat stripe is displaced anteriorly (3). Displacement of this fat stripe can be taken to indicate the presence of an underlying vertebral injury, but it is of limited value in the pediatric age group, for it is not readily visible in the infant and young child.

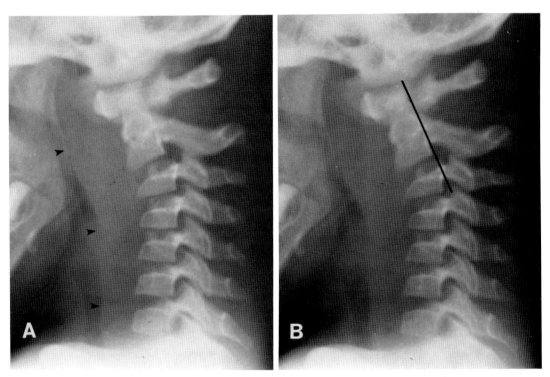

Figure 6.2. *C_2–C_3 angulation pseudoabnormality and pseudoprevertebral soft tissue thickening.* (**A**) Note that the prevertebral soft tissues appear thickened (*arrows*). Such thickening is due to poor roentgenographic technique (i.e., inadequate distension of the airway and hyperflexion of the spine). Also note that C_2 is angled forward on C_3. However, in (**B**) note that a line drawn along the posterior aspect of the dens and body of C_2 demonstrates that there is no associated anterior displacement of C_2 on C_3. In the absence of such displacement, angulation of C_2 on C_3 is of no particular consequence and can be seen with both voluntary and involuntary muscle spasm. Finally, note that the predental distance is wide (4–5 mm in this patient), and that the distance between the spinous tips of C_1 and C_2 also is unusually wide. Both of these findings are normal.

In terms of normal measurement guidelines for prevertebral soft tissue thickening in children, far too much variability exists for such measurements to be useful. Nonetheless, it has been suggested that above the glottis soft tissue thickness of 7 mm or more be considered abnormal, and that below the glottis over 14 mm of soft tissue space be considered abnormal (1). These measurements are reasonably dependable in the older child, but must be adjusted upward in younger children and infants in whom vertebral body ossification is incom-

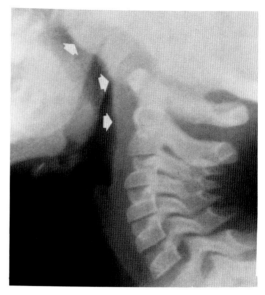

Figure 6.4. *Normal adenoidal prevertebral soft tissues.* Note prominent adenoidal prevertebral soft tissues extending into the retropharyngeal space (*arrows*). This type of soft tissue thickening should not be misinterpreted as pathologic thickening. Note preservation of the normal stepoff of the posterior walls of the hypopharynx and trachea. Compare with the smooth arcing configuration of these two walls with true soft tissue thickening seen in Figure 6.3.

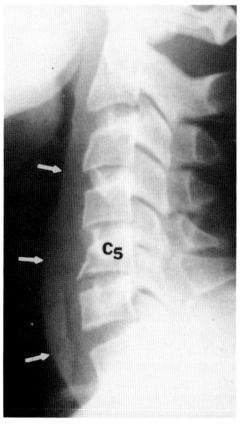

Figure 6.3. *Prevertebral soft tissue swelling.* Note prevertebral soft tissue swelling (*arrows*) anterior to a compression fracture of C_5. Not only are the tissues thickened but they also produce continuous, arcing anterior displacement of the airway. Compare these prevertebral soft tissues with the normal ones shown in Figure 6.4.

plete and even greater width variations occur. *In general, however, the measurements do define a rule that I have followed for years. This rule states that below the level of the glottis the normal soft tissues double in thickness (Fig. 6.4).* This occurs because below this level the esophagus separates from the airway and becomes part of the airless prevertebral soft tissue mass.

REFERENCES

1. Clark, W.M., Gehweiler, J.A., Jr., and Laib, R.: Twelve significant signs of cervical spine trauma. Skeletal Radiol. 3: 201–205, 1979.
2. Penning, L.: Prevertebral hematoma in cervical spine injury: Incidence and etiologic significance. A.J.R. 136: 553–561, 1981.
3. Whalen, J.P., and Woodruff, C.L.: The cervical prevertebral fat stripe. A.J.R. 109: 445–451, 1970.

Increase in the Predental Space (C_1 to Dens Distance). Before beginning any discussion of the predental distance, one must realize that normal variations are much more pronounced in children than in adults. In the adult, a distance >2.5 mm usually is considered abnormal, but in children distances of 3–4 mm are commonplace and normal. Indeed, a few children can demonstrate a predental distance of 5 mm and still be normal (Fig. 6.5). This was demonstrated by Locke et al. (6) a number of years ago, and duplicated in our own survey of 100 consecutive cervical spine roentgenograms in normal children (Table 6.1). In addition to these differences, it should be noted that the predental distance can widen significantly between flexion and extension (Fig. 6.6), often with variations of up to 2 mm (1). Consequently, one must be cautious not to overinterpret an *apparently* abnormally wide predental space in children.

Abnormal widening of the predental

Table 6.1
Normal Predental (C_1 to Dens) Distances

Predental Distance (mm)	No. of Patients
1–1½	7
2–2½	54
3–3½	27
4–4½	9
5	3
Total	100

space occurs when there is disruption of the transverse ligament between C_1 and the dens (3–5), but in actual fact, this is not such a common injury, even with dens fractures. The reason for this is that the dens and C_1 move as a unit, and thus the predental distance is not altered. Actually, widening of the predental space occurs more often with atlantoaxial instability due to underlying abnormalities such as rheumatoid arthritis (7) or congenital hypoplasia of the dens (2). In either case, these patients are prone to abnormal atlantoaxial ligament laxity and movement, and dislocation without fracture is more likely to occur. Other injuries that can be associated with an increase in the predental distance include rotatory subluxation of C_1 on C_2 and some Jefferson bursting fractures of C_1.

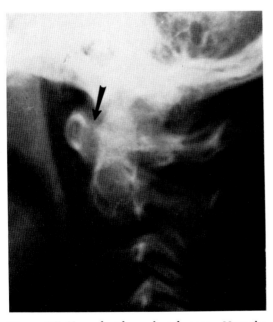

Figure 6.5. *Normal wide predental space.* Note the wide (4–5 mm) predental space (*arrow*) in this normal 8-year-old child.

REFERENCES

1. Cattell, H.S., and Filtzer, D.L.: Pseudosubluxation and other normal variations in the cervical spine in children. J. Bone Joint Surg. 47A: 1295–1309, 1965.
2. Dawson, E.G., and Smith, L.: Atlanto-axial subluxation in children due to vertebral anomalies. J. Bone Joint Surg. 61A: 582–587, 1979.
3. deBeer, J. deV., Hoffman, E.B., and Kieck, C.F.: Traumatic atlantoaxial subluxation in children. J. Pediatr. Orthop. 10: 397–400, 1990.
4. Floman, Y., Kaplan, L., and Elidan, J.: Transverse ligament rupture and atlanto-axial subluxation in children. J. Bone Joint Surg. 73B: 640–643, 1991.
5. Harouchi, A., Padovani, J.P., and Elandaloussi, M.: Atlanto-axial dislocation in children: A review of 9 cases. Chir. Pediatr. 25: 136–144, 1984.
6. Locke, G.R., Gardner, J.I., and Van Epps, E.F.: Atlas-dens interval (ADI) in children: A survey

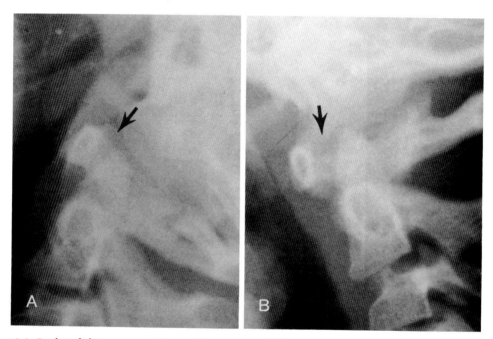

Figure 6.6. *Predental distance—variation with extension and flexion.* (*A*) On extension, note the normal appearance of the predental space (*arrow*). (*B*) With flexion, note how much widening has occurred (*arrow*). This patient was normal. A 2-mm increase in the predental space is normal.

based on 200 normal cervical spines. A.J.R. 97: 135–140, 1966.

7. Reid, G.D., and Hill, R.H.: Atlantoaxial subluxation in juvenile ankylosing spondylitis. J. Pediatr. 93: 531–532, 1978.

Hypermobility of C_1. In infants and young children, both during flexion and extension, C_1 tends to stay in close apposition to the base of the skull, and thus may appear hypermobile in relation to C_2. In extension, high positioning of the anterior arch of C_1 results but is normal (see Fig. 6.1). Similarly, an apparently wide intraspinous distance between the spinous tips of C_1 and C_2 seen on flexion also is normal (see Figs. 6.2 and 6.15B). However, both of these configurations, to the uninitiated, can appear very abnormal. In explaining this phenomenon, it might be recalled that the ligamentous attachments between the base of the skull and C_1 are very firm, while in the upper cervical spine, in general, they are quite lax. Therefore, if any excessive motion is to occur, it will occur from C_1 downwards.

Displacement of the Vertebral Bodies. In most instances, displacement of one vertebral body on another is a significant abnormal finding and reflects underlying instability of the spine. Anterior displacement is much more common than posterior displacement and usually occurs with flexion or rotational injuries. Almost invariably, anterior displacement of a vertebral body indicates a significant underlying injury, but caution must be exercised in the upper cervical spine of infants and young children in whom normal anterior displacement can occur.

Anterior displacement of the vertebral bodies in the upper cervical spine of infants and young children is a well-known phenomenon and is physiologic (1–3, 5–9). Such displacement may involve all upper four vertebral bodies or occur at the C_2–C_3 level only. In those cases where multiple vertebral bodies are involved, the findings are not difficult to interpret (Fig.

6.7), but when isolated anterior displacement of C_2 on C_3 occurs, interpretation can be a problem. Indeed, in some children, the degree of displacement is so pronounced that it is almost impossible to accept that it is physiologic (Fig. 6.8). Nonetheless, it is physiologic and results from the fact that the fulcrum for flexion of the upper cervical spine in the infant is at the C_2–C_3 level (see Fig. 6.71). The cervical spine generally is a lax structure in infants and children, and consequently a great deal of excessive normal motion can occur at this site.

As an aid to this problem, I devised the *posterior cervical line* (7), and this line has proven to be most helpful in differentiating physiologic from pathologic displacement of C_2 on C_3 (Fig. 6.8). The line is drawn from the anterior aspect of the cortex of the spinous process of C_1 to the same point on C_3 and its relationship to the anterior cortex of C_2 is noted. If it misses the anterior cortex of C_2 by 2.0 mm or more, a true

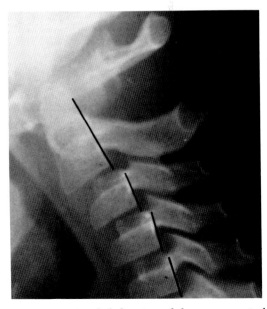

Figure 6.7. *Pseudodislocation of the upper cervical spine—multiple levels.* Note that each of the vertebral bodies from C_2 through C_5 demonstrates anterior displacement. Such displacement is normal and physiologic.

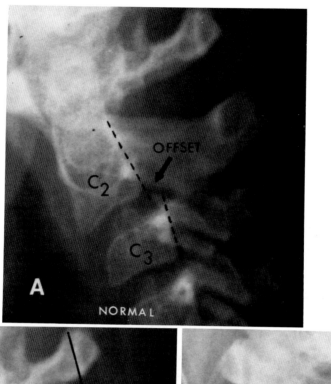

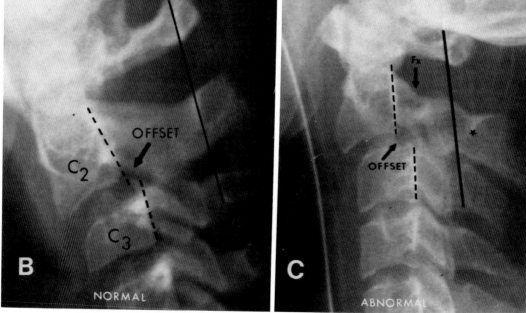

Figure 6.8. *Physiologic dislocation of C₂ on C₃—use of posterior cervical spine.* (*A*) Note that C₂ is anteriorly displaced on C₃ (*dotted lines*). (*B*) The posterior cervical line is drawn from the anterior cortex of the spinous process of C₁ to the anterior cortex of the spinous process of C₃. In this case, it passes directly through the anterior cortex of C₂. This is normal, and thus the findings represent physiologic displacement of C₂ on C₃ only. (*C*) Pathologic dislocation of C₂ on C₃ secondary to hangman's fracture—use of posterior cervical line. Note that the body of C₂ is displaced forward on the body of C₃ and that offsetting is present. Also note that the posterior cervical line is abnormal in that it misses the cortex of C₂ (*star*) by more than 2 mm. The actual measurement was 4 mm. (Reprinted with permission from L.E. Swischuk: Anterior displacement of C₂ in children—physiologic and pathologic: A helpful differentiating line. Radiology 122: 759–763, 1977.)

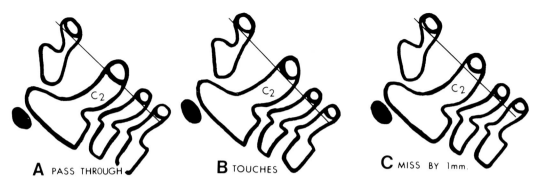

Figure 6.9. *Posterior cervical line—normal limits.* The posterior cervical line is normal when it: (*A*) passes through or just behind the cortex of C_2, (*B*) touches the anterior cortex of C_2, or (*C*) passes within 1 mm of the anterior aspect of the cortex of C_2. If it passes 1.5 mm in front of the cortex, it is borderline in significance, but if it misses the cortex by 2.0 mm or more, an underlying pathologic dislocation with an associated hangman's fracture should be present. (Reprinted with permission from L.E. Swischuk: Anterior displacement of C_2 in children—physiologic or pathologic: A helpful differentiating line. Radiology 122: 759–763, 1977.)

dislocation, associated with an underlying hangman's fracture, should be present. A measurement of 1.5 mm is borderline, but <1.5 mm the findings should represent physiologic displacement only (Fig. 6.8). A diagrammatic representation of the normal limits for the posterior cervical line is shown in Figure 6.9, but before one examines these limits, *it must be underscored that the posterior cervical line should be applied only in those cases where anterior displacement of C_2 on C_3 is present (7).* If there is mere angulation of C_2 on C_3, as demonstrated in Figure 6.2, the line may measure abnormal. The posterior cervical line is designed for use when there is actual anterior displacement of C_2 on C_3 (Fig. 6.10). In the neutral or extended position the spinous tip of C_2 lies posterior to both C_1 and C_3, and this is normal (7). This posterior positioning is retained when a hangman's fracture of C_2 occurs. *With this fracture, motion is transferred from the normal apophyseal joints at the C_2–C_3 level to the fracture site. As a result, C_1 and the anterior fracture fragment of C_2 move forward, while the posterior portion of the arch of C_2 remains in the extended position. It is for this reason that the posterior cervical line measures abnormal in these cases.* Anterior displacement of the body of C_2 results

from associated ligament disruption between the bodies of C_2 and C_3.

Conversely, however, *a normal posterior cervical line measurement does not exclude underlying ligamentous injury at the C_2–C_3 level.* Many times such injury becomes evident at a later date. In such cases, there is enough muscle spasm to keep the vertebral bodies in normal alignment and it is only in subsequent weeks when muscle spasm subsides that hypermobility due to the underlying ligament injury is appreciated (see Fig. 6.24). On the other hand, in some cases ligamentous injury is acute and there is clear-cut apophyseal joint separation (Fig. 6.11). However, because motion in these cases is not transferred from the C_2–C_3 apophyseal joint to the fracture site of the hangman's fracture, the posterior cervical line remains normal. *It is important to appreciate this potential pitfall when using the posterior cervical line.* The phenomenon of physiologic anterior displacement of C_2 on C_3 is common in childhood but tends to disappear around the age of 16 years. It has been documented in young adults (2), but generally it is a phenomenon of the early and midpediatric age group.

Pathologic posterior displacement of one vertebral body on another is not par-

Figure 6.10. *Pseudodislocation—C_2 on C_3.* Note that C_2 and C_3 are offset (*arrows*). Once this determination has been made, one can apply the posterior cervical line along the spinus tips of C_1 and C_3. In this case, the posterior cervical line measures normal.

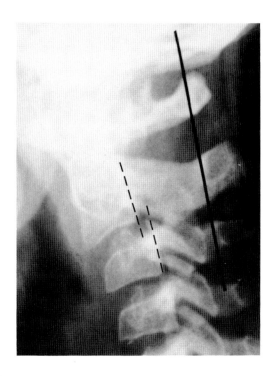

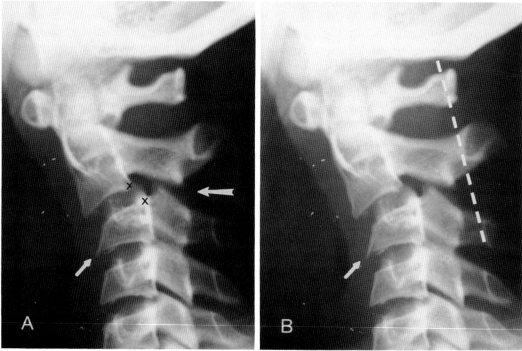

Figure 6.11. *Ligamentous injury: C2–C3.* (*A*) Note that C_2 and C_3 are offset (*X's*). In addition, **the apophyseal joint is V-shaped** (*arrow*) and subluxation is present. There may be a small teardrop fracture of C_3 present (*anterior small arrow*). The ring epiphysis seen on edge in this area commonly appears tipped and should not be misinterpreted for a fracture (see Fig. 6.69A). (*B*) The posterior cervical line measures normal. The reason for this is that flexion motion still is occurring through the apophyseal joint. The teardrop fracture of C_3 is a little more clearly visualized (*arrow*). The intraspinous distance between the spinous tips of C_2 and C_3 also is markedly increased, attesting to the hyperflexion injury. (Courtesy of A.M.O. Gorman, M.D., Montreal Children's Hospital.)

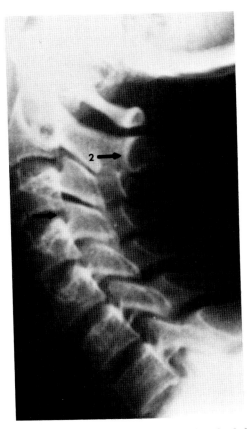

Figure 6.12. *Normal posterior vertebral body dislocation and posterior position of the spinous process of* C_2. Note the normal posterior displacement of C_3 on C_4 *(1)* and the normal posterior position of the spinous process of C_2 *(2)*. In the neutral or extended position, this is the normal location of the spinous process of C_2. With flexion, it moves forward and lines up with the spinous processes of C_1 and C_3. In so doing, it constitutes the basis for the application of the posterior cervical line as delineated in Figures 6.8 and 6.9.

ticularly common, but probably occurs during the acute phase of certain extension injuries. Such displacement, however, does not seem to persist for long, and the reason may be that with subsequent return to a more neutral position or with hyperflexion secondary to whiplashing, normal alignment tends to reestablish itself. Normal physiologic posterior displacement also is not particularly common (1, 4), but it does occur (Fig. 6.12). In such cases, I have not seen the displacement to result in

more than 1–2 mm of offsetting. Displacement of the vertebral bodies in a lateral direction also can occur, but usually is associated with severe fracture-dislocations with significant changes clearly visible on the lateral view.

Alterations in the Width of the Disc Space. In most normal patients, the width of the intervertebral disc spaces is the same from one level to another. This is most important to note, for if there is a level where gross discrepancy occurs, underlying longitudinal ligament injury with cervical spine instability should be inferred. Narrowing of the disc space occurs with flexion and rotation injuries (Fig. 6.13*A*), but widening of the disc space signifies the presence of an underlying extension injury (Fig. 6.13*B*). Disc space narrowing or widening is best assessed on lateral views of the cervical spine.

REFERENCES

1. Cattell, H.S., and Filtzer, D.L.: Pseudosubluxation and other normal variations in the cervical spine in children. J. Bone Joint Surg. 47A: 1295–1309, 1965.
2. Harrison, R.B., Keats, T.E., Winn, H.R., Riddervold, H.O., and Pope, T.L., Jr.: Pseudosubluxation in the axis in young adults. J. Can. Assoc. Radiol. 31: 176–177, 1980.
3. Jacobson, G., and Bleecker, H.H.: Pseudosubluxation of the axis in children. A.J.R. 82: 472–481, 1959.
4. Kattan, K.R.: Backward "displacement" of the spinolaminal line at C2: A normal variation. A.J.R. 129: 289–290, 1977.
5. Pennecot, G.F., Gouraud, D., Hardy, J.R., and Pouliquen, J.C.: Roentgenographical study of the stability of the cervical spine in children. J. Pediatr. Orthop. 4: 346–352, 1984.
6. Sullivan, C.R., Bruwer, A.J., and Harris, L.E.: Hypermobility of the cervical spine in children: A pitfall in the diagnosis of cervical dislocation. Am. J. Surg. 95: 636–640, 1958.
7. Swischuk, L.E.: Anterior displacement of C_2 in children: physiologic or pathologic? A helpful differentiation. Radiology 122: 759–763, 1977.
8. Teng, P., and Paptheodorou, C.: Traumatic subluxation of C_2 in young children. Bull. Los Angeles Neurol. Soc. 32: 197–202, 1967.
9. Townsend, E.H., Jr., and Rowe, M.L.: Mobility of the upper cervical spine in health and disease. Pediatrics 10: 567–572, 1952.

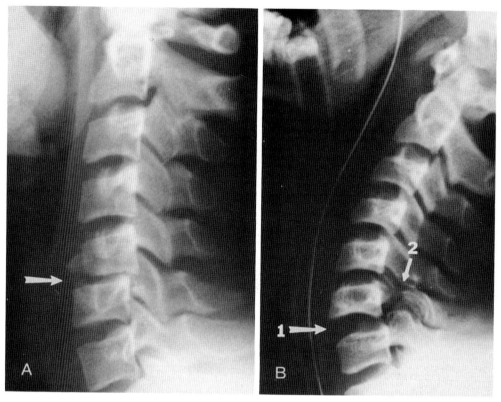

Figure 6.13. *Disc space abnormalities.* (*A*) Note the narrowed disc space (*arrow*) associated with a compression fracture of C_5. The vertebral body is retropulsed into the spinal canal and there is associated widening of the apophyseal joint and widening of the interspinous distance at the C_5–C_6 level. (*B*) Wide disc space (*1*) due to hyperextension injury, which also has resulted in bilateral fractures through the neural arch of C_6 (*2*).

Abnormal Apophyseal Joint Configurations. On a true lateral view of the cervical spine all of the apophyseal joints are superimposed on one another and clearly visualized (Fig. 6.14*A*), but with rotation the apophyseal joints are thrown one off the other. However, if all are rotated to the same general degree, rotation due to positioning only should be the cause (Fig. 6.14*B*). If, however, there is an abrupt discrepancy in the configuration of the joints at one level, that is, if the apophyseal joints are visualized in true lateral position to a certain point and then above that point they are visualized in oblique position, one should suspect rotatory subluxation with a locked facet (Fig. 6.14*C*).

In other cases, the apophyseal joints can be frankly dislocated or subluxed, and almost always this occurs with flexion-rota-

tion injuries. In such cases, the joints, in addition to being anteriorly dislocated also may appear unduly wide and/or V-shaped (Fig. 6.14*D* and *F*). Either configuration is abnormal and should infer ligamentous injury with instability.

Widening of the Joints of Luschka. On normal frontal projection, with lateral bending the contralateral joints of Luschka uniformly increase in width. This phenomenon is quite common and renders evaluation of the joints of Luschka somewhat difficult. However, if one sees undue widening at one or two levels, then one should suspect underlying ligamentous injury.

Interspinous Distance Widening. Widening of the interspinous distance is seen with hyperflexion injuries which result in tearing of the posterior spinal liga-

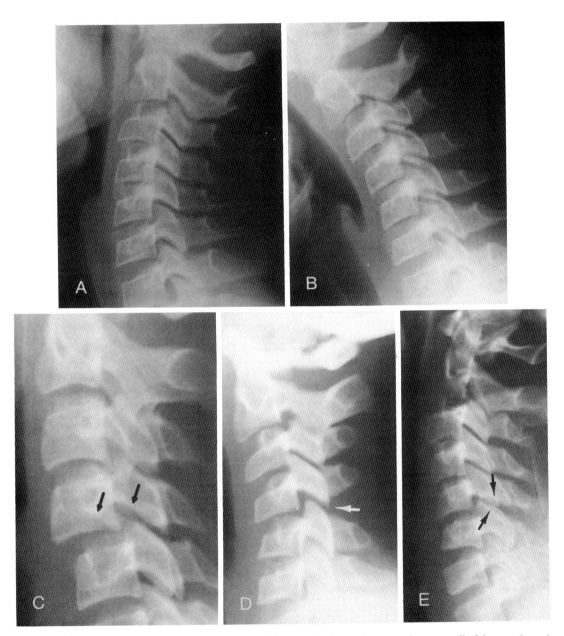

Figure 6.14. *Apophyseal joint alignment: normal and abnormal.*   (*A*) In this normal patient, all of the apophyseal joints are superimposed one on the other and all are normal. (*B*) With flexion, and slight rotation due to a stiff neck, universal offsetting of the apophyseal joints is seen. This still is normal. (*C*) Unilateral offsetting of the apophyseal joints (*arrows*) resulting from rotatory dislocation. Note that C$_4$ is anteriorly displaced on C$_5$. (*D*) Wide apophyseal joint (*arrow*) secondary to hyperflexion injury at the C$_4$–C$_5$ level. The interspinous distance also is increased. (*E*) Another patient with a hyperflexion injury leading to a V-shaped or "fanned" apophyseal joint (*arrows*). The interspinous distance at this level also is increased.

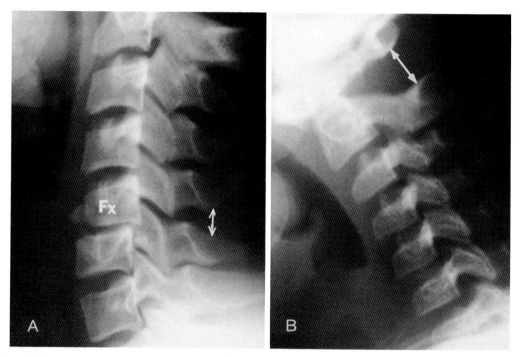

Figure 6.15. *Increased interspinous distance.* (**A**) Flexion injury. Note the increased interspinous distance (*arrows*) between the spinous processes of C_5 and C_6. The apophyseal joint through the same level is also a little widened, and there is a compression fracture of C_5 with retropulsion of the vertebral body into the spinal canal. The intravertebral disc space between C_5 and C_6 is narrowed. (**B**) Normally wide intraspinous distance between C_1 and C_2 (*arrows*).

ments. It is most important to determine whether such an increase in distance is present (Fig. 6.15A), for if it is, the injury is unstable. Such widening also can be appreciated on frontal views (2).

With flexion of the upper cervical spine, however, it should be noted that very commonly the distance between the spinous tip of C_1 and C_2 appears unusually wide and is entirely normal (Fig. 6.15B). In such cases, I believe that tight ligamentous attachments between the base of the skull and C_1 cause the pseudoabnormal configuration. It is a very common finding in children (1) and should not be misinterpreted as pathologic separation of the spinous processes of C_1 and C_2.

REFERENCES

1. Cattell, H.S., and Filtzer, D.L.: Pseudosubluxation and other normal variations in the cervical spine in children. J. Bone Joint Surg. 47A: 1295–1309, 1965.
2. Naidich, J.B., Naidich, T.P., Garfein, C., Liebeskind, A.L., and Hyman, R.A.: The widened interspinous distance: A useful sign of anterior cervical dislocation in the supine frontal projection. Radiology 123: 113–116, 1977.

Lateral Deviation of the Spinous Processes. On frontal view, in most normal patients the spinous tips are lined up in a straight line. As long as no anomalies such as bifid or unfused spinous tips are present, the tips are easy to visualize. If rotation secondary to positioning occurs, the spinous tips are deviated to the opposite side, but the degree of deviation is progressive and more pronounced in the upper spine. If deviation of the spinous tips is abrupt at one level, one should suspect underlying rotatory subluxation with a locked facet (see Fig. 6.51).

Interpedicular Space Widening. Widening of the interpedicular space occurs with bursting fractures of the vertebral bodies. In such cases, on frontal view, the pedicles are displaced laterally and the distance between them increased. In addition, the apophyseal joints also may widen.

Lateral Mass of C_1 to Dens Relationships. A number of offsetting abnormalities of the lateral masses of C_1 have been described (1–6), and to say the least the subject is confusing. One of the reasons for this is that almost any type of offsetting can be produced by varying degrees of rotation and tilting of the upper cervical spine in normal individuals. Because of this, I believe that the only significant abnormal configuration is that of bilateral or unilateral outward offsetting of the lateral masses as seen with Jefferson bursting fractures of C_1 (Fig. 6.16). This observation should be made on nonrotated films only. With rotation, one lateral mass may appear to be displaced outward and its mate inward, but this is not indicative of a fracture, only rotation. Such rotation may be positional only, due to spasm, or associated with rotatory dislocation of C_1 on C_2.

REFERENCES

1. Fielding, J.W., and Hawkins, R.J.: Atlanto-axial rotatory fixation (fixed rotatory subluxation of the atlanto-axial joint). J. Bone Joint Surg. 59: 37–44, 1977.
2. Jacobson, G., and Adler, D.C.: Examination of the atlanto-axial joint following injury with particular emphasis on rotational subluxation. A.J.R. 76: 1081–1094, 1956.
3. Jacobson, G., and Adler, D.C.: An evaluation of lateral atlanto-axial displacement in injuries of the cervical spine. Radiology 61: 355–362, 1961.
4. Shapiro, R., Youngberg, A.S., and Rothman, S.L.G.: The differential diagnosis of traumatic lesions of the occipito atlanto-axial segment. Radiol. Clin. North Am. 11: 505–526, 1973.
5. von Torklus, D., and Gehle, W.: *The Upper Cervical Spine.* Grune & Stratton, New York, 1972.
6. Wortzman, G., and DeWar, F.P.: Rotary fixation of the atlanto-axial joint: Rotational atlanto-axial subluxation. Radiology 90: 479–487, 1968.

Actual Fracture Visualization. I have left assessment of the cervical spine for the detection of fractures to the end, not because I feel it is unimportant, but because I think it is more important to first assess the spine in other ways. If one looks for fractures first, then one is more likely to miss the other, perhaps more important, findings. However, when one does get to looking for fractures in the cervical spine, it is most important to appreciate those that are associated with instability. Many of these fractures are clearly visible on regular views, but others may remain occult until a variety of oblique views, laminograms, or CT scans are obtained.

DETERMINING INSTABILITY OF A CERVICAL SPINE INJURY

In the final analysis, *one's most important mission in cervical spine injuries is to determine whether the injury is stable or unstable, and in this regard the lateral plain film of the cervical spine is the single most valuable study.* Instability results from severe ligamentous injury, with or without a bony fracture, and certain plain film findings should signify the presence of such injury. These findings are summarized in Table 6.2, and only a few pitfalls exist. These include: (a) the flexion injury that

Table 6.2
Signs of Instability of Cervical Spine Injuries[a]

Anterior, posterior or lateral dislocation of a vertebral body
Widened or narrowed intervertebral disc spaces
Widened, narrowed or dislocated apophyseal joint
Focally widened (dislocated) joints of Luschka
Bilateral or unilateral locked facets
Separation of the spinous processes with or without associated avulsion fractures[b]
Flexion or extension teardrop fractures
Anterior wedge compression fracture with posterior displacement of involved vertebral body
Widened predental (C_1-dens) space
Outward displacement of the lateral masses of C_1 (Jefferson fracture—especially unilateral)
Unilateral anterior displacement of one of the lateral masses of C_1 (rotatory dislocation)
Fracture of the dens, with or without displacement
Bursting fracture of vertebral body

[a]More than one may be present in any case.
[b]May require flexion views for demonstrable instability.

appears normal on extension (see Fig. 6.23), (b) the patient with a central cord syndrome and a normal appearing cervical spine (see Fig. 6.64), and (c) the patient with a nondisplaced or minimally displaced fracture through the base of the dens (see Fig. 6.28). In all of these cases, although a significant, even unstable injury is present, the cervical spine may appear remarkably normal on initial inspection. Other than under these circumstances, however, one should be able to correlate the abnormal findings listed in Table 6.2 with the presence of cervical spine instability.

TYPES AND MECHANISMS OF CERVICAL SPINE INJURIES

Injuries to the cervical spine range from minimal soft tissue and ligamentous injury to complete fracture-dislocation with spinal cord injury. Basically, however, the spine is subject to five forces: (a) flexion, (b) extension, (c) lateral flexion, (d) rotation, and (e) axial compression (2, 6, 12, 17, 19, 45). The types of injuries resulting when these forces become excessive are discussed in detail in the following paragraphs.

Flexion Injuries of the Lower Cervical Spine. These injuries usually produce abnormality in three areas: (a) the vertebral body and its ligaments, (b) the apophyseal joints and their ligaments, and (c) the spinous processes and their ligaments (Fig. 6.17). Overall, compressive forces are in effect anteriorly and distraction forces posteriorly. Anteriorly, this results in vertebral body compression (Fig. 6.18), and in many cases a triangular, corner, avulsion, or "teardrop" fracture (Fig. 6.19A). This fracture results from buckling of the anterior longitudinal ligament during hyperflexion, and most often it is the lower, anterior corner of the vertebral body that is avulsed (25, 26, 36). With extension injuries, the teardrop involves the upper anterior corner (see Fig. 6.35). When a tear-

drop fracture is noted, an unstable hyperflexion injury can be assumed. In children, the equivalent of the teardrop fracture often consists of displacement of a fragment of the normal vertebral epiphyseal ring (14, 24). An example of such an injury is seen in Figure 6.19C. In other cases, the corner fracture may be very subtle. In addition to the findings just noted, accompanying ligamentous injury in and around the disc space can lead to disc disruption and narrowing of the disc space (Fig. 6.20).

Prevertebral soft tissue swelling also is a common finding with flexion injuries, but does not occur in all cases. Indeed, often it is not present with mere anterior compression fractures. However, with more severe injuries, the soft tissues may appear thickened.

In those cases where significant vertebral body compression occurs, a vertical fracture (33) through the involved vertebra frequently is present (Fig. 6.19B). Actually this fracture attests to the presence of the vertebral compression forces. The presence of such forces causes the involved vertebra to become squashed or burst and the vertical fracture is one manifestation of this phenomenon. On lateral view, when anterior compression is pronounced there is associated posterior displacement of the compressed vertebral body into the spinal canal (Fig. 6.20). The various fractures of the vertebral body usually are vividly demonstrable with CT scanning, while posterior impingement of the spinal canal can be seen with both CT and MR scanning (Fig. 6.21). MR also is very useful in detecting associated spinal cord injury.

The posterior distracting forces associated with hyperflexion injuries lead to ligamentous injury through the apophyseal joints and between the neural arches and spinous processes. At the apophyseal joint level, this can lead to widening of the involved joints and variable degrees of subluxation (Fig. 6.22). Vertebral body dis-

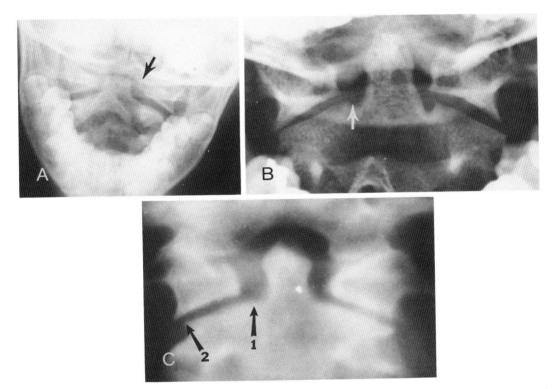

Figure 6.16. *Lateral mass of C₁ to dens distance.* (**A**) Tilting of the head due to a wry neck results in rotation of the spine and widening of the C₁ to dens distance *on the left* (*arrow*). (**B**) Another patient with neck spasm demonstrates a wide C₁ to dens distance *on the right* (*arrow*). Even though one might believe that displacement of the lateral mass should be present, there really is little if any present. There is, however, some narrowing of the atlantoaxial joint and on the contralateral side, note that the lateral mass has shifted medially. This type of arrangement usually is due to rotation or spasm. (**C**) True widening of the C₁ to dens distance (*1*) due to a unilateral Jefferson fracture of C₁ which has caused the lateral mass of C₁ *on the right* to be offset on the body of C₂ (*2*). The contralateral side shows no offsetting in either direction and is normal.

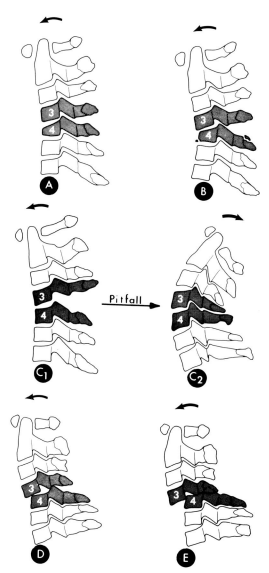

Figure 6.17. *Flexion injuries of the lower cervical space—diagrammatic representation.*   (*A*) Minimal flexion causes anterior compression of C_4. (*B*) More pronounced flexion causes dislocation of the apophyseal joints between C_3 and C_4, narrowing of the disc space between the two vertebral bodies, and widening of the interspinous distance between the two vertebrae. Also note an anterior inferior teardrop fracture of C_4 and an avulsion fracture of the spinous process of C_4. (*C*) Flexion injury pitfall. On flexion (*C1*) note that there is separation of the apophyseal joints between C_3 and C_4. Also note that the spinous processes have been separated. On extension (*C2*), however, note that the vertebrae align normally and that no injury is apparent. This is an important pitfall to avoid in the interpretation of flexion injuries and is illustrated in Figure 6.23. (*D*) More pronounced flexion causes marked dislocation of C_3 on C_4 and locking of the facets. (*E*) Severe anterior dislocation of C_3 on C_4, with locking of the vertebral bodies.

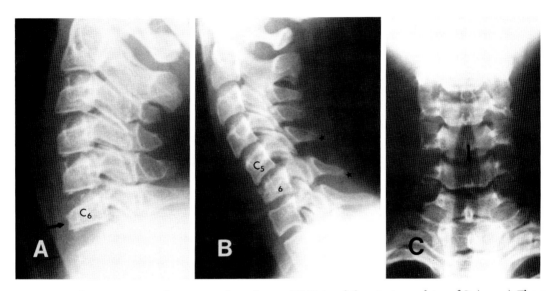

Figure 6.18. *Flexion injuries with compressed vertebrae.* (**A**) Note subtle anterior wedging of C$_6$ (*arrow*). There is no corresponding soft tissue swelling and no other findings of injury. (**B**) More severe injury demonstrates localized kyphosis at the level of C$_5$–C$_6$. The corresponding spinous processes are separated (°), leading to an increase in the interspinous distance. There is anterior apophyseal joint dislocation, narrowing of the intervening disc space, anterior compression and fragmentation of C$_6$, anterior dislocation of C$_5$ on C$_6$, and clear-cut prevertebral soft tissue swelling. In addition, note that the posterior portion of C$_6$ has been displaced into the spinal canal. (**C**) Frontal view demonstrating associated vertical fracture (*arrow*) through the body of C$_6$.

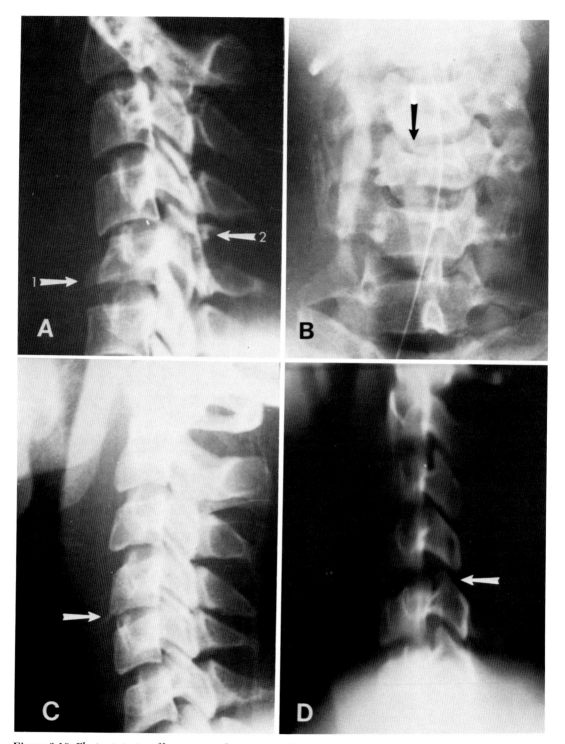

Figure 6.19. *Flexion injuries of lower cervical spine—teardrop and spinous process avulsion fractures.* (**A**) Note the large teardrop fracture (*1*) of C$_5$. Also note that C$_5$ is compressed anteriorly and that the disc space between C$_4$ and C$_5$ is narrowed. The interspinous distance between C$_4$ and C$_5$ also is increased and there is an associated avulsion fracture (*2*) of the posterior elements of C$_5$. (**B**) Frontal view demonstrating associated vertical fracture

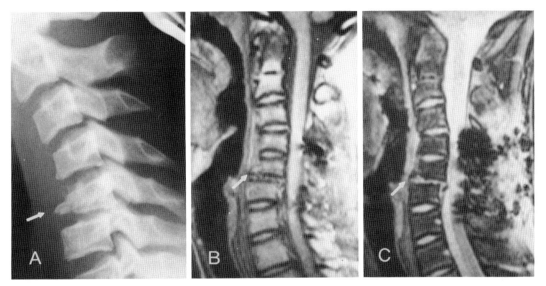

Figure 6.20. *Hyperflexion injuries with MR imaging.* (*A*) Note the compression and teardrop fracture of C_5 (*arrow*). There may be a small teardrop fracture of the inferior anterior corner of C_4. The disc space between C_5 and C_6 is narrowed and C_5 is retropulsed into the spinal canal. The apophyseal joints are widened. (*B*) T_1-weighted MR image demonstrates the compressed vertebra with the teardrop fracture (*arrow*). (*C*) T_2-weighted image more clearly identifies the teardrop fracture (*arrow*), compressed vertebra, narrowed disc space, and retropulsed vertebral body into the spinal canal. There also is a small posterior fragment of bone that has been avulsed off of the posterior aspect of C_6. There is minimal impingement of the spinal canal but no impingement of the cord. Extensive soft tissue edema and bleeding are seen in the posterior soft tissues.

(*arrow*) of the compressed and expanded body of C_5. Note again that the disc space between C_4 and C_5 is narrowed. (*C*) Small teardrop fracture along the inferoanterior aspect of C_4 (*arrow*). Actually, this fragment probably represents an avulsed fragment of the ring epiphysis. Also note marked prevertebral soft tissue swelling and narrowing of the disc space between C_4 and C_5. All of these findings should indicate the presence of an unstable flexion injury. (*D*) Subsequent laminography demonstrates associated anterior dislocation of the apophyseal joint (*arrow*) at the involved level, attesting to the presence of a hyperflexion injury.

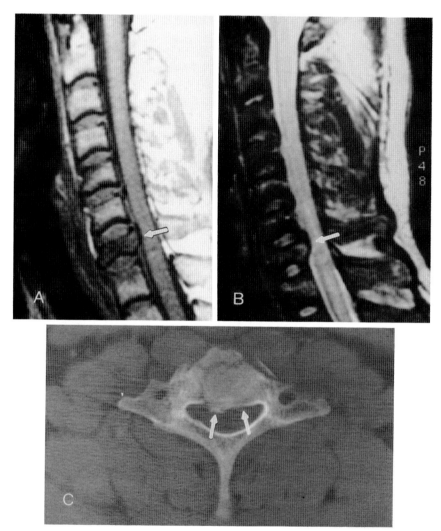

Figure 6.21. *Flexion injury with compression fracture: MR and CT findings.* (*A*) Patient with a compressed vertebra with retropulsion into the spinal canal (*arrow*)(T$_1$-weighted image). (*B*) T$_2$-weighted image more clearly identifies the bulging vertebra (*arrow*). There is minimal impingement on the spinal cord. (*C*) CT study in the same patient demonstrates the retropulsed fragment (*arrows*) and the other fractures of the vertebral body.

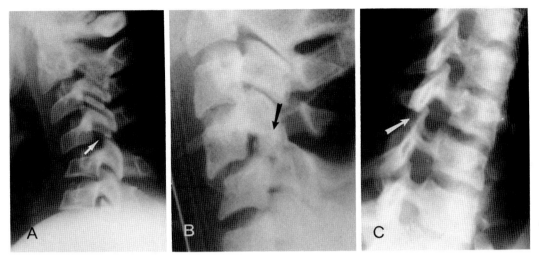

Figure 6.22. *Apophyseal joint dislocation.* Marked apophyseal joint dislocation (*arrows*) just short of a locked facet. Also note the increased interspinous distance. (*B*) Another patient with actual locked facets (*arrows*). Note that the interspinous distance also has increased and that the disc space between C_3 and C_4 is narrowed. C_3 is anteriorly displaced on C_4. (*C*) Oblique view in still another patient demonstrates apophyseal joint dislocation (*arrow*) with a so-called "perched" facet. With more flexion it would jump and lock.

placement can be minimal, and in terms of measurement, 3 mm or more definitely is considered abnormal (6). Correspondingly, anterior angulation of more than 12°–15° also is considered abnormal (6). Apophyseal joint dislocation also can be demonstrated with oblique views (Fig. 6.22C). Greater degrees of dislocation can lead to perched or frankly locked facets (Fig. 6.22B and C), or even locked vertebral bodies (see Fig. 6.17E).

At the neural arch and spinous process level, ligamentous injury results in separation of the involved spinous processes with widening of the interspinous distance (29) (Fig. 6.22), and in some cases, avulsion fractures of the posterior elements (Fig. 6.19A). Once all of these features of flexion injuries of the cervical spine are appreciated, it is easy to understand why the spine becomes unstable. Clearly, when there is damage to the anterior and posterior longitudinal ligaments, the ligaments of the apophyseal joints, neural arches, and spinous processes, instability must result.

A significant pitfall in the interpretation of flexion injuries of the lower cervical spine deals with the patient whose cervical spine shows little or no abnormality in the neutral or extended position (Fig. 6.23A). In these patients, until the spine is flexed (Fig. 6.23B), the lesion can escape detection completely. It is important to appreciate this pitfall, for the lesion is quite unstable (37).

In other patients, initial ligamentous injury may cause so much pain that the patient cannot flex the spine, and thus any ligamentous injury remains occult until later. Then, as mobility returns, evidence of the unstable ligamentous injury is seen (Fig. 6.24). All the while these patients continue to have pain, and thus it is very important that if such patients continue to have pain, they be reexamined. On follow-up studies of these patients, ossified avulsions along the posterior interspinous ligaments due to the previously occult avulsion injuries may be seen (22, 31) (Fig. 6.24C).

In addition to this pitfall, it should be re-

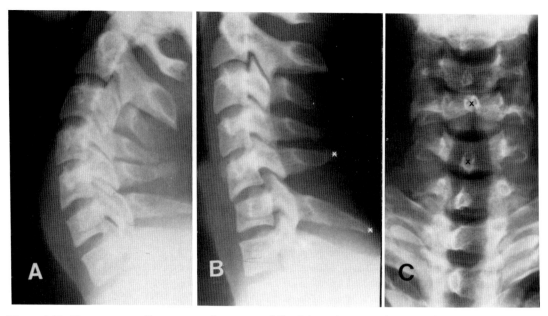

Figure 6.23. *Flexion injury of lower cervical spine—pitfall.* (*A*) On this neutral or extended view, there is little to see in the way of abnormality. Some soft tissue swelling over the anterior lower cervical spine might be suggested, but no fractures or dislocations are visualized. (*B*) With flexion, however, note that the interspinous distance between C_5 and C_6 has increased markedly (*asterisks*). In addition, the apophyseal joints at the same level show anterior dislocation and the disc space at the same level shows a little narrowing. Prevertebral soft tissue swelling again is suggested, but the finding still is equivocal. (*C*) On frontal view, note the increased distance between the involved spinous processes (*X's*). (Courtesy of C. Mott, M.D.)

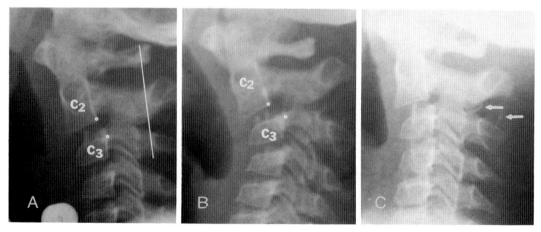

Figure 6.24. *Occult flexion injury C_2–C_3.* (*A*) Note normal alignment of the vertebral bodies. C_2–C_3 offsetting is minimal (*dots*) and appears physiologic. The posterior cervical line lies within normal range. There may be a little prevertebral soft tissue swelling. (*B*) After 2 months in a collar and 1 month out of a collar, the patient returned with chronic neck pain. Note acute kyphosis at the C_2–C_3 level, more pronounced anterior displacement of C_2 on C_3 (*dots*), widening of the intraspinous distance between C_2–C_3, and disruption of the apophyseal joint between the two vertebrae. (*C*) Another view, with less flexion, demonstrates some realignment of the vertebral bodies but also demonstrates evidence of two avulsion fractures (*arrows*). For another ligamentous injury at the C_2–C_3 level, see Figure 6.11.

called that physiologic displacement of the body of C_2 on the body of C_3 is a common phenomenon in childhood (see Fig. 6.8) and should not be misinterpreted as pathologic dislocation. These patients also often demonstrate normal wedging of C_3 (see Fig. 6.70).

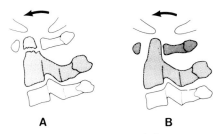

Figure 6.25. *Flexion injuries of the upper cervical spine—diagrammatic representation.* (*A*) Fracture through the base of the dens with slight anterior displacement. (*B*) Isolated atlantoaxial dislocation with no fracture of the dens. Note that the predental distance has increased.

Flexion Injuries of the Atlas and Axis. These injuries most commonly result in fractures through the base of the dens with anterior displacement of the dens (Fig. 6.25A). Widening of the predental distance may be present if there is associated anterior dislocation of the atlas on the axis (see Fig. 6.25B). In infants and young children, fractures through the base of the dens usually occur through the dens-body synchondrosis (15, 38) (Fig. 6.26). This synchondrosis remains open until late childhood and should not be misinterpreted as a fracture (Fig. 6.27). Lesser degrees of flexion injury may result in an undisplaced fracture of the dens which usually is more difficult to detect (Fig. 6.28). These or similar fractures usually require regular tomography (Fig. 6.28B) or computerized tomography with reconstruction for their complete demonstration (see Fig. 6.43).

In young infants, dens fractures may go

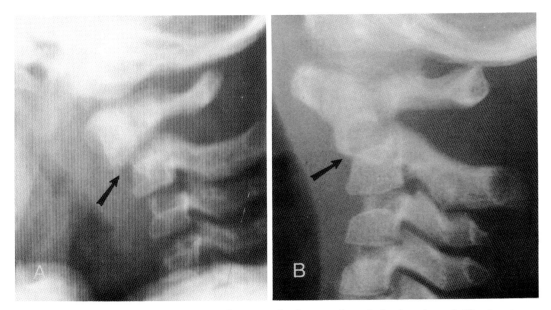

Figure 6.26. *Fracture of dens.* (*A*) In this infant, note the fracture through the dens (*arrow*). The dens is anteriorly tilted and anteriorly displaced. In addition, all of C_1 is anteriorly displaced on C_2. (*B*) Another patient with an anteriorly tilted dens resulting from a displaced fracture through the base of the dens (*arrow*). Again, all of C_1 is anteriorly displaced on C_2. In both of these cases, note how little prevertebral soft tissue swelling is present. (Part *B* courtesy of C. Keith Hayden, Jr., M.D., Fort Worth Children's Hospital, Fort Worth, Texas.)

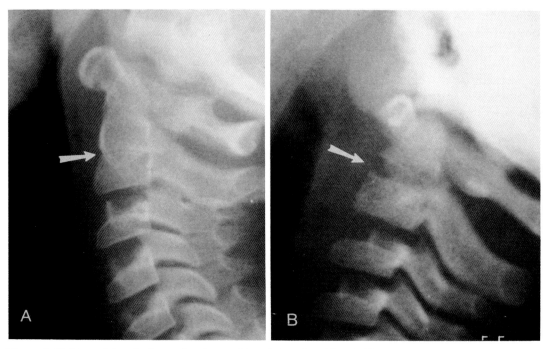

Figure 6.27. *Normal dens-body synchondrosis of C₂.* (*A*) In this older child, note the very thin dens-body synchondrosis (*arrow*). Its sclerotic edges should speak towards a normal synchondrosis. (*B*) An infant with a wide, but normal dens-body synchondrosis (*arrow*). In both of these cases note that the dens is not anteriorly tilted. It is in normal position.

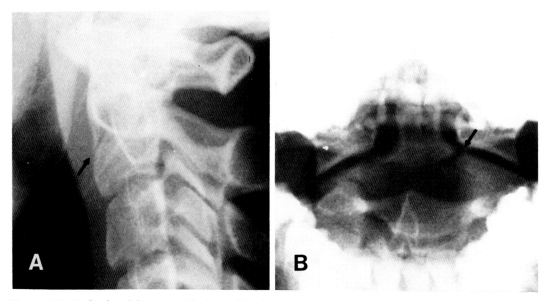

Figure 6.28. *Undisplaced fracture of the base of the dens—subtle findings.* (*A*) Note a subtle fracture through the base of the dens (*arrow*). There is no displacement of the dens, but the prevertebral soft tissues might be slightly widened. (*B*) Frontal view demonstrating the fracture more clearly (*arrow*) and subsequent laminography demonstrated the fracture to extend across the entire base of the dens. (Courtesy of T. Brown, M.D.)

unrecognized (38), until pain and persistent loss of normal motion bring the patient back for examination. At that time, some 1–2 weeks later, resorption of bone at the dens-body synchondrosis is seen (Fig. 6.29C and D). These dens fractures probably are more common than generally realized and, indeed, frequently are missed entirely. However, increased width and radiolucency of the synchondrosis (38) should signal their presence and one should be doubly suspicious when the dens is cocked anteriorly (Fig. 6.29A and B). *This latter finding is important, for while posterior tilting of the dens is a common, normal phenomenon (see Fig. 6.42B), anterior tilting is not and should suggest injury.* Similarly, mere increased width of the synchondrosis should not automatically infer injury, for it can be normal (see Fig. 6.27B). *It is widening and anterior tilting that is the most suggestive combination of findings.*

In other instances, blood supply to the entire dens may be disrupted and the dens slowly may be resorbed (13) and disappear (Fig. 6.30). In such cases, the normal os terminale overgrows in a compensatory fashion and results in the so-called "acquired os odontoideum" (11, 15, 18).

Anterior atlantoaxial dislocations generally are uncommon but do occur. They may be isolated injuries or injuries associated with other upper cervical spine injuries (Figs. 6.30 and 6.31). When gross, they usually are inconsistent with survival (Fig. 6.31). In terms of atlantoaxial instability and laxity, it is important to appreciate that in children such laxity most often is due to underlying problems such as

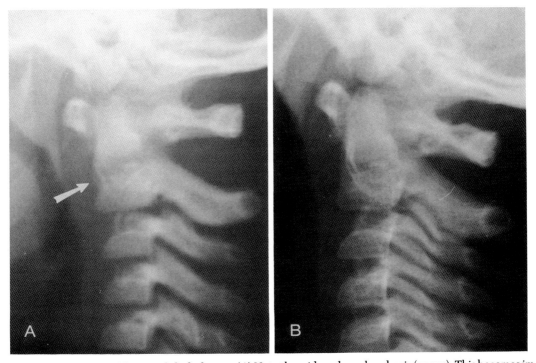

Figure 6.29. *Fracture of dens—subtle findings.* (A) Note the widened synchondrosis (*arrow*). This becomes important in view of the fact that the dens is also anteriorly tilted. The synchondrosis also is indistinct and there is some resorption of bone on either side. The reason for this is that the patient sustained this injury 3 weeks earlier in an automobile accident. (B) One year later the dens and body of C_2 have fused but the dens remains anteriorly tilted.

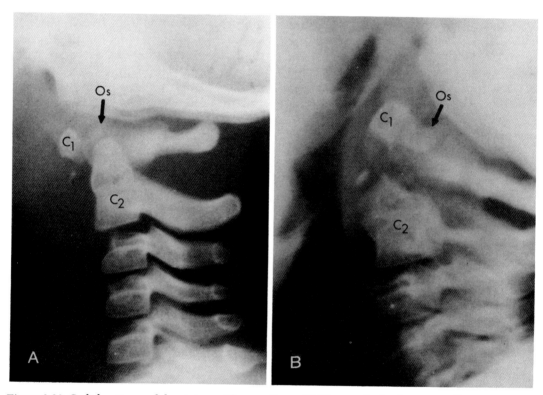

Figure 6.30. *C_1 dislocation, and dens injury with resorption.* (**A**) Note marked soft tissue swelling, anterior displacement of C_1 with an increased C_1-dens distance, and an avulsed bony fragment from C_1. Not clearly seen but also present is a dislocated os terminale (*Os*). (**B**) Years later, the dens has completely resorbed and the os terminale has overgrown to produce an acquired os odontoideum (*Os*). (From J.E. Ricciardi, H. Kaufer, and D.S. Louis: Acquired os odontoideum following acute ligament injury. J. Bone Joint Surg. 58A: 410–412, 1976.)

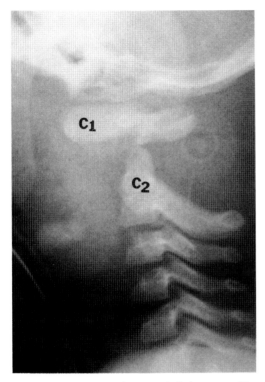

Figure 6.31. *Gross atlantoaxial dislocation.* Note that C_1 is completely separated and anteriorly displaced from C_2. There is extensive prevertebral edema. This patient was dead on arrival.

misinterpreted as being indicative of posterior ligamentous injury at this level.

Extension Injuries of the Lower Cervical Spine. These injuries, as opposed to flexion injuries, result in compressive forces posteriorly and distracting forces anteriorly (Fig. 6.33). Consequently, often there is little in the way of vertebral body fracturing, but considerable evidence of fracturing of the articular facets, pillars, and posterior elements (Fig. 6.34). Disc space widening due to anterior ligament disruption also can occur (3) and may be associated with an *extension type "teardrop" fracture (Fig. 6.35).* This fracture occurs anteriorly, and just as the flexion "teardrop" fracture indicates the presence of a significant ligamentous, unstable injury. However, as opposed to the flexion "teardrop" fracture, the extension "teardrop" fracture involves the upper anterior corner of the vertebral body (Fig. 6.35). It results from undue stretching or tearing of the anterior longitudinal ligament during hyperextension (see Fig. 6.33C) and, be-

rheumatoid arthritis and congenital hypoplasia of the dens (often in the trisomy 21 syndrome). Finally, with some hyperflexion injuries of the upper cervical spine, posterior element avulsion fractures may be seen (Fig. 6.32).

Roentgenographically, when anterior atlantoaxial dislocation is present, no matter what the cause, the predental distance is widened. However, it should be remembered that the predental distance in children normally is wider than in adults, and that it is not unusual for it to measure as much as 4 or 5 mm and still be normal (see Fig. 6.5). In addition to this finding, it should be recalled that the interspinous distance between C_1 and C_2 also frequently is unusually prominent in most normal children (see Fig. 6.15B) and should not be

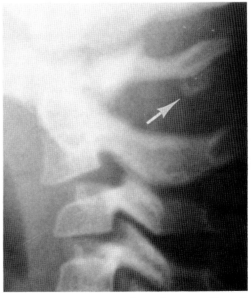

Figure 6.32. *Posterior avulsion fracture.* Note the posterior avulsion fracture (*arrow*) of C_1.

EXTENSION INJURIES
(Lower Cervical Spine)

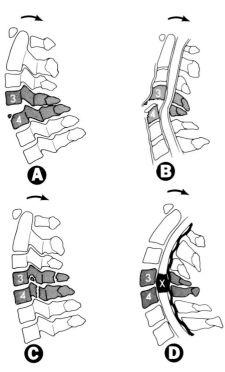

Figure 6.33. *Extension injuries of lower cervical spine—diagrammatic representation.* (*A*) Hyperextension causes widening of the disc space between C$_3$ and C$_4$, a characteristic upper anterior teardrop (corner) fracture of C$_4$, and alteration of the associated apophyseal joint. (*B*) Note how stretching and tearing of the anterior longitudinal ligament leads to the avulsion-teardrop fracture and how cord damage occurs with this type of injury. (*C*) Hyperextension also can produce a variety of posterior element fractures of the involved vertebrae. A combination of disruption of the disc space and posterior element fractures can lead to slight anterior displacement of the vertebral body (see Fig. 6.36*A*). (*D*) Central cord syndrome. In this type of injury no fracture occurs, but buckling of the ligamentum flavum during hyperextension causes compression and injury to the cord (*X*).

soft tissues remain normal. Posteriorly, with hyperextension injuries, a variety of fractures through the neural arches, pedicles, articular facets, pillars, spinous processes, etc., can occur. When these latter fractures are unilateral and not associated with any other injuries, the spine is not particularly unstable, but when they are bilateral and occur through the neural arch or pedicles, they result in an unstable injury. This injury, of course, is identical to

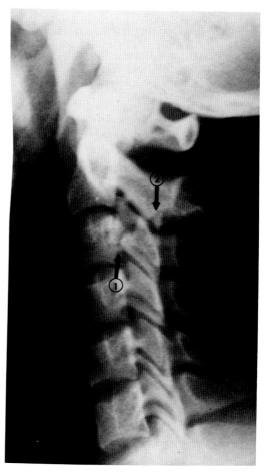

Figure 6.34. *Extension injury—multiple posterior element fractures.* Note fractures through the base of the articular facet of C$_3$ (*1*) and the posterior articulating facet of C$_2$ (*2*). The involved facet of C$_3$ is dislocated posteriorly to a slight degree, and probably rotated. Actually, the injury is most likely the result of a combination of extension and rotation forces.

cause of this, is associated with a widened disc space (3) (Figs. 6.35 and 6.36).

When an extension "teardrop" fracture is present, prevertebral soft tissue swelling usually also is present, but if there is no anterior ligamentous injury, the prevertebral

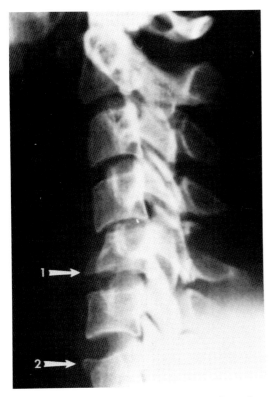

Figure 6.35. *Extension and flexion teardrop fractures.* This patient sustained a whiplash injury, and on this lateral view shows evidence of both flexion and extension injuries. A typical flexion teardrop fracture of C_5 is demonstrated at level *1*. Note that the vertebra above is anteriorly displaced and that the intervening disc space is narrowed. An extension teardrop fracture is demonstrated at level *2*. Note that it is located at the upper anterior corner of the involved vertebra, and that the disc space above is widened. Such widening is characteristic of extension injuries.

the injury which occurs with the classic hangman's fracture of C_2. In these cases, often it is not until laminography (in the past), and CT scanning (currently) are obtained that the posterior element fractures come to one's attention (Figs. 6.36 and 6.37). Anterior vertebral body displacement is not as common with extension injuries as with flexion injuries, but yet, if posterior arch fractures occur in association with ligament and disc disruption, a mild degree of anterior displacement can

be seen (Fig. 6.36A). An important pitfall in the evaluation of hyperextension injuries of the lower cervical spine occurs with the so-called "central cord syndrome." This syndrome (see Fig. 6.64) is discussed at a later point, but at the present time it should be noted that the cervical spine in these patients usually appears normal. What occurs is that rather than fracture-dislocation, there is buckling of the ligamentum flavum during hyperextension, and focal compression of the spinal cord (Fig. 6.33D). Consequently, while clinically there is definite evidence of cord injury, cervical spine films appear remarkably negative. In such cases MRI (5) is extremely useful in detecting spinal cord and soft tissue injury (see Fig. 6.64).

Extension Injuries of the Atlas and Axis. These injuries are quite common (Fig. 6.38), and among the most common are fractures through the posterior arch of C_1, fractures of the dens, and the classic hangman's fracture of C_2 (9, 28, 39, 44). Fractures through the posterior arch of C_1 can be bilateral or unilateral, and can be seen alone or in association with other fractures of C_1 or C_2 (Fig. 6.39). These fractures usually produce narrow defects through the posterior arch of C_1, and in this way can be differentiated from commonly occurring congenital defects of the arch. The latter usually are quite wide and associated with triangular, tapered, or otherwise peculiarly shaped residual, ossified fragments of the posterior arch of C_1 (Fig. 6.40). At the extreme end of this group of anomalies, posterior arch ossification is absent altogether (Fig. 6.41). Less commonly, extension injuries produce transverse fractures of the anterior arch of C_1 (Fig. 6.38A). These fractures usually remain occult until laminography or CT with reconstruction is performed.

Fractures of the dens secondary to extension injuries often are associated with a variable degree of posterior tilting or displacement (Fig. 6.42A). Minimal such dis-

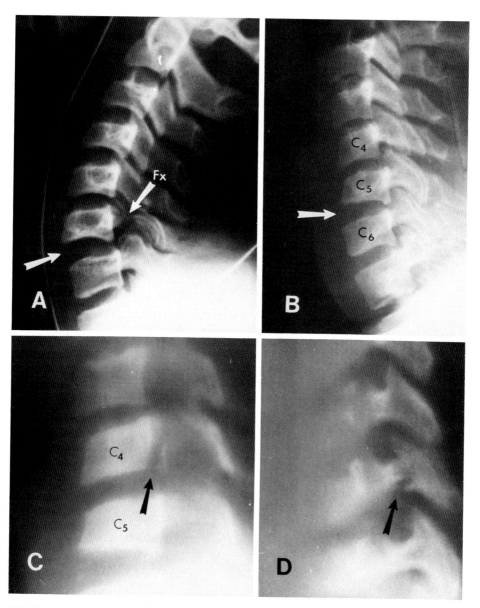

Figure 6.36. *Hyperextension injuries: lower cervical spine.* (*A*) Note the fracture through the posterior elements (*Fx*) and the widened disc space (*anterior arrow*). There is slight anterior displacement of the vertebra above the widened disc space. (*B*) Another patient with widening of the disc space between C_5 and C_6 (*arrow*). Fractures of the posterior elements are not visualized. An associated flexion injury is present at the C_4–C_5 level (i.e., anterior displacement of C_4 and apophyseal joint widening or fanning is seen). (*C* and *D*) Tomography, however, demonstrates a number of fractures through the posterior elements (*arrows*), consistent with a hyperextension injury.

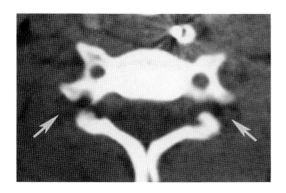

Figure 6.37. *Hyperextension injury: CT findings.* Note the bilateral fractures through the posterior pedicles (*arrows*) of the vertebrae. This is the same patient as shown in Figure 6.36A.

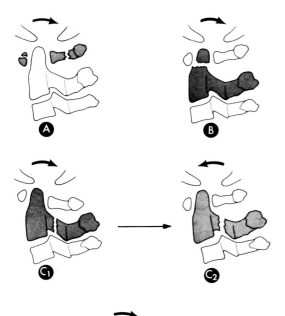

Figure 6.38. *Extension injuries of the upper cervical spine.* (**A**) Typical transverse fracture through the anterior arch of C_1 and vertical fracture through the posterior arch of C_1. (**B**) Fracture of the base of the dens with posterior displacement. (C_1 and C_2) Hangman's fracture of C_2. With initial extension bilateral fractures through the arch or pedicles of C_2 occur (C_1). With subsequent return to a more neutral position, abnormal motion through the fracture site occurs, and associated ligament disruption through the C_2–C_3 disc allows the body and dens of C_2, and all of C_1 to move forward (C_2). (**D**) Posterior atlantoaxial dislocation without fracture of the dens. This is a very uncommon injury.

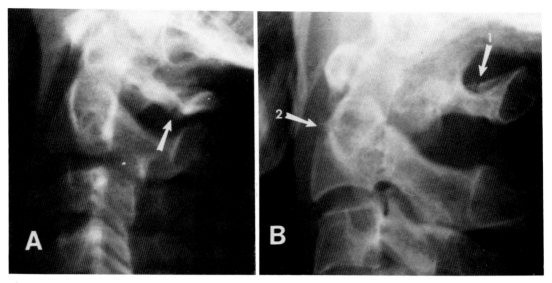

Figure 6.39. *Hyperextension, posterior arch of C_1 fractures.* (*A*) Note the typical thin radiolucent line of a fracture (*arrow*) through the posterior arch of C_1. Such fractures can be unilateral or bilateral. (*B*) Another patient demonstrating a vertical fracture through the posterior arch of C_1 (*1*), but in addition there is a fracture through the base of the dens (*2*). Note associated posterior tilting and angulation of the dens. Both of these injuries result from hyperextension.

placements or tilts must be differentiated from the normally tilted or lordotic dens (Fig. 6.42*B*) occurring with surprising frequency in many normal individuals (43). As with flexion injuries, some of these fractures are very subtle and come to light only with subsequent CT with reconstruction (Fig. 6.43).

With the hangman's fracture of C_2 initial hyperextension causes bilateral fractures through the neural arch and/or pedicles and disruption of the ligaments anteriorly (Fig. 6.44). Thereafter, with subsequent return to a more neutral position, abnormal motion through the fracture site and ligaments between C_2 and C_3, leads to slight anterior displacement of the body of C_2. In some of these cases, the fracture through the posterior element of C_2 is clearly visible, while in others it remains obscure. In these latter cases, if any degree of anterior displacement of C_2 on C_3 is suspected, one should apply the posterior cervical line, for it will be abnormal (i.e., it will miss the posterior arch of C_2 by 2 mm

or more [Fig. 6.44]). Unilateral neural arch fractures may be more difficult to detect, but usually are not associated with cervical spine instability (Fig. 6.45).

Congenital defects of the posterior arch of C_2 are not as common as those of C_1. However, they do occur and they tend to resemble fractures more than they do when they are seen through the posterior elements of C_1 (Fig. 6.46). Keys to recognizing these as normal synchondroses is their incidental discovery, sclerosis along their margins, and the fact that they do not change their configuration with flexion (i.e., no abnormal motion). Congenital defects of the lower cervical vertebra are even less common.

Another injury of the cervical spine sustained during hyperextension is the pure posterior atlantoaxial dislocation (Fig. 6.38*D*). This injury, however, is rare, for the strong transverse ligament usually causes a dens fracture to occur instead.

Lateral Flexion Injuries of the Cervical Spine. These injuries can result in simple

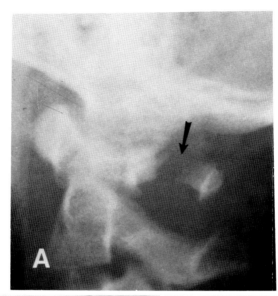

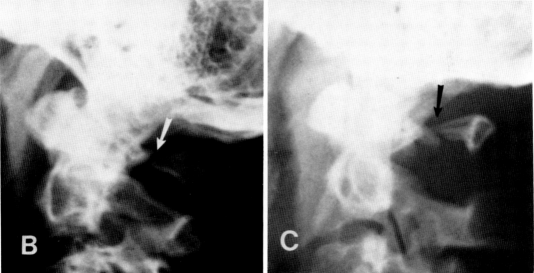

Figure 6.40. *Congenital defects of the posterior arch of C₁.*   (**A**) Wide defect (*arrow*) in a young girl who was in an automobile accident. Note the bizarre appearance of the remaining ossicles of the posterior arch of C₁. (**B**) Typical triangular posterior ossicle and tapered ossicle ends seen with congenital defects (*arrow*) of C₁. (**C**) Another patient demonstrating a generally thin and hypoplastic posterior arch of C₁ and typical tapering of the bone ends on either side of the congenital defect (*arrow*). These defects should not be misinterpreted as posterior arch fractures. (Part *C* courtesy of P.S. Kline, Jr., M.D.)

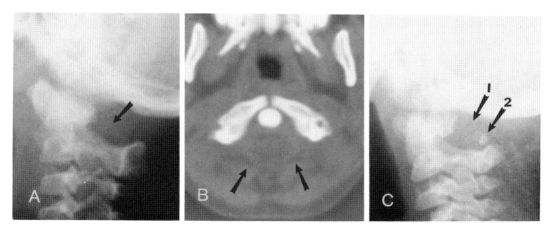

Figure 6.41. *Absence of posterior arch of C₁.* (**A**) Note complete absence of the bony posterior arch of C₁ (*arrow*). (**B**) CT study in the same patient demonstrates absence of the posterior arch (*arrows*). (**C**) Another patient with almost complete absence of the posterior arch (*1*) with only a small ossicle of the spinous tip (*2*) remaining.

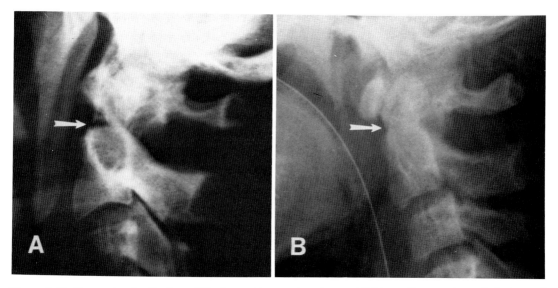

Figure 6.42. *Hyperextension fracture of the dens with posterior tilting.* (**A**) Note a fracture through the base of the dens (*arrow*), and readily visible posterior tilting of the dens. A similar fracture is shown in Figure 6.39*B*. (**B**) Normal posteriorly tilted dens. This patient was in an automobile accident and the normal posteriorly tilted dens was misinterpreted as a fractured dens. This type of misinterpretation often is enhanced by the presence of a slight notchlike defect at the base of the dens (*arrow*).

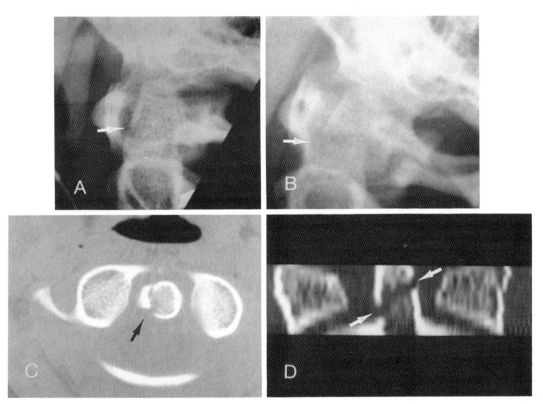

Figure 6.43. *Subtle dens fracture.* (*A*) On this view note a subtle fracture (*arrow*) of the dens. It probably would be entirely missed on this view. (*B*) Another view demonstrates a more suspicious appearing finding (*arrow*) at the base of the dens. Still, nothing is absolutely clear. (*C*) Axial CT demonstrates a clear-cut fracture through the dens (*arrow*). (*D*) Coronal reconstruction demonstrates the fracture (*arrows*) more clearly. The C_1 to dens distance on the right is widened due to rotation. (Courtesy of C. Keith Hayden, M.D., Fort Worth Children's Hospital, Fort Worth, Texas.)

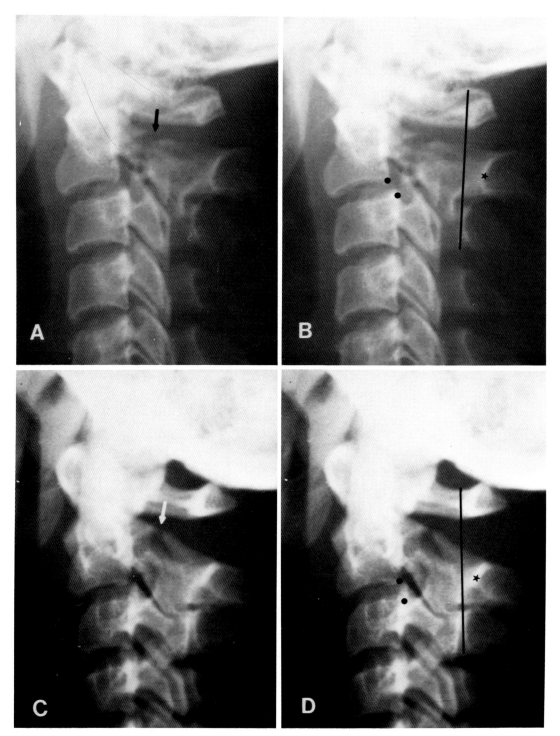

Figure 6.44. *Hangman's fracture of* C_2. (*A*) Typical location of the bilateral fractures through the neural arch-pedicle junctions of C_2 (*arrow*). (*B*) Same patient. Note that C_2 is displaced on C_3 (*dots*), and that the posterior cervical line lies more than 2 mm anterior to the cortex of the spinous process of C_2 (*star*). (*C*) Another patient with more subtle findings. However, note the characteristic location of the fracture (*arrow*). (*D*) Same patient as

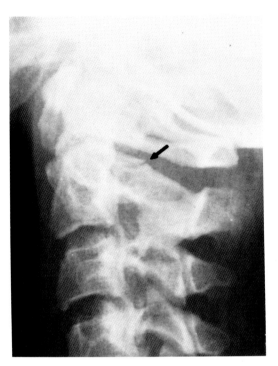

Figure 6.45. *Extension injury of C₂—unilateral arch fracture.* Note the fracture (*arrow*) through the neural arch-pedicle junction of C₂. This was a unilateral fracture and no instability was present.

ipsilateral vertebral body compression, contralateral fractures of the transverse or uncinate processes (34), and contralateral brachial plexus avulsions (Fig. 6.47).

With lateral flexion injuries, the contralateral joints of Luschka can be disrupted and appear widened. However, it should be noted that with normal lateral flexion some widening of the joints of Luschka occurs, and if such widening occurs at numerous adjacent levels, it most likely is normal. If, however, there is marked disparity at one or two levels, significant un-

derlying ligamentous injury with potential instability of the cervical spine should be suspected (Fig. 6.48). Indeed, very often when this finding is present, considerable injury to the cervical spine has occurred and significant findings also will be present on the lateral view. In the upper cervical spine, lateral flexion can produce fractures of the dens with associated lateral displacement of this structure (Fig. 6.45B). Normal lateral tilting of the dens is rare, and thus any lateral tilting should be treated with suspicion (Fig. 6.48C). Brachial plexus injuries are discussed later (see Fig. 6.63).

Rotation Injuries of the Cervical Spine. These injuries frequently are missed and can occur both in the upper and lower cervical spine (Fig. 6.49). Usually they are associated either with a flexion or extension injury, but most often it is the former. In the lower cervical spine, flexion-rotation injuries result in the so-called unilateral "locked" or "jumped" facet (35), and associated disruption of the intervening ligaments and disc space. This injury can be suspected on lateral views of the cervical spine either by noting that the rotated vertebral body is anteriorly displaced on the one below it, or that there is an abrupt change in alignment of the apophyseal joints at the level of injury (Fig. 6.50). Anterior displacement of the vertebral body, due to disc and ligament disruption, usually is not difficult to detect, and most often is associated with narrowing of the disc space and swelling of the soft tissues anterior to the site of injury. Abnormal alignment of the apophyseal joints, on the other hand, may be more difficult to detect and frequently is missed. *To avoid this, one*

in *C*. Very little anterior displacement of C₂ on C₃ is present (*dots*), but the fact that such displacement is present becomes significant. Under these circumstances, the posterior cervical line should be applied, and in this case it misses the anterior cortex of the spinous process of C₂ by more than 2 mm. Consequently, it is abnormal and should reflect the presence of pathologic dislocation of C₂ on C₃ secondary to a hangman's fracture. For more discussion of the posterior cervical line in normal and abnormal cases, see Figure 6.9.

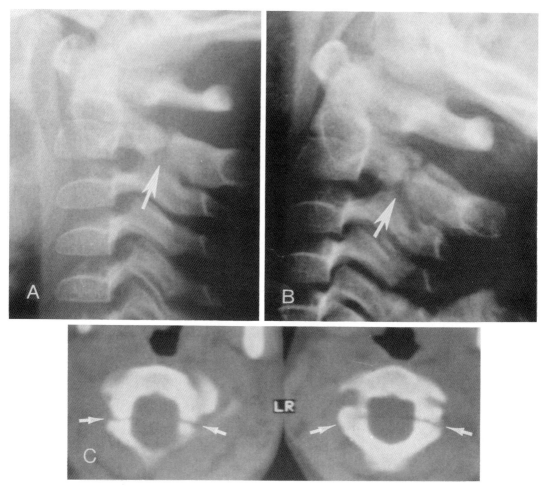

Figure 6.46. *Congenital defect through posterior arch of C₂.* (*A*) Note the fracture-like appearing defect (*arrow*) through the posterior arch of C₂. The edges are somewhat sclerotic. (*B*) Another view with slight rotation makes the defects (*arrow*) appear even more as though they were fractures. (*C*) Axial CT through C₂ demonstrates the smooth congenital defects (*arrows*).

should recall that for the apophyseal joints to be normal, they either should all be in true lateral projection or all rotated to the same degree. Therefore, if one notes an abrupt change in the alignment of the apophyseal joints at one level, one should suspect injury (Fig. 6.50). In addition, the space between the posterior cortex of the apophyseal joint and spinolaminar line (cortex of spinous process) remains normal

below the level of rotation. Above the level of rotation, it is reduced (Fig. 6.50).

In many of these cases, associated fractures through the articular facets, pillars, and posterior elements occur, and often there is associated lateral displacement of the upper vertebral body and localized widening and dislocation of the joints of Luschka (see Fig. 6.48). Actual demonstration of the associated fractures and the "locked" or "jumped" facet often is best accomplished with oblique views, laminography, or CT (Fig. 6.51). On frontal view, a unilateral locked facet can be suspected when it is noted that the spinous processes of the rotated vertebra and the vertebrae above it are shifted off midline (Fig. 6.51).

Extension-rotation injuries of the cervical spine usually result in fractures of the articular facets, pillars, and posterior elements (Fig. 6.49C). In this regard, the resulting injury is not particularly different from that seen with pure hyperextension injuries.

Rotation abnormalities of the atlas and axis consist of rotatory dislocation, rotatory subluxation, and rotatory fixation (8, 10, 20, 21, 23, 30, 32, 40, 47). Rotatory dislocation and subluxation probably represent different degrees of the same problem, but whereas rotatory subluxation usually is reversible with conservative measures, rotatory dislocation requires

proper surgical treatment for correction. Actually, rotatory subluxation of C_1 on C_2 is the classic problem in the typical wryneck or torticollis abnormality of childhood (7, 40). Clinically, these patients present with acute onset of a stiff neck, and often with a history of "catching a draft" or previous "minor trauma." Roentgenographically, lateral views of the cervical spine may be relatively normal or may demonstrate a peculiar cocking or dislocated appearance of C_1 on C_2 (Fig. 6.52). However, in spite of this disturbing appearance of C_1, there will be no evidence of true atlantoaxial dislocation in that the predental distance will be normal. On frontal view, however, a characteristic alignment of the spinous process of C_2 and the tip of the mandible occurs. Normally when the head is turned to one side, the spinous tips of the vertebral bodies rotate to the opposite side (i.e., opposite to the side to which the mandible has rotated or points). With torticollis, on the other hand,

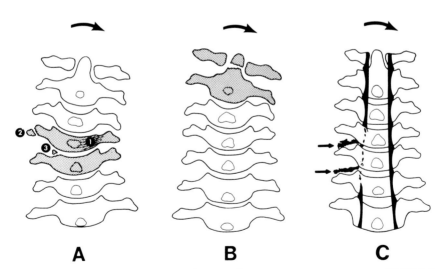

A   **B**   **C**

Figure 6.47. *Lateral flexion injuries of the cervical spine—diagrammatic representation.* (**A**) With flexion, a fracture (compression) can occur through the ipsilateral side of a vertebral body (*1*). On the contralateral side, avulsion fractures occur through the transverse process (*2*) or through the uncinate process (*3*). (**B**) Fracture of the base of the dens with some lateral displacement to the side of flexion. (**C**) Brachial plexus avulsion. These avulsions occur on the side opposite the side of bending and result in dural tears.

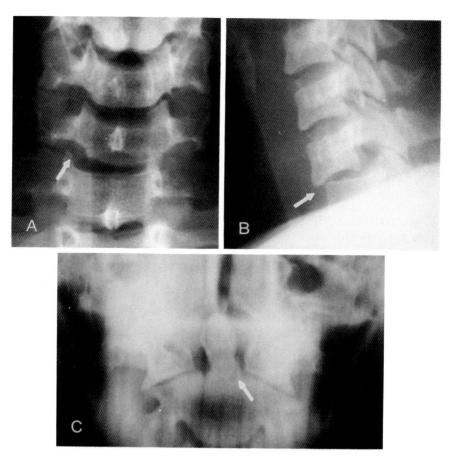

Figure 6.48. *Lateral flexion injuries of the spine.* (*A*) Note disruption of the joint of Luschka at the C_6–C_7 level *on the right* (*arrow*). (*B*) This was due to a rotatory dislocation at this level. Note the narrowed disc space (*arrow*) anteriorly displaced vertebral body of C_6 and the malaligned apophyseal joints at that level. (*C*) Laterally tilted dens due to fracture through the base (*arrow*). The C_1 to dens distance *on the right* is increased due to rotation.

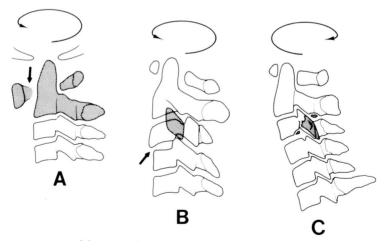

Figure 6.49. *Rotation injuries of the cervical spine—diagrammatic representation.* (*A*) Rotatory subluxation of C_1 on C_2. One of the anterior masses will be displaced forward and the predental distance (*arrow*) will be increased. (*B*) Unilateral locked facet. In these cases, the involved facet (*shaded*) comes to lie anterior to its mate. In addition, the involved vertebral body becomes anteriorly displaced on the one below it (*arrow*), and the disc space often is narrowed. (*C*) Associated extension forces usually result in a variety of fractures through the pillars, articular facets, and posterior elements. There also may be disc disruption.

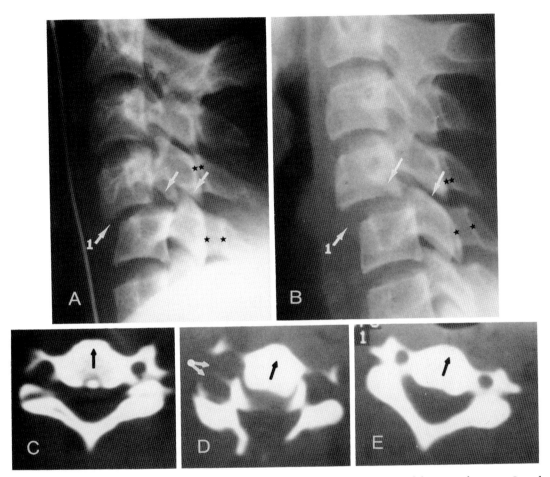

Figure 6.50. *Unilateral locked facet—rotation-flexion injury.* (*A*) Note the narrowed disc space between C$_4$ and C$_5$ (*1*). C$_4$ is anteriorly displaced on C$_5$ and the apophyseal joints are offset (*arrows*). Note that the distance between the posterior cortex of the apophyseal joint facet and anterior cortex of the spinous tip is wider below the level of dislocation than above the level (*stars*). (*B*) Another patient with similar findings demonstrating a disrupted disc space (*1*) with anterior displacement of the vertebral body above it. The apophyseal joints at the level are offset (*posterior arrows*), while the space between the posterior cortex of the articular facet and the anterior cortex of the spinous tip again is wider below the level of rotation than above the level (*stars*). (*C*) CT study in another patient with rotatory dislocation. Note the anteriorly pointing lower vertebral body (*arrow*). (*D*) Just above this level the upper vertebral body is rotated *to the left* (*arrow*). The two offset apophyseal joint facets are seen (*white arrows*). (*E*) Slightly higher cut demonstrates the upper vertebral body to be rotated *to the left* (*arrow*).

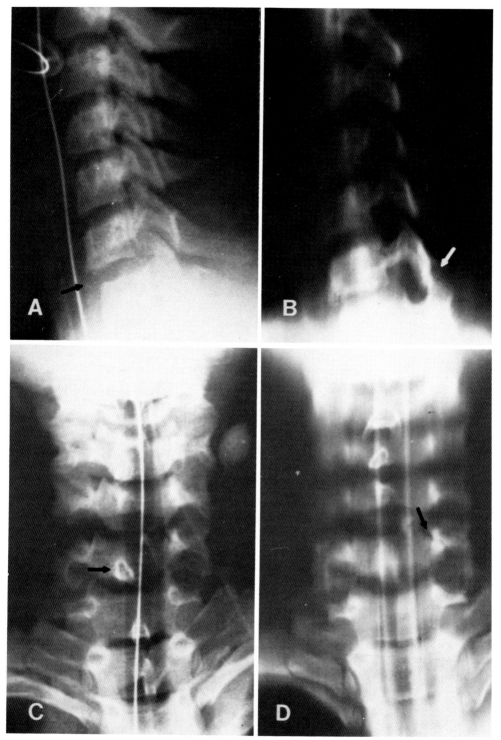

Figure 6.51. *Unilateral locked facet with associated fractures.* (*A*) Note that C_6 is anteriorly displaced on C_7 (*arrow*) and that while above this level the apophyseal joints are seen in pairs, at the level of dislocation only one joint is visualized (the posterior one). Once again, this should signify the presence of a unilateral locked facet. (*B*) Subsequent laminagram demonstrates the locked or jumped facet (*arrow*) at the C_6–C_7 level. (*C*) Frontal

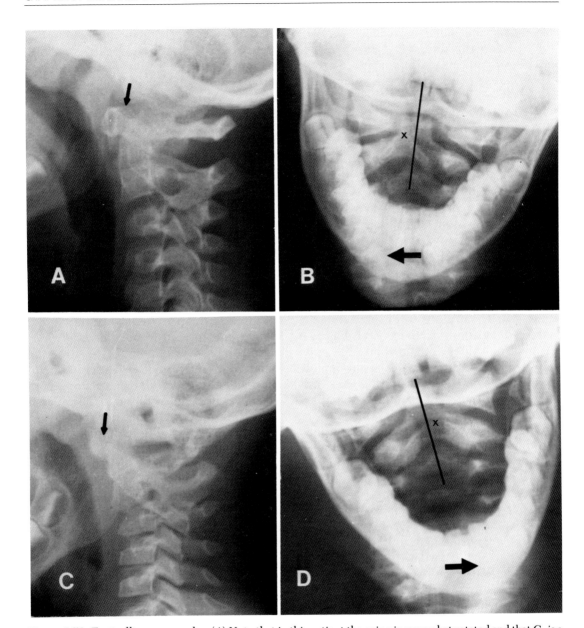

Figure 6.52. *Torticollis or wry neck.* (*A*) Note that in this patient the spine is somewhat rotated and that C_2 is a little cocked forward on C_3. However, the predental distance is normal (*arrow*). (*B*) Frontal view demonstrating that the spinous process of C_2 (*X*) lies to the same side of the midline as the mandible points (*arrow*). The lateral mass of C_1 to dens distance is narrow on the right and wide on the left. This is common with rotation. (*C*) Another patient with torticollis showing a completely scrambled-appearing upper cervical spine. However, the predental distance (*arrow*) is normal. (*D*) Frontal view demonstrating characteristic findings in that the spinous process of C_2 (*X*) lies to the same side of the midline as the mandible points (*arrow*).

view demonstrating the spinous process of C_6 to be displaced to the right (*arrow*). The spinous processes above this level all line up with C_6, while those below the level line up with C_7. This is characteristic of unilateral locked facet. (*D*) Subsequent laminagraphy demonstrates extensive fractures through the lateral aspect of C_6 (*arrow*). The bony ossicles just adjacent to the inner aspect of the ribs are normal secondary ossification centers.

the rotated anterior facet of C_1 becomes "locked" on the underlying facet of C_2, and because of this C_2 cannot rotate properly. The end result is that the spinous tip of C_2, rather than rotating to the side opposite to which the mandible has rotated, stays on the same side. This is demonstrable on frontal roentgenograms when a line is dropped from the tip of the dens through the midsagittal plane of the dens (Fig. 6.52). If rotatory subluxation does not spontaneously correct with conservative measures, the patient should be evaluated with dynamic CT for the presence of rotatory fixation (see Fig. 6.54).

With rotatory dislocation of C_1 on C_2, the same general abnormalities are visualized on frontal view, but on lateral view cocking of C_1 on C_2 is more pronounced and fixed. In addition, there is visible anterior displacement of the rotated lateral mass of C_1 and widening of the predental space (Fig. 6.53A and B). In this way, the findings are quite different from simple torticollis.

On frontal view, in addition to deviation of the spinous process of C_2 off the midline, it has been noted that inward offsetting of the rotated lateral mass of C_1 also occurs (20, 21). However, while there is no question that such a malalignment occurs in many cases, similar malalignment can be seen under normal circumstances (40). Furthermore, it is not uncommon for similar or other offsetting abnormalities of the lateral masses of C_1 to occur with simple torticollis (Fig. 6.52B). Consequently, *I have come to the conclusion that it is best to ignore what the lateral masses are doing in these cases, for there are other, more important, findings to assess.* Lateral masses should be assessed only on true anteroposterior films.

Rotatory fixation is a peculiar problem wherein there is persistent subluxation or offsetting of the involved lateral mass of C_1 (23, 30, 32, 40, 47). In these cases, no matter which way the patient turns his head, offsetting remains the same. The injury is believed to result from fixed invagination

of ligaments into the involved joint and, as such, differs from simple subluxation in that the problem is transient. Otherwise, I believe the two conditions are similar, if not the same. With rotatory fixation, as with rotatory subluxation, there is no widening of the predental distance on lateral view. This is different from rotatory dislocation where widening is present.

Once rotatory fixation is suspected, dynamic CT with neutral and right and left rotation is best for evaluating the problem (32). The study can be augmented with reconstructed images in the coronal, sagittal, or angled planes, where the actual apophyseal joints can be seen. However, the simple dynamic CT study usually serves to alert one to the problem. With this study, the patient, in neutral position, shows C_1 angled on C_2. C_1 will point in the direction of the rotation. Thereafter, with rotation to the unaffected side, C_1 rotates along with C_2. However, when rotation to the affected side is attempted, C_1 does not rotate with C_2 and remains fixed in its initially abnormal position (Fig. 6.54).

Axial Compression Injuries of the Cervical Spine. These injuries generally result in bursting of the involved vertebra (Fig. 6.55). In the upper cervical spine, the classic bursting fracture is the Jefferson fracture of C_1 (16, 40, 46). In the other vertebral bodies, including the body of C_2, axial compression injuries result in bursting and expansion of the vertebral body in all directions, including into the spinal canal (Fig. 6.55).

The Jefferson bursting fracture is unstable and is characterized by bilateral outward displacement of the lateral masses of C_1. Instability is more of a problem when less than four breaks (two on each side) are present for transverse ligament tears commonly are associated (27). The fractures through the anterior and posterior arches of C_1 usually are not visible unless laminography, in the past, and, currently, CT scanning are performed. Consequently, it is most important to detect C_1 lateral mass

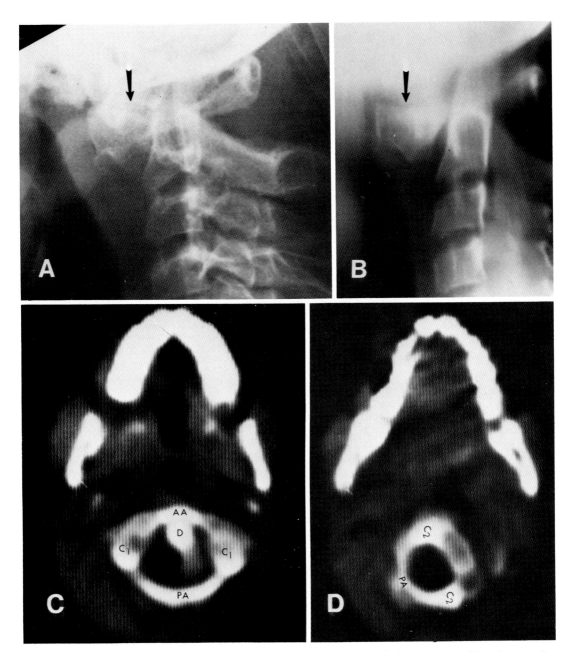

Figure 6.53. *Rotatory subluxation of C_1 on C_2.* (*A*) Note the peculiarly cocked appearance of C_1. Also note that the predental distance, although not clearly visualized, appears abnormally wide (*arrow*). A little prevertebral soft tissue swelling also is present. (*B*) Subsequent laminograms demonstrate the anterior position of the rotated lateral mass (*arrow*). (*C*) CT scan in another patient. Note the position of the lateral masses (C_1), the anterior arch (*AA*), and the posterior arch (*PA*) of C_1. The dens (*D*) is off the midline. (*D*) Lower cut. Note the position of the articular facets of C_2 (C_2) and the position of the posterior arch (*PA*). Almost 90° dislocation is present. (Courtesy of F.L.G. Rothman, M.D.)

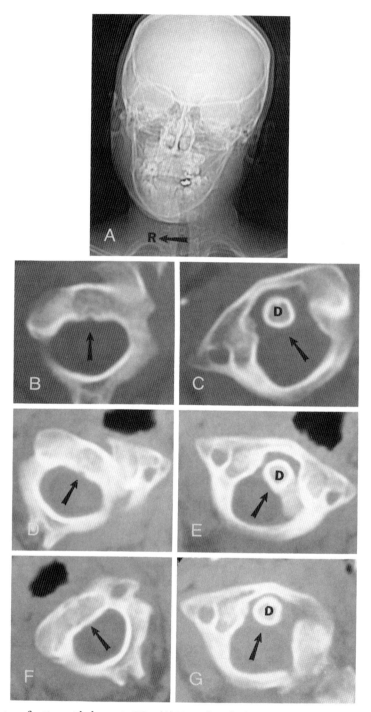

Figure 6.54. *Rotatory fixation with dynamic CT.* (*A*) Note that the head is tilted *to the right* (*R*). (*B*) In neutral position C_2 points anteriorly (*arrow*). (*C*) C_1, however, points *to the right* (*arrows*). Dens (*D*). (*D*) With rotation to the left, C_2 points *to the left* (*arrow*). (*E*) C_1 also points *to the left* (*arrow*). Dens (*D*). (*F*) With turning to the right, C_2 points *to the right* (*arrow*). (*G*) C_1, however, is fixed and cannot rotate to the right and still points *to the left* (*arrow*). Dens (*D*).

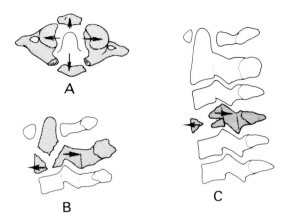

Figure 6.55. *Axial compression injuries of the cervical spine.* (*A*) Typical Jefferson bursting fracture of C_1. Fractures occur posteriorly and anteriorly, and the fracture fragments are displaced in all directions. (*B*) Bursting fracture of C_2. The findings are self-evident. (*C*) Similar findings in a bursting fracture of one of the lower cervical vertebrae.

displacements on frontal views. Most often, with four fracture sites (two on each side) both lateral masses are displaced (Fig. 6.56A). With unilateral lateral mass displacement, a unilateral or partial (two or three fracture sites) Jefferson fracture is present. On lateral view, all of these fractures basically are invisible (Fig. 6.57). Less commonly, with compression injuries of C_1, one may note an isolated fracture of the medial portion of the lateral mass (1). A normal variation in infants has been noted to mimic a Jefferson fracture (42). In these patients, on frontal view, the lateral masses appear widely displaced and, as such, suggest a Jefferson fracture (Fig. 6.56E). This is believed to occur because C_1 and its lateral masses grow faster than C_2 (42). In addition to this normal variation, occasionally one can encounter a normal individual with an increased dens to lateral mass distance (Fig. 6.58). In such cases, one is dealing with an anomaly of development of the lateral mass of C_1 and the underlying body of C_2. These patients are asymptomatic.

Axial compression injuries of the body and dens of C_2 cause vertical or oblique fractures, and expansion of the vertebral body in all directions (Fig. 6.59A and B). The same is true of axial fractures of the lower cervical vertebrae (Fig. 6.62C). The configuration of the expanded body of C_2

in these cases has been termed the "fat C_2" sign (41). It is most important not to confuse a similar configuration of C_2 occasionally seen in normal individuals (Fig. 6.60).

C^1-Occipital Injuries. These injuries, by and large, are not particularly common. Atlanto-occipital dislocations can result from both flexion or extension forces and both often are associated with sudden death (4). With anterior atlanto-occipital dislocations, the dens lies anterior to the anterior lip of the foramen magnum, while with posterior dislocations, the dens lies posterior to the anterior lip of the foramen magnum. Normally, of course, it lies just below the anterior lip of the foramen magnum. Complete atlanto-occipital dislocation also can occur (Fig. 6.61). Such injuries result from violent distracting-rotational forces and also can occur elsewhere in the spine (Fig. 6.61).

Other injuries of the cervical occipital junction consist of fractures through the occipital condyles, but often these fractures are not detected until subsequent laminography or CT scanning is performed (Fig. 6.62). The basic mechanisms through which these fractures occur are poorly understood, but since they can be associated with fractures of C_1, it might be that they result from axial compression and hyperextension forces.

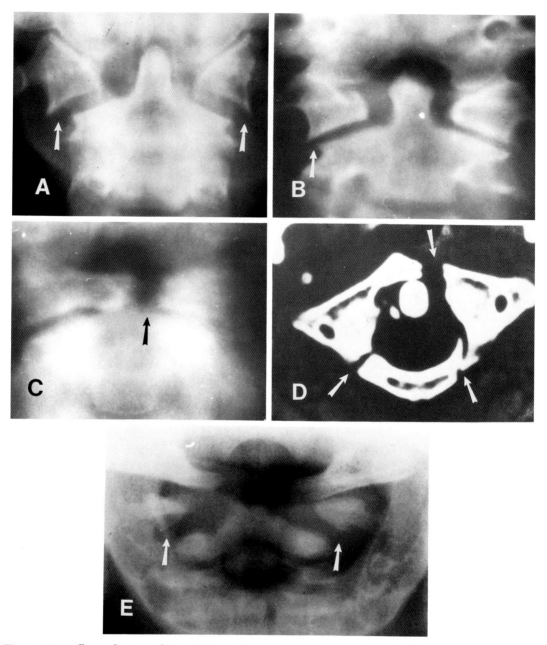

Figure 6.56. *Jefferson fracture of C₁.* (*A*) Typical outward displacement (*arrows*) of both lateral masses of C₁ (*arrows*). The one *on the right* is more displaced than the one *on the left*. Because of this, the distance between the dens and lateral mass on the right is greater than on the left. (*B*) Unilateral Jefferson fracture of C₁. Note unilateral outward displacement of the right lateral mass of C₁ (*arrow*). There is an associated increase in distance between the right lateral mass and the dens. (*C*) Laminogram demonstrates the associated fracture through the anterior arch of C₁ (*arrow*). (*D*) CT findings: partial fracture. Note how clearly the bursting phenomenon is depicted at the three fracture sites (*arrows*). (*E*) Pseudo-Jefferson fracture in an infant. Note how the lateral masses of C₁ (*arrows*) appear laterally displaced in this normal infant.

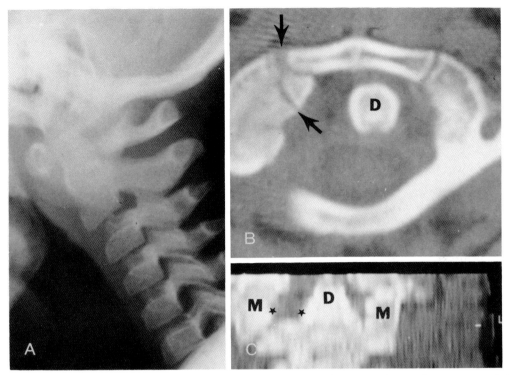

Figure 6.57. *Jefferson fracture of C1: CT detection.* (*A*) On this lateral view, no abnormality is suspected. The anterior C_1-dens distance is within normal range. (*B*) CT demonstrates a fracture through the lateral mass of C_1 (*arrows*). (*C*) Coronal reconstruction demonstrates the lateral masses of C_1 (*M*) and the dens (*D*). The space between the right lateral mass and dens is increased (*stars*).

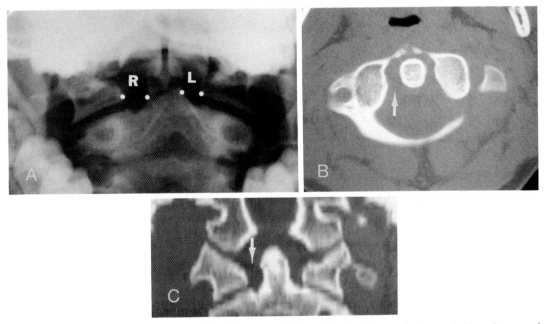

Figure 6.58. *Normally wide lateral mass-dens distance.* (*A*) Note that the distance between the lateral mass and the dens (*dots*) is greater on the right than on the left. This patient had minor cervical spine injury. (*B*) Axial CT demonstrates similar widening (*arrow*). Coronal reconstruction again demonstrates unilateral widening (*arrow*). Note, however, that there is no offsetting of the lateral mass on this view or in *A*. This patient had a full range of motion at this time and the dynamic CT was normal. No fractures or ligamentous injury was identified.

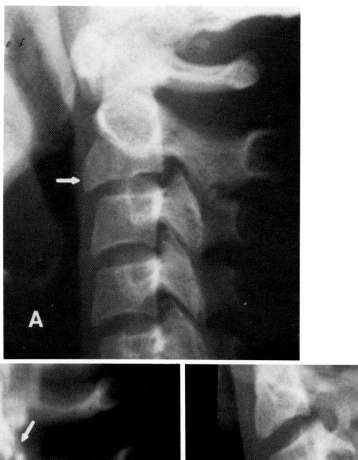

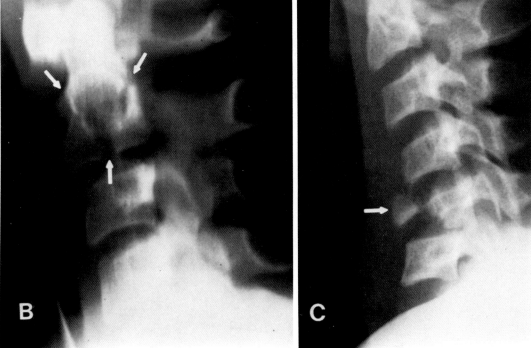

Figure 6.59. *Axial compression bursting fractures of the cervical vertebrae—fat vertebra sign.* (*A*) Fat C_2 sign. Note anterior displacement of the expanded body of C_2 (*arrow*). There is some associated disc space narrowing but clear-cut fractures are difficult to define. (*B*) Laminagraphy demonstrates a Y-shaped bursting fracture (*arrows*) involving the body and lower aspect of the dens of C_2. (*C*) Bursting fracture of C_5 (*arrow*). The findings represent a combination of an axial compression fracture of C_5 and a hyperflexion injury at this level. In this regard, note that there is kyphosis at the level of injury, and marked narrowing of the disc space between C_5 and C_6. Prevertebral soft tissue swelling is extensive. Very often axial compression injuries of the lower cervical spine are accompanied by a flexion component.

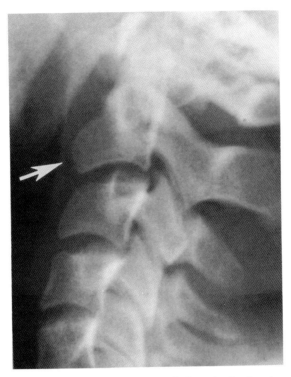

Figure 6.60. *Pseudofat C_2 sign.* Note the normally wide and plump body of C_2 (*arrow*) in this patient with no injuries.

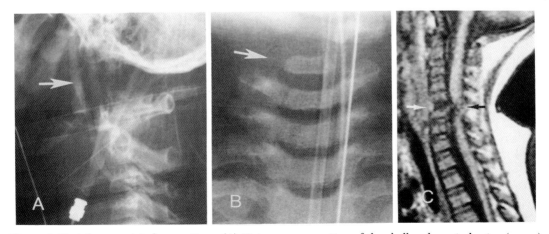

Figure 6.61. *Atlanto-occipital separation.* (*A*) Note gross separation of the skull and cervical spine (*arrow*). There probably also is some dislocation at the C_1–C_2 level: i.e., note the markedly increased C_1–C_2 interspinous distance. (*B*) Another patient with avulsion of the neural arch from the body of C_5 (*arrow*). (*C*) Same patient. Sagittal, T_1-weighted MR study demonstrates cord compression and virtual transection of the cord (*black arrow*). The completely destroyed disc and altered vertebral bodies in the area also are noted (*white arrow*).

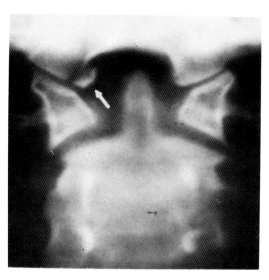

Figure 6.62. *Occipital condyle fracture.* Note the fracture *(arrow)* of the occipital condyle *on the right.* Also note that the right lateral mass of C₁ is displaced outwardly, suggesting the associated presence of a unilateral Jefferson fracture.

REFERENCES

1. Barker, E.G., Krumpelman, J., and Long, J.M.: Isolated fracture of the medial portion of the lateral mass of the atlas: A previously undescribed entity. A.J.R. 126: 1053–1058, 1976.
2. Beatson, T.R.: Fractures and dislocations of the cervical spine. J. Bone Joint Surg. 45B: 21–35, 1963.
3. Cintron, E., Gilula, L.A., Murphy, W.A., and Gehweiler, J.A.: The widened disk space: A sign of cervical hyperextension injury. Radiology 141: 639–644, 1981.
4. Cohen, A., Hirsch, M., Katz, M., and Sofer, S.: Traumatic atlanto-occipital dislocation in children: Review and report of five cases. Pediatr. Emerg. Care 7: 24–27, 1991.
5. Davis, S.J., Teresi, L.M., Bradley, W.G., Jr., Ziemba, M.A., and Bloze, A.E.: Cervical spine hyperextension injuries: MR findings. Radiology 180: 245–250. 1991.
6. Dolan, K.D.: Cervical spine injuries below the axis. Radiol. Clin. North Am. 15: 247–259, 1977.
7. Donaldson, J.S.: Acquired torticollis in children and young adults. J.A.M.A. 160: 458–461, 1956.
8. El-Khoury, T.Y., Clark, C.R., and Grabbett, A.W.: Acute traumatic rotatory atlanto-axial dislocation in children. J. Bone Joint Surg. 66A: 774–777, 1984.
9. Elliott, J.M., Jr., Rogers, L.F., Wissinger, J.P., and Lee, J.F.: The hangman's fracture: Fractures

10. of the neural arch of the axis. Radiology 104: 303–307, 1972.
10. Fielding, J.W., and Hawkins, R.J.: Atlanto-axial rotatory fixation (fixed rotatory subluxation of the atlanto-axial joint). J. Bone Joint Surg. 59: 37–44, 1977.
11. Fielding, J.W., and Griffin, P.O.: Os odontoideum: An acquired lesion. J. Bone Joint Surg. 56A: 187–190, 1974.
12. Forysth, H.F.: Extension injuries of the cervical spine. J. Bone Joint Surg. 46A: 1792–1797, 1964.
13. Freiberger, R.H., Wilson, P.D., Jr., and Nicholas, J.A.: An acquired absence of the odontoid process: A case report. J. Bone Joint Surg. 47A: 1231–1236, 1965.
14. Gooding, C.A., and Hurwitz, M.E.: Avulsed vertebral rim apophysis in a child. Pediatr. Radiol. 2: 265–268, 1974.
15. Griffiths, S.C.: Fracture of odontoid process in children. J. Pediatr. Surg. 7: 680–683, 1972.
16. Han, S.Y., Witten, D.M., and Musselman, J.P.: Jefferson fracture of the atlas: Report of six cases. J. Neurosurg. 44: 368–371, 1976.
17. Hanafee, W., and Crandall, P.: Trauma of the spine and its contents. Radiol. Clin. North Am. 4: 365–382, 1966.
18. Hawkins, R.J., Fielding, J.W., and Thompson, W.J.: Os odontoideum—congenital or acquired: A case report. J. Bone Joint Surg. 58A: 413–414, 1976.
19. Holdsworth, F.W.: Fractures, dislocations, and fracture-dislocations of the spine. J. Bone Joint Surg. 52A: 1534–1551, 1970.
20. Jacobson, G., and Adler, D.C.: Examination of the atlantoaxial joint following injury with particular emphasis on rotational subluxation. A.J.R. 76: 1081–1094, 1956.
21. Jacobson, G., and Adler, D.C.: An evaluation of lateral atlanto-axial displacement in injuries of the cervical spine. Radiology 61: 355–362, 1961.
22. Jones, E.T., and Hensinger, R.N.: C₂-C₃ dislocation in a child. J. Pediatr. Orthop. 1: 419–422, 1981.
23. Kawabe, N., Hirotani, H. and Tanaka, O.: Pathomechanism of atlantoaxial rotatory fixation in children. J. Pediatr. Orthop. 9: 569–578, 1989.
24. Keller, R.H.: Traumatic displacement of the cartilaginous vertebral rim: A sign of intervertebral disc prolapse. Radiology 110: 21–24, 1974.
25. Kim, K.S., Chen, H.H., Russell, E.J., and Rogers, L.F.: Flexion teardrop fracture of the cervical spine: Radiographic characteristics. A.J.R. 152: 319–326, 1989.
26. Lee, C., Kim, K.S., and Rogers, L.F.: Triangular cervical vertebral body fractures; diagnostic significance. A.J.R. 138: 1123–1132, 1982.

27. Lee, C., and Woodring, J.H.: Unstable Jefferson variant atlas fractures: An unrecognized cervical injury. A.J.R. 158: 113–118, 1992.

28. McGrory, B.E., and Fenichel, G.M.: Hangman's fracture subsequent to shaking an infant. Ann. Neurol. 2: 82, 1977.

29. Naidich, J.B., Naidich, T.P., Garfein, C., Liebeskind, A.L., and Hyman, R.A.: The widened interspinous distance: A useful sign of anterior cervical dislocation in the supine frontal projection. Radiology 123: 113–116, 1977.

30. Ono, K., Yonenobu, K., Fuji, T., and Okada, K: Atlantoaxial rotatory fixation: Radiographic study of its mechanism. Spine 10: 602–608, 1985.

31. Pennecot, G.F., Leonard, P., Des Gachons, S.P., Hardy, J.R., and Pouliquen, J.C.: Traumatic ligamentous instability of the cervical spine in children. J. Pediatr. Orthop. 4: 339–344, 1984.

32. Phillips, W.A., and Hensinger, R.N.: The management of rotatory atlanto-axial subluxation in children. J. Bone Joint Surg. 71: 664–665, 1989.

33. Richman, S., and Friedman, R.L.: Vertical fracture of cervical vertebral bodies. Radiology 62: 536, 1954.

34. Schaaf, R.E., Gehweiler, J.A., Jr., Miller, M.D., and Powers, B.: Lateral hyperflexion injuries of the cervical spine. Skeletal Radiol. 3: 73–78, 1978.

35. Scher, A.T.: Unilateral locked facet in cervical spine injuries. A.J.R. 129: 45–48, 1977.

36. Scher, A.T.: "Tear-drop" fractures of the cervical spine—radiological features. S. Afr. Med. J. 61: 355–356, 1982.

37. Scher, A.T.: Anterior cervical subluxation: An unstable position. A.J.R. 133: 275–280, 1979.

38. Seimon, L.P.: Fracture of the odontoid process in young children. J. Bone Joint Surg. 59A: 943–948, 1977.

39. Seljeskog, E.L., and Chou, S.N.: Spectrum of the hangman's fracture. J. Neurosurg. 45: 3–8, 1976.

40. Shapiro, R., Youngberg, A.S., and Rothman, S.L.G.: The differential diagnosis of traumatic lesions of the occipitoatlanto-axial segment. Radiol. Clin. North Am. 11: 505–526, 1973.

41. Smoker, W.R.K., and Dolan, K.D.: The "fat" C_2: A sign of fracture. A.J.R. 148: 609–614, 1987.

42. Suss, R.A., Zimmerman, R.D., and Leeds, N.E.: Pseudospread of the atlas: False sign of Jefferson fracture in young children. A.J.R. 140: 1079, 1983.

43. Swischuk, L.E., Hayden, C.K., Jr., and Sarwar, M.: The posteriorly tilted dens (a normal variation mimicking a fracture of the dens). Pediatr. Radiol. 8: 27–28, 1979.

44. Weiss, M.H., Kaufman, B.: Hangman's fracture in an infant. Am. J. Dis. Child. 126: 268–269, 1973.

45. Whitley, J.E., and Forsyth, H.F.: The classification of cervical spine injuries. A.J.R. 83: 633–644, 1960.

46. Wirth, R.L., Zatz, L.M., and Parker, B.R.: Case report: CT detection of a Jefferson fracture in a child. A.J.R. 149: 1001–1002, 1987.

47. Wortzman, G., and DeWar, F.P.: Rotary fixation of the atlanto-axial joint: Rotational atlanto-axial subluxation. Radiology 90: 479–487, 1968.

CERVICAL CORD AND NERVE ROOT INJURIES

Brachial Plexus Injuries (1–4). These injuries are avulsion injuries of the brachial plexus resulting from excessive lateral flexion-rotation of the spine. They also can result from excessive posterior stretching of the arm. In either case, there is paralysis of the affected limb and with C_5–C_7 root injuries, a Duchenne-Erb's paralysis of the shoulder and upper arm results, while a Klumpke's paralysis of the hand results from C_7–T_1 injuries. With C_7–T_1 injuries, Horner's syndrome also may be present. The diagnosis usually is made clinically, for without myelography, CT, or MR there is little in the way of roentgenographic abnormality. Typical myelographic findings consist of extravasation of contrast material along the nerve roots in so-called "traumatic meningoceles" or "cysts" (Fig. 6.63).

Central Cord Syndrome. The central cord syndrome usually results from hyperextension injuries of the cervical spine. Clinically, there is a definite cord level with neurologic deficit clearly apparent (5–8). The roentgenograms, however, usually show no fracture or dislocation, but in spite of these rather negative findings, the lesion should be considered unstable and the neck should be properly immobilized. Cord injury results from pinching or squeezing of the cord between the anterior and posterior walls of the spinal canal secondary to buckling of the ligamentum flavum during hyperextension (see Fig. 6.33C). Currently MR scanning readily detects the subsequent contusion to the spinal cord (Fig. 6.64).

Figure 6.63. *Brachial plexus avulsion.* Myelogram. Note characteristic extravasation of contrast material along a nerve root (*arrow*).

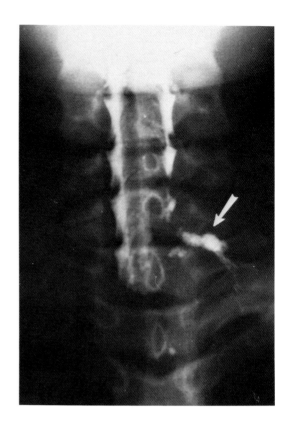

Figure 6.64. *Central cord syndrome.* This patient had no bony abnormalities visible but **MR** scanning demonstrates an area of cord contusion (low signal areas) in the midcervical cord (*arrows*).

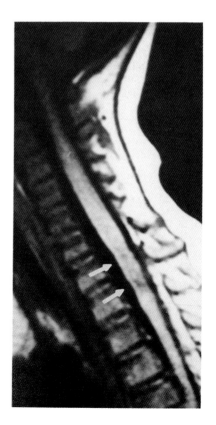

REFERENCES

1. Davies, E.R., Sutton, D., and Blight, A.S.: Myelography in brachial plexus injury. Br. J. Radiol. 39: 362–371, 1966.
2. Lester, J.: Pantopaque myelography in avulsion of the brachial plexus. Acta Radiol. 55: 186–192, 1961.
3. Murphey, F., Hartung, W., and Kirklin, J.W.: Myelographic demonstration of avulsing injury of the brachial plexus. A.J.R. 58: 102–105, 1947.
4. Murphey, F., and Kirklin, J.: Myelographic demonstration of avulsing injuries of the nerve roots of the brachial plexus—a method of determining the point of injury and the possibility of repair. Clin. Neurosurg. 20: 18–28, 1972.
5. Rand, R.W., and Crandall, P.H.: Central spinal cord syndrome in hyperextension injuries of the cervical spine. J. Bone Joint Surg. 44A: 1415–1422, 1962.
6. Schneider, R.C., Cherry, G., and Pantek, H.: The syndrome of acute central cervical spinal cord injury. J. Neurosurg. 11: 546–577, 1954.
7. Taylor, A.R., and Blackwood, W.: Paraplegia in hyperextension cervical injuries with normal radiographic appearances. J. Bone Joint Surg. 30B: 245–248, 1948.
8. Taylor, A.R.: The mechanism of injury to the spinal cord in the neck without damage to the vertebral column. J. Bone Joint Surg. 33B: 543–547, 1951.

NORMAL FINDINGS AND ANOMALIES OF THE CERVICAL SPINE CAUSING PROBLEMS

Most of the significant normal findings in the cervical spine have been covered at appropriate points in previous sections, but a few others should be discussed for completeness. In this regard, one of the most common normal findings to be misinterpreted for a fracture is the *dens-arch synchondrosis of* C_2 (3, 6). Actually, this synchondrosis is part of a triad of synchondroses between the dens, body, and arch of C_2 (Fig. 6.65). All of these synchondroses lie anterior and are seen only on oblique views of the cervical spine. In the injured child, this most commonly occurs fortuitously on skull roentgenograms. In such cases, while the head is in lateral position, the cervical spine is in the rotated, oblique position (Fig. 6.66).

In assessing these synchondroses, it is important to appreciate that they are an-terior structures, and thus visible only when the spine is obliqued. Once this is appreciated, they can be differentiated from fractures through the neural arch of C_2 with ease, for these fractures are visible on both oblique and lateral views (Fig. 6.67). Indeed, if one notes a defect in the neural arch of C_2 on lateral view, it should be considered a fracture until proven otherwise. Congenital defects in this region are extremely rare (1) (see Fig. 6.45). The synchondroses between the bodies and arches of the lower cervical vertebrae are less of a problem (Fig. 6.68).

Other normal findings causing problems include the *transverse processes* being projected through the intervertebral disc spaces and the normal *ring epiphysis* of the growing vertebral body. These ring epiphyses can be misinterpreted for corner (teardrop) fractures of the vertebral bodies, for often they may appear "tilted" (Fig. 6.69A). The transverse processes can be misinterpreted as intervertebral disc calcifications (Fig. 6.69B).

Wedging of C_3 is a normal phenomenon in infants and young children that often is confused with a compression fracture (7). In some of these cases the wedging deformity is quite pronounced (Fig. 6.70). Although it is not precisely known why this occurs, it is believed that it results from the normal hypermobility that occurs at the C_2–C_3 level in young children (7). It has been suggested that the chronic subclinical impaction of the upper anterior corner of C_3 leads to impaired bone growth and variable degrees of wedging (7). The phenomenon may occur at the C_4 level, but basically does not occur at the other levels. Furthermore, it disappears with increasing age. Interestingly enough, with increasing age, as the wedging deformity disappears, there is an associated change in the apex of the flexion curve of the cervical spine. In other words, in infancy the apex occurs in the upper cervical spine, at the C_2–C_3 level (Fig. 6.71), while in the older child the curve is more uniform and curving and the

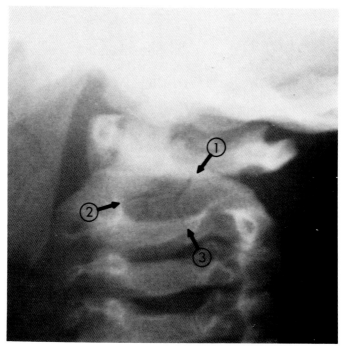

Figure 6.65. *Normal synchondroses of C2.* Synchondrosis between the dens and arch (*1*), synchondrosis between the dens and body (*2*), and synchondrosis between the body and arch (*3*). The synchondrosis between the dens and arch is the one most commonly misinterpreted as a fracture of C_2.

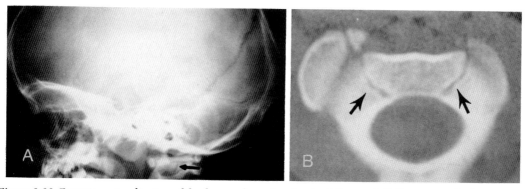

Figure 6.66. *Fortuitous visualization of the dens-arch synchondrosis of C_2 on a skull film.* Note the fracture-like appearance of the synchondrosis between the dens and arch of C_2 (*arrow*). This synchondrosis is visible on oblique views of the cervical spine in infants and young children because it is anterior in location. It is not visible on lateral view. (*B*) CT scan demonstrates the anterior position of the synchondroses (*arrows*). Also note the small accessory ossicle *on the right.*

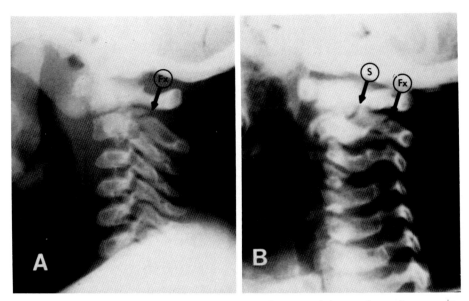

Figure 6.67. *Dens-arch synchrondrosis of C₂ versus hangman's fracture.* (*A*) Lateral view demonstrating a defect (*Fx*) through the arch of C₂. This should be a hangman's fracture. (*B*) Oblique view demonstrates the posterior position of the fracture (*Fx*) and the anterior position of the normal dens-arch synchrondrosis (*S*) of C₂.

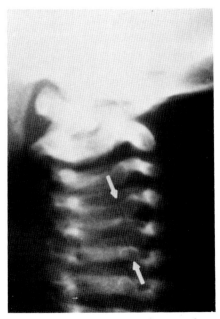

Figure 6.68. *Synchrondroses of lower cervical vertebrae.* Note the typical appearance of the synchrondroses between the bodies and arches of the lower cervical vertebrae (*arrows*).

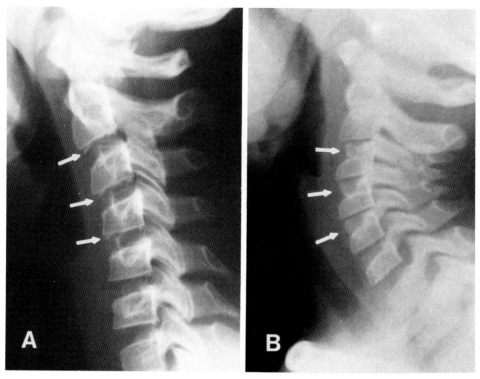

Figure 6.69. (*A*) *Ring epiphyses.* Note normal ring epiphyses (*arrows*). The one off C₃ appears tilted and avulsed. This, however, is a normal appearance. (*B*) Transverse processes projected through intervertebral discs. Note the transverse processes of the cervical vertebrae (*arrows*) projected through the intravertebral discs. They should not be confused with intravertebral disc calcifications.

apex is located in the midcervical spine (Fig. 6.71*D*). It is believed that the apex occurs in the upper cervical spine in infancy and childhood because of normal hypermobility in this area (7). In any case, if there is doubt as to the presence of a fracture one can perform CT scanning of the cervical spine. In cases where wedging is normal no fracture is seen (Fig. 6.72).

In terms of anomalies causing problems, although a number exist, the most important is the *hypoplastic dens associated with an os odontoideum* (2, 4, 6). In these cases, the os odontoideum can appear as though it were a fractured dens. Actually, the os odontoideum probably is an overgrown os terminale, and it overgrows when the dens is hypoplastic (9). The os terminale is a small ossicle occurring in all children, just

at the tip of the dens and seated in a V-shaped notch (Fig. 6.73*A*). By adolescence, the os terminale becomes fused with the dens. Ordinarily it is not seen on lateral view, because it is seated deeply in the notch. In some cases, however, it is located higher and then becomes visible (Fig. 6.73*B*).

When the os terminale becomes the os odontoideum, it is associated with dens hypoplasia and usually some degree of hypermobility at the C₁–C₂ area (Fig. 6.74). Indeed, in advanced cases, the entire lesion is quite unstable and frequently requires surgical stabilization. Occasionally an os odontoideum can be acquired (2, 5), resulting from pronounced dens resorption (interrupted blood supply) after dens injuries in infancy (see Fig. 6.30).

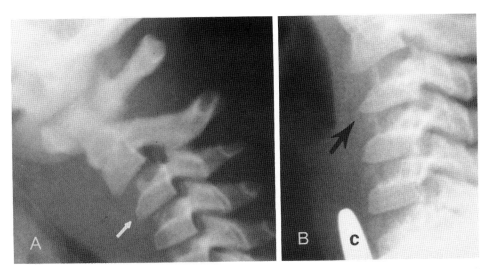

Figure 6.70. *Normal wedging of C₃.* (*A*) Note the wedged appearance of C₃ (*arrow*). In this patient, also note other normal findings often misinterpreted as pathology. The C₁ to dens distance is wide but normal. The interspinous distance from C₁–C₂ also is wide but is normal. The apophyseal joint at the C₂–C₃ level shows considerable anterior displacement but this is also normal. (*B*) Note the wedged appearance of C₃ (*arrow*). A compression fracture might be suggested; however, this patient was examined for a coin (*C*) in the esophagus. (Reproduced with permission from L.E. Swischuk, P.N. Swischuk, and S.D. John: Wedging of C₃ in infants and children: Usually a normal finding and not a fracture. Radiology 188:523–526, 1993.)

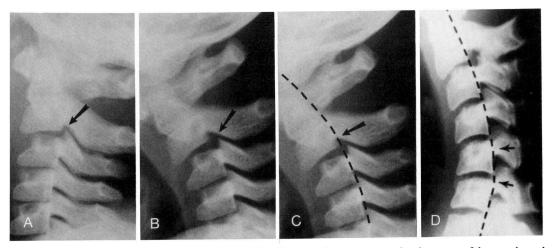

Figure 6.71. *Physiologic motion through C₂–C₃.* (*A*) In the neutral position note the alignment of the apophyseal joints of the various vertebrae. Specifically, note the configuration of the joints at the C₂–C₃ level (*arrow*). Also note that C₃ is slightly wedged. (*B*) With flexion, most motion occurs through the C₂–C₃ level (*arrows*). (*C*) The apex of the curve during flexion is at the C₂–C₃ level. (*D*) In older children and adults it is located in the mid-cervical spine (*arrows*).

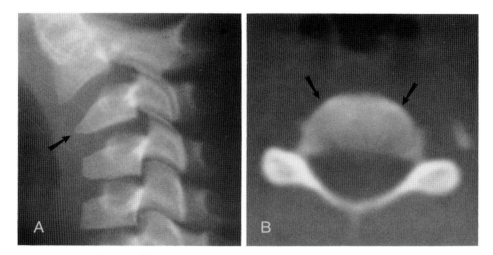

Figure 6.72. *Wedging of C₃.* (*A*) Note marked wedging of C₃ (*arrow*). Is a fracture present? Angulation of C₂ on C₃ is normal (see Fig. 6.2). (*B*) CT scan through C₃ demonstrates no fracture (*arrows*). (Reproduced with permission from L.E. Swischuk, P.N. Swischuk, and S.D. John: Wedging of C₃ in infants and children: Usually a normal finding and not a fracture. Radiology 188: 523–526, 1993.)

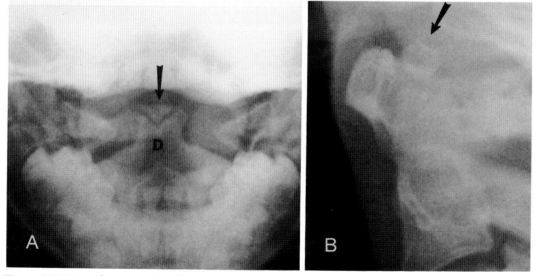

Figure 6.73. *Normal os terminale.* (*A*) Frontal, open-mouth odontoid view demonstrates the typical normal os terminale (*arrow*) seated in the wedge at the top of the dens (*D*). (*B*) On lateral view, the os terminale usually is not visible but in some cases it is located high, and above the wedge of the dens and then becomes visible (*arrow*).

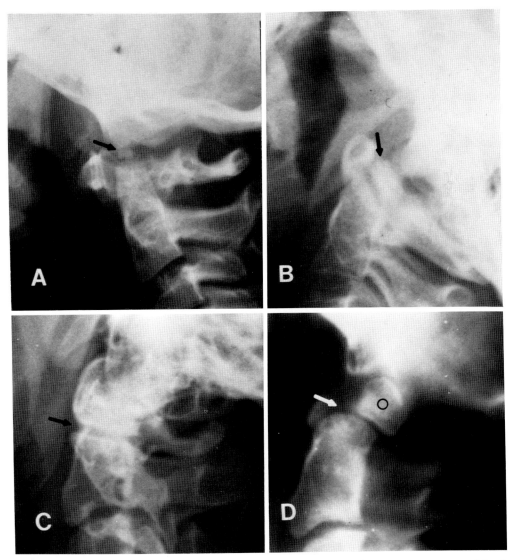

Figure 6.74. *Os terminale-os odontoidium anomalies.* (**A**) Normal os terminale (*arrow*) at the tip of the dens.
(**B**) Large os odontoideum (*arrow*). This actually is an overgrown os terminale associated with a hypoplastic dens.
(Courtesy of D. Binstadt, M.D.) (**C**) This 15-year-old boy was in an automobile accident and at first the defect
through the base of the dens (*arrow*) was thought to represent a dens fracture. However, note how smooth it
appears and note that considerable anomalous development of the upper cervical spine is present. More specifically, C_1 is markedly hypoplastic and deformed. (**D**) Subsequent laminography demonstrates that the defect is
not a fracture, but rather a persistent congenital defect between the hypoplastic dens and overgrown os terminale or os odontoidium (*O*). The os odontoidium shows marked posterior displacement, attesting to the instability
of this lesion.

REFERENCES

1. Harwood-Nash, D.C., and Fitz, C.R.: *Neuroradiology in Infants and Children*, p. 1094. C.V. Mosby, St. Louis, 1976.
2. Hawkins, R.J., Fielding, J.W., and Thompson, W.J.: Os odontoideum-congenital or acquired: A case report. J. Bone Joint Surg. 58A: 413–414, 1978.
3. Keats, T.: *Normal Roentgen Variants that May Simulate Disease.* Year Book, Chicago, 1973.
4. Ricciardi, J.E., Kaufer, H., and Louis, D.S.: Acquired os odontoideum following acute ligament injury: Report of a case. J. Bone Joint Surg. 58A: 410–412, 1976.
5. Shapiro, R., Youngberg, A.S., and Rothman, S.L.G.: The differential diagnosis of traumatic lesions of the occipito-atlanto-axial segments. Radiol. Clin. North Am. 11: 505–526, 1973.
6. Swischuk, L.E., Hayden, C.K., Jr., and Sarwar, M.: The dens-arch synchondrosis versus the hangman's fracture. Pediatr. Radiol. 8: 100–102, 1979.
7. Swischuk, L.E., Swischuk, P.N., and John, S.D.: Wedging of C_3 in infants and children: Usually a normal finding and not a fracture. Radiology 1993 (in press).
8. von Torklus, D., and Gehle, W.: *The Upper Cervical Spine: Regional Morphology, Pathology and Traumatology: An X-ray Atlas.* Grune & Stratton, New York, 1972.

THORACOLUMBAR SPINE TRAUMA

In the thoracolumbar spine, much as in the cervical spine, injuries can result from flexion, extension, lateral flexion, rotation, and axial compression forces.

Flexion Injuries. Most often flexion injuries of the thoracolumbar spine result in anterior compression of the vertebral bodies (Figs. 6.75 and 6.76). However, the more severe the injury the greater is the likelihood that there will be posterior ligament injury, widening of the interspinous distance, and associated spinous tip or neural arch avulsion fractures. Actually, the mechanics of injury are exactly the same as those encountered in flexion injuries of the cervical spine, and in addition to the preceding fractures, teardrop fractures also can be seen (Fig. 6.76). In the lumbar spine, teardrop fractures often are referred to as limbus fractures. If the injury is severe enough, patients with these frac-

tures also will demonstrate anterior subluxation through the apophyseal joints, and once this finding, or widening of the interspinous distance is present, the fracture is considered unstable.

Extension Injuries. Extension injuries of the thoracolumbar spine are not as common as flexion injuries. In some cases, nothing more than nondisplaced neural arch and spinous process fractures result, but in other cases a hangman's type fracture mechanism is at play.

Another fracture that might be sustained when excessive extension forces are applied to the thoracolumbar spine is the so-called "corner" fracture of the vertebral body. Actually, this is the same fracture as the extension, teardrop fracture seen in the cervical spine, and should indicate underlying ligamentous injury with instability. In addition, there may be asso-

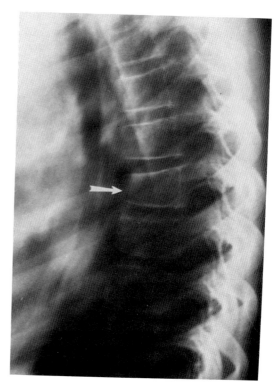

Figure 6.75. *Compression fracture-thoracic vertebra.* Note the typical appearance of the anteriorly compressed vertebra (*arrow*).

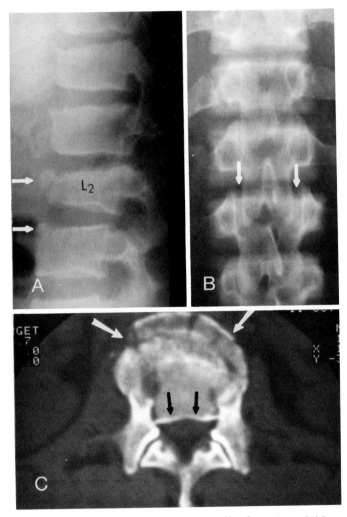

Figure 6.76. *Combined hyperflexion-axial compression injury of lumbar spine.* (*A*) Lateral view demonstrating marked anterior compression of L_2, anterior teardrop fractures of L_2 and L_3 (*arrows*), and minimal anterior compression of T_{12}. Also note that the posterior portion of L_2 is minimally displaced posteriorly into the spinal canal. (*B*) Frontal view demonstrating widening of the apophyseal joints of L_2 (*arrows*) and some widening of the corresponding interpedicular distance. These findings result from the compression-induced bursting of the vertebra. This patient fell directly on his buttocks and sustained an axial compression-hyperflexion injury of the thoracolumbar spine. (*C*) CT scan demonstrating the compression fracture of the lumbar vertebra (*white arrows*) and protrusion of the posterior fragment (*black arrows*) into the spinal canal.

ciated disc space widening and actual posterior displacement of the involved vertebral body.

Lateral Flexion Injuries. As in the cervical spine, lateral flexion injuries can result in ipsilateral compression fractures of the vertebral bodies or contralateral transverse process fractures. Most often, these injuries are not particularly serious if lateral flexion is the sole force involved. If other forces are involved, more serious injuries can occur. Transverse process fractures must be differentiated from rudimentary lumbar ribs or bipartite transverse processes (see Fig. 6.90).

Rotation Injuries. These are either rotation-flexion or rotation-extension injuries. The upper thoracic spine is especially prone to severe wrenching injuries and considerable spinal damage can result (Fig. 6.77).

Axial Compression Injuries. Axial compression results in a "burst" vertebra, and often this type of injury is associated with some degree of hyperflexion injury (see Fig. 6.76). When axial compression is a prominent component of these injuries, the vertebral body bursts and spreads outward in all directions. Once again, the mechanics are the same as those seen in the cervical spine. On frontal view, one may note widening of the interpedicular distance and/or widening of the apophyseal joints. On lateral view, the compressed vertebra will be squashed, and the posterior portion of it will protrude into the spinal canal. When significant associated interspinous ligament laxity or tearing occurs, the lesion becomes unstable.

Other Injuries of the Thoracolumbar Spine. The transverse fracture of the vertebral body with anterior or lateral dislo-

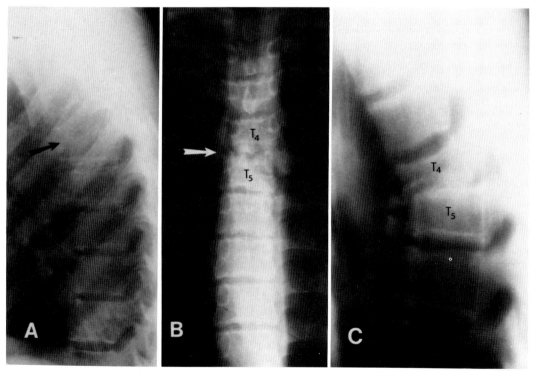

Figure 6.77. *Wrenching injury of thoracic spine.* (**A**) Note acute kyphosis at the T$_4$–T$_5$ level (*arrow*). The vertebral bodies and intervening disc space are difficult to identify. (**B**) Frontal view demonstrating obliteration of the disc space between T$_4$ and T$_5$ (*arrow*) and lateral displacement of T$_4$ on T$_5$. (**C**) Subsequent laminography demonstrates the extensive nature of the rotation-flexion injury of T$_4$ and T$_5$.

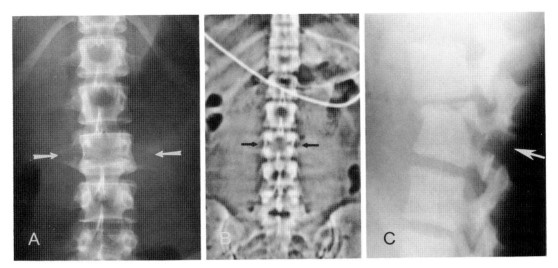

Figure 6.78. *Chance fracture of lumbar vertebra body.* (**A**) Note the transverse fracture through the third lumbar vertebra (*arrows*) in this teenager who was in a car accident. Actually the film was obtained because of abdominal pain. However, note that the vertebra and its transverse processes are completely fractured. Also note that the pedicles of the involved vertebra are distorted because of the fracture. (**B**) Topogram in another patient demonstrating suspicious findings involving L₃ (*arrows*). (**C**) Lateral view demonstrates a classic Chance fracture through the pedicles and vertebral body (*arrows*). There is some associated compression of the anterior aspect of the third lumbar vertebra.

cation of the upper half of the fractured vertebra is a well-known injury occurring in patients wearing lap seatbelts (2, 3, 6, 12–15, 17, 18). These are termed "Chance" fractures (3) and can be detected on frontal views (Fig. 6.78). However, it is not uncommon for the fracture to remain undetected for some time, for often in these patients supine roentgenograms for abdominal pain are obtained, and not enough attention is paid to the lumbar spine. In addition, these fractures often are ignored in cases of multiple body injuries, especially when CT studies are first obtained (16). It is important to examine the topogram of these CT studies, for it often provides the clue to the underlying fracture (Fig. 6.78*B* and *C*).

Another unusual fracture of the vertebral body is the fracture of the ring epiphysis (4, 7, 8, 11, 14). With flexion injuries the superior ring is involved, while with extension injuries the inferior ring is involved (7). In addition, these fractures can be associated with disc herniation. The fracture fragment can be seen to be dis-

placed into the spinal canal and this can be demonstrated both with CT scanning and MRI (Fig. 6.79).

Still another relatively uncommon injury of the thoracolumbar spine is the anterior chronic compression injury or anterior Schmorl's node (5, 18). In these cases, chronic trauma leads to disc damage and herniation of nuclear material into the anterior superior corner of the vertebral body with a resultant triangular teardrop-like fracture fragment (Fig. 6.80). In some cases, considerable sclerosis is seen at the site, indicating a chronic problem with attempt at healing. The condition is a source of chronic back pain and is usually seen in the lower thoracic and upper lumbar regions. The fact that disc material herniates into the vertebral body is now clearly demonstrable with MR scanning (Fig. 6.80).

Spinal injuries in the battered child syndrome also can be encountered. Although they are not particularly common, one can see simple compression fractures, compression fractures with notched vertebrae,

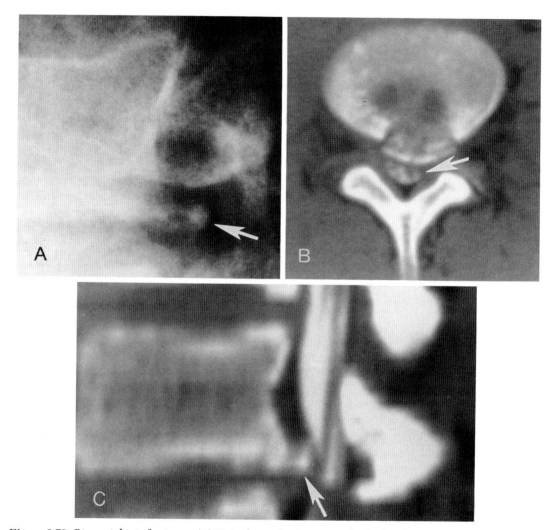

Figure 6.79. *Ring epiphysis fracture.*   (*A*) Note the avulsed, posteriorly displaced, ring epiphysis (*arrow*). (*B*) CT scan demonstrates the posteriorly displaced fracture fragment and avulsed ring epiphysis (*arrow*). (*C*) Sagittal reconstruction demonstrates the displaced ring epiphyseal fragment (*arrow*) causing spinal canal compression.

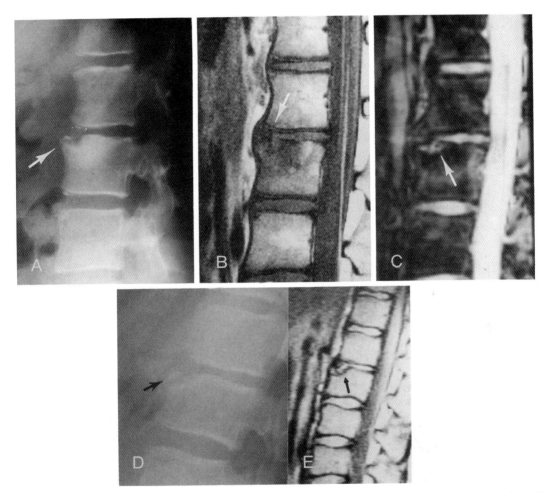

Figure 6.80. *Anterior Schmorl's nodes.* (*A*) Note the classic appearance of a chronic anterior Schmorl's node (*arrow*) of the involved lumbar vertebra. The adjacent disc space shows narrowing and there is reactive sclerosis in the vertebral body. (*B*) T$_1$-weighted sagittal **MRI** demonstrates loss of signal in the disc anteriorly, narrowing of the disc, and loss of signal in the vertebral body because of the sclerosis. (*C*) T$_2$-weighted image demonstrates how the nuclear material has extruded into the upper anterior corner of the vertebral body (*arrow*). (*D*) Another patient with similar findings (*arrow*). (*E*) T$_1$-weighted sagittal **MR** scan demonstrates extrusion of disc material into the upper anterior corner of the vertebral body (*arrow*). The involved disc space is narrower than normal. This also has been called a limbus vertebra.

actual fracture dislocations, and spinous tip avulsions (1, 9, 10, 16).

SACROCOCCYGEAL SPINE TRAUMA

Injuries of the coccyx are quite uncommon except in older children who might fall on their buttocks, and if the injury is severe enough, the lateral view will demonstrate tilting of the fractured coccyx. Sacral fractures have been dealt with in the section on pelvic injuries.

REFERENCES

1. Caffey, J.: The whiplash shaken infant syndrome; manual shaking by the extremities with whiplash-induced intracranial and intraocular bleedings, linked with residual permanent brain damage and mental retardation. Pediatrics 54: 396–403, 1974.
2. Carroll, T.B., and Gruber, F.H.: Seat belt fractures. Radiology 91: 517–518, 1968.
3. Chance, G.Q.: Note on type of flexion fracture of spine. Br. J. Radiol. 21: 452–453, 1948.
4. Gooding, C.A., and Hurwitz, M.E.: Avulsed vertebral rim apophysis in a child. Pediatr. Radiol. 2: 265–268, 1974.
5. Greene, T.L., Hensinger, R.N., and Hunter, L.Y.: Back pain and vertebral changes simulating Scheuermann's disease. J. Pediatr. Orthop. 5: 1–7, 1985.
6. Hayes, C.W., Conway, W.F., Walsh, J.W., Coppage, L., and Gervin, A.S.: Seat belt injuries: Radiologic findings and clinical correlation. RadioGraphics 11: 23–36, 1991.
7. Jonsson, K., Niklasson, J., and Josefsson, P.O.: Avulsion of the cervical spine ring apophyses: Acute and chronic appearance. Skeletal Radiol. 20: 207–212, 1991.
8. Keller, R.H.: Traumatic displacement of the cartilaginous vertebral rim: A sign of intervertebral disc prolapse. Radiology 110: 21–24, 1974.
9. Kleinman, P.K., and Zito, J.L.: Avulsion of the spinous processes caused by infant abuse. Radiology 151: 389–392, 1984.
10. McGrory, B.E., and Fenichel, G.M.: Hangman's fracture subsequent to shaking an infant. Ann. Neurol. 2: 82, 1977.
11. Ogden, J.A., Buchotz, R.W., Hughes, S.A.: Physeal injuries of the cervical spine. J. Pediatr. Orthop. 7: 428–435, 1987.
12. Rogers, L.F.: The roentgenographic appearance of transverse or chance fractures of the spine: The seat belt fracture. A.J.R. 111: 844–849, 1971.
13. Smith, W.E., and Kaufer, H.: Patterns and mech-

anisms of lumbar injuries associated with lap-seat belts. J. Bone Joint Surg. 51A: 239, 1969.
14. Sovio, O.M., Bell, H.M., Beauchamp, R.D., and Tredwell, S.J.: Fracture of the lumbar vertebral apophysis. J. Pediatr. Orthop. 5: 550–552, 1985.
15. Steckler, R.M., Epstein, J.A., and Epstein, B.S.: Seat belt trauma to lumbar spine: Unusual manifestation of seat belt syndrome. J. Trauma 9: 508–513, 1969.
16. Swischuk, L.E.: Spine and spinal cord trauma in battered child syndrome. Radiology 92: 733–738, 1969.
17. Taylor, G.A., and Eggli, K.D.: lap-belt injuries of the lumbar spine in children: A pitfall of CT diagnosis. A.J.R. 150: 1355–1358, 1988.
18. Walters, G., Coumas, J.M., Akins, C.M., and Ragland, R.L.: Magnetic resonance imaging of acute symptomatic Schmorls' node formation. Pediatr. Emerg. Care 7: 294–296, 1991.

MISCELLANEOUS PROBLEMS OF THE SPINE

Infections of the Spine. Generally speaking, infections of the spine consist of osteomyelitis and so-called "spondyloarthritis" or "discitis" of childhood (1–5, 7, 9, 14). In all of these conditions, the hallmark of radiographic diagnosis is disc space narrowing with destruction of the two adjacent vertebral body surfaces (Fig. 6.81). Most often these patients present with back pain, hip pain, or a limp, but abdominal pain also has been noted (8). The degree of systemic reaction is variable, and the underlying organism usually is *Staphylococcus aureus*. In some of these cases, however, an infectious agent is not demonstrable, and this has prompted some to consider such cases as traumatic rather than infectious in origin. Bone scanning is very worthwhile in the detection of these infections (5, 10, 14), especially since the roentgenographic changes are somewhat late in onset (Fig. 6.81). CT and MRI (6, 11–13) also are excellent in demonstrating the disc and bony changes, but MRI is probably the more informative of the two (Fig. 6.82). With MRI, the disc loses its normal signal, either in its entirety or in part. In addition, on T_1-weighted images, signal loss also often is seen in the vertebral

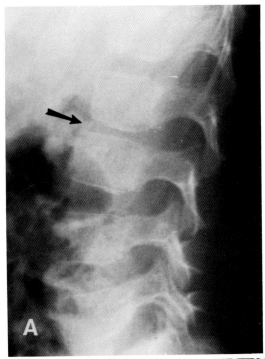

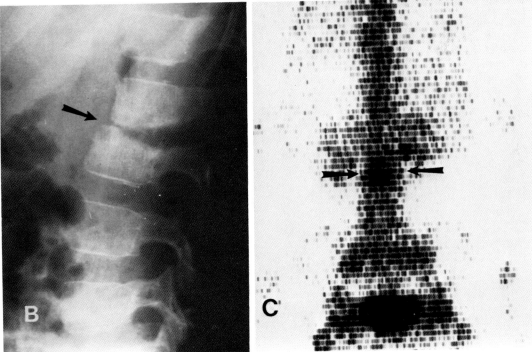

Figure 6.81. *Discitis or spondyloarthritis.* (*A*) Typical early changes consisting of disc space narrowing only (*arrow*). (*B*) Two weeks later, note how much destruction has occurred at the site of infection (*arrow*). In addition, there has been some posterior displacement of the upper vertebral body. (*C*) Bone scan obtained after the first roentgenogram demonstrates increased activity over the lesion (*arrows*).

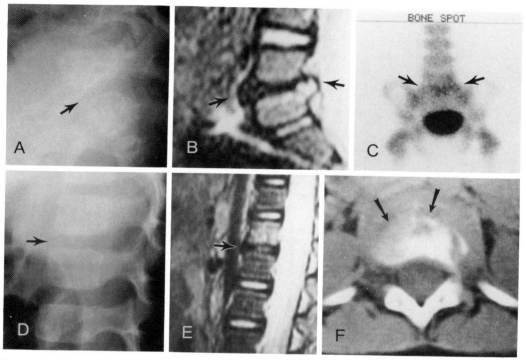

Figure 6.82. *Discitis: MR and CT findings.* (*A*) Note subtle suggestion of narrowing of the disc space between L$_5$ and S$_1$ (*arrow*). (*B*) Sagittal T$_1$-weighted MRI demonstrates loss of signal in the disc, bulging of the ligament anteriorly (*anterior arrow*), and bulging of the posterior ligament with a portion of the disc protruding (*posterior arrow*) into the spinal canal. (*C*) Nuclear scintigraphy demonstrates increased activity at the L$_5$-S$_1$ level (*arrows*). (*D*) Another patient with virtually normal findings at the involved disc space (*arrows*). (*E*) Sagittal MR T$_1$-weighted study demonstrates loss of signal in the involved disc (*arrow*) and increased signal in the vertebral body above it, on this T$_2$-weighted image. (*F*) CT scan in another patient demonstrates vertebral body destruction (*arrows*).

bodies (Fig. 6.82). On T$_2$-weighted images, there is increased signal in the involved areas of the vertebral bodies (Fig. 6.82). In some cases, disc material may herniate beyond the confines of the normal disc space. These herniations may be anterior or posterior (Fig. 6.82).

REFERENCES

1. Alexander, C.J.: The aetiology of juvenile spondyloarthritis (discitis). Clin. Radiol. 21: 178–187, 1970.
2. Brass, A., and Bowdler, J.D.: Non-specific spondylitis of childhood. Ann. Radiol. 12: 343–354, 1969.
3. Bolivar, R., Kohl, S., and Pickering, L.K.: Vertebral osteomyelitis in children: Report of four cases. Pediatrics 62: 549–553, 1978.
4. Childe, A.E., and Tucker, F.R.: Spondyloarthritis in infants and children. J. Can. Assoc. Radiol. 12: 47–51, 1961.
5. Fischer, G.W., Popich, G.A., Sullivan, D.E., Mayfield, G., Mazat, B.A., and Patterson, P.H.: Diskitis: A prospective diagnosis analysis. Pediatrics 62: 543 548, 1978.
6. Forster, A., Pothmann, R., Winter, K., and Baumann-Rath, C.A.: Magnetic resonance imaging in non-specific discitis. Pediatr. Radiol. 17: 162–163, 1987.
7. Gates, G.F.: Scintigraphy of discitis. Clin. Nucl. Med. 2: 20–25, 1977.
8. Leahy, A.L., Fogarty, E.E., Fitzgerald, R.J., and Regan, B.F.: Diskitis as a cause of abdominal pain in children. Surg. 95: 412–414, 1984.
9. Moes, C.A.F.: Spondyloarthritis in childhood. A.J.R. 91: 578–587, 1964.
10. Norris, S., Ehrlich, M.G., Keim, D.E., Guitermann, H., and McKusick, K.A.: Early diagnosis of disc-space infection using gallium-67. J. Nucl. Med. 19: 384–386, 1978.

11. Price, A.C., Allen, J.H., Eggers, F.M., Shaff, M.I., and James, A.E., Jr.: Work in progress: Intervertebral disk space infection: CT changes. Radiology 149: 725–730, 1983.

12. Sartoris, D.J., Moskowitz, P.S., Kaufman, R.A., Ziprkowski, M.N., and Berger, P.E.: Childhood diskitis: Computed tomographic findings. Radiology 149: 701–708, 1983.

13. Szalay, E.A., Green, N.E., Heller, R.M., Horev, G., and Kirchner, S.G.: Magnetic resonance imaging in the diagnosis of childhood discitis. J. Pediatr. Orthop. 7: 164–167, 1987.

14. Wenger, D.R., Bobechko, W.P., and Gilday, D.L.: The spectrum of intervertebral disc-space infection in children. J. Bone Joint Surg. 60A: 100–108, 1978.

Pathologic Fractures. Pathologic fractures of the spine are an occasional cause of acute back pain. In this regard, the most commonly encountered condition is eosinophilic granuloma or histiocytosis X. However, metastatic neuroblastoma, other metastatic disease, or underlying solitary primary bone lesions such as aneurysmal bone cysts, interosseous hemangiomas, etc., also can lead to pathologic compression. Histiocytosis X and eosinophilic granuloma differ a little from these latter conditions in that they produce a very flat vertebra, the so-called vertebra "plana" (Fig. 6.83). Patients with leukemia or lymphoma also can present with compression fractures of the vertebrae, but most often these patients also are receiving steroid therapy. Compression fracture secondary to poorly mineralized bone such as might be seen with hyperparathyroidism, rickets, and osteogenesis imperfecta also can be encountered, especially if the children with these conditions are active and ambulant.

The roentgenographic hallmark of all these fractures is loss of vertebral body height due to compression. The adjacent intervertebral discs, however, remain normal. This is a most important point, for the configuration is completely opposite to that which is seen with osteomyelitis or discitis. The only exception to this rule is coccidioidomycosis or other fungal disease, which can be associated with retention of the integrity of the disc space.

Calcified Intervertebral Discs. Commonly this condition occurs in the cervical spine (Fig. 6.84), but it also can be seen in the thoracic spine. Usually, it is associated with neck pain and stiffness, but the etiology is unknown (1–3, 6–8). There is debate as to whether the calcification results from trauma or inflammation, but even though no conclusive data to support either etiology are currently available, inflammation seems more plausible. Systemic response in these patients is variable, and while some show signs of marked inflammation and muscle spasm, others are less symptomatic. Continuing observation shows that these calcifications eventually disappear, and little in the way of residual vertebral bony change remains (11). In the interval, however, some of these discs have been noted to herniate and protrude either anteriorly or posteriorly (4, 9). Of course, those protruding

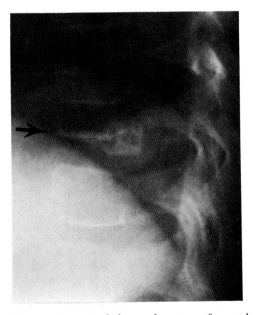

Figure 6.83. *Pathologic fracture of vertebral body.* Note typical flat vertebra (vertebra plana) associated with pathologic compression secondary to histiocytosis X (*arrow*).

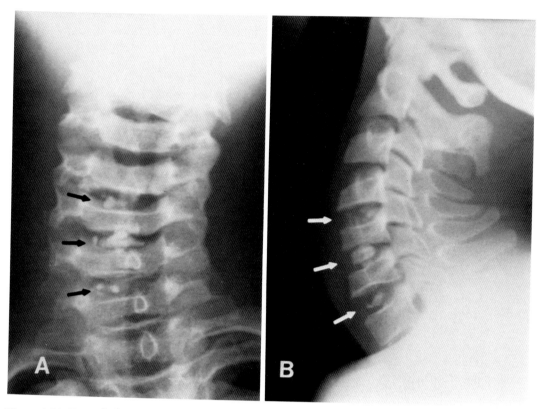

Figure 6.84. *Disc calcifications.* (*A*) Frontal view demonstrating acute scoliosis and multiple disc calcifications (*arrows*). This boy presented with acute neck pain and torticollis. (*B*) Lateral view demonstrating characteristic appearance of the calcified intervertebral discs (*arrows*). Note that the spine is normal in other respects.

posteriorly will do so into the spinal canal, but they do not seem to cause cord injury (4, 9). MRI is useful in delineating this generally benign entity (5), and can even show changes before calcification occurs (10)(Fig. 6.85).

REFERENCES

1. Blomquist, H.K., Lindqvist, M., and Mattsson, S.: Calcification of intervertebral disc in childhood. Pediatr. Radiol. 8: 23–26, 1979.
2. Girodias, J.-B., Azouz, E.M., and Marton, D.: Intervertebral disk space calcification: A report of 51 children with a review of the literature. Pediatr. Radiol. 21: 541–546, 1991.
3. Henry, M.J., Grimes, H.A., and Lane, J.W.: Intervertebral disk calcification in childhood. Radiology 89: 81–84, 1967.
4. Mainzer, F.: Herniation of the nucleus pulposus: A rare complication of intervertebral disk calcification in children. Radiology 107: 167–170, 1973.
5. McGregor, J.C., and Butler, P.: Disc calcification in childhood: Computed tomographic and magnetic resonance imaging appearances. Br. J. Radiol. 59: 180, 1986.
6. Melnick, J.C., and Silverman, F.N.: Intervertebral disk calcifications in childhood. Radiology 80: 399–408, 1963.
7. Mikity, V.G., and Isenbarger, J.: Intervertebral disk calcification in children. A.J.R. 95: 200–202, 1965.
8. Sonnabend, D.H., Taylor, T.K.F., and Chapman, G.K.: Intervertebral disc calcification syndromes in children. J. Bone Joint Surg. 64B: 25–31, 1982.
9. Sutton, T.J., and Turcotte, B.: Posterior herniation of calcified intervertebral discs in children. J. Can. Assoc. Radiol. 24: 131–136, 1973.
10. Swischuk, L.E., and Stansberry, S.D.: Calcific discitis: MRI changes in discs without visible calcification. Pediatr. Radiol. 21: 365–366, 1991.

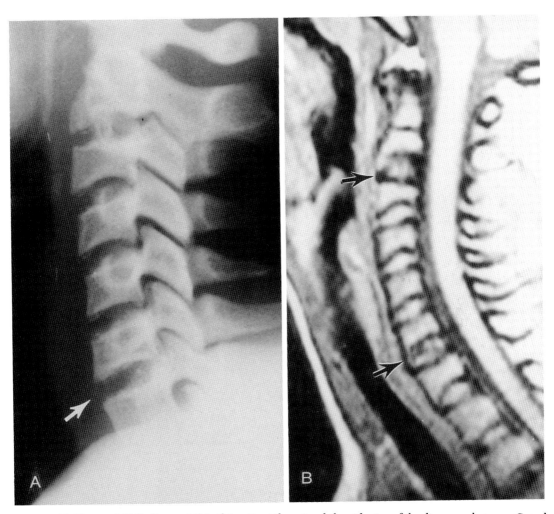

Figure 6.85. *Discitis: MR findings.* (*A*) In this patient there is subtle widening of the disc space between C_6 and C_7 (*arrow*). In addition, there is some suggestion of widening of the disc space between C_2 and C_3. These findings are subtle. There is no evidence of calcification. (*B*) Proton density MRI demonstrates loss of signal in the disc space between C_2 and C_3 (*upper arrow*) and the disc space between C_6 and C_7 (*lower arrow*). The discs also are expanded. (From L.E. Swischuk and S.D. Stansberry: Calcific discitis: MRI changes in discs without visible calcification. Pediatr. Radiol. 21: 365–366, 1991.)

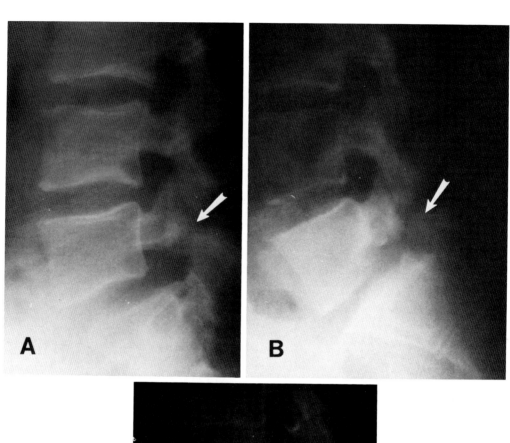

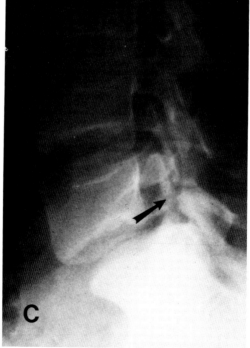

11. Urso, S., Colajacomo, M., Migliorini, A., and Fassari, F.M.: Calcifying discopathy in infancy in the cervical spine: Evaluation of vertebral alterations over a period of time. Pediatr. Radiol. 17: 387–391, 1987.

Spondylolysis and Spondylolisthesis.

Generally not a cause of acute pain, spondylolysis occasionally can result from acute trauma. Nonetheless, most cases are chronic in nature and generally accepted opinion is that most are acquired (1, 5–8). In this regard, there is considerable feeling that the initial problem may be a fatigue fracture (8). Some familial tendency toward the problem has been documented (1), but most cases are sporadic. In support of a traumatic etiology is the prevalence of the problem in adolescent athletes (2, 3). In early cases, the defect is rather straight and subtle (Fig. 6.86A), but later on, bony resorption occurs and a more dysplastic appearance results (Fig. 6.86B). This has prompted dividing the condition into those cases with a small defect and those with a dysplastic-appearing pedicle, but probably both represent the same problem, merely representing different stages of abnormality (1). Since in many cases findings may be subtle on roentgenograms, positive studies have been obtained with SPECT scintigraphy in problematic cases (2).

Spondylolysis usually is associated with spondylolisthesis (anterior displacement of the upper vertebral body) and spondylolisthesis is generally graded on the basis of degree of anterior slippage of the vertebral body. The grades usually consist of I through IV, and reflect anterior slippage as related to quarters of the underlying vertebral body (Fig. 6.86).

REFERENCES

1. Albanese, M., and Pizzutillo, P.D.: Family study of spondylolysis and spondylolisthesis. J. Pediatr. Orthop. 2: 496–499, 1982.
2. Bellah, R.D., Summerville, D.A., Treves, S.T., and Micheli, L.J.: Low-back pain in adolescent athletes: Detection of stress injury to the pars interarticularis with SPECT. Radiology 180, 509–512, 1991.
3. Letts, M., Smallman, T., Afanasiev, R.., and Gouw, G..: Fracture of the pars interarticularis in adolescent athletes: A clinical biomechanical analysis. J. Pediatr. Orthop. 6: 40–46, 1986.
4. Libson, E., Bloom, R.A., Dinari, G., and Robin, G.C.: Oblique lumbar spine radiographs: Importance in young patients. Radiol. 151: 89–90, 1984.
5. McKee, B.W., Alexander, W.J., and Dunbar, J.S.: Spondylosis and spondylolisthesis in children. J. Can. Assoc. Radiol. 22: 100–109, 1971.
6. Oakley, R.H., and Carty, H.: Review of spondylolisthesis and spondylolysis in paediatric practice. Br. J. Radiol. 57: 877–885, 1984.
7. Wertzberger, J., and Peterson, H.: Acquired spondylolysis and spondylolisthesis in the young child. Spine 5: 437, 1980.
8. White, L.L., Widell, E.H., and Jackson, D.W.: Fatigue fracture: The basic lesion in isthmic spondylolisthesis. J. Bone Joint Surg. 57A: 17–22, 1975.

Intervertebral Disc Herniation.

Disc herniations are extremely uncommon in infants and young children, but are not so uncommon in the active adolescent (1–5). Roentgenographically, there is little to see except for muscle spasm causing straightening or curvature of the spine. For the most part, these patients require CT scanning or MRI for final diagnosis (Fig. 6.87). In some cases disc herniation is associated with fractures of the ring epiphysis (1).

REFERENCES

1. Banerian, K.G., Wang, A.-M.F, Samberg, L.C., Kerr, H.H., and Wesolowski, D.P.: Association of vertebral end plate fracture with pediatric lumbar

---

Figure 6.86. *Spondylolisthesis.* (A) Note typical spondylolysis (*arrow*) with minimal spondylolisthesis. (B) More extensive lytic changes producing a dysplastic appearance through the pedicle (*arrow*). Also note bone resorption along the posterior aspect of the vertebral bodies, some disc space narrowing, and an at least grade II spondylolisthesis (i.e., 50% or ½ of the vertebral body). (C) Acute spondylolysis. Patient in car accident with acute back pain. Note defect in the pedicle (*arrow*). On this oblique view, spondylolisthesis is suggested, but on true lateral view, none was present.

Figure 6.87. *Disc herniation: MR findings.* Note posteriorly herniated discs at two levels (*arrows*). The disc spaces are irregular and the discs themselves have lost some signal.

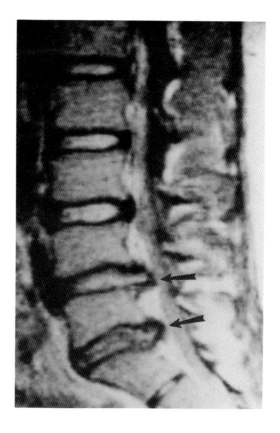

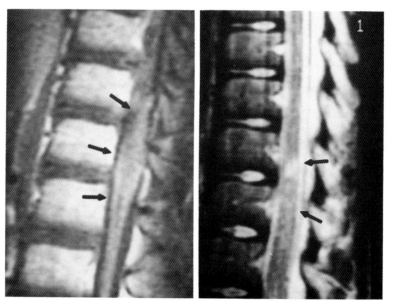

Figure 6.88. *Cord contusion.* (*A*) Note the swollen, expanded spinal cord (*arrows*) in this patient who sustained a back injury with no visible bony fractures. The patient, however, had significant neurologic deficit in the lower extremities. (*B*) T$_2$-weighted image demonstrates the areas of contusion and hemorrhage as patchy areas of increased white signal (*arrows*).

intervertebral disk herniation: Value of CT and MR imaging. Radiology 177: 763–765, 1990.

2. Clarke, N.M.P., and Cleak, D.K.: Intervertebral lumbar disc prolapse in children and adolescents. J. Pediatr. Orthop. 3: 202–206, 1983.

3. Hashimoto, K., Fujita, K., Kojimoto, H., and Shimomura, Y.: Lumbar disc herniation in children. J. Pediatr. Orthop. 10: 394–396, 1990.

4. Kurihara, A., and Kataoka, O.: Lumbar disk herniation in children and adolescents. Spine 5: 443, 1980.

5. Zamani, M.H., and MacEwen, G.D.: Herniation of the lumbar disc in children and adolescents. J. Pediatr. Orthop. 2: 528–533, 1982.

Miscellaneous Thoracolumbar Spine Problems. Occasionally patients can present to the trauma center with intraspinal or bony tumors. These are relatively rare, however, and a complete discussion of them is beyond the scope of this book. Similarly, patients may present with spinal epidural abscesses. Metastatic disease leading to vertebral compression has been discussed elsewhere. Almost invariably, spine and spinal cord lesions such as those just mentioned are best evaluated with MRI. Plain film findings usually are absent with epidural abscesses, while with bony tumors they usually are present. With intraspinal tumors, the plain films may be normal or may show evidence of intracannulicular expansion consisting of scalloping of the posterior vertebral bodies and erosion of the medial aspects of the pedicles.

Spinal Cord Injury without Bony Injury. This occurs in the thoracolumbar spine (1, 2), just as it does in the cervical spine with the central cord syndrome. Usually injuries sustained are quite significant (i.e., football injuries, motor vehicle accidents, etc.). These patients have clear-cut neurologic deficit and yet no bony abnormality. However, MRI now clearly identifies the underlying contusion present in these patients (Fig. 6.88).

REFERENCES

1. Pang, D., Wilberger, J.E., Jr.: Spinal cord injury without radiographic abnormalities in children. J. Neurosurg. 57: 114–129, 1982.

2. Yngve, D.A., Harris, W.P., Herndon, W.A., Sullivan, J.A., and Gross, R.H.: Spinal cord injury without osseous spine fracture. J. Pediatr. Orthop. 8: 153–159, 1988.

NORMAL VARIATIONS CAUSING PROBLEMS IN THE THORACOLUMBAR SPINE

One of the most common normal variations causing problems is the normal *ring epiphysis* of the vertebral body (Fig. 6.89). These ring-like growth plates of the vertebral bodies occur throughout the entire spine in childhood, and to the uninitiated can suggest a corner, avulsion, teardrop, or limbus fracture. This, however, is not to say that the ring epiphysis never is involved in this type of fracture, for, in chil-

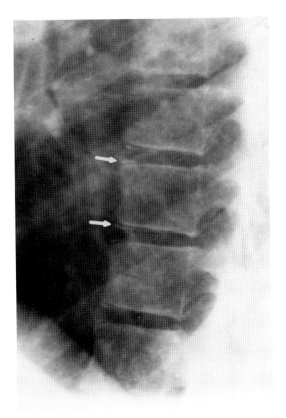

Figure 6.89. *Ring epiphyses.* Note the sliver-like appearance of the normal ring epiphyses of the vertebral bodies (*arrows*). These should not be misinterpreted for teardrop fractures.

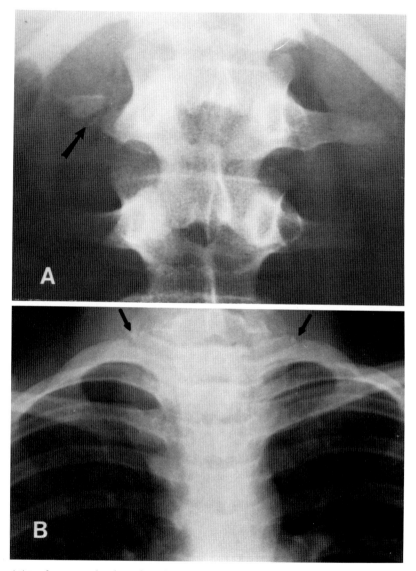

Figure 6.90. (*A*) Rudimentary lumbar rib or bipartite transverse process (*arrow*). This finding should not be misinterpreted for a fracture. (*B*) Normal secondary ossification centers of the upper thoracic transverse processes (*arrows*).

dren, a portion of the ring epiphysis can be avulsed with certain flexion or extension injuries. In these cases, the ring epiphysis fragment constitutes a true teardrop fracture (see Fig. 6.79). However, when this occurs it will not be located in its normal place.

The *apparently bipartite transverse process, but really a rudimentary rib* of a lumbar vertebra can be misinterpreted as a fracture (Fig. 6.90A), and a similar problem can arise in the upper thoracic spine where *accessory ossicles of the transverse processes* also are prone to misinterpretation (Fig. 6.90B).

REFERENCES

1. Azouz, E.M., Kozlowski, K., Marton, D., Sprague, P., Zerhouni, A., and Asselah, F.: Osteoid osteoma and osteoblastoma of the spine in children. Pediatr. Radiol. 16: 25–31, 1986.
2. Kricun, R., Shoemaker, E.I., Chovanes, G.I., and Stephens, H.W.: Epidural abscess of the cervical spine: MR findings in five cases. A.J.R. 158: 1145–1149, 1992.
3. Schweich, P.J., Hurt, T.L.: Spinal epidural abscess in children: Two illustrative cases. Pediatr. Emerg. Care 8: 84–87, 1992.

Index